Medical Management of the Violent Patient

Medical Psychiatry

Series Editor

William A. Frosch, M.D.

Cornell University Medical College
New York, New York

1. Handbook of Depression and Anxiety: A Biological Approach, *edited by Johan A. den Boer and J. M. Ad Sitsen*
2. Anticonvulsants in Mood Disorders, *edited by Russell T. Joffe and Joseph R. Calabrese*
3. Serotonin in Antipsychotic Treatment: Mechanisms and Clinical Practice, *edited by John M. Kane, H.-J. Möller, and Frans Awouters*
4. Handbook of Functional Gastrointestinal Disorders, *edited by Kevin W. Olden*
5. Clinical Management of Anxiety, *edited by Johan A. den Boer*
6. Obsessive-Compulsive Disorders: Diagnosis • Etiology • Treatment, *edited by Eric Hollander and Dan J. Stein*
7. Bipolar Disorder: Biological Models and Their Clinical Application, *edited by L. Trevor Young and Russell T. Joffe*
8. Dual Diagnosis and Treatment: Substance Abuse and Comorbid Medical and Psychiatric Disorders, *edited by Henry R. Kranzler and Bruce J. Rounsaville*
9. Geriatric Psychopharmacology, *edited by J. Craig Nelson*
10. Panic Disorder and Its Treatment, *edited by Jerrold F. Rosenbaum and Mark H. Pollack*
11. Comorbidity in Affective Disorders, *edited by Mauricio Tohen*
12. Practical Management of the Side Effects of Psychotropic Drugs, *edited by Richard Balon*
13. Psychiatric Treatment of the Medically Ill, *edited by Robert G. Robinson and William R. Yates*
14. Medical Management of the Violent Patient: Clinical Assessment and Therapy, *edited by Kenneth Tardiff*

ADDITIONAL VOLUMES IN PREPARATION

Medical Management of the Violent Patient

Clinical Assessment and Therapy

edited by

Kenneth Tardiff

Cornell University Medical College
New York, New York

MARCEL DEKKER, INC. NEW YORK • BASEL

Library of Congress Cataloging-in-Publication Data

Medical management of the violent patient : clinical assessment and
therapy / edited by Kenneth Tardiff.
p. cm. — (Medical psychiatry : 14)
Includes bibliographical references and index.
ISBN: 0–8247–9906–2 (alk. paper)
1. Violence. 2. Violence in psychiatric hospitals. I. Tardiff,
Kenneth. II. Series.
[DNLM: 1. Dangerous Behavior. 2. Violence—prevention & control.
3. Crime Victims—psychology. 4. Patients—psychology. W1 ME421SM
v. 14 1999 / WM 600 M489 1999]
RC569.5.V55M43 1999
616.85′82–dc21
DNLM/DLC 99-26167
for Library of Congress CIP

This book is printed on acid-free paper.

Headquarters
Marcel Dekker, Inc.
270 Madison Avenue, New York, NY 10016
tel: 212-696-9000; fax: 212-685-4540

Eastern Hemisphere Distribution
Marcel Dekker AG
Hutgasse 4, Postfach 812, CH-4001 Basel, Switzerland
tel: 41-61-261-8482; fax: 41-61-261-8896

World Wide Web
http://www.dekker.com

The publisher offers discounts on this book when ordered in bulk quantities. For more information, write to Special Sales/Professional Marketing at the address above.

Current printing (last digit):
10 9 8 7 6 5 4 3 2 1

PRINTED IN THE UNITED STATES OF AMERICA

Series Introduction

Many years ago I reviewed a symposium on aggressive behavior (1). At the time I wrote: "On May 2, 1968, the front page of *The New York Times* dealt importantly with the war in Vietnam and disruption of college campuses. In Vietnam, the previous year's presidential peace candidate was arrested for having urged the formation of a coalition government as a step toward peace; American military officials were reported arguing for resumption of American bombing of North Vietnam; six youths and five policemen were hurt in a clash on the Columbia campus . . . . On these same dates a symposium on aggressive behavior was held in Milan. . . ." (2). Thirty years later our daily headlines are similar: a child dead from parental abuse and/or neglect in New York City, ongoing massacres and genocidal warfare in central Africa, a band of homeless children shot and killed in South America, road-rage killings in California, and a breakdown of the peace processes in the Middle East and in what used to be Yugoslavia. The world does not seemed to have changed. Violence has not gone away, and the lives of all of us are touched by it.

Thirty years ago my review concluded that "We certainly seem far from sufficient knowledge." This volume, *Medical Management of the Violent Patient: Clinical Assessment and Therapy*, shows us that we have advanced our knowledge in many areas. We are now better able to help those who are violent to control themselves, or if necessary, to impose control in humane ways; and to assist in the recovery of those who are victims of violence. It is also clear, unfortunately, that our knowledge is still insufficient to the magnitude of the problem. As many of the chapter authors stress, our ability to predict future dangerousness is poor, at best limited to the short-term behavior of several days; lasting behavioral change is difficult to achieve; and aspects of our society work against the control of aggression or reward violent acts. Continuing basic and clinical research is essential to our childrens' futures. While we wait for that additional basic and applied knowledge, this book will help us to deal with the difficult problems clinicians face in emergency rooms, in inpatient units, and in our offices: it will help us to do what needs to be done as well as one can, and to do it without unnecessary physical or legal risk to ourselves.

REFERENCES

1. Aggressive Behaviour, S. Garattini and E. B. Sigg, eds. Excerpta Medica Foundation, Amsterdam, 1969.
2. *Journal of Clinical Pharmacology and New Drugs, 11*, 1971, pp. 74–75.

William A. Frosch, M.D.

Preface

Over the past 25 years, violence has increased, particularly in the United States and Europe. Violence is defined in this book as behavior aimed at intentionally harming or attempting to harm another person. A major portion of this violence is related to crime such as robberies and drug dealing. Some violence is committed by persons because of psychiatric and medical disorders. Although the portion of violence due to psychiatric and medical problems is smaller than that due to crime, it is of great importance to us as health professionals because we have the responsibility to treat these disorders and because violence by patients can be directed at us.

This book is intended primarily to be a clinical resource for psychiatrists, other physicians, psychologists, social workers, and all other professionals who are involved in the care of patients. We anticipate that it will be of interest to the legal profession since violence by patients is the subject of numerous legal proceedings in cases of malpractice and advocacy for proper standards of medical care. This book covers causes of violence by patients, guidelines for the evaluation of patients, guidelines for the treatment of violent patients, issues related to victims of violence, and special concerns such as legal issues, violence in the workplace, and the link between suicide and violence by patients.

Causes of violence are addressed in six chapters. In Chapter 1, Dr. Shulamit Glaubach discusses the role of developmental factors in violent behavior, including maltreatment, neurochemical/neuroendocrine factors, and prenatal causes. She presents vignettes and a discussion of prevention and treatment of violent behavior, providing strategies to minimize the risk factors that increase the propensity for violence.

In Chapter 2, Dr. Robert Phillips discusses social and environmental causes of violence. Although certain factors, such as race and the criminal justice system, are particularly significant for the United States, other factors are relevant to Europe and other areas of the world—for example, poverty, social disorganization, the media, and substance abuse.

In Chapter 3, Dr. Serena-Lynn Brown reviews research on the role of neurotransmitters in violence. She discusses the serotonin system and how low levels of this neurotransmitter are related to violence and suicide. Although the literature on other systems is not as voluminous as that on serotonin, she reviews studies of the norepinephrine, dopamine, GABA/benzodiazepines, and cholinergic systems.

In Chapter 4, Dr. Karen Anderson and Dr. Jonathan Silver review the literature on a number of neurological and medical disorders that can result in violence by patients. These include dementia, traumatic brain injury, congenital brain disorders, epilepsy, encephalitis, AIDS, movement disorders, brain tumors, stroke, hypoglycemia, sleep disorders, endocrine disorders, vitamin deficiencies, electrolyte imbalance, hypoxia and toxins.

In Chapter 5, Dr. Leslie Citrome and Dr. Jan Volavka describe the association of psychiatric disorders and violence by patients. They focus on schizophrenia and other psychotic disorders, personality disorders, mood disorders, anxiety disorders, and mental retardation. Their conclusions are based on a review of epidemiological studies of violence in relation to these disorders, for patients in hospitals and in the community as well as for prisoners. They describe psychopathology in each disorder as it relates to violence, and provide case vignettes.

In Chapter 6, the final chapter on causes, Dr. Jan Volavka and I present studies of violence-associated alcohol and drug abuse. We discuss possible mechanisms by which alcohol and drugs cause violence and describe how violence is manifested in various intoxication and withdrawal states. In addition to the pharmacological effects on violence, we describe how violence is involved in drug-dealing and other criminal activities.

There are two chapters on the evaluation of violent patients. In Chapter 7, Dr. William Reid discusses the comprehensive evaluation of violent patients. He begins with important issues that surround the evaluation, such as safety, confidentiality, the allegiance of the examiner, and the purpose of the evaluation. He describes the content of the evaluation, including a history of violence and other psychopathology as well as the social, medical, and developmental histories. He discusses laboratory and psychometric testing. He briefly talks about how to evaluate the risk of future violence by a patient. In Chapter 8, I continue a discussion of how to predict violence—that is, whether a patient poses a significant risk of violence in the near future. Some of the information that should be considered in making a decision about the risk of violence includes degree of formulation of threats or thoughts of violence and the presence of intent, availability of the targeted person, past history of violence, psychosis, alcohol or drug abuse, personality disorders, organicity, and noncompliance with treatment. I present some malpractice cases in which prediction of violence was an issue.

The next five chapters deal with the treatment of violent patients. In Chapter 9, Dr. William Dubin presents information on clinician safety and violence by patients. He reviews the literature on the frequency and patterns of violence by patients aimed at clinicians. He presents guidelines for dealing with threats of violence made by patients and discusses the significance of threats toward clinicians. He provides suggestions about how to increase the safety of clinicians with verbal means of de-escalation, physical defense techniques, and the physical design of the office and hospital settings. In Chapter 10, I discuss the acute management of violence by patients. This includes how to determine instantly what type of patient the clinician is facing. Issues of safety are addressed. I present guidelines for the use of medication, seclusion, and restraint to manage violence as it is occurring. Attention is paid to alternatives such as one-to-one observation and verbal interventions.

In Chapter 11, Dr. Burr Eichelman and I present guidelines for the long-term treatment of violent patients. We review the literature on the use of antipsychotics, benzodiazepines, lithium, anticonvulsants, beta-blockers, and other medications. In Chapter 12, Dr. Gary Maier gives a detailed discussion on the emotions generated in the treatment of violent patients. He reviews transference and countertransference, in other words, the patient's emotional reactions to the clinician and the clinician's emotional reactions to the patient. He describes phases in the violent episode and how interventions should be planned accordingly. He illustrates this with case examples. Techniques to address inappropriate and/or negative feelings of the staff are also presented. In Chapter 13, Dr. Marilyn Lanza reviews the literature on the psychotherapeutic treatment of violent patients using individual, couples/family, and group modalities. She discusses selection of patients, setting of goals, and techniques. For group psychotherapy, she discusses the role of the leader, phases of group development, and the structure of groups.

There are four chapters that focus more on the victims of violence than on the perpetrators. In Chapter 14, Dr. Matthew Friedman presents information on the consequences of violence from the perspective of the victim, particularly for posttraumatic stress disorder (PTSD). He discusses the clinical phenomena necessary for a diagnosis of PTSD, its prevalence, and factors that increase the risk of PTSD among victims of violence. He describes the treatment of PTSD using dynamic and cognitive-behavior therapy as well as medication. In Chapter 15, Dr. Leah Dickstein writes about domestic violence. She calls our attention to the seriousness and pervasive nature of the problem of spouse abuse, especially toward women. She provides information that will be useful to all health providers in the recognition of spouse and child abuse. She outlines treatments available for victims as well as perpetrators of domestic violence.

Dr. Dawn Hughes and Dr. Marylene Cloitre, in Chapter 16, discuss rape and sexual assault of adult women. They review the literature of the prevalence of rape and sexual abuse in society and the factors related to an increased risk of being a victim of rape and sexual assault. They describe the psychological sequelae and present guidelines for the assessment and treatment of victims. In Chapter 17, the final chapter on victims of violence, Dr. Arthur Green focuses on children who are victims of physical or sexual abuse. He discusses the consequences of abuse such as aggression, criminality, depression and self-destructive behavior, and sexual problems. He presents theories of why these consequences of abuse occur and describes the parents who sexually abuse their children. Finally, he discusses treatment for abused children.

Three chapters address special issues related to violence. Dr. James Beck and Mr. Pat Cerundolo discuss in Chapter 18 the legal aspects of assessing and treating violent patients. These include the duty of the clinician to protect persons foreseeably endangered by their patients, issues concerning breaches of confidentiality, and the nature of malpractice suits in the treatment of violent patients. They also review recent court decisions on the duty of clinicians to protect potential victims of violence. In Chapter 19, Dr. Carol Wilkinson discusses the problem of violence in the workplace, presenting data on the magnitude and nature of violence in the workplace. She gives suggestions about the development of programs to prevent such violence, and how to intervene with employees who have been violent, as well as discussing legal considerations in addressing violence in the workplace. In Chapter 20, Dr. Peter Marzuk discusses a link between violence and suicide. He reviews the literature on the occurrence of both violence and suicide among psychiatric patients and prisoners, as well as the literature on possible reasons for a link between violence and suicide. He stresses that suicide should be adequately assessed for perpetrators as well as victims of violence.

I wish to express my gratitude to the contributors, who agreed to write about their areas of expertise, and to the staff of Marcel Dekker, Inc., for their patience and assistance in the development of this book. I hope readers will find this book to be helpful as they face one of the most distressing aspect in the care of patients: violence.

Kenneth Tardiff

Contents

Contributors

Karen E. Anderson, M.D. Department of Psychiatry, Columbia University College of Physicians and Surgeons, New York, New York

James C. Beck, M.D., Ph.D. Associate Professor of Psychiatry, Harvard Medical School, and Associate Chair, Department of Psychiatry, Cambridge Hospital, Cambridge, Massachusetts

Serena-Lynn Brown, M.D., Ph.D. Department of Psychiatry, Albert Einstein College of Medicine, Bronx, New York

Pat Cerundolo, J.D. Associate, Foley, Hoag & Eliot, L.L.P., Boston, Massachusetts

Leslie Citrome, M.D., M.P.H. Clinical Associate Professor of Psychiatry, New York University, New York, and Director, Clinical Research and Evaluation Facility, Nathan S. Kline Institute for Psychiatric Research, Orangeburg, New York

Marylene Cloitre, Ph.D. Assistant Professor of Psychology in Psychiatry and Director of Training in Psychology, Cornell University Medical College, New York, New York

Leah J. Dickstein, M.D. Professor of Psychiatry and Behavioral Sciences and Associate Dean for Faculty and Student Advocacy, University of Louisville School of Medicine, Louisville, Kentucky

William R. Dubin, M.D. Vice President of Health Services, AmeriChoice Behavioral Healthcare, and Clinical Professor of Psychiatry, Jefferson Medical College, Philadelphia, Pennsylvania

Burr S. Eichelman, M.D., Ph.D. Clinical Professor of Psychiatry, University of Wisconsin–Madison, Madison, Wisconsin

Matthew J. Friedman, M.D., Ph.D. Executive Director, National Center for Posttraumatic Stress Disorder, White River Junction, Vermont, and Professor of Psychiatry and Pharmacology, Dartmouth Medical School, Hanover, New Hampshire

Shulamit Glaubach, M.D. Private Practice, Seattle, Washington

Arthur H. Green, M.D.[†] Clinical Professor of Psychiatry and Medical Director, Therapeutic Nursing, Columbia University College of Physicians and Surgeons, New York, New York

Dawn H. Hughes, Ph.D. Research Associate, Trauma Recovery Service, Payne Whitney Clinic, Cornell University Medical College, New York, New York

Marilyn Lewis Lanza, D.M.S.C., A.R.N.P., C.S. Associate Chief, Nursing Service for Research, Edith Nourse Rogers Memorial Veterans Hospital, Bedford; Associate Professor of Psychiatry, Boston University School of Medicine, Boston; and Associate Professor of Epidemiology and Biostatistics, Boston University School of Public Health, Boston, Massachusetts

Gary J. Maier, M.D. Forensic Program, Mendota Mental Health Institute, Madison, Wisconsin

Peter M. Marzuk, M.D. Associate Professor of Psychiatry, Department of Psychiatry, Cornell University Medical College, New York, New York

Robert T. M. Phillips, M.D., Ph.D. Adjunct Associate Professor of Psychiatry, University of Maryland Schools of Medicine and Law, and Medical Director, Forensic Consultation Associates, Annapolis, Maryland

---

[†]Deceased.

William H. Reid, M.D., M.P.H. Clinical Professor of Psychiatry, University of Texas Health Science Center, San Antonio, Texas

Jonathan M. Silver, M.D. Clinical Professor of Psychiatry, Columbia University College of Physicians and Surgeons, New York, New York

Kenneth Tardiff, M.D., M.P.H. Professor of Psychiatry and Public Health, Cornell University Medical College, New York, New York

Jan Volavka, M.D., Ph.D. Professor of Psychiatry, New York University, New York, and Chief, Clinical Research Division, Nathan S. Kline Institute for Psychiatric Research, Orangeburg, New York

Carol W. Wilkinson, M.D., M.S.P.H. Regional Medical Director, IBM Corporation, Armonk, New York

1
Developmental Factors of Violence

Shulamit Glaubach
Private Practice, Seattle, Washington

> Kip Kinkel spoke to his classmates at Thurston High of bombs and guns and of killing deer and torturing pets. He filled his essays in a freshman English class with stories of killings. But few took the 15-year-old seriously even Wednesday, when the high school suspended him after finding a pistol in his locker.
>
> Yesterday, Kiplan Phillip Kinkel, the only son of two schoolteachers, proved true to his word. Just before 8 a.m., Kinkel, dressed in a hat and black trench coat, walked calmly into a school cafeteria where hundreds of students had gathered.
>
> Armed with three guns, including a .22-caliber rifle, witnesses said, Kinkel began shooting, spraying bullets throughout the room and stopping to reload.
>
> When the carnage had ended, one student was dead and twenty-three were wounded. Four students remained in critical condition last night. Other injuries ranged from minor to serious (1). (A second student died a day later from gunshot wounds.)

Before Springfield, Oregon, there was Fayetteville, Tennessee; Enidoboro, Pennsylvania; and Jonesboro, Arkansas—a sad litany of towns where disturbed teenagers had opened fire on their teachers and fellow students. Kinkel's rampage was another extreme display of how violence can manifest itself in today's youth. More disturbing than this shooting and the others is that, against a backdrop of society's outcry and handwringing, precious little is now being done to prevent the next Kip Kinkel from pulling the trigger. Given the growing list of wounded and deceased not only on school grounds but also in low-income housing projects and dysfunctional families, preventing violence is no longer an option—it is a necessity.

Kip Kinkel exhibited certain behaviors and concerns early that were neither addressed soon nor adequately enough. The fact is that the earlier violence manifests itself in a person, the more likely he or she will act in this manner into and through adulthood (2). Therefore, since violent behavior is often rooted in early stages of personal development, it is imperative that we identify the possible variables contributing to such conduct.

By understanding the developmental factors that lead to violence, we can institute programs that identify significant risk factors and advance preventive measures. The earlier risk factors are identified and addressed in a child's development, the more likely it is that preventive programs will be successful. This means an enhanced sense of well-being for the child, enabling him to identify his own feelings, and thereby empathize with others. The critical ability to empathize with others can increase the likelihood that a child will interact with others and communicate his thoughts and feelings in more productive, nonviolent ways.

To this end, what is needed is a comprehensive approach that recognizes how the child, the family, the community, and the larger social environment contribute to the child's overall health and well-being. A comprehensive approach utilizes prevention and intervention. While prior research studies have suggested that interventions are unsuccessful (3–6) the poor results were likely due to faulty methodology in failing to address the child in a comprehensive manner. Given the damaging consequences that violence offers to at-risk children in Springfield, Oregon, and elsewhere, a comprehensive approach is not only appropriate but also imperative.

I. A WINDOW OF UNDERSTANDING

What factors determine whether one will go on to become a violent person? Understanding the psychological and development factors that influence violent behavior begins with recognizing the long-standing debate between nature versus nurture. On the "nature" side, Lombroso (7) concluded that criminals were born with distinct physical features such as sloping foreheads, long arms, and flat feet (8). In contrast, "nurture" proponents believe that one's environment ultimately causes violent behavior. In actuality, a person possesses a complex array of factors that may potentiate or diminish his or her likelihood of becoming violent. Nature and nurture are *both* at work; natural and environmental factors are entwined in the developmental process.

In Kip Kinkel's case the media have made us aware of clear warning signs. However, it is likely that other risk factors lurked in Kip's makeup. Even before Kip began to torture animals, he likely experienced a number of difficulties—for example, problems establishing healthy attachments, similar to those of children carrying the diagnosis of Reactive Attachment Disorder (RAD) (9) (the inhibited type of RAD, in which the child cannot trust or connect with others). Kip likely had problems identifying his own feelings and conveying them to others, which may have contributed to his unempathetic, disrespectful behavior. By the time he began torturing animals, it was essentially too late for intervention.

The following composite case study not only gives us a window to see what major environmental and biological factors come into play (underlined below) but also exemplifies the many different variables that can contribute negatively to violent behavior into adulthood.

II. JANE'S STORY . . .

Jane was a 14-year-old adolescent living in low-income housing. Her mother had *dropped out in ninth grade*. While growing up, Jane *moved around frequently* to places where her parents could find work. The house Jane lived in was not well maintained and *exposed her family to undue dangers*.

Jane had a history of *major depressive symptoms*, which had never been diagnosed or adequately treated. Jane began *to use recreational drugs* with her peers; alcohol was her drug of choice. She began having *unprotected sex* at age 13 and got pregnant a year later. Jane was *unaware of her pregnancy* and continued to *drink alcohol, smoke cigarettes, and use other recreational drugs*. She *did not seek prenatal care*. During the course of her pregnancy, she was *severely beaten* by her boyfriend on numerous occasions.

Jane went into *labor prematurely* after she *used cocaine*. Her baby was of *low birth weight* and had a *low Apgar score*. After the immediate medical needs of both Jane and her baby, Robin, were met, mother and daughter were discharged. Robin became yellow, and given Jane's *lack of knowledge*, she did not seek medical treatment for her *child's jaundice* until Robin was unresponsive (when high billirubin levels led to *kernicterus*).

Jane would adequately feed, bathe, and clothe her child. However, her *supervision* of Robin was *less than adequate*, as Robin took subsequent *serious falls* and ingested *paint chips*. Jane would wear a Walkman while caring for Robin. This characterized Jane's *limited social interaction*, both in quality and quantity, with her daughter.

Jane's parenting included *inconsistent limit setting* and *overall unresponsiveness* to her child's needs. Jane's depressive symptoms and alcohol abuse would influence her interaction with Robin. At times, when she was frustrated or irritated, Jane would *shake her child vigorously*. Robin also *witnessed her mother being beaten* by her boyfriend.

As time passed, Robin appeared to *exhibit developmental delays*. Upon entering school, she exhibited a significant amount of *learning difficulty*, was *unable to express herself verbally*, and exhibited temper tantrums and aggressive behavior in an attempt to communicate her needs. She *was unable to sit still* and focus, and *exhibited oppositional defiant behavior*. This behavior led to her teachers' repeated reprimands as they conveyed their view that Robin was a "bad girl."

Through her early years Robin *felt bad about herself* and *her ongoing failures at school*. She was laughed at and mocked by her peers when called on to read. She began to *cut classes* with some other children at school. Robin would watch *television shows* and *movies*, which *depicted many violent scenes*. She started to *use drugs* and *joined a gang*.

By *age 9*, Robin had already been *arrested for mugging* someone. She began to feel accepted by the gang. Robin felt good that she belonged in a group that did not demand that she perform tasks she knew she would fail at, such as schoolwork. She achieved respect from her peers by behaving in a tough, threatening manner. She was encouraged by her peers to be more and more destructive and aggressive. Subsequently she *obtained a gun*. When Robin was thirteen, while drunk, she got into an argument and shot someone.

(See Section VIII, "A Comprehensive Plan," which outlines the various stages in the lives of Jane and Robin where society could have intervened on their behalf.)

III. CHILDHOOD DEVELOPMENT

If the above case study illustrates the reality of environmental and biological factors at work, then a brief summary of childhood development (below) offers a necessary and helpful context within which to appreciate how these factors can influence violent behavior—even prior to birth.

A. Prenatal/Neonatal

Prenatal factors include far more than propr nutrition and adequate medication, which start with conception. In utero, both biological and environmental factors affect the development of the fetus. For instance, alcohol and rubella (environmental) can cause significant congenital defects (biological), which will have a long-standing impact on the child. Babies born prematurely due to a mother's smoking, drinking, or using crack cocaine have a higher rate of morbidity and mortality (8,10–15). Studies have shown that there is a link between perinatal events and the development of behavioral disorders (16,17), particularly acts of violence and property crime. Delivery events predicted adult violent offending, particularly for recidivistically violent offenders (18). Raine et al. here has demonstrated that the combination of maternal rejection and birth complications predisposes to violent crime (19).

A longitudinal study found that "low lead levels may have deleterious effects on levels of achievement in children" (8). Children born prematurely and already at risk for developmental delays will, when exposed to lead, experience compounding, negative effects. Adequate parental attention and stimulation are necessary to minimize the brain damage that may result from lead toxicity (20).

B. Temperament

A child's perception of how his needs are being met will establish a foundation of how he perceives himself and others and how he relates to the world around him. This foundation can, ideally, help a child establish a secure sense of self and further the child's ability to identify and communicate his needs. Chess and Thomas (21) found that a child's temperament plays a role in later behavioral disturbances. A child whose temperament complements the temperaments of his parents is more likely to thrive and reach his potential than a child whose temperament clashes with those of his caregivers (22).

A child's temperament is going to influence a parent's responsiveness, and that responsiveness, in turn, will have a direct impact on healthy or unhealthy attachment. A mother's mental health and degree of commonsense intelligence can, for instance, greatly influence her ability to protect her child from abuse and the environment. A mother's history of depression can increase her risk for ending up in abusive situations, thereby increasing her risk for future depression as well as decreasing her ability to protect herself and her child (23). Her capacity to react socially and interact with the child can be markedly jeopardized, along with her ability to set firm, consistent limits without being overly harsh to her child.

Psychoanalysts from Freud to the present have emphasized the centrality of positive and negative interaction in the mother-child relationship and their consequent internalizations and representations as central to the child's development (24).

At about the same time a child strives to achieve autonomy (at approximately 9 months), there is evidence of increased aggression. During this time, a child begins to gain the capacity to inhibit some of his actions. Example: A child has been observed arresting the motion of his raised arm, pulling back, and not following through to strike out. Or, a child threatens his mother with a wooden block. The child, recognizing that the mother is his caretaker, strikes out at another person, thereby displacing his hostile feelings for his mother onto the other individual. These behaviors suggest that the child is making an effort to cope with his hostile, destructive feelings toward his mother. This ability to inhibit the acting out of one's frustrations in a destructive and/or violent manner is crucial to setting the important boundaries between acceptable and maladaptive behavior (24).

Such boundaries are not inborn. They are only achieved only after a child has mastered a number of skills that have been built on preceding, foundational abilities. Changes in the child's developmental course are always possible as a result of new experiences and reorganizations. Early achievements of competence tend to facilitate later successful adaptation. However, a child's difficulties in meeting the challenges of adaptation may impede later efforts at adjustment and consequently lead to the emergence of psychopathological outcomes (25).

From infancy through childhood, there are specific developmental tasks that must be achieved and integrated with skills acquired earlier so that the child can progress to the next developmental stage (26,27). The degree of success achieved at each stage influences the way in which subsequent developmental issues will likely be negotiated. In this way, individuals begin to proceed down different developmental pathways (25,28).

In optimal circumstances, a growing child progresses through various stages, in an "average expectable environment," (29) becoming increasingly competent and adaptive. However, children exposed to and victims of maltreatment experience significant environmental failures. These negative settings are likely to have a substantially deleterious impact on the child's capacity to negotiate the progression through the developmental stages (25).

C. Affect Regulation

One of the early developmental tasks an infant must master is the ability to regulate and differentiate affective experience. Early parent-child interaction is essential in facilitating competency in this area (25,30). Children who experience maltreatment exhibit numerous difficulties in their emotional self-regulation (25,31). Maltreated infants have been shown to experience distortions in their patterns of affect differentiation. These include excessive amounts of negative affect or blunted patterns of affect expression (25,32). At 3 to 4 months of age, maltreated infants lack the cognitive ability to process fear-inducing stimuli appropriately. The infant's lack of capacity to cognitively process the fear, along with distorted affective communication with its caregivers, is likely to result in severe problems in the regulation and organization of affect (25,33,34). At later stages of development, maltreated preschool-age children have exhibited problems regulating their affect. Once they reach school age, these children have shown impaired ability to interact with their peers (25,35).

D. Attachments

Achieving security in an attachment relationship provides an infant with a secure base, from which he begins to explore his surrounding more actively (25,36,37). Some 70 to 100% of maltreated infants have been shown to have insecure attachment organizations (25,38–41). These patterns of insecure attachments persist, even after the negative stimuli cease. The difficulties maltreated children are apt to experience in attaining a secure attachment relationship with a primary care provider can lead to continued disturbances in interpersonal relationships as their development proceeds (25).

Hirschi established a theory of social control in 1969 and proposed that there are four bonds that ensure normative conduct and "control" the potential for delinquent behavior: attachment, commitment, involvement, and belief (8,42).

Attachment refers to a person's sensitivity to the opinions and judgments of others, expressed, for example, as empathy, or obligation in personal relationships. *Commitment* is the rational side of bonding, determined by weighing the potential gains versus losses that may result from conforming or nonconforming behavior. *Involvement* is the degree of time and energy devoted to conventional activities; it not only gives the child a sense of purpose and accomplishment but also displaces the energy that would otherwise be available for deviant behavior. *Belief* is the moral component of the bond, reflecting the degree of which a person agrees with the legal rules. According to Hirsch, the stronger a youth's attachments, commitments, involvements, and beliefs within institutions of social control, such as family and schools, the lower the likelihood or later deviant behavior (4,42).

E. Autonomous Functioning

Maltreated toddlers experience greater difficulty in making the transition to autonomous functioning (25,40). As a result of their impaired states, these children find it difficult to identify their own feelings and experiences (which bodes poorly for achieving meaningful social interaction through understanding oneself and others.) Their inability to identify their true feelings leads these children to inhibit negative affect and exhibit a false-positive affect as a means to please the parent. This false reality perpetuates an inaccurate perception of their surroundings and relationships (25,43–45).

F. Symbolic and Representational Development

In the toddler and preschool years, symbolic capacities—including language, play, representational models, and social information processing—emerge and become differentiated. Studies show that maltreated children, particularly those who have been neglected, exhibit delays n developing receptive and expressive language (25,46–48). They produce less contingent speech and less internal-state language (25,49,50). Their symbolic play also tends to lag behind that of children who have not been abused or neglected. Compared with normal controls, maltreated children show more restriction in the types of themes they portray as well as in the degree of affect expressed in their play. Because their play is so limited, they are unable to explore different avenues to help them process their life experiences (25,51). A person's cognitive ability and social processing skills directly impact his or her effectiveness to perceive social situations accurately and respond appropriately. The basis of one's social processing is rooted in early experiences with the primary caregiver. A child who has experienced harsh maltreatment is likely to exhibit deficits in social information processing, resulting in excessive aggressive behavior and difficulties in social interactions (25,52–54).

G. Peer Relations

Maltreated preschoolers have been shown to exhibit heightened levels of aggression and avoidance in peer interactions (25,55). Children who have not been maltreated respond to distress in peers with prosocial behavior. However, maltreated children respond with fear, threats, and angry behavior, vacillating with attempts to comfort. Maltreated children have been found to respond with anger and aggression to both friendly behavior and distress in their peers. Some maltreated children have been shown to exhibit heightened levels of both aggression and withdrawal (25,56–59).

H. Adaptation to School

As noted above, maltreated children have difficulty balancing comfort with others while exploring aspects of the world through learning. Maltreated children exhibit numerous difficulties adapting to school. They perform poorly on standardized tests, achieve lower grades, exhibit greater dependence on their teachers, experience more discipline referrals and suspensions, and demonstrate lower social competence (25,60–62).

Neglected children were shown to exhibit the most severe difficulties in school. They are anxious and inattentive as well as dependent on their teachers and uncooperative with them. They were aggressive or withdrawn from peers as well as insensitive and unempathetic. More than half of the children identified as being neglected or physically abused were either held back in first grade or referred for services (63).

A child unable to identify his own feelings and fearful of others' responses to his own actions and words will have difficulty "reading" what others are thinking and feeling. This can limit the child's interaction with peers. The inability to empathize with others will facilitate a lack of respect for individuals, which can contribute to a lack of self-restraint and a tendency toward aggressive violence. Often poor self-esteem, along with a lack of respect for self, is at the root of negative behavior. This behavior is in response to the child's perception of the need for his own physical and emotional preservation (25).

A person who shows an inability to empathize often shows no remorse because he lacks the wherewithal to perceive the impact of his violent actions on another person. This deficiency can mean that the child will take part in more aggressive, violent behavior without realizing the impact on both self and society. Successful rehabilitation, therefore, becomes more difficult (25).

IV. INTELLIGENCE/MORAL DEVELOPMENT

It is important to distinguish moral development from IQ. Although intellectual maturity plays a role in a person's behavior and perception of the world, it is not a given that one's moral reasoning will match the level of his intelligence. Although the acquisition of higher stages of moral development is related to intelligence, longitudinal research on mental retardates indicates that developmental gains in moral reasoning, conduct, and judgment are evident throughout adolescence (64–66). In turn, halts or delays in moral development among individuals of average intelligence may be influenced by the environment (65). Campagna and Harter have found that in comparing IQ-matched normal individuals with sociopathic children, the latter displayed a lower stage of moral development (67).

It is thought that this lower level of moral development is due to the lack of opportunities for role taking in sociopaths' families (67). Other comparisons have suggested that parents of delinquent children may discourage mature moral reasoning (68,69). One of the ways parents may inhibit mature moral reasoning is through their own behavior—by engaging in violence, such as domestic violence, showing anger (70), or through other unlawful acts (4).

Simons et al. have emphasized that poor parenting contributed to early onset delinquency (not late onset) (71). Poor parenting methods, such as inadequate supervision and inconsistent response to the child's actions (including being too harsh and too lenient), were also found to contribute to the development of conduct problems (4,71). Other investigators add poor marital relations (72), poor supervision, lack of parental involvement, and poor parent-child interactions as correlates of delinquency (4,70–74). Often, such behavior is not due to an absence of punishment but rather to the fact that a child has, at times, been treated very harshly. Such children have been subjected to inconsistent, illogical consequences of their behavior because of the parents' own poorly controlled anger, immature impulsiveness, or drunkenness. The relational skills (or lack thereof) in such children have been based largely on what they have observed in their "role models" (4,70,74,75).

Numerous studies have raised an ongoing controversy over the degree to which intellectual capabilities influence delinquent, criminal, and violent behavior. Early studies that link lower IQ scores to delinquency in youth have been found to have a number of flaws. For example, concern has been raised partly because the intelligence tests have been standardized with white middle-class children, who do not adequately reflect abilities of minorities or those from lower socioeconomic levels (4).

Lipsitt et al. reviewed earlier studies linking delinquency to intelligence. After comparing children at three different ages, they found that at 8 months of age there was no significant difference in mental or motor skills (tested by the Bayley Scale). At 4 years of age, the Stanford-Binet scores were significantly lower among the delinquent sample, and at 7 years of age, the delinquent sample scored lower on the Wechsler Intelligence Scale for Children (WISC) for both verbal and performance measures. Based on these findings, the investigators found support for the view that intelligence score at an early age is a factor in the vulnerability of children toward future delinquency. These findings are relevant when schools and families identify children who are experiencing academic difficulties. Appropriate intervention is indicated if these children are to be kept out of the juvenile justice system (76).

Danish adolescents who later become delinquents have lower tested intelligence than nondelinquents and eventually perform more poorly in school (77). While taking into account socioeconomic factors, subsequent analyses of Danish samples continue to suggest a lower intelligence for delinquents (78). Studies by Wolfgang (79), West (80), and Farrington (81) have supported this conclusion (8).

Denno points out a significant distinction between violent offenders and other offenders. Compared with nonoffenders, violent offenders scored 17% lower on vocabulary, 16% lower on total reading, and 10 to 12% lower on total language, the total battery, comprehension, mechanics, usage, and structure. As children progress to and through adolescence, their deficiencies in language and verbal communication become more magnified (8).

Learning disabilities appear paramount in the emergence of delinquency (8,81,82). Waldie et al. found that certain personality characteristics, such as impulsivity and poor judgment, discriminate between persisting and nonpersisting delinquency in youth with learning disabilities. Not surprisingly, there is a hypothesis that learning disabilities produce academic failure, which leads to a poor self-image, which in turn results in school dropout and delinquent behavior (83).

Foley's study of adolescents with reading disabilities reveals a significant association with the later manifestation of Conduct Disorder (CD) in boys and increased police contact in both girls and boys (4,84). Behavioral disorders originate in the preschool years, with evidence of deficits in social skills, motor control, and cognitive skills. These deficits are often obvious in kindergarten and in first grade (85). White et al. found that displaying behavioral problems in preschool was the single best predictor of antisocial disorders at age 11 (86). Carig and Glick found that family characteristics when the child was 6 years old were both the earliest and among the best predictors of future delinquency, and from 9 yeas of age onward, problematic behaviors appear as predictors, with antisocial referrals, aggressiveness, and predelinquency being the pest predictive triad (87,88). At 10 years of age, parent criminality appears to be predictive of later child delinquency. At 15 years of age, grade point average becomes predictive, and at 16 years of age, high self-reported delinquency and officially recorded delinquency become predictive (88,89).

In both sexes, violent offenders—compared with nonviolent offenders and nonoffenders—had lower test results from language, reading, and spelling achievement. These discrepancies were significantly more prominent in females (4,8).

IQ test scores measure more than just intellectual capabilities. We can surmise that a child's ability to get along with teacher and peers, sit quietly, concentrate, and learn, will be reflected in the test results. In addition, a child's conduct will clearly influence the ability to learn and participate in classroom projects and activities.

In summary, research indicates that violent, repeat, and chronic offenders of both genders have a significantly higher incidence of learning difficulties, particularly in their decreased verbal ability. This deficit resulted in more disciplinary placement programs for violent, chronic, and repeat offenders compared with nonviolent offenders and nonoffenders. The problems faced by offenders in school may be behavioral as well as intellectual (4,8).

Brain laterality has also been suggested as a factor in the etiology of violence. Some research (8,90) points to a right-hemisphere deficit, whereas other investigators (8,91) point to a left-hemisphere deficit when discussing delinquency. Left-handed persons have been found to be less analytical and more impulsive, thereby explaining why left-handers and delinquents experience greater deficits in tasks such as reading and language. The skills to analyze, read, and know language are circuited through the left hemisphere, whereas the more emotional and impulsive characteristics are circuited through the right hemisphere. Of note, the right hemisphere has been shown to function as their dominant hemisphere in left-handed persons (8).

The success with which a child strides through the developmental stages will set up a trajectory for her future developmental course. The child's failure to achieve a basic foundational aptitude will be evident in her struggle to tackle another more complex skill that relies on previous, more fundamental abilities.

V. CYCLE OF VIOLENCE

Widom, in her study on *The Cycle of Violence*, initially set out to review the unfounded premise that violence begets violence. She points out that the studies had significant flaws, one of which, in the majority of research, was the lack of a comparison/control group. Widom then proceeded to conduct her own study with a control group. Her research showed that both abused and neglected children were more likely to be arrested for delinquency, adult criminality, and violent criminality than their matched controls (92).

Although males have a higher rate of delinquency, adult criminality, and violence, abused or neglected females also had higher rates of these crimes compared with their gender- and age-matched controls (92).

The girls who had been the victims of physical and/or sexual abuse were at risk for developing delinquent behavior. It has been hypothesized that their behavior is a modeling of what had been done to them by continuing to violate the rights of others. Children who were abused significantly enough to have been removed from their parents' home showed a greater prevalence of Attention-Deficit Hyperactivity Disorder (ADHD) and CD (4,93).

While African Americans had higher rates for violent criminal behavior, only Caucasians had increased rates of having a criminal records as both juveniles and as adults. Caucasians did not have higher rates of violent criminality (92).

In all of the abused and neglected children in Widom's study, there was no difference between the continuity of delinquent behavior and criminal behavior as an adult. Victims of physical abuse were at the highest risk of violent criminal behavior, whereas neglect was the next highest risk. This provides strong support for the cycle-of-violence hypothesis. Once a child commits a crime or becomes a delinquent, whether it is due to abuse, neglect, or neither, their risk of continuing as a criminals into adulthood is the same (92).

To understand violence in adults, it is important to understand the etiology of juvenile delinquency. Some 55% of all crimes and 15% of all violent crimes are committed by juvenile delinquents (4).

Negative emotions and weak constraint have been linked to delinquency. Caspi et al. explain that persons with low-level constraint might be inclined to translate their negative emotions into action more readily (4,94).

Studies revealed that peer relationships with other delinquents were more important than school performance in predicting delinquent behavior. Not only do delinquents attract delinquents, they also cause each other to act in delinquent ways, thereby having an interactional effect, each influencing the other (4,95).

Environmental factors contributing to delinquency have been addressed with socioeconomic status (SES). Williams and McGee attribute the source of delinquency to a disadvantaged background as well as early antisocial behavior (4,84). However, Strouthamer-Loeber and Loeber found SES to be "only weakly related" (4,96), and Simons et al. saw an "indirect" relationship between SES and delinquency (4,71). Of importance, even in deteriorated neighborhoods, McCord found that "competent mothers seem to insulate a child against criminogenic factors" (97). Consequently, the impact of SES in the development of delinquency has yet to be determined (4). In his genetic review, Dinwiddle stresses that there is a genetic basis only for property offenses and no such link for violent offenses. In addition, he notes that lower SES was only an increased risk for those already biologically at risk (98).

In a study by Kemph et al. there were more similarities than differences between juvenile delinquents who had committed violent crimes and juveniles who had committed nonviolent crimes. There were no statistically significant differences with regard to the following: the Beck Hopelessness Scale, the IQ scale, the MMPI scores, job stability, and whether they were treated by a psychiatrist or not. The significant differences were that the violent group was younger and those with a diagnosis of paranoid schizophrenia committed violent crimes, while those with a diagnosis of dysthymia committed nonviolent crimes (99).

Kemph found in the youth offender program that treating aggressive offenders with medication and counseling proved to be helpful. However, there were frequent requests to discontinue the medications once symptoms were under control. Once symptoms recurred, requests were made to restart the medication. The majority of patients seen had mood, adjustment, or psychotic disorders (100).

Both CD and ADHD are commonly thought to be associated with and to represent risks for juvenile delinquent behavior. Controversy exists as to whether each of these disorders alone is, in fact, a strong predictor of juvenile delinquency. Approximately 90% of juvenile offenders meet criteria for CD, the most common diagnosis associated with delinquency (4,101,102).

Klein and Mannuzza reviewed several longitudinal studies and found the link between ADHD and criminality was questionable (4,103). Another extensive study found that ADHD did, in fact, lead to an increased risk of subsequent antisocial behavior. However, when the effects for CD were controlled for, CD alone, and not ADHD, was found to increase the risk of juvenile delinquency (4).

Children with ADHD and CD are more likely to go on and commit crimes as adults. A 14-year longitudinal study found that ADHD and antisocial behavior were among the most important predictors of later offending behavior at age 32 (4,104). Eyestone and Howell found that 25½% of the inmates they studied had ADHD as children and still had the disorder as adults (4,105).

Children with ADHD who had high levels of aggression and defiance had higher offending rates than ADHD children with low levels of aggression and defiance. However, even ADHD children with lower levels of aggression and defiance still had a higher offending rate than their matched controls (4,106,107). Of note, CD is present in 50% of people diagnosed with ADHD (4,5,106). Forehand et al. reported that comorbidity of ADHD and CD is associated with more arrests and more antisocial behavior, which tend to start at a younger age (4,108). The earlier a child exhibits significant behavioral disturbances, such as conduct behavior disorder, the more likely this behavior will persist and lead to adult criminality (4,109–111). Ferguson et al. concluded that 13-year-olds who exhibited conduct problems at 6, 8, and 10 years of age continued to exhibit offending behavior (4,112). Early onset of criminal behavior is a strong predictor of long-term criminality (4,109–112).

Rogers et al. identified late onset of conduct disorder as a good prognostic indicator and noted that it is frequently time-limited. Absence of certain symptoms such as physical cruelty, stealing, truancy, forced sex, and breaking and entering is also a positive indicator. If the symptoms are overt and nondestructive, that is also a good indicator (4,113).

Most studies have shown that those with ADHD are at higher risk for committing criminal acts. However, as noted, ADHD is not as great a predictor as CD. There does not seem to be one form of treatment that has been proven to be successful in treating children with ADHD and CD (3,4,5,107). Research done on ADHD and its risk for delinquent/aggressive behavior has not distinguished, identified, or likely included subjects who were adequately treated for their ADHD symptoms. The lack of adequate treatment early on may increase the development of CD and thereby significantly increase the risk of delinquency. It is critical for research to distinguish and separate out CD children from ADHD children so as to determine if a particular group would be responsive to treatment and thereby have less likelihood of progressing and developing into juvenile delinquents.

Monhahan found that there is an association between acts of violence in childhood and later acts of violence (2,111). The earlier a child manifests violent behavior patterns, the greater the correlation with a more extensive criminal career of violence in later years (72). Nearly all violent adult criminals have histories of juvenile violence. However, not all aggressive juveniles become violent adults (114), and it has been reported that aggression at 8 years of age was predictive of future aggression. Wolfgang et al. reported that early antisocial behavior and being black were predictive of ongoing criminality (8,79).

According to Dorothy Lewis, early aggression can only predict adult violence and has no implication for our understanding of its causes, treatment or prevention. Juvenile violence alone, as noted, did not offer a clear distinction between those who would or would not go on to commit violent crimes as adults. Some 77% of the more violent juveniles and 61% of the less violent juveniles committed adult aggressive offenses (114).

Lewis concluded there are combinations of intrinsic vulnerabilities and environmental stressors that help to explain which delinquents will proceed to commit crimes as adults. She found that the combined interactions of cognitive, psychiatric, and neurologic factors along with a history of abuse and/or violence were predictors of adult violent crime (114,115).

Although organic factors are clearly important, family and psychological issues may be more important. A 20-year study in Hawaii found that the perinatal difficulties (birth difficulties, delayed breathing, and neonatal instability) are associated with delinquency only if the parents later deprive or neglect the child (116).

The link between prenatal and perinatal complications and intellectual and behavioral deficits is potentially strong in poor environments. Children who have experienced prenatal or perinatal complications but were fortunate to have been raised in advantaged families had negligent or nonexistent long-term effects, whereas a child with the same vulnerabilities raised in a disadvantaged family had, "significant retardations in later functioning" as well as intellectual deficits (8,114,117).

Mednick et al. did find that perinatal factors seem to play a role in predisposing individuals toward violence. The effect of such factors was found to be strongest when combined with an unstable family environment (118).

A. Maltreatment

The impact of preschoolers who observe violence, along with their response to trauma, is reason for grave concern. Girls who have witnessed marital aggression between parents have an increased risk of being victims in their own marriages. Boys who witness marital aggression find themselves at increased risk of becoming perpetrators of marital violence (23,119–121).

Studies of child witnesses of spousal abuse find significant difficulties in their behavioral, emotional, social, and academic functioning. These children exhibit a significant increase of anxiety, depression, somatic complaints, aggressive behavior, inattention, impulsivity, and academic difficulties. They also have difficulty empathizing, and they exhibit deficiencies in their social problem-solving abilities (120–126).

Possible mechanisms of the development of behavioral problems in children who witness spousal abuse are seen in children who model aggressive parental behavior, become "triangulated" in parental conflict, and are exposed to inconsistent or ineffectual child-rearing practices (120,127).

Sons who witness spousal abuse tend to view it as "normal." Therefore they tend to view domestic violence as an acceptable means of "conflict resolution" (120).

Children who witness domestic violence, even if they are not in danger, could still experience symptoms of Posttraumatic Stress Disorder (PTSD). A substantial number of children who witness domestic violence are victims of abuse. Therefore both witnessing and being a victim of abuse puts the child at particular risk for family violence when the child, in turn, begins a family (120,121, 128,130). Girls tend to become withdrawn, depressed, and passive. (In contrast, boys tend to respond with externalizing behavior, such as fighting, delinquency, and attacks on their mothers) (120,130). In order to escape both witnessing and being victims of abuse, girls tend to marry early (23). They have children before they have processed their own experiences and are therefore at higher risk to end up in the same victim roles as their mothers.

In a study by Hilberman, most battered women report an increase in their husbands' violence during their pregnancies, violence that led to subsequent miscarriages and premature births (23,131). As a result of being beaten in utero, the developing fetus is vulnerable to subsequent neurologic sequelae. Women between the ages of 17 and 28 were found to be at increased risk for assault at the hands of their partners (23).

Ladoucer and Temple found that alcohol was related to adolescent violence in social settings (23,132–134). Illicit drug use has also been associated with interpersonal violence among adults as well as maltreatment of children in the families of drug users (23,132). Mothers of repeat offenders and one-time offenders have been shown to have significantly lower educational levels. Fathers of repeat offenders have had significantly longer periods of unemployment and have moved frequently between birth and age 7 (8).

VI. NEUROCHEMICAL/NEUROENDOCRINE FACTORS

There are a number of biological markers that have been shown to be altered in a violent person (8,135–137). It helps to understand how we can treat people who are violent by understanding the various shifts in biological markers in a violent adult, including neurotransmitters, receptor sensitivity, etc. Serena-Lynn Brown addresses the research findings on receptor, neurochemical, and treatment findings. The causes that may lead to these shifts in neurochemical and neuroendocrine are factors of interest for treatment but more importantly for prevention. These shifts have been studied in children. De Bellis and Putnam studied the psychobiology of childhood maltreatment and found that maltreatment had an impact that persisted on the neurochemical neuroendocrine systems long after the maltreatment had stopped. They found maltreatment to cause a shift in the catecholamine system, the serotonin system, the benzodiazepine receptor system, the endogenous opiate system, and the neuroendocrine systems, including the hypothalamic-pituitary-adrenal axis, the hypothalamic-pituitary-thyroid axis, the hypothalamic-pituitary-growth hormone axis, and the immune system (138).

Cannon was the first to demonstrate the flight-or-fight reaction in response to life-threatening stressors. This flight-or-fight phenomenon involves activation of the peripheral sympathetic nervous system, a part of the autonomic nervous system (138,139). The primary physiological mechanisms for coping with stress and trauma are the neurotransmitter, the neuroendocrine, and the immune systems. These systems are interconnected at many different levels, coordinating a person's individual responses and adaptation to acute and chronic environmental stress (138).

A. Catecholamine System

Norepinephrine (NE), epinephrine, and dopamine are the three catecholamines involved in arousal, stress reactions, regulation of mood, and thinking/perception (138,140). In experimental animal models, unpredictable and uncontrollable stress is known to increase arousal via brainstem mechanisms. This increase in arousal produces fear and increases the responsiveness of neurons in the locus coeruleus (LC) to excitatory stimulation (138,141). The LC is the major norepinephrine nucleus in the brain (138,142); when there is increased responsiveness in the LC neurons, there is, in turn, increased turnover in the hypothalmus, hippocampus, amygdala, and cerebral cortex. These brain regions have been found to be associated with regulation of stress reactions, memory, and emotion in experimental animals (138,143,144). Increased central NE turnover activates the sympathetic nervous system, leading to the biological fight-or-flight response (138,145).

Dopamine (DA) release and metabolism has been shown to be enhanced in the prefrontal cortex by exposure to stress (138,146). This region of the brain has been shown to be involved in coping responses to stress. Chronic stress enhances DA release in other brain areas (138,147). Drugs such as amphetamines and cocaine cause an increase in presynaptic DA, which results in hypervigilance (138,148). Therefore, elevated DA metabolism may be an adaptive response to environmental stress. Preclinical studies of the effects of trauma during early development have demonstrated permanent changes in the sympathetic nervous system and the hypothalmic-pituitary-adrenal axis of development mammals. An example of this is found in the traumatic separation of infant rhesus monkeys and laboratory rats from their mothers, which was shown to cause behavioral agitation, elevated levels of plasma adrenocorticotropic hormone (ACTH), elevated plasma cortisol, and hyperactivity of the sympathetic nervous system to stress experienced later in life (138,149,150).

Combat veterans with PTSD have heightened sympathetic nervous system (SNS) arousal, with correlated symptoms (138,146). Vietnam veterans with PTSD have been shown to have elevated excretion of DA, NE, and E (138,151–153).

There are a few studies involving the alterations in the catecholaminergic systems of child abuse victims. Catecholamine activity is similar for sexually abused girls as it is for combat veterans with PTSD (138,146,153). [Only one of the sexually abused girls in the study met DSM III-R criteria for PTSD of the *Diagnostic and Statistical Manual of Mental Disorders*, 3d ed. (DSM-III).] It has been noted to be difficult to determine whether the preliminary data of the dysregulation of the catecholamine system in the sexually abused girls reflects primary effects of stress and abuse or secondary effects of dysthymia and depression (138,154).

A preliminary study by Galvin et al. found evidence of low dopamine–beta-hydroxylase activity in psychiatrically hospitalized boys with a diagnosis of conduct disorder and a history of abuse and neglect (further research indicated) (138).

B. Serotonin System

This system plays an important role in the regulation of mood, aggression, impulsivity, and compulsive behaviors. It has also been linked to suicidal behavior and a number of psychiatric disorders (138,155,156). Lower levels of 5-hydroxytryptamine have been associated with suicidal behavior, which is common in victims of childhood maltreatment (further research indicated) (138,157,158).

C. Benzodiazepine Receptor System

Studies have shown that animals exposed to unpredictable, uncontrollable, inescapable shock develop decreases in benzodiazepine receptor binding. These binding sites regulate gamma-aminobutyric (GABA) type A, an inhibitory neurotransmitter system. Decreases in these receptor sites have been demonstrated in a genetically fearful strain of Maudsley rats and in rats who have been fear-conditioned (138,140). One can speculate that initially the decrease in benzodiazepine receptor binding sites may be adaptive in an acutely stressful situation. However, a chronic decrease in these receptor binding sites may contribute to the hyperarousal symptoms seen in PTSD patients and possibly maltreated children (138).

D. Endogenous Opiate System

Exposure to stress causes endogenous opiates to increase and also contributes to the development of analgesia to pain (138,140,159). Opiates dampen the stress response and decrease the firing rate of the LC neurons (138,140). Persons with PTSD have reduced pain sensitivity during exposure to traumatic reminders of war (138,159). This analgesic response is reversed by naloxone, an opiate antagonist (138,160). This system has not yet been studied in maltreated children, but it may be postulated that the effect on these children's opiate systems may be a contributing factor to the constricted affect and high incidence of self-injury reported in maltreated children and in adults who have experienced abuse or neglect as children (138,157,158).

E. Neuroendocrine Systems

With regard to the hypothalamic-pituitary-adrenal (HPA) axis, behavioral agitation and elevated plasma ACTH and cortisol responses to stress were shown in infant rhesus monkeys and rats traumatically separated from their mothers. These responses to stress are continued later on in life (138,149). Elevated levels of glucocorticoid activity may have neurotoxic effects and result in learning impairments secondary to hippocampal damage (138,161). After sustained social stress, hippocampal degeneration was noted in monkeys (138,162). Animal studies in which animals were administered exogenous glucocorticoids showed significant hippocampal damage (138,163,164). Children with a diagnosis of depression who have been maltreated were shown to have abnormalities in cortisol secretion (138,165).

The data in abused children differ from that in adults with depression and are most similar to adults with a diagnosis of PTSD. Thus child abuse is not only a traumatic event that causes an increase in psychiatric morbidity but also one that is associated with sustained changes in the HPA axis in these children (138).

F. Hypothalmic-Pituitary-Thyroid Axis

Preclinical studies have demonstrated that activation of the LC neurons, which occurs when a child is exposed to stress, results in direct stimulation of the hypothalamic neurons secreting thyrotropin-releasing hormone (138,166). Thyrotropin-releasing hormone (TRH) stimulates the secretion of pituitary thyrotropin (TSH), which stimulates the thyroid to secrete thyroid hormone. In addition, during acute stress, direct stimulation by NE through postganglionic sympathetic innervation of the thyroid also stimulates release and increased synthesis of thyroid hormone through the production of cyclic adenosine monophosphate (cAMP) (138,167). During an episode of acute stress, the increased metabolic rate caused by the increase in the thyroid hormone provides "emergency" energy. Thyroid hormones are necessary for the growth and differentiation of brain neurons and glial cells throughout fetal, child, and adolescent development (138,168). Thyroid hormone inhibits TSH release (138,167). Therefore, chronic TRH secretion secondary to prolonged stress will not cause sustained release of TSH because of downregulation of pituitary TRH receptors (132,169). Thus chronic stress is associated with decreased production of TSH and inhibition of conversion of thyroxine to triiodothyronine (the more biologically active form) in peripheral tissues (138,170). This mechanism tends to conserve energy during periods of chronic stress. Thus, chronic stress such as childhood neglect or abuse may lead to physiologically normal central suppression of the HPT axis. Since the HPT axis is extremely important for physical growth and cognitive development, additional studies of HPT axis functioning in maltreated children is warranted. Lower TSH levels can result in a reduced set point for metabolic rate, and this may be contributory to the higher rates of obesity reported in women with a history of sexual abuse (138,171). There is also speculation that childhood maltreatment may lead to profound changes in the child's brain development, and this may lead to decreased intelligence (138).

G. Hypothalmic-Pituitary-Growth Hormone (HPG) Axis

Growth hormone, which is critical in the development of a child, is also affected by stress. During acute stress, the HPG axis is initially activated, causing increased growth hormone secretion. However, in chronic stress, secretion of corticotropin-release hormone directly inhibits secretion of growth hormone (138, 170,172). Disruption of the infant–primary caretaker relationship, as in maternal deprivation, rejection, and abuse, has been shown in animals to contribute to physiological and behavioral abnormalities in the offspring as a result of changes in HPG secretion (138,173).

The linear growth and final adult stature in humans depends on genetic constitution, nutrition, hormones, the presence or absence of systemic diseases, and a nurturing phychosocial environment (138,174). In infants and toddlers, there are two syndromes that parallel the above-mentioned animal studies: one is the Nonorganic Failure to Thrive (NOFTT) and the other is Psychosocial Dwarfism (PD) (138).

NOFTT has various causes and is primarily a condition of malnutrition. A disturbed primary caregiver–infant relationship is thought to be the most common cause. Controlled investigations have shown that when the primary caretaker–infant interactions during feeding and play are of poor quality, there are more struggles for control as well as more conflict, less dyadic reciprocity, more negative affects, fewer positive vocalizations, and less ability of the primary caretaker to read the infant's cues and signals in a contingent, sensitive manner (138,175).

Studies have shown that NOFTT infants and children are more likely to grow up with various forms of psychosocial adversity, such as being the child of an unemployed, poor, depressed, suicidal, or alcohol-dependent parent(s). Other adversities that these infant and children may be exposed to include living in inadequate housing, where there is social isolation, marital discord, or domestic violence. Controlled studies have shown that these infants are usually cachectic, have developmental delays, and may be behaviorally disturbed. These behavioral disturbances may consist of the following behavior: restlessness, listlessness, irritability, apathy, wariness, hypervigilance, and hypertonicity or hypotonicity as compared with the behavior of thriving infants. They also tend to have a higher incidence of learning disabilities and behavioral problems (138,175).

A disruption in the bond between an infant and its primary caretaker can also lead to PD, also known as abuse dwarfism or psychologically determined short stature (138,176–178). Unlike NOFTT, PD occurs independently of malnutrition. A severely disturbed primary caretaker–infant relationship is thought to be the primary etiological factor. Child abuse, neglect, marital discord, and psychopathology in caretakers are common found in association with both of the above disorders. Onset is usually between 2 and 4 years of age, and some of these children have histories of NOFTT (138,176).

The syndrome of PD has been characterized by three primary reversible impairments: (a) growth disturbance (subnormal growth rate after a period of normal growth or normal birth weight); (b) endocrine dysfunction [fasting plasma growth hormone (GH) levels and GH response to insulin induced hypoglycemia are abnormally low]; and (c) behavioral and developmental disturbances, such as polyphagia, gorging and vomiting, polydipsia, social immaturity, social withdrawal, developmental delays, mental retardation, pain agnosia, and self-injury. Sleep disturbances also occur, most notably in stage 4 on the polysomnograph, during which GH is usually secreted. The reduction of stage 4 sleep leads to a corresponding reduction in the secretion of GH. Once a child with PD is placed in a more favorable environment, these symptoms—including GH abnormalities, sleep disturbances, and delays in bone growth—rapidly normalize (138,176).

One study has investigated the effects of maltreatment on the HPG axis. Sexually abused boys had a statistically significant elevated ratio of GH response to clonodine versus L-dopa, whereas physically abused boys were found to have lower clonidine/L-dopa GH responses compared with controls (138,179). GH plays an important role in pubertal development, and children with GH deficiency have delayed onset of puberty (138,180). Delayed growth can be one of many psychobiological sequelae of neglect, physical abuse, and chronic life stress (138).

H. Immune System

Immunosuppression secondary to chronic stress may lead to increased rates of medical illness in neglected or abused children. This may subsequently lead to serious morbidity from medical illness in maltreated children (138).

The examples, noted above, of the effect of environment on biological health and vice versa emphasize the critical nature of a comprehensive treatment plan. As described, children wh are victims and/or witnesses of violence experience a shift in their neurochemical production and receptor sensitivity that will significantly impact the rest of their lives. The effects can be seen both in the emotional stability of a person as well as their physical well-being. Research has shown that these neurochemical shifts persist long after the maltreatment has ceased (138). This shift in a person's neurochemical makeup may contribute to an increased risk of becoming violent and/or impulsive and deserves further investigation.

VII. A COMPREHENSIVE PLAN

Violence affects society in so many ways—whether we walk our child to school, avoid certain neighborhoods, or obtain security systems to protect ourselves and those we love. To effectively address the violence in our society, we need a comprehensive plan that looks at the whole person and considers many necessary combined avenues of intervention. This includes the person's physical well-being, mental health, education, relationships, family interactions, employment, living circumstances, and community. To address only one of these and abandon the others is likely to lead to failure of the intervention.

Every facet of a person's life—strengths, weaknesses, and vulnerabilities that contribute to potentially violent behavior—needs to be (and is) addressed in a comprehensive plan. The goal is for parents to be healthy and stable, both emotionally (and to some extent, financially), so that they can provide adequately for their sons and daughters. For example, the amount of time the father is unemployed, the amount of time the child is exposed to lead intoxication, and the number of times the family relocates all contribute to an increased risk of juvenile delinquency (8). A comprehensive plan can best be understood in a chronological overview.

It is unlikely that a teenage mother who has only begun to establish her own autonomy, can do what is in the best interest of her child. Therefore we need to address teenage pregnancy. Jane, for instance, became pregnant when she was 14. She had not finished school, was using drugs, was in an unhealthy relationship, and had a history of depression that was not adequately addressed. Jane does not have what is needed to be even an adequate parent.

When society fails with respect to a teen becoming pregnant—and if she chooses to carry the baby to term—she must become aware of her pregnancy as early as possible in order to seek appropriate prenatal care. This includes proper nutrition and abstaining from toxic substances such as recreational drugs or medications. And she must protect her fetus from physical abuse. In order for a teenager to seek out prenatal care, she needs to be educated comprehensively about how all of her decisions, such as to use cocaine, can contribute to premature birth. If Jane is not educated about the care for her fetus, plus the specific ramifications of her actions, both she and her baby will remain at risk. Jane needs to understand that if she takes cocaine, she risks premature birth, leading to low birth weight as well as neurologic and developmental delays, which, as noted above, are contributing risk factors for violence.

After the child is born, we need to educate the mother thoroughly because, owing to managed care, mothers and infants are being discharged earlier than ever. Therefore a mother needs to be educated on numerous topics, from how to hold the baby to ensuring that all of the child's medical and emotional needs are met. The child, for instance, may develop jaundice, which, without proper medical treatment, will lead to kernicterus. Although Jane showed that she could feed, clean, and clothe the baby, which are all critical to the infant's health, she seemed to lack the ability to supervise and protect her child from serious falls and ingestion of paint chips. She also did not appreciate the value and importance of social interaction with her child and instead remained isolated from the child by wearing a Walkman.

Jane's inadequate parenting skills, including inconsistent limit setting—which vacillated between overly harsh and overly permissive—plus overall unresponsiveness to her child's needs, made it unlikely that Robin begin to develop secure attachments and a secure sense of self. As noted earlier, attachment is crucial in establishing healthy peer relationships. Given Jane's lack of education and attention to her daughter, it is unlikely that Robin will experience secure attachments, through which a child gains a sense of self as well as respect for others, and develop a capacity to empathize, which enhances the quality of one's relationships.

In feeling frustrated and irritated, Jane would shake Robin, not leaving any open wounds or marks. It is unlikely that she appreciated the damage she inflicted on her child. By addressing Jane's psychiatric difficulties, such as depression and teaching her more adaptive ways to cope with her frustrations as a parent as well as helping her to appreciate the benefits of consistent limits for both her and her child, Jane might be helped to feel more confident as a parent. Ideally, her child would reap the benefits.

One of the particular risks faced by Jane's child was observing the abuse her mother sustained at the hands of her boyfriend. As a result of witnessing the abuse, Robin's neuroendocrine system was likely shifted for life. In later life, this can affect Robin's ability to cope with stress, lower her resistance to illness, and put her at increased risk for drug use. (Alteration of benzodiazepine receptors due to trauma will likely increase her risk for alcohol and benzodiazepine abuse.)

Witnessing violence in an everyday manner will facilitate the child's tendency to view abusive behavior as "normal" (120). Biological vulnerabilities tend to be expressed with significant detriment to the child raised in a dysfunctional, abusive family. Conversely, biological vulnerabilities in children raised in healthy, nurturing environments are lessened to varying degrees (8,21,107,109). Even the best parent will make mistakes, and a child can withstand bad decisions without long-term effects on his or her emotional and physical well-being. Children with preexisting biological, behavioral, intellectual, neurological, or psychiatric vulnerabilities may have more difficulty succeeding in bad conditions without suffering deleterious effects. However, certain children succeed regardless of the circumstances of their early environment. If those resilient features could be identified and promoted in other children, their chances of withstanding unfortunate circumstances without deleterious effect might be improved (116,182). For some children, the support that comes from individuals and institutions outside of the family can counteract the negative effects of a bad family environment.

One way society could have intervened would have been to help Jane understand the abusive structure of her relationship with her boyfriend and its damaging long-term effects on her and her child. Helping Jane to establish a sense of pride in herself and in her work, such as helping her achieve adequate employment, could give her the strength to value herself enough to not tolerate abusive treatment. In this way, she could become a role model and teach her daughter that one must respect oneself and demand respect from others.

Jane failed to identify and address her daughter's developmental delays. Upon entering school, Robin's developmental delays impeded her ability to learn and created a sense of failure. This contributed to Robin's poor self-image and yearning to be accepted and appreciated despite her failures—a process led Robin away from the educational system and into the tragic world of gangs.

It is critical for us to address a child's developmental weaknesses and strengths so that, in the end, the child will feel good about himself or herself and not seek out negative (and potentially violent) alternatives in yearning to feel accepted and loved. Children who have not experienced a stable, consistent relationship with a caregiver (i.e., children who have lived in multiple foster homes or experienced sexual or physical abuse and/or neglect) are likely to suffer from reactive attachment disorder. Children with this disorder have significant difficulty forming healthy attachments. Children who have the disinhibited type of reactive attachment disorder (9) will, in the void of a healthy primary caregiver–child relationship, attach themselves to anyone, including strangers, thereby putting themselves at significant risk for abuse—and, possibly, violence. Children with inhibited reactive attachment lack the sense of empathy and moral responsibility that stems from a healthy caregiver-child attachment. Children suffering from the inhibited type of reactive attachment disorder could be expected to have an increased risk of becoming delinquent and perpetrating violence. Although further study is needed, my clinical experience in evaluating and treating children who suffer from reactive attachment disorder supports the above hypotheses. I theorize that by improving the emotional environmental and interactions of children and caregivers, children can establish healthy attachments from infancy on and thereby lessen their risk of becoming victims or perpetrators.

Jane was not successful in providing Robin with a stable parent-child attachment, and Robin exhibited symptoms of reactive attachment disorder. As noted above, Jane's behavior as a parent prevented the nurturing interaction that is a necessary part of establishing healthy attachments.

Robin had difficulty communicating verbally and tried to get her needs met acting out with temper tantrums, hitting, and banging. If Robin had received adequate help with verbal communication skills, perhaps she would have been able to express her needs in more acceptable, effective ways. If Robin had not seen violence glorified as an easy form of conflict resolution and had found access to a firearm more difficult, perhaps she would not have resorted to assault with a deadly weapon.

One of the factors that impeded Robin's ability to learn in school was her inability to sit still, focus, and concentrate. Perhaps if Robin had received appropriate diagnosis and treatment in conjunction with attention to her verbal weaknesses, she would have felt more comfortable learning and more at home at school. Addressing ADHD, school, and verbal communication, each on its own is inadequate for meeting Robin's overall needs as a whole person—needs that only a comprehensive plan can address.

VIII. PREVENTION/TREATMENT

Obviously prevention would be ideal; however, at this point in time, prevention for all is unrealistic. It is therefore critical that we address the issue of treatment. It is helpful to identify those most likely to respond positively to treatment and to distinguish which treatment is most appropriate for which behaviors and age groups. For example, Baily points out the importance of certain strengths in a child's nature that make some interventions more successful for particular people. Baily discusses how the capacity to form emotional attachments with others and the ability for self-examination and insight are good indicators for social skill intervention programs. Therapeutic gains emerge slowly, given the frequently chaotic and abusive backgrounds of the young offenders and severe past aggression. She also identifies low intelligence and poor capacity as being associated with poor outcomes. Baily points out that the majority of child and adolescent offenders initially disassociate themselves from the reality of their offense and situation. Depending upon their stage of emotional and psychological development, many will eventually engage in treatment despite their initial disassociation (181). Baily addresses one treatment option, but clearly there are a variety of treatment and intervention options that deserve further exploration.

IX. CONCLUSION

Clearly we have identified that the earlier a child exhibits violent behavior, the worse the long-term prognosis. *The earlier interventions are made, the more likely that they will be successful in decreasing a person's maladaptive ways and enhancing productive communication and behavior.* Effective measures that can predict risk and outcome are vital if we are to make the much-needed interventions at the appropriate time.

One of the main obstacles to implementing preventive measures is the lack of approved funding. Unfortunately, the government, responding to public pressure to keep violent offenders locked up, is more prone to build jails than to initiate ultimately more efficacious preventive measures designed to focus predominantly on the causes of violence. One intervention in Washington State, called "blended funding," is implemented to help children who have failed every other system. How tragic that we wait until children fail all interventions before we implement what they needed all along—coordination of care with school, family, community, and psychiatric services. A genre of treatment that targets individual risk factors rather than the child's comprehensive environment is a contributing factor to the failure of many studies of delinquency treatments.

The need for a comprehensive plan is imperative: if we are going to be effective in decreasing violence, we need to take every possible measure that can lessen the likelihood of risk factors that increase the propensity for violence. How?

By decreasing brain neurological developmental delays
By decreasing abuse and negative role models
By decreasing harmful effects of drug use in utero
By decreasing teen pregnancy
By eliminating the ingestion of lead chips
By decreasing child injury due to poor supervision
By preventing inconsistent parenting
By addressing each child's educational needs
By improving a child's poor sense of self
By minimizing media glorification of violence
By addressing each child's psychiatric risk and needs
By decreasing the availability of drugs and guns (183)

Decreasing these risk factors through a comprehensive plan can help decrease the propensity for violence in children. Will all beatings, domestic rage, and schoolyard shootings be eliminated for good? Not likely. Yet if a comprehensive plan could have made a difference in the life of person like Jane or Kip Kinkel, why not try? The alternative is captured by the plea one student wrote on a small sign propped up at the impromptu memorial of flowers at Thurston High in Springfield, Oregon: "Will we ever learn?"

ACKNOWLEDGMENTS

Thanks to Mark Cutshall and Vanessa Raymond for helping me write this chapter.

REFERENCES

1. S. Sunde and S. Miletich, Teens Rage Turns Deadly, *Seattle Post-Intelligencer*, May 22, 1998, p. 1.
2. J. Monahan, *Predicting Violent Behavior, an Assessment of Clinical Technique 14*, Sage Library of Social Research, Beverly Hills, CA, 1981.
3. R. Cohen, D. Parmalee, L. Irwin, et al., Characteristics of children in adolescence in a psychiatric hospital and a corrections facility, *J. Am. Acad. Child Adolesc. Psychiatry 29*:909 (1990).
4. H. Foley, C. Carlton, and R. Howell, The Relationship of Attention Deficit Hyperactivity Disorder and Conduct Disorder to Juvenile Delinquency: Legal Implications, *Bull. Am. Acad. Psychiatry Law 24 (3)*:333 (1996).
5. R. O'Shaughnessy, Clinical aspects of forensic assessment of juvenile offenders, *Psychiatr. Clin. North Am. 15*:721 (1992).
6. J. Satterfield, J. Swanson, A. Schell, and F. Lee, Prediction of antisocial behavior in attention-deficit hyperactivity disorder boys from aggression/defiance scores, *J. Am. Acad. Child Adolesc. Psychiatry 33*:185 (1994).
7. C. Lombroso, *L'Uomo delinquente*, Hoepli, Milan, 1876.
8. D. Denno, *Biology, Crime and Violence: New Evidence*, Cambridge University Press, Cambridge, England, 1989.
9. *American Psychiatric Association: Diagnostic and Statistical Manual of Mental Disorders (ed. 4)*, APA, Washington DC, 1994.
10. S. Litt, A study of perinatal complications as a factor in criminal behavior, *Criminology 12 (1)*: 125 (1974).
11. R. Naeye, Causes of perinatal mortality in the U.S. Collaborative Perinatal Project, *J.A.M.A. 238 (3)*: 228 (1977).
12. R. Naeye, Placenta previa: Predisposing factors and effects on the fetus and surviving infants, *Am. Coll. Obstet. Gynecol. 52*:521 (1978).
13. National Center for Health Statistics, *Factors Associated with Low Birth Weight: United States, 1976*, U.S. Department of Health, Education and Welfare, Washington, DC, 1980.
14. K. Niswander, E. Friedman, D. Hoover, H. Pietrowski, and M. Westphal, Fetal morbidity following potentially anoxigenic obstetric conditions, *Am. J. Obstet. Gynecol. 95*:853 (1966).

15. K. Niswander and M. Gordon, *The Women and their Pregnancies*, U.S. Department of Health, Education, and Welfare, Washington, DC, 1972.
16. T. McNeil, R. Wiegerink, and J. Dozier, Pregnancy and birth complications in the births of seriously, moderately, and mildly behaviorally disturbed children, *J. Nerv. Ment. Dis. 151*:24–34 (1970).
17. M. Rogers, A. Lilienfeld, and B. Pasamanick, *Prenatal and Paranatal Factors in the Development of Childhood Behavior Disorders*, Ejnar Munksgaard, Copenhagen, 1955.
18. E. Kandel and S. Mednick, Perinatal complications predict violent offending, *Criminology 29*:519–529 (1991).
19. A. Raine, P. Brennan, and S. Mednick, Birth complications combined with early maternal rejection at age 1 year predispose to violent crime at age 18 years, *Arch. Gen. Psychiatry 51*:984–988 (1994).
20. D. Fergusson, J. Fergusson, L. Horwood, and N. Kinzett, A longitudinal study of dentine lead levels, intelligence, school performance and behaviour, *J. Child Psychol. Psychiatry Allied Disc. 29*:811–824 (1988).
21. S. Chess and A. Thomas, *Origins and Evolution of Behavior Disorders*, Brunner/Mazel, New York, 1984.
22. S. Chess and A. Thomas, *Temperament in Clinical Practice*, Guilford Press, New York, 1986.
23. M. Lystad, M. Rice, and S. Kaplan, Domestic violence, *Family Violence—A Clinical and Legal Guide* (S. Kaplan, ed.), American Psychiatric Press, Washington, DC, 1996, pp. 145–150.
24. H. Parens, A view of the development of hostility in early life, *Affect: Psychoanalytic Perspectives* (T. Shapiro and R. Emde, eds.), International Universities Press, New York, 1992.
25. D. Cicchetti and F. Rogosch, The toll of child maltreatment on the developing child—Insights from developmental psychopathology, *Child Adolesc. Psychiatry Clin. North Am. 3 (4)*: 759 (1994).
26. L. Sroufe and M. Rutter, The domain of developmental psychopathology, *Child Dev. 55*:17 (1984).
27. H. Werner and B. Kaplan, *Symbol Formation: An Organismic-Developmental Approach to Language and the Expression of Thought*, John Wiley & Sons, New York, 1963.
28. D. Cicchetti and N. Garmezy, (eds.), Milestones in the development of resilience [special issue], *Dev. Psychopathol. 5*:497 (1993).
29. H. Hartmann, *Ego Psychology and the Problem of Adaptation*, International Universities Press, New York, 1958.
30. D. Cicchetti and K. Schneider-Rosen, An organizational approach to childhood depression, *Depression in Young People: Clinical and Developmental Perspectives* (M. Rutter, C. Izard, and P. Read, eds.), Guildford Press, New York, 1986, pp. 71–134.
31. D. Cicchetti, J. Ganiban, and D. Barnett, Contributions from the study of high-risk populations to understanding the development of emotional regulation (N. Frude, ed.) *The Development of Emotion Regulation and Dysregulation* (J. Garber and K.A. Dodge, eds.), Cambridge University Press, New York, 1991, p. 15–48.

32. T. Gaensbauer, D. Mrazek, and R. Harmon, Emotional expression in abused and/or neglected infants, *Psychological Approaches to Child Abuse*, Rowman & Littlefield, NJ, 1981, pp. 120–135.
33. D. Cicchetti and M. Lynch, Failures in the expectable environment and their impact on individual development: The case of child maltreatment, *Developmental Psychopathology 2: Risk, Disorder, and Adaptation* (D. Cicchetti and C. Cohen, eds.), John Wiley, New York. In press.
34. T. Gaensbauer, The differentiation of discrete affects, *Psychoanal. Study Child 37*:29 (1982).
35. A. Shields, D. Cicchetti, and R. Ryan, The development of emotional and behavioral self-regulation and social competence among maltreated school-age children, *Dev. Psychopathol. 6*:57 (1994).
36. J. Bowlby, *Attachment and Loss: Vol 1: Attachment*, Basic Books, New York, 1969/1982.
37. L. Sroufe, The coherence of individual development, *Am. Psychol. 34*:834 (1979).
38. D. Cicchetti, How research on child maltreatment has informed the study of child development: Perspectives from developmental psychopathology, *Abuse and Neglect* (D. Cicchetti and V. Carlson, eds.), Cambridge University Press, New York, 1989, pp. 377–341.
39. P. Crittenden, *Relationships at Risk. Clinical Implications of Attachment Theory* (J. Belsky and T. Nezworski, eds.), Lawrence Erlbaum Associates, Hillsdale, NJ, 1988, pp. 136–174.
40. B. Egeland and L. Sroufe, Developmental sequelae of maltreatment in infancy, *New Dir. Child Dev. 11*:77 (1981).
41. K. Schneider-Rosen and D. Cicchetti, The relationship between affect and cognition in maltreated infants: Quality of attachment and the development of visual self-recognition, *Child Dev. 55*:648 (1984).
42. T. Hirschi, *Causes of Delinquency*, University of California Press, Berkeley, CA, 1969.
43. P. Crittenden and D. DiLalla, Compulsive compliance: The development of an inhibitory coping strategy in infancy, *J. Abn. Child Psychol. 16*:585 (1988).
44. M. Main and J. Solomon, Procedures for identifying infants as disorganized/disoriented during the Ainsworth Strange Situation, *Attachment in the Preschool Years* (M. Greenberg, D. Cicchetti and E. Cumming, eds.), University of Chicago Press, Chicago, 1990, pp. 121–160.
45. D. Winnicott, The Maturational Processes and the Facilitating Environment: Studies, *Theory of Emotional Development*, International Universities Press, New York, 1965.
46. R. Allen and J. Oliver, The effects of child maltreatment on language development, *Child Abuse Neglect 6*:299 (1982).
47. R. Culp, R. Watkins, H. Lawrence, et al., Maltreated children's language and speech development: Abused, neglected, and abused and neglected, *First Lang. 11*:377 (1991).
48. L. Fox, S. Long, and A. Langlois, Patterns of language comprehension deficits in abused and neglected children, *J. Speech Hear. Disord. 53*:239 (1988).
49. M. Beehgly and D. Cicchetti, Child maltreatment, attachment, and the self system:

Emergence of an internal state lexicon in toddlers at high social risk, *Dev. Psychopathol. 6*:5 (1994).
50. W. Coster, M. Gersten, M. Beeghly, et al., Communicative functioning in maltreated toddlers, *Dev. Psychol. 25*:1020 (1989).
51. S. Alessandri, Play and social behavior in maltreated preschoolers, *Dev. Psychopathol. 3*:191 (1991).
52. N. Crick and K. Dodge, A review and formulation of social information-processing mechanisms in children's social adjustment, *Psychol. Bull. 115*:74 (1994).
53. K. Dodge, G. Pettit, and J. Bates, Effects of physical maltreatment on the development of peer relations, *Dev. Psychopathol. 6*:43 (1994).
54. B. Weiss, K. Dodge, J. Bates, et al., Some consequences of early harsh discipline: Child aggression, and a maladaptive social information processing style, *Child Dev. 63*: 1321 (1992).
55. C. George and M. Main, Social interactions of young abused children: Approach, avoidance, and aggression, *Child Dev. 50*:306 (1979).
56. C. Howes and R. Eldredge, Responses of abused, neglected, and non-maltreated children to the behaviors of their peers, *J. Appl. Dev. Psychol. 6*: 261 (1985).
57. C. Hoews and M. Espinosa, The consequences of child abuse for the formation of relationships with peers, *Child Abuse Neglect 9*:397 (1985).
58. B. Klimes-Dougan and J. Kistner, Physically abused preschoolers' response to peers' distress, *Dev. Psychol. 26*:599 (1990).
59. M. Main and C. George, Responses of abused and disadvantaged toddlers to distress in age-mates: A study in the daycare setting, *Dev. Psychol. 21*: 407 (1985).
60. J. Eckenrode, M. Laird, and J. Doris, School performance and disciplinary prob lems among abused and neglected children, *Dev. Psychol. 29*: 53 (1993).
61. B. Egeland, L. Sroufe, M. Erickson, The developmental consequences of different patterns of maltreatment, *Child Abuse Neglect 7*:459 (1983).
62. F. Rogosch and D. Cicchetti, Illustrating the interface of family and peer relations through the study of child maltreatment, *Social Dev.* In press.
63. M. Erickson, B. Egeland, and R. Pianta, The effects of maltreatment on the development of young children, *Child Maltreatment: Theory and Research on the Causes and Consequences of Child Abuse and Neglect* (D. Cicchetti and V. Carlson, eds.), Cambridge University Press, New York, 1989, pp. 647–684.
64. J. Aronfreed, Discussion: Developmental gains in moral judgement, *Am. J Mental Defic. 79*:113 (1974).
65. D. Goleman, *Emotional Intelligence*, Bantam Books, New York, 1995.
66. H. Gardner and T. Hatch, Multiple intelligences go to school: Educational implications of the theory of multiple intelligences, *Educ Res 18(8)*:4 (1989).
67. A. Campagna and S. Harter, Moral Judgments in sociopathic and normal children, *J. Personal. Soc. Psychol. 31*:199 (1974).
68. N. Prentice and F. Kelly, Intelligence and delinquency: A reconsideration, *J. Soc. Psychol. 60*:327 (1963).
69. G. Jukovic, The juvenile delinquent as a moral philosopher: A structural-developmental perspective, *Psychol. Bull. 88*:709 (19).
70. M. Fraser, Aggressive behavior in childhood and early adolescence: An

ecologicaldevelopmental perspective on youth violence, *Social Work 41*:347 (1996).
71. R. Simons, C. Wu, R. Conger, and F. Lorenz, Two routes to delinquency: differences between early and late starters in the impact of parenting and deviant peers, *Criminology 32*: 247 (1994).
72. M. Stouthamer-Loeber and R. Loeber, The use of prediction data in understanding delinquency, *Behav. Sci. Law 6*:333 (1988).
73. R. Loeber, M. Stouthamer-Loeber, W. Van Kammen, and D. Farrington, Initiation, escalation, and resistance in juvenile offending and their correlates, *J. Crim. Law Criminol. 82*:36 (1991).
74. A. Johnson, Sanctions for superego lacunae of adolescents, *The Psychology of Adolescence: Essential Readings*, International Universities Press, New York, 1974, pp. 267–283.
75. J. McCord and W. McCord, The effects of parental role model on criminality. *Readings in juvenile delinquency* (R. Cavan, ed.), Lippincott, Philadelphia, 1975.
76. P. Lipsitt, S. Buka, and L. Lipsitt, Early intelligence scores and subsequent delinquency: A prospective study, *Am. J Fam. Ther. 18*(2): (1990).
77. L. Kirkegaard-Sorenson and S. Mednick, A prospective study of predictors of criminality: 4. School behavior, *Biosocial Bases of Criminal Behavior* (S. Mednick and K. Christiansen, eds.), Gardner Press, New York, 1977.
78. T. Moffitt, W. Gabrielli, and S. Mednick, Socioeconomic status, IQ, and delinquency, *J. Abn. Psychol. 90(2)*:152 (1981).
79. M. Wolfgang, R. Figlio, and T. Sellin, *Delinquency in a Birth Cohort*, University of Chicago Press, Chicago, 1971.
80. D. West and D. Farrington, *Who Becomes Delinquent?* Heinemann, London, 1973.
81. D. Farrington, Offending from 10 to 25 years of age, *Prospective Studies of Crime and Delinquency* (K. Van Dusen and S. Mednick, eds.), Kluwer-Nijhoff, Boston, 1983.
82. D. Crawford, The link between delinquency and learning disabilities, *Judges J. 24*:23 (1985).
83. K. Waldie and O. Spreen, The Relationship Between Learning Disabilities and Persisting Delinquency, *J. Learn. Disabil. 26*:417 (1993).
84. S. Williams and R. McGee, Reading attainment and juvenile delinquency, *J. Child Psychol. Psychiatry 35*:441 (1994).
85. J. Meeks, Behavioral and antisocial disorders, *Handbook of Child Psychiatry* (J. Noshpitz, ed.), Basic, New York, 1979.
86. J. White, T. Moffitt, F. Earls, L. Robins, and P. Silva, How early can we tell?: Predictors of childhood conduct disorder and adolescent delinquency, *Criminology 28*: 507 (1990).
87. M. Craig and S. Glick, Ten years experience with the Glueck Social Prediction Table, *Crime Delinq. 9*: 249 (1963).
88. R. Loeber and T. Dishion, early Predictors of male delinquency: A review, *Psychol. Bull. 94*:68 (1983).
89. L. Robins, P. West, and B. Herjanic, Arrests and delinquency in two generations:

A study of black urban families and their children, *J. Child Psychol. Psychiatry 16*:125 (1975).
90. L. Yeudall, A neuropsychosocial perspective of persistent juvenile delinquency and criminal behavior, *Ann. N.Y. Acad. Sci. 347*:349 (1980).
91. J. Andrew, Are left-handers less violent? *J. Youth Adolesc. 9 (1)*:1 (1980).
92. C. Widom, The cycle of violence, *Science 244*:160 (1989).
93. R. Famularo, R. Kinscherff, and T. Fenton, Psychiatric diagnoses of maltreated children: Preliminary findings, *J. Am. Acad. Child Adolesc. Psychiatry 31*:863 (1992).
94. A. Caspi, T. Moffitt, P. Silva, M. Stouthamer-Loeber, R. Kruger, P. Schmutte, Are some people crime-prone? Replications of the personality-crime relationship across countries, genders, races, and methods, *Criminology 32*:163 (1994).
95. T. Thornberry, A Lizotte, M. Krohn, M. Farnsworth, and S. Jang, Delinquent peers, beliefs, and delinquent behavior: A longitudinal test of interactional theory, *Criminology 32*:47 (1994).
96. M. Stouthamer-Loeber and R. Loeber, The use of prediction data in understanding delinquency, *Behav. Sci. Law 6*:333 (1988).
97. J. McCord, Family relationships, juvenile delinquency, and adult criminality, *Criminology 29*:397 (1991).
98. S. Dinwindle, Psychiatric genetics and forensic psychiatry: A review, *Bull. Am. Acad. Psychiatry Law 22 (3)*:323 (1994).
99. J. Kemph, R. Braley, and P. Ciotola, A comparison of youthful inmates who have committed violent versus nonviolent crimes. *J. Am. Acad. Psychiatry Law 26 (3)*:67 (1998).
100. J. Kemph, R. Braley, and P. Ciotola, Description of an outpatient psychiatric population in youthful offender's prison, *J. Am. Acad. Psychiatry Law 25(2)*:149 (1997).
101. T. Eppright, J. Kashani, B. Robinson, and J. Reid, Comorbidity of conduct disorder and personality disorders in an incarcerated juvenile population, *Am. J Psychiatry 150*:1233 (1993).
102. R. Milin, J. Halikas, J. Meller, and C. Morse, Psychopathology among substance abusing juvenile offenders, *J. Am. Acad. Child Adolesc, Psychiatry 30*:569 (1991).
103. R. Klein and S. Mannuzza, Long-term outcome of hyperactive children: A review, *J. Am. Acad. Child Adolesc. Psychiatry 30*:383 (1991).
104. D. Farrington, Implications of criminal career research for the prevention of offending, *J. Adolesc. 13*:93 (1990).
105. L. Eyestone and R. Howell, An epidemiological study of attention-deficit hyperactivity disorder and major depression in a male prison population, *Bull. Am. Acad. Psychiatry Law 22*:181 (1994).
106. R. Barkley, M. Fischer, C. Edelbrock, and L. Smallish, The adolescent outcome of hyperactive children diagnosed by research criteria I: An 8-year prospective follow-up study, *J. Am. Acad. Child Adolesc. Psychiatry 29*:546 (1990).
107. J. Satterfield, C. Hoppe, and A. Schell, A prospective study of delinquency in 110 adolescent boys with attention deficit disorder and 88 normal adolescent boys, *Am. J Psychiatry 139*:795 (1982).
108. R. Forehand, M. Wierson, C. Framce, T. Kempton, and L. Armisted, Juvenile delin-

quency entry and persistence: do attention problems contribute to conduct problems? *J. Behav. Ther. Exp. Psychiatry 22*:261 (1991).
109. T. Moffitt, Juvenile delinquency and attention deficit disorder: boys' developmental trajectories, from age 3 to age 15, *Child Dev. 61*:893 (1990).
110. J. Weisz, S, Martin, B. Walter, and G. Fernandez, Differential prediction of young adult arrests for property and personal crimes: Findings of a cohort follow-up study of violent boys from North Carolina's Willie M. Program, *J. Child Psychol. Psychiatry 32*:783 (1991).
111. J. Monahan, *The Clinical Prediction of Violent Behavior*, Department of Health and Human Services, Rockville, MD, 1981.
112. D. Fergusson, J. Horwood, and M. Lynskey, The effects of conduct disorder and attention deficit in middle childhood on offending and scholastic ability at age 13, *J. Child Psychol. Psychiatry 34*:899 (1993).
113. R. Rogers, J. Johansen, J. Chang, and R. Salekin, Predictors of adolescent Psychopathy: Oppositional and conduct disordered symptoms, *J. Am. Acad. Psychiatry Law 25*:261 (1997).
114. D. Lewis, R. Lovely, C. Yeager and D. Della Femina, Toward a theory of genesis of violence: A follow-up study of delinquents, *Americ. Acad. Child Adolesc. Psychiatry 28 (3)*:431 (1989).
115. D. Lewis, J. Pincus, B. Bard, E. Richardson, L. Prichep, M. Feldman, and C. Yeager, Neuropsychiatric, psychoeducational, and family characteristics of 14 juveniles condemned to death in the United States, *Am. J. Psychiatry 145*:584 (1988).
116. E. Werner and R. Smith, *Vulnerable But Invincible*, McGraw-Hill, New York, 1982.
117. A. Sameroff, Early influences on development: Fact or fancy, *Merrill-Palmer Q 21(4)*:267 (1975).
118. S. Mednick, T. Moffitt, and S. Stack, *The Causes of Crime: New Biological Approaches*, Cambridge University Press, New York, 1987.
119. S. Kaplan, D. Pelcovitz, S. Salzinger, et al., Psychopathology of nonviolent women in violent families, *The Child in His Family* (E. Anthony and C. Chiland, eds.), John Wiley & Sons, New York, 1988.
120. D. Pelcovitz and S. Kaplan, Child witnesses of violence between parents: Psychological correlates and implications for treatment, *Child Adolesc. Psychiatry Clin. North Am. 3 (4)*:745 (1994).
121. M. Straus, *Violence in the Lives of Adolescents*, W.W. Norton & Company, New York, 1994, pp. 1–30.
122. E. Hilberman and K. Munson, Sixty battered women, *Victimol. Int. J. 2*:460 (1977).
123. E. Jouiles, J. Barling, and K. O'Leary, Predicting child behavior problems in maritally violent families, *J. Abn. Child Psychol. 15*:165 (1987).
124. M. Rosenberg, Children of battered women: The effects of witnessing violence on their social problem-solving abilities, *Behav. Ther. 4*:85 (1987).
125. B. Westra, H. Martin, Children of battered women, *Matern. Child Nurs. J. 10*:41 (1981).

126. S. Wildin, W. Williamson, and G. Wilson, Children of battered women: Developmental and learning profiles, *Clin. Pediatr. 30*:299 (1991).
127. G. Holden and K. Ritchie, Linking extreme marital discord, child rearing and child behavior problems: Evidence from battered women, *Chid Dev. 62*:311 (1991).
128. P. Jeffe, D. Wolfe, and S. Wilson, *Children of Battered Women*, Sage, Newbury Park, CA, 1990.
129. D. Kilpatrick, B. Saunder, A. Amick-McMullan, et al., Victim and crime factors associated with the development of crime-related post-traumatic stress disorder, *Behav. Ther. 20*:199 (1989).
130. J. Fantuzzo and C. Lindquist, The effects of observing conjugal violence on children: A review and analysis of research methodology, *J. Fam. Violence 4*:77 (1989).
131. E. Hilberman, Overview: the "wife-beater's wife" reconsidered, *Am. J. Psychiatry 137*:1336 (1980).
132. A. Campbell and J. Gibbs (eds.), *Violent Transactions*, Basil Blackwell, New York, 1986.
133. G. Hotaling and D. Sugarman, An analysis of risk makers in husband to wife violence: The current state of knowledge, *Victims Violence* 101 (1986).
134. P. Ladoucer and M. Temple, Substance abuse among rapists, *Crime Delinq. 31*:269 (1985).
135. S. Brown, Pathogenesis of violence and aggression: Neurotransmitter data *Violence: Causes and Medical Management* (K. Tardiff, ed.), Marcel Dekker, New York. In press.
136. L. DiLalla and I. Gottesman, Heterogeneity of causes for delinquency and criminality: Lifespan perspectives, *Dev. Psychopathol. 1*:339 (19).
137. J. Oliver, Successive generations of child maltreatment: The children, *Br. J. Psychiatry 153*:543 (19).
138. M. De Bellis and F. Putnam, The psychobiology of childhood maltreatment, *Child Adolesc. Psychiatry Clin. North Am. 3 (4)*:663 (1994).
139. W. Cannon, The wisdom of the body, *Physiol. Rev. 9*:399 (1929).
140. J. Bremner, M. David, S. Southwick, et al., Neurobiology of posttraumatic stress disorder, *Review of Psychiatry* (J. Oldham, M. Riba, and A. Tasman, eds.), American Psychiatric Press, Washington, DC, 1993, pp. 183–205.
141. P. Simson and J. Weiss, Altered activity of the locus coeruleus in an animal model of depression, *Neuropsychopharmacology 1*:287 (1988).
142. R. Chronister and J. DeFrance, Functional organization of monoamines, *Neuropharmacology Central Nervous System and Behavioral Disorders* (G. Palmer, ed.), Academic Press, New York, 1981, pp. 435–462.
143. G. Glavin, Stress and brain noradrenaline: A review, *Behav. Neurosci, Rev. 9*:233 (1985).
144. A. Tsuda and M. Tanaka, Differential changes in noradrenaline turnover in specific regions of rat brain produced by controllable and uncontrollable shocks, *Behav. Neurosci. 99*:802 (1985).
145. G. Aston-Jones, M. Shipley, G. Choevet, et al., Afferent regulation of locus coer-

uleus neurons: Anatomy, physiology, and pharmacology, *Progr. Brain Res. 88*:47 (1991).
146. D. Charney, A. Deutch, J. Krystal, et al., Psychobiological mechanisms of post-traumatic stress disorder, *Arch. Gen. Psychiatry 50*:294 (1993).
147. A. Deutch, R. Roth, The determinants of stress-induced activation of the prefrontal cortical dopamine system, *The Pre-Frontal Cortex: Its Structure, Function, and Pathology*. (H. Uylings, C. VanEden, and M. DeBruin, eds.), Elsevier Science Publishers, Amsterdam, 1989, pp. 367–403.
148. S. Satel, S. Southwick, and F. Gawin, Clinical features of cocaine-induced paranoia, *Am. J. Psychiatry 148*:495 (1991).
149. S. Suomi, Adolescent depression and depressive symptoms: Insights from longitudinal studies with rhesus monkeys, *J. Youth Adolesc. 20*:273 (1991).
150. E. Thomas, E. Levine, and W. Arnold, Effects of maternal deprivation and incubation rearing on adrenocortical activity in the adult rat, *Dev. Psychobiol. 1*:21 (1968).
151. T. Kosten, J. Mason, E. Giller, et al., Sustained urinary norepinephrine and epinephrine elevation in posttraumatic stress disorder, *Psychoneuroendocrinology 12*:13 (1987).
152. B. Lerer, A. Bleich, E. Bennett, et al., Platelet adenylate cyclase and phospholipase C activity in posttraumatic stress disorder, *Biol. Psychiatry 27*:735 (1990).
153. R. Yehuda, M. Lowy, S. Southwick, E. Giller, et al., Urinary catecholamine excretion and severity of PTSD symptoms in Vietnam combat veterans, *J. Nerv. Ment. Dis. 180*:321 (1992).
154. M. Galvin, A. Shekhar, J. Simon, et al., Low dopamine-beta-hydroxylase: A biological sequelae of abuse and neglect? *Psychiatry Res. 39*:1 (1991).
155. C. Benkelfat, Serotonergic mechanisms in psychiatric disorders: New research tools, new ideas, *Int. Clin. Psychopharmacol. 8 (suppl 2)*:53 (1993).
156. L. Siever, R. Trestman, The serotonin system and aggressive personality disorder, *Int. Clin. Psychopharmacol. 8 (suppl 2)*:33 (1993).
157. B. van der Kolk, J. Perry, and J. Herman, Childhood origins of self-destructive behavior, *Am. J Psychiatry 148*:1655 (1991).
158. H. Yeo and W. Yeo, Repeated deliberate self-harm: A link with childhood sexual abuse? *Arch. Emerg. Med. 10*:161 (1993).
159. B. van der Kolk, M. Greenberg, S. Orr, et al., Endogenous opoids, stress induced analgesia, and posttraumatic stress disorder, *Psychopharmacol. Bull. 25*:417 (1989).
160. P. Pittman, B. van der Kolk, S. Orr, et al., Naloxone-reversible analgesic response to combat-related stimuli in postraumatic stress disorder, *Arch. Gen. Psychiatry 47*:541 (1990).
161. E. Edwards, K. Harkins, G. Wright, et al., Effects of bilateral adrenalectomy on the induction of learned helplessness, *Behav. Neuropsychopharmacol. 3*:109 (1990).
162. H. Uno, R. Tarara, J. Else, et al., Hippocampal damage associated with prolonged and fatal stress in primates, *J. Neurosci. 9*:1705 (1989).

163. R. Sapolsky and P. Plotsky, Hypercortisolism and its possible neural bases, *Biol. Psychiatry 27*:937 (1990).
164. R. Sapolsky, H. Uno, C. Rebert, et al., Hippocampal damage associated with prolonged glucococorticoid exposure in primates, *J. Neurosci. 10*:2897 (1990).
165. J. Kaufman, Depressive disorders in maltreated children, *J. Am. Acad. Child Adolesc. Psychiat. 30*:257 (1991)
166. G. Gillette, J. Garbutt, and A. Prange, Anxiety and the thyroid axis, *Handbook of Anxiety* (G. Burrows, M. Roth, and R. Noyes, eds.), Elsevier, New York, 1990.
167. F. Delange, Part B: Thyroid hormones: biochemistry and physiology, *Pediatric Endocrinol.: Physiol., Pathophysiol., and Clin. Aspects, ed. 2.* (J. Bertrand, R. Rappaport, P. Sizonenko, eds.), Williams & Wilkins, Baltimore, 1993, pp. 242–252.
168. P. Czernichow, Thyrotropin and thyroid hormones, *Pediatric Endocrinology: Physiology, Pathophysiology, and Clinical Aspects, ed 2.* (J. Bertrand, R. Rappaport, and P. Sizonenko, eds.), Williams & Wilkins, Baltimore, 1993, pp. 79–88.
169. M. Rabello, P. Snyder, and R. Utiger, Effects of pituitary-thyroid axis in prolactin secretion of single and repetitive oral doses of thyrotropin-releasing hormone (TRH), *Clin. Endocrinol. Metab. 39*:571 (1974).
170. C. Chrousos and P. Gold, The concepts of stress and stress systems disorders: Overview of physical and behavioral homeostasis, *J.A.M.A. 267*:1244 (1992).
171. V. Felitti, Childhood sexual abuse, depression and family dysfunction in adult obese patients: A case control study, *South Med. J. 86*:732 (1993).
172. C. Rivier and W. Vale, Involvement of corticotropin-releasing factor and somatostatin in stress-induced inhibition of growth hormone secretion in the rat, *Endocrinology 117*:2478 (1985).
173. S. Schanberg and T. Field, Maternal deprivation and supplemental stimulation. *Stress and Coping Across Development* (T. Field, P. McCabe, and N. Schneiderman, eds.), Erlbaum, Hillsdale, NJ, 1988, pp. 3–25.
174. E. Johnson, T. Kamilaris, G. Chrousos, et al., Mechanisms of stress: A dynamic overview of hormonal and behavioral homeostasis, *Neurosci. Biobehav. Rev. 16*:115 (1992).
175. D. Benoit, Phenomenology and treatment of failure to thrive, *Child Adolesc. Psychiatr. Clin. North Am. 2*:61 (1993).
176. W. Green, A theoretical model for classical psychosocial dwarfism (psychosocially determined short stature), *Psychoneuroendocrinology: Brain, Behavior, and Hormonal Interactions* (C. Holmes, ed.), Springer-Verlag, New York, 1990, pp. 92–112.
177. J. Money, C. Annecillo, and J. Kelly, Abuse-dwarfism syndrome: After rescue, statural and intellectual catchup growth correlate, *J. Clin. Child Psychol. 12*:279 (1983).
178. G. Powell, J. Brasel, and R. Blizzard, Emotional deprivation and growth retardation stimulating idiopathic hypopituitarism: Clinical evaluation of the syndrome, *N. Engl. J. Med 276*:1271 (1967).
179. J. Jensen, J. Pease, R. Ten Bensel, and B. Garfinkel, Growth hormone response

patterns in sexually or physically abused boys, *J. Am. Acad. Child Adolesc. Psychiatry 30*:784 (1991).

180. J. Ducharme and M. Forest, Normal pubertal development, *Pediatric Endocrinology: Physiology, Pathophysiology, and Clinical Aspects* (J. Bertrand, R. Rappaport, and P. Sizonenko, eds.), Williams & Wilkins, Baltimore, 1993, pp. 372–386.
181. W. Baily, Young Offenders, Serious Crimes, *Br. J. Psychiatry 167*:5 (1995).
182. J. Flesman and G. Vaillant, Resilient children as adults: A 40-year study, *The Invulnerable Child* (E. Anderson and B. Cohen, eds.), Guilford Press, New York, 1987.
183. A. Blumstein, Youth violence, guns, and the illicit-drug industry, *J. Crim. Law Criminol. 86 (1)*:10 (1995).

2

Violence in America: Social and Environmental Factors

Robert T. M. Phillips
University of Maryland Schools of Medicine and Law, and Forensic Consultation Associates, Annapolis, Maryland

I. POSING THE PROBLEM

The most enigmatic question that is before us today concerns the violent individual. Given what we know about the origin and nature of violence, what might be reasonable approaches to its prevention and management within clinical or other social settings? This question is of immediate practical concern for those whose lives may be affected by violence and is no less profound for the communities in which violence occurs. The answer continues to elude social, ethical, and legal scholars, in large measure because their respective paradigms have been intellectually isolated and have failed to take into account broader interdisciplinary constructs. The politics of violence—its occurrence and its prevention—are uniquely human and therefore lends itself to social and behavioral analysis. Only recently has there been any sustained scholarly interest in this subject except among those psychiatric practitioners who find themselves immersed in the forensic world of evaluation and treatment.

Violence is pandemic in the United States and has emerged as our premier public health crisis. The effects of violence are measured not only in its human carnage but also in its devastation to our communities and destruction of the lives of our citizens. Violence is everywhere in America. It is not just an "inner-city" problem. It is not unique to racial or ethnic minorities, and, despite efforts to the contrary, no such causal linkages have been established. Violence is manifested not only by the act of murder but also overtly and covertly by acts committed against others as well as against self, such as physical and sexual assault, rape, arson, child abuse, spousal abuse, elder abuse, and suicide. Efforts to bolster law enforcement's response to violence is both laudable and essential, but in the absence of informed public policy that addresses the root causes of violence, it is destined to fail.

Violence is not a diagnosis, nor is it a disease. It is, however, a behavioral manifestation of a human condition as old as time itself. Plato once said "Poverty is the mother of crime." Aristotle taught us that "The chief universal cause of the revolutionary impulse is the desire for equality." Socrates mused, "The existence of such persons is to be attributed to the want of education, ill training and evil constitution of the state." While poverty, lack of opportunity, and discrimination are intimately associated with violence, It would be reductionistic to view such socioeconomic conditions as the sole cause. Yet the sociology of violence and the related economics are the key to understanding causality and cure.

Children have increasingly become not only the victims of violence but also its fastest-growing segment of perpetrators. Juveniles accounted for 17% of all violent crimes in calendar year 1991. The juvenile arrest rates for murder increased by 85% between the years 1987 and 1981. Three out of every ten juvenile murder arrests in this country involve a victim under the age of 18. There is no hope of getting violence off our streets until we figure out how to get the guns out of the hands of our young children. Between 1987 and 1991, the juvenile arrest rates for weapons violations increased by 62%. In 1991, one out of every five weapons arrest was a juvenile arrest. Most disturbing to me as an African-American psychiatrist is the fact that black youth were arrested for weapons law violations at a rate triple that of white youth in 1991. Black youth were the victims of homicide at a rate six times higher than that of whites.

Snyder et al. recently updated much of the data on juvenile violence and victimization (1). The following summarizes their data and the fact sheet. In 1994, the juvenile violent crime arrest rate in the United States reached its highest level ever, totaling 514 arrests per 100,000 juveniles between the ages of 10 and 17 years, continuing the sharp increase begun in 1988. Of the 2.7 million arrests of persons under age 18, over 150,000 were for violent crimes (murder, rape, robbery, and aggravated assault) and nearly 160,000 were for drug abuse violations. One of every five violent crime arrests in 1994 was of a juvenile, which represents a 54% increase in the juvenile crime arrest rate. While these data are sobering, it is also reassuring to note that less than one-half of 1% of juveniles (about 1 in every 200) were arrested for a violent crime in 1994.

Nonetheless, juvenile homicide rates are growing exponentially. Between 1984 and 1994 the number of juvenile murderers known to police tripled. The number of juveniles who killed with a gun quadrupled. Murders by juveniles both acting alone and with others in groups have increased substantially since 1984. Some 2800 juveniles were responsible for killing an estimated 2300 people—

more than 2½ times the number killed by juveniles in 1984. Among juveniles who killed, 8 in 10 used a gun, compared with 5 in 10 in 1980. More than half of the juveniles who killed did so with at least one other accomplice; while 3 in 10 juveniles had an adult accomplice.

The data concerning juvenile victimization are equally staggering. In 1994, an estimated 2660 juveniles were murdered—a rate of seven killed per day. One in five murdered juveniles was killed by another juvenile. More than half of the victims were teens between 15 and 17 years old. Between 1984 and 1994, while the number of juveniles murdered dropped for the first time in a decade in 1994 (down 6% from 1993), the number was nearly double that in 1984 (up 82%). The number of firearm-involved murders of juveniles nearly tripled, while those involving other weapons remained constant. The increases in murders of juveniles stem largely from rising teen murders.

Distressing to parents and students alike is the pervasive evidence of violence in our schools. In a national sample of sixth- through twelfth-graders surveyed in 1993, more than 1 in 3 students reported gangs in their school. More than 4 in 10 reported that they knew of students bringing weapons to school.

More than half of the students had witnessed violence in school. One-quarter of students said they worried about becoming victims of violence at school. A new analysis of law enforcement data from South Carolina, gathered for 1991–1992 as part of the FBI's National Incident-Based Report System, shows that one in six of all violent juvenile crimes occurred between the "curfew hours" of 10 p.m. and 6 a.m. weekdays and midnight to 6 a.m. weekends, while one in five occurred from 2 p.m. to 6 p.m. on days when school was in session. A comparison of the frequency of crimes per hour shows that violent juvenile crime is four times greater during the after-school period than during curfew hours. The efficacy of public policy attempts to "solve" the problem by taking children off the streets is obviously questionable.

While juvenile crime is predominantly a male problem, female delinquency has recently been noted to be increasing more than that of males. Again, Poe-Yamagata and Butts have provided the field with vital data compiled through their work at the U.S. Department of Justice (2). Their statistical summary shows that in 1993, some 570,100 arrests were made of females under the age of 18. In the 10 years between 1989 and 1993, the number of arrests involving females increased by 23%, compared with an 11% increase in arrests of their male counterparts. The offenses in the juvenile violent crime index increased by 55% for females, and the proportion of all juvenile female arrests increased from 21 to 24% during this same period. In 1993 the juvenile courts handled an estimated 1,489,700 delinquency cases nationally, 20% of which involved females, with the 5-year trend increasing by 31% for females as compared with 21% for males. Crimes against persons increased among female juvenile offenders between 1989 and 1993, representing a shift from 16 to 29% of the custody population and from

23 to 31% of the committed population. Most strikingly, female delinquency cases were less likely to be processed formally, more likely to receive probation as the most restrictive disposition, and less likely to result in detention or out-of-home placements.

Among our young today, in particular our minority young, anger, anger, frustration, hopelessness, and rage fuel the fires that inevitably are manifested in violence. The compounding problems of substance abuse, teenage pregnancy, illiteracy, truancy, and dropping out have provided fertile soil for the seeds of discontent that have been sown for generations in this country (3–6). Although the homicide rates are disproportionately and exponentially higher among young male African Americans and Hispanics in the United States as compared to their white counterparts, controlling for socioeconomic status yields no statistically significant differences among the groups (7). The operational conclusion is that the only color that is of determinative importance in understanding the sociocultural demography of violence is colloquially "green," or more precisely low socioeconomic status, not race or ethnicity (8). The deterioration of the family unit and the absence of strong and consistent male and female role models only begin to help us understand of the origins of this dilemma and further underscore the futility of trying to effect solely clinical solutions.

Child protective services received over 2 million reports of child maltreatment in 1993; a total of 1028 children were known to have died as a result of abuse or neglect. Between 1980 and 1993, reports of child maltreatment increased by 155%. Juvenile drug use is unfortunately back on the rise. In 1995 more than 1 in 5 twelfth graders, more than 1 in 6 tenth graders, and nearly 1 in 10 eighth graders reported using marijuana in the previous month. Between 1993 and 1994, juvenile arrests for drug abuse rose by 42%; the majority of these were marijuana-related, according to FBI analysts. While illicit drug use by juveniles declined substantially during the 1980s, it has increased steadily since 1992.

The prosecution of juvenile offenders has also become a focus of great attention an controversy. In 1993, an estimated 11,800 delinquency cases were judicially waived to criminal court for prosecution. No national data exist on other methods of transfer of juvenile cases to criminal court by prosecutorial discretion or statutory exclusion of selected offenses. For the first time since 1975, personal offense cases waived to criminal court outnumbered property offense cases. Between 1989 and 1993, the number of juvenile court cases judicially waived to criminal court rose by 41%.

This issue is extremely challenging and has recently been somewhat harder to evade. Over the course of the past 15 years, there has been a progressive movement away from the rehabilitative model toward a more punitive construct. The 106th Congress received legislation introduced by the chairman of the House Judiciary Subcommittee on Crime that would largely end federal mandates requiring states to segregate juveniles from adults in jails and prisons. Over the course of the past 15 years, there has been a growing movement away from the rehabilitative model in the juvenile justice system and toward a more punitive construct. Some contend that this movement is accelerated by angry and fearful responses from middle-class Americans and intensified when the offender is nonwhite (9).

II. VIOLENCE AND MENTAL ILLNESS

Conventional wisdom has relegated to myth the belief that there is a direct link between mental illness and violent behavior. Yet despite voluminous research, no one has been able to firmly establish such causality. In fact, the percentage of mentally ill and mentally disabled individuals who act out violently is small in comparison to the total number of individuals who suffer from such illness. While the vast majority of those who are mentally ill are no more or perhaps even less dangerous than the general population, there is a small group that do become violent toward themselves or others. These beliefs, while scientifically valid, were based primarily on research conducted on institutionalized populations. Recent inquiry has challenged these assumptions.

Swanson et al. demonstrated, by reanalysis of NIMH ECA data, that persons suffering schizophrenia had statistically significantly higher rates of violence than those without mental illness (11 to 13% versus 2%) and that persons suffering from substance-abuse disorders were more likely to exhibit violent behavior [alcohol abuse 25%, drug abuse 35% (10)]. The comorbidity of substance abuse, dependence, or intoxication; hallucinations and delusions; poor impulse control; and character pathology alone or in tandem appear also to increase the risk of violent behavior (11,12). Additionally, Link and Stueve proffer that "threat-control-override symptoms" (three characteristics of psychotic thought process: paranoia, thought control, and thought insertion) appear to be more frequently associated with violent behavior (11,12).

Monahan has functionally reframed the issue by questioning whether there is a fundamental link between mental disorder and violence, and if so, can people with mental disorders who will be violent be distinguished from those who will not (13).

No one has mastered the ability to predict future violent behavior. It is clear, however, that the risk of violence is increased among *all* individuals in society who abuse substances, are victims of violence, or are socioeconomically deprived (15). Among those who are mentally ill, the risk increases if violence has been a symptom of their illness. Statisticians and epidemiologists tell us that violence is not uniformly distributed in the population and that individuals differ in their thresholds for acting out their violent impulses. Several older studies demonstrated that patients released from psychiatric hospitals had lower arrest rates than the general population. Newer studies utilizing similar methods came to opposite conclusions. But when comparisons were made with the arrest rates of released criminal offenders, the ex-prisoners had a subsequent arrest rate six times higher than that of former patients.

Monahan and Steadman—in an earlier work (16) and more recently via the risk-assessment study sponsored by the Research Network on Mental Health and the Law of the John D. and Catherine T. MacArthur Foundation and the National Institute of Mental Health—are currently examining over 1000 patients released from psychiatric hospitals in Massachusetts, Missouri, and Pennsylvania. Departing from the traditional attempts to codify predictions of an individual's future dangerousness, the researchers have instead sought to identify those psychotic symptoms and related factors that could predict the occurrence of violent behavior. They postulate that in a public health framework, the risk factors for violence can be classified into four categories: personal/dispositional factors, developmental/historical factors, contextual factors, and clinical factors. The findings of the MacArthur risk-assessment study are expected to help us better understand whether and to what extent mental illness is associated with violence in the general population.

III. CRIMINALITY AS A MANIFESTATION OF "SOCIAL ILLNESS"

Jails have always been the repository for society's unwanted. Historically, the trends in America were similar to the one that had become evident in Europe in the late seventeenth century. As in Europe, the aim was to remove and isolate not only the mentally ill but also the outcasts of society, such as criminals and vagrants. There is, in fact, not a single culture in organized society in the history of the planet that has not ultimately sought to remove from its midst and sequester at a distance those who suffer from mental illness. Why then, in the twentieth century, is our attention still riveted on the plight of the mentally ill and their entrapment in jails and prisons? Perhaps it is because, over a hundred years following the systemized efforts by Dorothea Dix and other activists to address the social plight of incarcerated persons suffering from mental illness, approximately 1.1 million persons currently reside in the nation's jails and prisons, up to one-third of them suffering from serious mental illness.

For the purposes of our discussion, serious mental illnesses comprise schizophrenia, unipolar and bipolar illness, major depression inclusive of suicidality, organic syndrome with psychotic features, and substance abuse. The use of jail for the confinement of mentally ill persons in America is commonplace (17).

The criminal justice system is incapable of keeping up with the expanding number of mentally ill persons within it. With the doubling of the prison population in this past decade, the United States has quietly created a new form of entitlement for indigent citizens, paradoxically providing them with social services such as housing and education when, in years gone by, would have been external to the prison walls and based in their communities of origin. Ironically, had these services been available, they might have prevented some of these individuals from turning to crime.

It is almost as if the United States had concluded that the problems of the urban poor were intractable and that it has therefore invested in a vast network of prisons rather than seeking solutions to the social problems that plague its communities—in particular, the communities in which a disproportionate number of racial and ethnic minorities reside. Tragically, this country appears to be quite willing to spend millions on prisons but seems to have a greater deal of difficulty in developing programs that would improve conditions for the urban poor and decrease the incidence of crime. We seem to be unwilling to move forward and address the social needs of our citizens. I would submit that the jails and the prisons of this country have become the ghettos of our society. They are the new tenements for the urban poor, and for those of us who provide mental health services in correctional and forensic mental health settings, they are the new asylums. It is in our prisons that we provide the highest degree of medical and psychiatric coverage to the poor—in particular the urban poor. Facilitated by constructs of law and failed public policy, we have "transinstitutionalized" a segment of our society from psychiatric hospitals and their communities of origin.

IV. MENTAL ILLNESS AND CRIMINALITY

In our criminal code, a crime is more than an objectionable act. It must be accomplished by a "criminal intent." We distinguish between accidents and intentional behavior. A small percentage of the mentally ill or disabled are so impaired that they may meet the threshold of not knowing or appreciating the wrongfulness of their actions or being able to conform their behavior to the requirements of the law. This group makes up less than 1% of all crimes nationally, In most states, the maximum-security forensic hospital is the repository for persons whose mental illness is manifested by extreme forms of violence. The forensic hospital is saddled with a difficult dual mandate that society imposes, central to the treatment and custody of mentally ill offenders (18). The press, politicians, and courts have made clear their desire to have "criminally insane" individuals removed from the community and thus prevented from harming innocent citizens. The courts have made it clear that long-term restrictions on a person's liberty place several heavy burdens on the state, not the least of which is the provision of adequate psychiatric treatment.

The dual mandate is made more difficulty by several complicating factors. There is a strong data base casting doubt upon the ability of forensic hospitals to make long-term predictions about the dangerousness of individual patients upon release. This inability to predict dangerousness is compounded by fiscal restraints limiting the number of patients who can be housed in maximum-security settings without overcrowding them and endangering both staff and patients. The forensic patient is clinically indistinguishable from other citizens with chronic mental illnesses. As the mental health disciplines have improved in their ability to provide treatment for the chronically ill, there has been an increasing acknowledgment of the incapacitating effect of years of institutionalization. Logically, the best treatment may also often require movement to a less structured, more independent setting. In addition, many clinicians in this field believe that the best way to ensure an eventual safe return to freedom is to allow patients to experience graduated decreases in structure and increases in freedom and responsibility.

Such clinical and fiscal pressures to move patients to less secure settings often run in direct contradiction to the advocates of public safety who demand that the system "cure" these patients in the hospital before they are released. Clinicians respond that in order to "cure" (i.e., properly treat) such individuals, it may be necessary to release them. Finally, the stakes in this conflict of interests are raised astronomically by the fact that occasionally patients released from forensic hospitals will again commit highly publicized, violent acts. The fact that these incidents are infrequent rarely diminishes the effect on public perceptions about the dangerousness of the mentally ill, especially those with prior histories of violent crime who have been institutionalized in a forensic setting.

In its extreme form, this dilemma can result in a class of "political prisoners" who have exhausted the benefits of treatment in a forensic hospital, whose psychotic illnesses have long since disappeared, yet whose prior crimes are perceived as so heinous as to permanently preclude release. Presented in this context, this reality seems unfair and unenlightened. Thus, in the case of a man who has murdered and mutilated the bodies of multiple young children, the public asks, "How can you even think of releasing this person when you cannot assure that he is no longer dangerous?" More to the point, state officials are likely to be precluded from doing so, whether through the courts, political influence, or public pressure mounted by the media. Yet, given our inability to make long-term individual predictions about dangerousness, we are also unable to make predictions about who will *not* pose a danger if released.

One way of looking at what we do know, what we can predict, is to view it as a risk-benefit analysis. Arguably, there are three kinds of data about an individual patient that are of value in making release decisions: (a) prior acts, (b) response to treatment, and (c) necessary conditions of release. Prior acts, especially the offense that led to the current hospitalization, tend to define the possible costs of failure. Therefore, the risk of inappropriately releasing a person found guilty of murder is seen as greater than that in the case of an individual who had committed a simple assault. A second type of data is descriptive of ways in which the patient has changed, especially in response to treatment. This information serves to lessen the perceived risk and obviously needs to be more substantial with more serious offenses. Included are the general course of hospital treatment and successful adaptations to *less* structured situations. The third type of data involves managing the risk, which is to say the conditions under which the proposed release is to be accomplished and supervised. Thus, patients who have committed more severe offenses need to demonstrate higher degrees of clinical improvement prior to release. Upon release, they will likely receive a greater degree of scrutiny and, hopefully, supervision and support, than those whose offenses have been less serious.

V. RACE, ETHNICITY AND THE VIOLENCE OF CRIMINAL JUSTICE AS A SOCIAL SYSTEM

The Rev. Jesse Jackson has eloquently pointed out that, "for many black youngsters, jail is a step up." That's a pretty powerful statement coming from an African American, and a more disturbing statement when you realize its accuracy. Conceptually, once a young African-American male is arrested, if he was homeless, he is no longer homeless. If he has not been eating, he is now going to receive three well-balanced meals. Once incarcerated, those African-American males who come from broken or dysfunctional families of who have been abandoned now have an institutional surrogate parent. Those youths who have not had adult supervision will now be supervised. That supervision may not be and will most often not be ethnocentric but will be rather distorted in a way that perpetuates the kind of racially targeted genocide which has been perpetrated upon African Americans and other persons of color in this country for centuries. Such practices in the service delivery arena produce the disturbingly attractive illusion that people are, in fact, better off in jail than they were in their communities of origin. There are data supporting this premise. In 1991, we spent $20.1 billion on building and operating jails and prisons in this country. If you were to add the support costs for this national system, that $20.1 billion rises to about $26.2 billion to take care of 1.1 million prisoners. In comparison, in the same calendar year, we spent $22.9 billion on Aid to Families with Dependent Children to support 13.5 million women and children. Spending on prisons has become the second fastest growth industry in state budgets in this country after Medicaid, climbing to 13% of the state budgetary expenditures, on average, since 1986. In times of great fiscal restraint, the expenditures, both state and federal, on the construction and operation of correctional institutions then diverts substantive resources from programs for education, health, and job training. It would appear that all we have done is to transinstitutionalized this population. We are spending the dollars for education, for health, and for job training in the correctional institutions rather than in the community.

Equally troubling is the fact that African Americans represent only 12% of the national population yet account for better than 40% of all those individuals who are incarcerated. This kind of disproportionality may be understood as one of the most clear-cut examples of institutionalized racism that exists in our society. The proportion of African-American inmates has been rising since 1920. In 1920, African-Americans represented 21% of those incarcerated. That figure has more than doubled in the last 70 years. The data for other racial and ethnic minorities are similarly disproportionate.

The color of one's skin, the amount of money one has for an attorney, and the passions of the moment play a much greater role in determining who dies than the circumstances of the crime involved or the background of the person on trial[1]. There are nearly 3000 persons on death row throughout the Untied States today[2], a disproportionate number of them are persons of color[3], and almost all are poor[4]. The quality of legal assistance, or the lack of it, is a critical problem for the poor who make up the vast majority of those sentenced to die[5]. The issues of race and poverty are at play whenever the state seeks the dcath penalty[6]. While African Americans are disproportionately represented among the number of individuals on death row for the commitment of capital crimes, there appears to be another rather striking disproportionality if you look at who their victims were. More simply put, a value judgment appears to be placed on white victims, suggesting that if it is a white person who is murdered, there is a much higher probability, if you are black, that you will be sentenced to die[7].

It is my belief that this is a profound example of an inherently violent institutional racism. Racism is a form of violence. That it is institutionalized racism is shown by the disproportionate way in which we entrap African-American males and females in the criminal justice system. It is institutionalized racism because we have failed to meet the needs of not only African Americans but all Americans in this society, which leads them to seek those services in a rather curious way through the criminal justice system rather than the social welfare system. But, more importantly, it is institutionalized racism because the basic tools of life are not provided to those within these institutions. Exposed to all the ravages of correctional life, including the kind of institutional violence that the system perpetuates and the social violence that is rampant in the criminal justice system, the young offender ultimately returns to the streets with more anger, rage, hopelessness, and fear.

The task for american psychiatry is to define its role in this complicated system. I can think of no more timely an issue deserving of the focus of our collective attention. Tardiff states "From a clinical perspective, violence can best be described as an obscure and confusing subject. Its definition remains unclear and, at best, controversial. The causes of violence and, in particular, violent behavior of human beings, remain largely unknown. Predictions of a discharged patient's involvement in violence are often not better than pure chance. The treatment of violent actions, as well as violent individuals, is submerged in such controversy that may define it as violence by psychiatry under the guise of providing help"[8].

VI. VIOLENCE AND THE AMERICAN MEDIA

We are a society that is infatuated with violence in a clinically obsessive way. We romanticize violence in film. We glorify violent sports and pay homage to its gladiators *with adoration*, and attach to such sport the financial rewards and spoils of our society. We feed our addition to violence in television news trailers for the 5, 6, 10, and 11 p.m. broadcasts. We sensationalize violence with special reports and special editions in both the electronic and print media. From Los Angeles to Lillehammer, violence has emerged as the strongest currency in a marketplace that just cannot get enough.

Singer's 1982 description of growing up in a television environment remains poignant: "A major advance in the research approaches to television in the 1970s has been reflected in the increasing recognition that this medium must be understood more broadly in relation to the natural cognitive and affective development of the growing child. In view of the evidence that children are already attentive to the television medium by the age of 6 to 9 months, it is no longer useful to talk of the television set as an extraneous and occasional intruder into the life of a child. Rather, we must recognize that children are growing up in an environment in which they must learn to organize experiences and emotional responses not only in relation to the omnipresent big 21-inch screen that talks, sings, dances, and encourages the desire for toys, candies, and breakfast foods.

It is increasingly clear that children, as they grow up, must learn to decode the verbal utterances of parents and friends or to establish schemes for the meanings of the smiles and frowns of adults around them. They must also learn the special codes of the television medium, its smaller-than-life frame, its appearances and disappearances of characters, intrusions of irrelevant commercials to otherwise engrossing story material, as well as the meanings of zooms, fadeouts, miraculous superhero leaps, and flashbacks. As children are clearly spending more time watching television than, in most cases, engaging in conversation with adults or siblings and certainly more time than they will spend in school, what happens to their cognitive growth? To what extent are the structural properties of the television medium likely to be influencing the way new information from other environments is processed? Is it perhaps the very nature of thinking itself, modified by the much heavier component of visual stimulation, that characterizes regular television viewing in comparison with reading?" (25).

In 1996, The National Television Violence Study completed and released its first year findings of the most thorough scientific survey of violence on television ever undertaken and the most complete contextual analysis done to date[9]. The study examined the largest, most extensive body of television programming ever collected for the purpose of contact analysis. Its conclusions are based on a sample of 2693 programs collected over the course of 9 months to construct a representative week of television content seen on 23 U.S. broadcast and cable channels. The study found that more than half of all entertainment programming sampled contained violence, the violent interactions occurred in multiple numbers, and that perpetrators engaged in repeated acts of violence. In 75 % of programming sampled, perpetrators of violence went unsanctioned. This is especially disturbing in the light of widely accepted research that has established that the most effective way of reducing the likelihood of young viewers imitating violent behavior is to show such behavior being punished. The body of additional research has also concluded that when violent scenes ignore consequences of violence or depict them unrealistically, viewers are apt to become desensitized and fearful while at the same time learning violent behaviors and attitudes.

The study found, in its analysis, that fewer than 16% of all victims show any long-term negative consequences, very few experience financial or emotional consequences of physical harm done to them, and most targets appear to feel little pain or suffering. Similarly, high numbers were reported for nonfiction entertainments, all of which contributed to desensitization, fear, and the learning of violent behaviors and attitudes.

Careful content analysis of the programming sample produced more disturbing findings: there are large numbers of violent interactions per program in which the majority of the perpetrators engage in repeated acts of violence; in more than half of all violent scenes, perpetrators go unpunished; and in more than half of all violent scenes, consequences are unrealistically portrayed. Less than 16% of all victims appeared to feel little pain or suffering and experienced no financial or emotional consequences as a result of the harm done to them. Finally, only 4% of all violent programs sampled emphasized any kind of strong antiviolence theme.

The report of year 2, released in March 1997, further underscored the findings of the earlier work, reaffirming that certain contextual features have potentially harmful effects on younger viewers, particularly those that fail to show harmful consequences of violent behaviors[10]. Most notable were the findings related to animated programming aimed at children. The data reveal that cartoon programming intended for young viewers contained alarmingly high rates of violence and that these portrayals were contextually conveyed in ways that increased the likelihood of harmful learned behaviors. The significance of these findings is paramount in light of the limited ability of some younger children to distinguish fantasy from reality, thereby increasing the likelihood of their being affected as much by animation as by reality-based programming. The greatest risk the study points to is the increased risk of learning violent or aggressive behaviors to due repeated exposure to cartoon violence that goes unpunished and is perpetrated by an attractive character in a justifiable manner with minimal consequence for the victim.

Coterminous with the 2 years of seminal research was the passage of extraordinary legislation by the Congress of the United States mandating the installation "V-Chip" technology in all manufactured television sets beginning in 1998. President Bill Clinton and Vice President Al Gore's leadership, supported by the grounds well of legislative activity in the U.S. Senate led by Senators Kent Conrad, Joseph Liebermann, Ernest Hollings, John McCain and in the House of Representatives by Congressmen Edward Markey, Jim Moran, Jim Spratt, and others created the unprecedented opportunity for the television industry to voluntarily develop a rating system for use with this technology. The first iteration of the TV Parental Guidelines released in December 1996 was met with strong opposition due to its apparent overreliance on age-based rating criteria. Subsequent collaborative efforts in concert with parents, educators, media advocacy groups, and medical and mental health professionals led to a revised system that combines specific content descriptors: V, violence; S, sexual content; L, offensive language; D, suggestive dialogue with age-based ratings; TV-Y, TV-Y7, TV-G, TV-PG, TV-14, and TV-MA, modified from the Motion Picture Association of America (MPAA) system utilized by American movie industry for the past 25 years. The modified TV Parental Guideline System—collectively endorsed and submitted for approval to the Federal Communications Commission in July 1997 by the American Medical Association, American Academy of Pediatrics, American Psychological Association, Center for Media Education, Children's Defense Fund, Children Now, National Association of Elementary School Principals, National Education Association, National Parents Teachers Association, Motion Picture Association of America, National Association of Broadcasters, and the National Cable Television Association—became operational on October 1, 1997. The impact and efficacy of these new ratings will need to be carefully examined through independent scientific research once the V-Chip sufficiently penetrates the marketplace.

While much recent attention has been focused on the effects of violent television programming on children and adolescents. The American Psychiatric Association joined with Senator Kent Conrad and the Citizens' Task Force on TV Violence in 1993 and is already on record regarding this issue. Clinically our attention appropriately must include the recording industry and the impact of sexually explicit musical lyrics on the physical and emotional well-being of our young. If television and movies are the window through which we see the reflections of art imitating life, then music is clearly the honing device of language by which we track the cultures and mores of our society.

Numerous studies have clearly established the relationship between actual exposure to violence and its negative consequences on normal childhood development. A substantial body of research has also demonstrated the association of violent or aggressive behaviors with repeated exposure to televised violence. Simply put, the more violent programming children view, the greater is the risk that they will behave violently or aggressively.

The same paradigm holds true for music and its potential effect on listeners. Rock music has always been viewed as representative of a "counterculture" by many adults. Nonetheless, it has firmly established itself as a powerful art form, particularly among the young. As each generation matures, what was considered "the norm" becomes passé as new contemporary themes emerge. Recently, there has an appropriate decrying of a form of rap music referred to as "gansta rap" whose lyrics contain some of the most violent and derogatory verbal assaults on women. We seem, however, to have forgotten that this is only the latest iteration of a theme that long predated rap music. Other forms of contemporary rock music, in particular certain segments of heavy metal and hard core punk, have persistently demonstrated substantial deviation, even from the norm of current contemporary themes. This type of music has been described by critics and researchers alike as "alienated, negativistic, nihilistic, and pornographic" at its best. A review of the lyrics of this kind of contemporary rock music reveals themes of homicide, suicide, and satanic practices that promote sex, sadomasochism, rape, and murder. There have also been clear examples in which lyrics have promoted the act of suicide. Haennelerswass et al., in their review of adolescent interests and destructive themes in rock music, provide us with some sample lyrics released since 1980 by heavy metal bands:

> ". . . No apparent motive/Just kill and kill again/Survive my brutal slashing/ I'll hunt you till the end . . . ."[11]
> ". . In goes my knife/Pull out his life/Consider that bastard dead . . . "[12]
> ". . . Ripping flesh, drawing blood/I live to eat your bones . . . "[13]
> ". . . I am possessed by all that is evil/The death of your God I demand/I spit at the virgin you worship/And sit at Lord Satan's right hand . . ."[14]
> ". . . Holy hell, death to us/Satan fell, unholy lust/Devil's water starts to flood/God is slaughtered, drink his blood . . . Satan's right hand . . ."[15]

The lyrics of "gansta rap" and misogyny in rap clearly then evolve from the same shameful and repugnant tradition.

> So if you at a show in the front row
> I'm a call you at bitch or a dirty-ass ho

You probably get mad like bitch is supposed to . . .
. . . So what about the bitch who got shot?
F_her
You think I give a damn about a bitch . . . [16]
Bitch . . . . I just want to f___ you and cut
Treat ya like a trampy slut.[17]
Her body's beautiful so I'm thinking rape
Shouldn't have had her curtains open so that's her fate . . .
Slit her throat and watched her shake[18]
Cause we're like the outlaws stridin' while suckers are hiding' . . . Jump behind
the bush when you see me drivin' by.
Hanging out the window with my magnum taking out some putas. Act kind of local, I'm
just another local kid from the street getting paid for my vocals.[19]

The effect of such music and music videos is best understood in the context of childhood development. Children are born with the innate capacity and desire to imitate adult human behavior. Whether the behavior imitated is triggered by a visual image, an audio image, or by combined audiovisual imagery, the cognitive impact is overwhelming. Violence is powerful, tantalizing, charismatic, and intoxicating.

Research on the impact of music and music videos on normal child development has been consistent with similar research that has examined the impact of repeated exposure to televised violence. Approximately 700 middle- and high-school students from central Florida completed a survey about rock music preferences. Nearly one-fifth of the students named as favorites those performers whose music describes homicide, suicide, and satanism. The majority of these fans were male. Among those studied, fans of heavy metal and punk rock were more likely than fans of other rock music to report knowing the lyrics to favorite songs.[20]

A content analysis of music videos was conducted by the *Journal of Broadcasting & Electronic Media*. The study found that violence and crimes were depicted in more than half of a random sample of 62 music videos shown on MTV. Violent videos features destruction of property, physical aggression against self and others, and use of weapons such as chains, guns, knives, and axes (19).

The effects of sexually violent rock music on men's acceptance of violence against women was reported in *Psychology of Women Quarterly*. Seventy-five male college students participated in an experiment to compare the effects of exposure to sexually violent heavy metal rock, Christian heavy metal rock, and easy-listening music on attitudes about women. The study found that men who listened to only 17 minutes of heavy metal music (regardless of sexually violent or Christian themes) expressed greater endorsement of sexual stereotypes, negative attitudes, and prejudicial beliefs about women than did men who heard easy-listening music (20). In another study designed to examine the influence of erotic and violent content on men's attitudes about violence against women, 144 male college students watched music videos featuring either erotic violent, erotic nonviolent, nonerotic violent, or nonerotic, nonviolent content. Those who watched the nonerotic violent videos expressed the most callous and antagonistic attitudes toward women (21).

In a 1990 study published in *Communication Research*, approximately 400 college students watched music videos containing either a low, moderate, or high level of visual violence. For both males and females, increasing the level of video violence decreased the appeal of the music and the visual content. The more violent videos made viewers fell less happy, more angry, more fearful, more anxious, less sexual, and more aggressive than did less violent videos. (22)

Sherman and Dominick viewed 166 videos sampled from MTV, WTBS's *Night Tracks*, and NBC's *Friday Night Videos*. They found that violence was reported in 57% of the sample. Aggression more often involved wrestling, punching, and grabbing than use of weapons. Men were three times more likely than women to be victims of violence. Nonwhite characters more often than white characters used weapons and had weapons used against them (23).

Finally, a random sample of 139 music videos from MTV showed an average of 10 acts of violence per hour, almost twice the amount of violence found in prime-time programming. An act of violence was defined as "force or the compelling threat of force that may result in harm to life or to valued objects" (22).

These data are clear convincing and overwhelming. The repeated exposure to violent imagery desensitizes us to violence and greatly increases the risk that we will manifest violence in our own behavior. We must educate parents to the risks of exposure to media violence in the same way we have educated them to the risks of exposure to infectious diseases.

Freedom of speech does not relieve artists, recording executives, or broadcasters of their responsibility to serve the public interest. More importantly, one's constitutionally guaranteed First Amendment right to free speech does not give license to do harm to others.

The repeated exposure to free and gratuitously violent media has a deleterious effect on our youth and places at grave risk their mental health and welfare as well as that of our communities.

VII. SUMMARY

Historically we have focused on research efforts attempting to determine whether mental illness was linked with violence. Only recent have we considered the social and environmental factors that confound such an analysis. The social indicia of familial dysfunction, community disorganization, the absence of structure and/or supervision, social dyscontrol, and poverty are causally related more to low socioeconomic status than to race. An extraordinary number of individuals are entrapped in our criminal justice system, many of whom belong there. But there is also a very large number of individuals entrapped in the criminal justice system who are simply there because they are mentally ill, because they are viewed as nuisances, because society has failed them, and because we have failed to meet the needs of our fellows citizens.

While I have focused on the plight of African Americans in sections of this chapter, let me underscore that these things are true for all persons in American society, particularly if they are socioeconomically disadvantaged. I think the data and the discussion contained herein illustrate, at the very least in my opinion, how we have unwittingly created a social welfare system that exists not in people's communities of origin, but in correctional institutions that have managed to sequester a disproportional number of racial and ethnic minorities and have inappropriately incarcerated the mentally ill. Not terribly dissimilar from what we saw in the sixteenth, seventeenth, and eighteenth centuries. We in America, I maintain, have neglected our responsibility to those who are largely disenfranchised from and are not in a position to speak out for themselves—namely children, the mentally ill, and the poor.

As we approach the turn of the century, we see all around us the inhumane results of shortsighted government policies and "quick fix" solutions calling for the building of more institutions and essentially creating new asylums. Our society has concluded by its actions that the problems of the urban poor are intractable and that it is cheaper to invest in a vast system of network prisons to remove the unwanted from society than to remedy the social problems plagueing our communities—in particular, the communities in which African Americans and other persons of color reside. We have quietly created a new class of entitlements through which we have paradoxically provided services that, if they were available in these individuals' communities of origin, might have had an impact in preventing them from turning to crime.

As psychiatrists, I think we have many duties, including a duty to provide care and to recognize that care must be provided no matter where the recipient of that care resides. We have a duty to advocate for community-based services and programs to address the urban problems of our American communities. And we have a duty to improve the mental health, not just treat the mental illness of those individuals that we serve. If we fail this duty, it is very clear—and I think the data support this conclusion—that the social problems in our country will not be remedied and there will be little hope of preventing our young from acting out violently and becoming inmates instead of productive citizens.

REFERENCES

1. *The Juvenile Offenders and Victims: A National Report*, NCJ 153 569, Washington, DC, 1996.
2. *Female Offenders in the Juvenile Justice System*, U.S. Department of Justice, OJJDP, Washington, DC, June 1966.
3. S.F. Messner and K. Tardiff, Economic inequality and levels of homicide: An analysis of urban neighborhoods, *Criminology 24*:197 (1986).
4. S.F. Messner and K. Tardiff, The social ecology of urban violence: An application of the "routine activities" approach, *Criminology 23*:241 (1985).
5. D.J. Sherman, The neglected health care needs of street youth. *Public Health Rep. 107*:433, (1992).
6. Sampson, R.J., Community structure an crime: Testing social-disorganization theory. *Am. J. Sociol. 94*:774 (1989).
7. R.M. McGahey, Economic conditions, neighborhood organization and urban crime, *Communities and Crime*, (A.J. Riess and M. Tonry, eds.). University of Chicago Press, Chicago, 1986, pp. 231–270.
8. K. Tardiff, P. Marzuk, A. Leon, C. Hirsch, M. Stajic, L. Portera, and N. Hartwell, A profile of homicides on the streets and in the homes of New York City, *Public Health Rep. 110*: 13 (1995).
9. Jailhouse Separation of Juvenile Offenders from Adult Offenders, memorandum from Herbert S. Sachs, M.D., president-elect, American Psychiatric Association, Washington, DC, June 1996
10. D.A. Regier, M.E. Farmer, D.S. Rae, B.Z. Locke, S.J. Keith, L.L. Judd, and F.K. Goodwin. Comorbidity of mental disorders with alcohol and other drug abuse: Results from the Epidemiologic Catchment Area (ECA) Study. *J.A.M.A. 264*:2511 (1990).
11. L. Citrome, and J. Volavka, Psychiatric disorders and violence, *Medical Management of the Violent Patient: Clinical Assesment and Therapy* (Tardiff, K., ed.). Marcel Dekker, New York (1999).
12. J. Monahan, Mental disorder and violent behavior: Perceptions and evidence. *Am. Psychol. 47*:511 (1992).
13. B.G. Link, and A. Stueve, Psychotic symptoms and the violent/illegal behavior of mental patients compared to community controls, *Violence and Mental Disorder: Developments in Risk Assessment* (J. Monahan and J.H. Steadman eds.), University of Chicago Press, Chicago, 1994, pp. 137–159.
14. J. Monahan, Mental illness and violent crime, *National Institute of Justice Research Preview*, U.S. Department of Justice OJP. NIJ. October 1996.
15. K. Tardiff, Prediction of violence, *Medical Management of the Violent Patient: Clinical Assesment and Therapy* (K. Tardiff, ed.). Marcel Dekker, New York (1999).
16. J. Monahan, and H. Steadman (eds). *Violence and Mental Disorder: Developments in Risk Assessment*. University of Chicago Press, Chicago, 1994.
17. E.F. Torrey, J. Steiber, J. Ezekiel, S. Wolfe, J. Sharfstein, J.H. Noble, and L.M.

Flynn, Criminalizing the seriously mentally ill: The abuse of jails as mental hospitals. *Joint Report of the National Alliance for the Mentally Ill and Public Citizen's Health Research Group*, Public Citizens' Health Research Group/National Alliance for the Mentally Ill, Washington, D.C. 1992.
18. R.T.M. Phillips, and C. Caplan, Administrative and staffing problems for psychiatric services correctional and forensic settings, *Principles and Practice of Forensic Psychiatry* (R. Rosner, ed.), Chapman and Hall, New York, 1994, pp. 388–392.
19. R. Baxyter, C. DeRiemer, A. Landine, L. Leslie, and M. Singletary, *J Broadcast Electr Media 29(3)*:333 (1995).
20. J. St. Lawrence and D. Joyner, *Psychol. Women Q. 15*:49 (1991).
21. D. Peterson and K. Pfost, *Psychol. Rep. 64*:319 (1989).
22. C. Hansen and R. Hansen, *Commun. Res. 17(2)*:212 (1990).
23. B. Sherman and J. Dominick, *J. Commun. 36*:79 (1986).
24. R. Caplan, *Journal. Q. 62(1)*:144 (1985).
25. J. L. Singer, Introductory Comments on Cognitive and Behavioral Aspects of Television in *Television and Behavior*, vol 2. Technical Reviews, National Institutes of Mental Health, U.S. Department of Health and Human Services, Washington, D.C. 1982.

ENDNOTES

[1]See Douglas W. Vick, Poorhouse justice: Underfunded indigent defense services and arbitrary death sentences, 43 *Buffalo L. Rev. 329*:410 (1995) (discussing the relationship between socioeconomic factors, such as race and poverty, and death sentencing); see also Stephen B. Bright, counsel for the poor: The death sentence not for the worst crime but for the worst lawyer, 103 *Yale Law J.* 1835, 1836 (1994) (noting that "[p]oor people accused of capital crimes are often defended by lawyers who lack the skills, resources, and commitment to handle such serious matters").

[2]See bureau of Justice Statistics, U.S. Dept of Justice, Sourcebook of Criminal Justice Statistics - 1994, at 587-99 (Maguire, K. & Pastor, A.L. eds.). 1995.

[3]See id.

[4]See Vick, supra note 63, at 410-12.

[5]See id.

[6]See id. At 335 & n.24.

[7]Phillips, R.T.M., The psychiatrist as evaluator: Conflicts and conscience, *The New York Law School Law Review*, XLI, p 198, (1996).

[8]K. Tardiff, Prediction of violence, *Medical Management of the Violent Patient: Clinical Assesment and Therapy* (K. Tardiff, ed.). Marcel Dekker, New York (1999).

[9]National Television Violence Study, Sample of programs for content analysis 1994-1995, MediaScope, Inc., 1995.

[10]National Television Violence Study, Volume 2, Executive Summary, (Federman, J. ed.), University of California, Santa Barbara 1997.

[11]By Slayer in album "Hell Awaits," Metal Blade Records, 1986.
[12]By Motley Crue, in album "Shout At The Devil," Electra/Asylum, 1983.
[13]By Metal Church, in album "The Dark," Electra/Asylum, 1986.
[14]By Venom, in album "Welcome To Hell," Power Metal/Neat Music, 1985.
[15]By Seven Churches, in album "Possessed," Combat Records, 1985.
[16]"Straight Outta Compton,"? N.W.A.
[17]"Hoes," Too Short.
[18]"Mind of a Lunatic" The Ghetto Boys.
[19]"How I Could Just Kill A Man" Cypress Hill.
[20]Omegao, 19(3), 177-186. Wass, H., Raup, J., Cerullo, K., Martel, L., Mingione, L., Sperring, A. (1989).

3
Neurotransmitters and Violence

Serena-Lynn Brown
Albert Einstein College of Medicine, Bronx, New York

I. INTRODUCTION

The incidence of interpersonal aggression in the United States is alarmingly high (1). Reports of assault, child abuse, and homicide are commonplace, and aggression is becoming an increasing burden to society, with costs not only to the perpetrator and victim but also to families, communities, and society as a whole. Accordingly, a great deal of effort has been given to the attempt to understand and modify human aggressive behavior through psychological, social, and—more recently—biological models and interventions.

The biological substrate of aggression has been extensively studied in animals as well as humans. Primary areas of investigation include neuroanatomical (2), genetic (3,4), and neurotransmitter (5,6) involvement in aggressive behavior. Psychopharmacologists have extensively studied the role of the various neurotransmitters in aggression in an attempt to understand the biochemical regulation of aggression and thus to be better able to develop specific drugs designed to selectively target dysfunctional aggressive behaviors. However, much remains to be learned and understood about the role neurotransmitter systems play in the regulation of aggression and violence.

II. THE SEROTONIN SYSTEM

Serotonin (5-HT) has been repeatedly implicated as a major neurotransmitter modulating aggressive behavior in invertebrates and in mammals (for review, see

Ref. 2). In fish, it has been found that the 5-HT system exerts an inhibitory influence on the regulation of aggressive behavior (7–10). In fact, it has been shown that there is a direct negative correlation between position in a dominance hierarchy and level of 5-HT (10). In rhesus monkeys, cerebrospinal fluid (CSF) 5-hydroxyindoleacetic acid (5-HIAA), the major metabolite of 5-HT, has been shown to have a significant negative correlation with severe and violent aggression and impulsivity, although not with milder, more functional aggressive acts (11).

In mice and rats, behaviors such as pup killing (12), shock-induced fighting (13,14) and muricidal behavior (15) have been demonstrated to increase when 5-HT function is diminished by pharmacological or neuroanatomical means. A number of investigators have shown isolation-induced aggression correlating with decreased 5-HT neurotransmission (16–18). Others have demonstrated that decreasing central 5-HT levels using a tryptophan-free diet or tryptophan hydroxylase inhibitors causes an increase in aggression in rats (14,19). Bonson et al. (20) have also shown that anabolic steroid–induced aggression in rats may be mediated by the 5-HT system and particularly by 5-HT1a receptors (20).

Alternatively, increasing 5-HT function tends to decrease many types of aggressive behavior (12–22). Unfortunately, some of these data are confusing, since both 5-HT reuptake inhibitors (23,24) and 5-HT receptor antagonists (25,26) have been shown to inhibit isolation-induced aggression in mice.

When receptor subtypes have been further studied in mice, however, it has been shown that both nonspecific 5-HT1 and 5-HT1a receptor agonists inhibit aggressive behavior to a greater extent than compounds acting on other receptor subtypes and that the antiaggressive effect may be directly related to the affinity for 5-HT1a receptor binding (27–29). The association between serotonergic activation and decreased aggression has been shown in species ranging from fish to lizards to monkeys (6,10,30).

Although the data indicate a connection between aggressive behavior and 5-HT using multiple paradigms in numerous animal species, it remains unclear whether the serotonergic system has a role in the initiation of the expression of the aggressive act or whether it functions instead as a regulator of threshold for the expression of aggression (i.e., a gatekeeper function). For instance, it is interesting to note that Marks et al. (31) and Vergnes et al. (32) have demonstrated that the previous exposure of rats to mice could inhibit the muricidal effect produced by chemical damage to serotonergic neurons of the central nervous system (CNS). Their conclusion was that 5-HT plays a major role as a facilitator rather than an initiator of aggressive behavior. In a similar vein, Korte et al. (33) demonstrated decreased function of 5-HT1a receptors in male rats following social defeat by a more dominant male rat.

A. Biochemical Data

1. CSF 5-HIAA Studies

The role of CNS 5-HT in human behavior was initially studied in major depression (34), and a bimodal distribution of CSF 5-HIAA was noted. Asberg et al. (35) confirmed the presence of a bimodal distribution of CSF 5-HIAA in depressed individuals and made the important observation that the number of suicide attempts was markedly higher in patients with decreased CSF 5-HIAA as compared with depressives who had normal CSF 5-HIAA levels (40 versus 15%). Moreover, those patients who attempted suicide by more "violent" means (e.g., hanging or drowning) had lower CSF 5-HIAA levels than those attempting suicide by "nonviolent"methods (e.g., drug overdose or superficial wrist cuts). Since suicide is conceptualized as a form of inwardly directed or autoaggression, this finding provided initial evidence suggesting involvement of the serotonergic system with human aggression.

A number of other studies over the ensuing years have confirmed the presence of low CSF 5-HIAA in depressed suicide attempters (36–40). Other researchers have also found CSF 5-HIAA to be low in nondepressed, nonpsychotic personality-disordered suicide attempters (37,41–44), as well as in nondepressed psychotic schizophrenics who attempted suicide in response to command auditory hallucinations (45,46).

Numerous studies have also suggested that 5-HT is involved in the modulation and expression of outwardly directed aggression in humans. Brown et al. (41) were the first to report abnormalities of central 5-HT in aggressive individuals. In military servicemen with personality disorders, CSF 5-HIAA was significantly negatively correlated with current and/or past aggressive behavior. Those diagnosed with personality disorders associated with increased impulsivity (i.e., antisocial, explosive, immature, and hysterical) had lower CSF 5-HIAA than those with disorders associated with less impulsivity (i.e., passive-aggressive, passive-dependent, schizoid, obsessive-compulsive, and inadequate). Histories of suicide attempts were also associated with low CSF 5-HIAA levels. Subsequently, Brown et al. (47) studied individuals diagnosed with borderline personality disorder and found that those with low CSF 5-HIAA had significantly higher aggression scores. Those patients with histories of suicide attempts also had significantly decreased CSF 5-HIAA as well as higher aggression scores as compared with those patients without such histories of suicide attempts.

Other studies have also shown significant associations between decreased CSF 5-HIAA and increased outwardly directed aggression. In six men with an extra Y chromosome and histories of arson and/or assaultive behavior, postprobenecid CSF 5-HIAA was decreased as compared with normal controls (48). Baseline CSF 5-HIAA was not different, however. Treatment with 5-

hydroxytryptophan (5-HTP, the immediate metabolic precursor of 5-HT) resulted in decreased aggression in five of six patients. Rydin et al. (49) also found a significant negative correlation between CSF 5-HIAA levels and both traits of impulsivity and sensation seeking as well as the hostility score on the Rorschach.

Lidberg et al. (50) reported that three individuals who had murdered or had attempted to murder one of their own children had histories of suicide attempts and were found to have low CSF 5-HIAA levels. Lidberg et al. (51) also found low CSF 5-HIAA levels in men who had murdered sexual partners. These levels were similar to those in suicide attempters. Interestingly, other murderers (most of whom had histories of alcoholism) did not have low levels. The authors speculate that since, according to case record review, the murders of the sexual partners occurred during periods of intense negative affect, low CSF 5-HIAA may be related to the tendency to lose control or to use violent means during periods of emotional arousal. Kreusi et al. (52) have also shown a negative correlation between CSF 5-HIAA and self-ratings of aggression in prepubertal and adolescent boys with disruptive behavior disorders, although opposite findings have also been reported (53). Finally, in a study by Roy et al. (54), a significant negative correlation was observed between CSF 5-HIAA and the "urge to act out hostility" subscale of the Foulds Hostility and Direction of Hostility Questionnaire in normal volunteers.

As mentioned above in regard to animal models of aggression, the specific aspects of aggressive display that are linked to low CSF 5-HIAA remain to be definitively determined. Linnoila et al. (55) assessed differences between violent criminals who committed "impulsive" crimes (i.e., nonpremeditated) and those who committed "nonimpulsive" crimes (i.e., premeditated). Those who committed impulsive offenses had lower CSF 5-HIAA levels than those committing nonimpulsive offenses. Individuals who committed multiple murders had lower CSF 5-HIAA levels than those committing single murders.

Impulsive offenders with histories of suicide attempts had the lowest levels of all. Also, impulsive offenders had more evidence of disturbed childhood behavior (consistent with diagnoses of attention deficit disorder or antisocial personality disorder) as well as increased histories of alcohol abuse. The authors have suggested that alcohol might lower the threshold for impulsive violent behavior in predisposed individuals (56). In fact, in a prospective follow-up study, low CSF 5-HIAA and blood glucose nadir were found to predict recidivism in over 84% of these impulsive offenders (57). Virkkunen et al. have also done several studies suggesting a link between poor impulse control and low CSF 5-HIAA levels. They have consistently shown that impulsive offenders, such as arsonists—many of whom carry the diagnoses of borderline personality disorder or intermittent explosive disorder—have significantly lower CSF 5-HIAA levels than habitually violent nonimpulsive offenders or normal controls (58,59).

Finally, as mentioned above and as we have elaborated in other work, inwardly directed aggression appears to be highly associated with outwardly directed aggression; that is, violent individuals are likely to make suicide attempts and suicidal individuals are likely to engage in violent behavior (41,47,50, 51,55,60–64). Low CSF 5-HIAA appears to be related to both forms of aggression and is found in individuals with histories of suicide attempts and violent acts. This relationship is not restricted to a particular psychiatric diagnosis but rather is found across a wide variety of diagnostic categories. As the above data suggest, it also appears that impulsivity or impulsive, nonpremeditated aggression may be the specific behavioral correlate of decreased 5-HT function.

2. Treatment Studies

The potentiation or inhibition of 5-HT function has also been examined in the study of violence and aggression. Tryptophan, the dietary amino acid 5-HT precursor, has been utilized in several such studies. Data are contradictory, however, showing both decreased aggressive behavior as well as no response to the administration of tryptophan in aggressive psychiatric patients (65,66). Another paradigm, involving the use of tryptophan depletion and using tryptophan-deficient amino acid mixtures, has also produced mixed results. While initially tryptophan depletion was not found to increase aggressive responses in humans in a laboratory study (67), the same group subsequently showed increased aggression in a similar laboratory study (68). Salomon et al. (69) have also shown no change in hostility during acute tryptophan depletion in impulsive inpatients. Hypotryptophanemia in impulsive adolescents has also been reported (70).

It has been suggested that drugs that increase central 5-HT function may be helpful in treating aggressive behavior (71). It should also be noted that several drugs are now in development—the piperazine derivatives eltoprazine and fluprazine as well as amperozide—which have been shown in animals and humans to decrease aggression and induce more sociable behavior while not causing sedation (24,72,73). Such drugs are primarily 5-HT1a and 5-HT1b mixed agonists (27).

3. Platelet and Whole Blood Studies

Investigators have used the human blood platelet as a peripheral model for the study of presynaptic 5-HT function (74). Decreased platelet and whole-blood 5-HT levels have been demonstrated to be associated with autoaggression, hostility, and lifetime history of aggression (75–78). Platelet MAO (monoamine oxidase) activity, associated with CSF 5-HIAA, has been found to show a negative correlation between MAO activity and impulsivity (79,80). Imipramine, a tricyclic antidepressant, has been shown to block platelet uptake of 5-HT through specific binding to a high-affinity 5-HT transporter receptor site (81). In a study of platelet ^{3}H-imipramine binding and MAO-B activity, Castrogiovanni et al. (19) found that while there was some indication for a correlation between increased 5-HT activity and decreased aggressive behavior, the more impressive significant correlation was between MAO-B activity and aggression. However, Sarne et al. (82) have reported increased platelet ^{3}H-imipramine binding in violent offenders compared with controls and in hostile schizophrenics compared with nonhostile matched patients.

4. Cholesterol and 5-HT

The association between serum cholesterol, 5-HT levels, and violence has also been an area of research interest. In the investigation of the relationship between increased cholesterol levels and cardiac disease, it was serendipitously found that individuals with low serum cholesterol levels had significantly increased mortality rates from suicides, homicides, and accidents (83–87). In a similar vein, it was found that criminals with histories of violence and aggression had correspondingly low levels of cholesterol (86). However, other investigators have not replicated these findings (88,89). It appears that a number of other variables such as the use of alcohol, drugs, and nicotine, psychiatric symptomatology, socioeconomic level, and other illnesses have probably influenced these findings (85). Even so, these results are striking enough to have generated several hypotheses concerning the relationship between cholesterol and 5-HT. For instance, it has been proposed that decreased blood cholesterol levels may cause an alteration of cell membrane permeability and viscosity, resulting in a change in 5-HT receptor activity (85,90). There are also some data from 5-HT metabolite challenge studies in monkeys that provide evidence for an association between cholesterol reduction and decreased serotonergic activity (91) as well as increased aggression (92).

Finally, it has been shown more recently that, among a large sample of male psychiatric inpatients, those with low cholesterol levels had twice the likelihood of having made a serious suicide attempt than those with higher cholesterol levels, even after controlling for both depression and alcohol use (93).

B. 5-HT Challenge Studies

As reviewed above, most of the studies associating 5-HT with human aggression have examined 5-HIAA obtained via lumbar puncture. While levels of this CSF metabolite yield a measure of overall 5-HT metabolism, information cannot be obtained about the functional state of specific 5-HT receptors. In addition, obtaining samples of CSF from psychiatric patients is often problematic, especially on a repeated basis. In an effort to develop a reliable, relatively noninvasive means of assessing the status of central 5-HT neuronal function, our group and other have developed the "neuroendocrine challenge paradigm." This paradigm involves peripheral administration of a direct or indirect monoamine (MA) agonist or antagonist and subsequent measurement of hormones under central monoaminergic regulation. The magnitude of the hormonal response is considered to be a measure of the responsivity of the MA system involved (94). Thus, such a technique allows us to give an agent orally and to inferentially assess CNS neuronal function.

We have noted elsewhere that the consistent finding of decreased CSF 5-HIAA in inwardly or outwardly directed aggression must be taken into account in any hypothesis concerning 5-HT receptor sensitivity and aggression, although decreased 5-HT metabolism might be unrelated to 5-HT receptor sensitivity. We have proposed that the most likely possibility is that decreased 5-HT metabolism is related to postsynaptic 5-HT receptor hypersensitivity for either of two reasons: (1) primary hypometabolism of 5-HT with secondary receptor hypersensitivity or (2) primary receptor hypersensitivity with secondary 5-HT hypometabolism (95).

The 5-HT challenge literature can be examined with these alternate hypotheses in mind. The release of cortisol and prolactin (PRL) has been shown to be serotonergically mediated in humans (96); thus these are the two hormones primarily measured in 5-HT challenge studies. Using the 5-HT challenge paradigm, Meltzer et al. (97) found an increased cortisol response to the 5-HT precursor 5-HTP in depressed and manic suicide attempters, as compared with nonsuicidal patients or normal controls. Since it has been shown that 5-HTP-induced cortisol release is negatively correlated with concentrations of CSF 5-HIAA, this suggests that decreased 5-HT metabolism may have been related to increased 5-HT receptor sensitivity in the suicide attempters.

1. The Fenfluramine Challenge Test

Fenfluramine acts as a presynaptic 5-HT releaser and 5-HT reuptake blocker in addition to directly stimulating the 5-HT receptor. In human subjects, this agent produces a dose-dependent rise in PRL (98), which is blocked by the 5-HT antagonists metergoline and cyproheptadine (99,100).

Unfortunately, challenge studies utilizing fenfluramine have produced inconsistent results. Fishbein et al. (101) challenged abstinent substance abusers with fenfluramine and found increased cortisol and PRL levels in individuals with aggressive and impulsive behaviors. Cortisol and PRL responses were correlated with measures of impulsivity and aggressiveness. However, Gerra et al. (102) did not replicate this finding in detoxified heroin abusers, while Coccaro et al.

(103) noted a blunted PRL response to fenfluramine in patients with major affective disorders and personality disorders. PRL levels were particularly reduced in patients with histories of suicide attempts. In patients with personality disorders, significant inverse correlations were noted between blunted PRL response and measurements of impulsivity and aggression. Similarly, O'Keane et al. (104) also found a blunted PRL response to fenfluramine in nine men with antisocial personality disorder convicted of murder, while Siever et al. (105) also showed reduced 5-HT function in aggressive patients with borderline personality disorder. Finally, in a challenge study of prepubertal and adolescent male patients with disruptive behavior disorders, Stoff et al. (106) found no correlation between fenfluramine-induced cortisol or PRL release and aggression and no difference between normal controls and patients.

There are several possible explanations for these discrepancies. Recent substance abuse or withdrawal may have influenced 5-HT receptor function in the subjects in the Fishbein et al. (101) study. In addition, the discrepancies between the 5-HTP and the fenfluramine studies may be due to the fact that these two compounds act on different aspects of the 5-HT system. Stoff et al. (106) have also suggested that these discrepancies may be due to individual differences in the way that the racemic mixture (DL-fenfluramine) used in these studies (less selective than pure D-fenfluramine, and therefore also causing release of DA and NE) is metabolized, or gender and age differences. Other challenge studies measuring 5-HT function, such as that of Moeller et al. (107), showing increased aggression significantly correlated with buspirone (a 5-HT1a agonist) induced increase in growth hormone in cocaine-dependent subjects, suffer from the same difficulties. Note that Coccaro (108) also has preliminary data suggesting a negative correlation between impulsivity and PRL response to buspirone challenge in personality-disordered patients.

There are several problems with the use of 5-HTP and fenfluramine as 5-HT challenge agents. Neither 5-HTP nor fenfluramine is 5-HT selective. High doses of 5-HTP cause formation of 5-HT in catecholaminergic neurons, which may then act as a false transmitter or by CA displacement. Similarly, fenfluramine has also been shown to increase DA metabolites and to block striatal DA receptors. It is therefore difficult to interpret to what extent the neuroendocrine responses are related to specific abnormalities in 5-HT function. Furthermore, since 5-HT–releasing agents depend on intact presynaptic mechanisms, a blunted hormonal response does not necessarily indicate decreased postsynaptic 5-HT receptor sensitivity; it may be due to decreased presynaptic 5-HT availability (109).

2. The MCPP Challenge Test

m-Chlorophenylpiperzine (MCPP), a metabolite of the antidepressant trazodone, has been used as a more reliable challenge agent for the study of central 5-HT receptor function. MCPP is a direct postsynaptic 5-HT receptor agonist which has pronounced 5-HT1 activity as well as some 5-HT2 activity (110) and 5-HT3 affinity (111). It stimulates the release of several hormones including PRL, cortisol, and growth hormone, which are partially regulated by 5-HT (112).

Recently, radioligand binding studies have indicated equipotent binding of MCPP at 5-HT1a, 5-HT2 as well as alpha-2-adrenergic receptor sites (113), suggesting that this agent may not be specific for the 5-HT system. However, in vitro receptor binding may not reflect actual in vivo receptor function. In addition, evidence suggests that the selectivity of MCPP for the serotonergic system appears to depend upon the dosage used. In animal studies, Invernizzi et al. (114) have shown that a dose of 1 mg/kg MCPP reduces 5-HIAA levels in rats, while higher doses (3 to 10 mg/kg) also raise levels of CSF 3-methoxy-4-hydroxyphenylglycol (MHPG), the primary noradrenergic metabolite, and homovanillic acid (HVA), the primary dopaminergic metabolite. These doses are considerably higher than those employed in human challenge studies. Finally, the serotonergic selectivity of MCPP in inducing neuroendocrine effects is supported by studies using 5-HT antagonists. MCPP-induced release of ACTH, cortisol, and PRL in rodents (115,116), monkeys (117), and in humans (118,119) has been shown to be blocked by the mixed 5-HT1/5-HT2 antagonist metergoline, suggesting that this release may be 5-HT-mediated (116,117,120,121).

The MCPP challenge paradigm has been employed to examine serotonergic function across different diagnostic patient groups, resulting in interesting data on aggression and impulsivity. Coccaro (103) has reported pilot data from five depressed and personality-disordered patients showing a negative correlation between MCPP-induced PRL response (0.5 mg/kg PO) and measures of impulsive aggression. Moss et al. (122) found a significant negative correlation between MCPP-induced PRL release (0.5 mg/kg) and measures of impulsive aggression, and augmented cortisol release among antisocial substance-abusing patients in a non-placebo-controlled design. Insel (123) has suggested that increased obsessive-compulsive (OC) symptoms found in OC patients but not normal subjects during MCPP challenge (124) may relate to altered aggression regulation, with OC symptoms emerging as the OC patient attempts to deal with this heightened state of aggression. They propose that this 5-HT receptor hypersensitivity compensates for a functional presynaptic deficit; OC patients thus lie at the opposite end of the spectrum from impulsively disordered patients (125). However, there are significant design problems with these studies, so that it is premature to conclude from them that impulsive aggression is related to 5-HT receptor hyposensitivity.

Our group has utilized a lower dose of MCPP (0.25 mg/kg) to investigate the hypothesis of 5-HT receptor hypersensitivity, rather than hyposensitivity, in aggression. In a group of patients with major depression or panic disorder and a matched group of normal controls, we found that MCPP did not induce hostility during the challenge test, that patients rated as being more hostile did not have significantly greater MCPP-induced cortisol or PRL release than patients rated as being less hostile, and that MCPP-induced hormonal release was unrelated to measures of aggression and hostility in these patients (126). Given the well-documented relationship between 5-HT and aggression, it might have been expected that MCPP would decrease aggressive indices in these patients, but no reduction of hostility was found either. While such findings do not support the 5-HT theory of aggression, it is also possible that MCPP does not stimulate the specific 5-HT receptor subtypes associated with aggression. However, it should be noted that patients were not chosen for this study on the basis of aggressive or hostile behavior and did not show a wide range of differences on these measures. Therefore it is quite possible that those classified as "more hostile" were not significantly different from those classified as "less hostile" on these significant serotonergic parameters.

III. THE NOREPINEPHRINE SYSTEM

Norepinephrine (NE), or noradrenaline, has also figured prominently in decades of research seeking a chemical model for arousal, aggression, and impulsivity. However, it has only been recently that this neurotransmitter has been linked to 5-HT in an interactive model of aggression that has been the focus of increasing research.

Early studies showed a direct relationship between behavioral arousal and increased NE as well as between aggression (foot shock–induced fighting) and increased NE synthesis in animals (127). Sham rage in cats and rats (induced by electrical stimulation of the amygdala) has been shown to be associated with increased central NE, while agents that cause a decrease in central NE function also stop this behavior (128). Increasing NE metabolism through the use of drugs such as monoaminergic antidepressants has also been shown to increase such aggressive behavior in rats (129). Matsumoto et al. (130) have shown that lesioning central noradrenergic nerve terminals markedly decreased desipramine-induced aggressive behavior in mice. Compounds such as rubidium, which increase NE turnover, have been shown to cause an increase in aggressive behavior in rats (131,132), while clonidine, which causes a decrease in NE function, decreases aggression (shock-induced fighting) (133). Investigators have also consistently demonstrated a reduction in aggressive behavior in animals after administration of beta blockers such as propranolol and nadolol (26,134,135). Summers and Greenberg (30) have also shown decrease in NE metabolites, although not in NE concentration itself, in subordinate versus dominant male lizards after the fight determining dominance.

A number of investigators have examined the relationship between stress, NE, and aggression. Rats subjected to environmental stress show increased aggression and irritability associated with two measures of increased NE metabolism, increased brainstem tyrosine-hydroxylase activity (the rate-limiting enzyme for the synthesis of NE), and downregulation of beta-adrenergic receptors in the cortex (136).

Eichelman (136) has pointed out, however, that it is important to differentiate animal aggression into affective and predatory components. While laboratory studies all confirm the relationship between increased NE in affective aggression, NE appears to have an inhibitory effect on predatory aggression.

Based upon such studies, it was initially proposed that, in contrast to 5-HT, increased central NE function mediates increased arousal and aggressive response (137).

A. Biochemical Data

1. CSF MHPG Studies

The primary metabolite of NE measured in the CSF is 3-methoxy-4-hydroxyphenylglycol (MHPG). Studies examining the relationship between CSF MHPG concentrations and aggression or impulsivity have produced contradictory results, however. While Brown et al. (41) found a positive correlation between CSF MHPG concentration and history of impulsive aggressive behavior in military personnel with personality disorders, Linnoila et al. (55) found no difference between impulsive and nonimpulsive violent offenders in CSF MHPG levels. While Redmond et al. (138) found no relationship between CSF MHPG concentration and hostility, they found a positive relationship between CSF MHPG and anxiety and agitation in depressed and manic patients and normal controls. Castellanos et al. (53) also reported a significant positive correlation between aggression, impulsivity, and CSF MHPG in boys and adolescents with attention-deficit hyperactivity disorder.

Studies of CSF MHPG in violent versus nonviolent suicide attempters have provided mixed and inconclusive results (37,43,139–141). Interestingly, several investigators have shown a direct correlation between increased CSF MHPG and increased aggression in nonhuman primates (142,143).

2. Treatment Studies

Subsequent studies in humans have provided more evidence for this hypothesis. Drugs that increase NE activity, such as the tricyclic and monoamine oxidase inhibitor antidepressants, which decrease beta-adrenergic receptor number, have been demonstrated to increase behavioral aggression (144–147), while drugs that decrease NE activity, such as propranolol and nadolol, have been shown to decrease behavioral aggression (148–151). Lithium, which is thought to decrease central NE availability (152), has been shown to decrease impulsive aggressive behaviors in chronically aggressive prisoners (153) as well as personality-disordered and/or psychotic patients (152). Hypertyrosinemia in impulsive adolescents has also been reported (70).

B. NE Challenge Studies

As discussed above, neuroendocrine challenge studies have been developed to provide a "window" on central monoaminergic function. Clonidine is an alpha-2-adrenergic receptor agonist that stimulates anterior pituitary hormone release, and has been shown to consistently cause growth hormone (GH) release through the activation of postsynaptic NE receptors (154–156). Studies in animals have suggested that this response is mediated by alpha-2-adrenergic receptors (157,158).

Coccaro et al. (159) challenged depressed and normal males with clonidine and found a significant correlation between GH rise and irritability but not assultiveness in both groups, heightened in healthy volunteers or in patients with personality disorders.

IV. THE DOPAMINE SYSTEM

Many studies have found significant correlations between indices of dopamine (DA) activity and aggressive behavior. Increasing DA levels or stimulating DA metabolism increases aggressive behavior in animals. The administration of levodopa or a DA agonist such as apomorphine causes increased aggression in rats (160,161). Shock-induced aggression in rodents has been shown to increase after administration of dopamine, levodopa, or D2 agonists such as apomorphine, bromocryptine, and pergolide, although other reports have found contradictory effects (162).

Summers and Greenberg (30) have also shown decrease in DA concentration in subordinate versus dominant male lizards immediately after a fight for dominance.

Numerous studies have examined the effects of DA antagonists (generally antipsychotics that block D2 receptors) and have found consistent suppression of aggressive behavior in both rodents and primates (152,163). However, these drugs lack behavioral specificity and cause sedation and suppression of a wide range of nonaggressive behaviors as well (163,164).

A. Biochemical Data

1. CSF HVA Studies

Homovanillic acid (HVA) is the primary DA metabolite measured in the CSF. In the studies by Brown et al. (41,47) cited above, while significant negative correlations were shown between CSF 5-HIAA and aggression and significant positive correlations were shown between CSF MHPG and aggression, no correlation was shown between CSF HVA and measures of aggression. Banki et al. (165) examined CSF metabolites in violent and nonviolent suicide attempters and showed no direct correlation between indices of aggression and CSF HVA. In the study cited above by Castellanos et al. (53), a significant positive correlation between aggression, impulsivity, and CSF HVA in boys and adolescents with attention-deficit hyperactivity disorder was also found, while Linnoila et al. (55) found no difference in CSF HVA in impulsive arsonists versus normal controls.

Finally, as with the results of CSF MHPG cited above, it should be noted that studies of CSF HVA in violent versus nonviolent suicide attempters have provided inconclusive results (37,43,139–141,166).

2. Treatment Studies

Numerous investigators have shown decrease in aggressive behavior in humans after administration of neuroleptics that are DA antagonists (144,152,164). However, as discussed above, these drugs lack behavioral specificity; they also cause sedation and suppression of a wide range of nonaggressive behaviors as well (163,164).

V. THE GABA/BENZODIAZEPINE SYSTEM

The role of the gamma-aminobutyric acid (GABA)/benzodiazepine system has also been studied in both animal and human aggression. Aggressive behavior has been shown to be inversely correlated with central GABA concentration in mice (167). GABA levels have been shown to be decreased in aggressive versus nonaggressive rodents (168–170). Increasing GABA availability through the use of aminooxyacetic acid or gamma-acetylenic GABA has been shown to inhibit or suppress aggression in animal models (171), while GABA antagonists such as picrotoxin or allylglycine increase aggression in rats (168–170).

Benzodiazepines (BZs) act on the GABA/benzodiazepine receptor to increase central GABAergic function. BZs have been shown to decrease aggression in animals across a variety of parameters (164), although, interestingly, chronic administration of GABA/benzodiazepine receptor agonists such as diazepam can increase aggression in mice (172), while acute administration of diazepam or chlordiazepoxide has also been shown to increase maternal and intruder-provoked aggression in rats (173,174).

A. Biochemical Data

1. Treatment Studies

Numerous investigators have reported on the use of BZs to decrease aggression in many diagnostic subgroups of patients (152,175–177). However, others have noted "paradoxical" rage reactions (177–179).

VI. OTHER NEUROTRANSMITTER SYSTEMS

A. Acetylcholine

The cholinergic system has also been implicated in aggressive behavior. Acetylcholine increases aggressive behavior in animals. Increasing cholinergic function through the use of agonists such as carbachol or the cholinesterase inhibitor physostigmine has been shown to induce aggressive behavior in rodents and cats, while decreasing cholinergic function (e.g., using atropine) reduces aggression (136,180). However, human studies in this area have not been published.

B. Opiates

Little work has been done in the area of opioid peptides and their receptors. Miczek et al. (164) have suggested that the preclinical paradigm of morphine withdrawal in mice, with high levels of resultant aggression, can be explained by interactions with the DA system increasing mesolimbic or striatal DA. Siegel and Schubert (1981) have also described opioid peptide mediation of suppression of defensive rage behavior in the cat.

VII. CONCLUSION

Biological abnormalities identified in psychiatric patients have been traditionally correlated with syndromes or disease entities rather than with psychological dysfunctions. Our group has argued that, as more work is done in the realm of neurochemical correlates of psychological phenomena, the latter approach may well supersede the former (109). For example, as described above, the specific variable of low CSF 5-HIAA level has been shown to be diagnostically nonspecific, having been identified in apparently dissimilar disorders (e.g., mood disorders, schizophrenia, and personality disorders). In fact, as the data were further developed, low CSF 5-HIAA appears to be more specifically related to particular psychopathological dimensions, such as increased aggression and/or impulsivity, as discussed above. Thus we have emphasized the need for biological research to include extensive and reliable psychometric measurement of a number of dimensions of psychological functioning across diagnostic categories, a method which Van Praag has termed the functional/dimensional approach (63,109) as contrasted to the nosological/categorical approach.

From an examination of the data presented in this chapter, it is clear that decreased 5-HT function has consistently been shown to be highly correlated with impulsive aggression. We have proposed that the 5-HT system may modulate aggression through the inhibition of behavioral responses to environmental stimuli (63,109). In fact, in animals, decreased 5-HT indices have been consistently shown to cause increased irritability and excitability (2), suggesting disinhibition in those areas.

Although there is pharmacological evidence that raising brain 5-HT levels reduces aggressive behavior (48,65,152,182) the relationship is surely more complicated than a simple linear one. Aggression is far from being a simple unidimensional psychological concept; thus it makes such data more difficult to interpret. For instance, anxiety, another important psychopathological dimension that has rarely been controlled for in studies of aggression, is also associated with dysregulation of 5-HT (see Brown and van Praag, Ref. 63). As discussed above, impulsivity, another psychological dimension often involved in aggressive behavior, is not only associated with abnormalities in 5-HT metabolism but in fact may the critical psychopathological entity associated with such 5-HT dysfunction.

As more work has been published linking aggressive behaviors with other neurotransmitters, the picture of interacting neurotransmitter systems in the regulation of impulsive aggression has begun to provide a more complex view of how these behaviors are modulated. While measures of central 5-HT are inversely correlated with aggression, central NE levels appear to be directly correlated with aggression. It is not clear as yet what role the other neurotransmitter systems may play in the development or expression of aggression. Coccaro et al. (183) have proposed that, since NE appears to regulate arousal and detection of environmental stimuli, release of central NE onto postsynaptic alpha-2 receptors may cause an increase in the "signal-to-noise" ratio, alerting the animal to outside stimuli. They propose that this would cause increased "irritability," particularly when the outside stimuli are adverse, and when combined with decreased central 5-HT function, behavioral disinhibition would occur (109), and the animal would respond aggressively. Thus, the hypothesis is that an interaction occurs between the strength of an adverse stimulus, threshold for detection of such stimuli, and behavioral disinhibition, which then triggers an aggressive response (159).

In a similar vein, Hollander et al. (184) have described impulsive disorders as resulting from an abnormal decrease in serotonergic activity, causing a defect in harm avoidance, coupled with abnormal noradrenergic activity, causing a malfunction of anticipatory anxiety. Candito et al. (70) have suggested that their studies showing hypotryptophanemia and hypertryosinemia in impulsive adolescents provide some evidence for this hypothesis.

It has also been proposed that the effect of NE on aggression occurs through the action of NE on 5-HT, and that NE and 5-HT interact through reciprocal modulation (185), which may include the DA system as well. Studies in animals have shown that noradrenergic drugs such as beta-adrenergic antagonists influence 5-HT-mediated behavior (135,186,187), while there are some data also suggesting DA influence on serotonergic responses as well (186,188). It has been found that the NE system must be intact in order for serotonergic lesions to cause aggression in animals (78,182). Ongoing studies by Siever and Trestman (78) highlighting the importance of NE in impulsivity and environmental reactivity also provide more evidence for the proposal by Coccaro et al. (183) suggesting a critical role for NE in the initial recognition of external stimuli, before 5-HT causes behavioral disinhibition and aggressive response.

One question which is being currently addressed involves the role of substance abuse, and particularly alcoholism, in impulsive violence. Linnoila and Virkkunen (56,189) have suggested that a heritable disorder called "low-serotonin syndrome" exists in a subgroup of habitually violent criminal offenders. This disorder is driven by 5-HT deficit, and involves early onset of both alcohol abuse and impulsive, violent behavior, with a family history of type II alcoholism, low CSF 5-HIAA associated with irritability and impulsiveness, and an associated propensity toward mild hypoglycemia and increased risk of suicide. They see the primary deficit as 5-HT dysfunction at the level of the raphe nuclei, leading to hypoglycemia, which then lowers the threshold for impulsive aggressive behavior. These authors suggest that chronic alcohol use worsens the 5-HT deficit, and increases the incidence of impulsive violent behavior, while serotonergic medication may at least partially treat this problem. Virkkunen et al. (190) have identified a polymorphism of the tryptophan hydroxylase (TPH) gene as a potential marker for this group.

Genetic studies are also yielding new information about the role of neurotransmitters in aggression and impulsivity. Mice with deleted genes for 5-HT1b receptors show increased aggressive behavior (191). Roubertoux et al. (192) have suggested that the gene encoding the enzyme steroid sulfatase, located on the Y chromosome, may be involved in the regulation of aggressive behavior.

Recently, a Dutch family with X-linked borderline mental retardation and unusual impulsive aggressive behaviors was found to have a genetic point mutation in Xp11-21 causing a deficiency in MAOA (monoamine oxidase-A is an enzyme involved in the metabolism and degradation of 5-HT, NE, and DA) (193).

In mice, deletion of the gene encoding MAOA produced severe aggressive behavioral alternations (194). The meaning of these data is not clear, since MAOA inhibitors cause an increase in 5-HT levels and have been shown to cause decreased rather than increased aggressive behavior on their own. Hen (4) has suggested that compensatory changes occurring during development might include downregulation of 5-HT receptors, resulting in a net appearance of low-HT activity or neuroanatomical changes involving 5-HT innervation. The resultant net decreased 5-HT activity then would correlate with the increased aggression in these individuals.

Continuing research into the role of neurotransmitters and impulsive aggression is needed to elucidate these relationships further and to aid in the development of pharmacological treatments for individuals with disturbances in the regulation of aggression. Genetic strategies hold promise of a direct means of examining specific enzymes and receptor systems. This field is complicated by the fact that such data will probably not provide the whole picture. It is becoming increasingly apparent that a higher level of integration will be required in order to examine reciprocal interactions between the different neurotransmitter systems, and particularly between the serotonergic and noradrenergic systems, in the regulation of aggression.

REFERENCES

1. *Vital Statistics Report*, 33 (suppl 22):27 (1984).
2. L. Valzelli, *Psychobiology of Aggression and Violence*, Raven Press, New York, 1981.
3. F.A. Elliott, Neuroanatomy and neurology of aggression, *Psychiatr. Ann. 17*:385 (1987).
4. R. Hen, Mean genes, *Neuron 16*:17 (1996).
5. S.L. Brown, A. Botsis, and H.M. van Praag, *Serotonin and Aggression. The Psychobiology of Aggression*, Haworth Press, New York, 1994, pp. 27–39.
6. M.J. Raleigh, M.T. McGuire, G.L. Brammer, D.B. Pollack, and A. Yuwiler, Serotonergic mechanisms promote dominance acquisition in adult vervet monkeys, *Brian Res. 559*:181 (1991).
7. H. Avis, The neuropharmocology of aggression: A critical review, *Psychol. Bull. 81*:47 (1974).
8. L. Maler and W.G. Ellis, Inter-male aggressive signals in weakly electric fish are modulated by monoamines, *Behav. Brain Res. 25:*75 (1987).
9. A.D. Munro, Effects of melatonin, serotonin, and naloxene on aggression in isolated cichlid fish (*Aequidens pulcher*). *J. Pineal Res. 3:*257 (1986).
10. S. Winberg, G.E. Nilsson, and H. Olsen, Changes in brain serotonergic activity during hierarchic behavior in Arctic charr (*Salvelinus alpinus L.*) are socially induced, *J. Comp. Physiol. A. 170*:93 (1992).

11. P.T. Mehlman, J.D. Higley, I. Faucher, A.A. Lilly, D.M. Taub, J. Vickers, S.J. Suomi, and M. Linnoila, Low CSF 5-HIAA concentrations and severe aggression and impaired impulse control in nonhuman primates. *Am. J. Psychiatry 10*:1485 (1994).
12. J.H. Copenhaver, R.L. Schalock, and M.J. Carver, Para-chloro-D, 1phenylalanine induced filicidal behavior in the female rat, *Pharmacol. Biochem. Behav. 8*:263 (1978).
13. K.M. Kantak, L.R. Hegstrand, and B. Eichelman, Facilitation of shock-induced fighting following intraventricular 5,7-dihydroxytryptamine and 6-hydroxy-DOPA, *Psychopharmacology 74*:157 (1981).
14. K.N. Kantak, L.R. Hegstrand, and B. Eichelman, Dietary tryptophan modulation and aggressive behavior in mice, *Pharmacol. Biochem. Behav. 12*:675 (1981).
15. R.J. Katz, Role of serotonergic mechanisms in animal models of predation. *Prog. Neuropsychopharmacol. Biol. Psychiatry 4*:219 (1980).
16. E. Kempf, S. Puglisi-Allegra, S. Cabib, C. Schleef, and P. Mandel, Serotoning levels and turnover in different brain areas of isolated aggressive or non-aggressive strains of mice, *Prog. Neuropsychopharmacol. Biol. Psychiatry 8*:365 (1984).
17. L. Valzelli, Serotonergic inhibitory control of experimental aggression, *Pharmacol. Res. Comm. 14*:1 (1982).
18. L. Valzelli, and S. Bernasconi, Aggressiveness by isolation and brain serotonin turnover changes in different strains of mice, *Neuropsychobiology 3*:35 (1979).
19. P. Castrogiovanni, M.R. Capone, I. Maremmani, and D. Marazziti, Platelet serotonergic markers and aggressive behaviour in healthy subjects, *Neuropsychobiology 29*:105 (1994).
20. K.R. Bonson, R.G. Johnson, D. Fiorella, R.A. Rabin, and J.C. Winter, Serotonergic control of androgen-induced dominance, *Pharmacol. Biochem. Behav. 49*:313 (1994).
21. S.R.G. Beckett, A.J. Lawrence, C.A. Marsden, and P.W. Marshall, Attenuation of chemically induced defense response by 5-HT1 receptor agonists administered into the periaqueductal gray, *Psychopharmacology 108*:110 (1992).
22. P. Broderick, and V. Lynch, Behavioral and biochemical changes induced by lithium and L-tryptophan in muricidal rats, *Neuropharmacology 21*:671 (1989).
23. S.-O. Ogren, A.-C. Holm, A.L. Renyi, and S.B. Ross, Antiaggressive effect of zimelidine in isolated mice, *Acta Pharmacol. Toxicol. 47*:71 (1980).
24. B. Olivier, J. Mos, J. van der Heyden, and J. Hartog, Serotonergic modulation of social interactions in isolated male mice, *Psychopharmacology 97*:154 (1989).
25. J.B. Malick, and A. Barnett, The role of serotonergic pathways in isolation-induced aggression in mice, *Pharmacol. Biochem. Behav. 5*:55 (1976).
26. M. Weinstock and C. Weiss, Antagonism by propranolol of isolation-induced aggression in mice: Correlation with 5-hydroxytryptamine receptor blockade, *Neuropharmacology 49*:653 (1980).
27. B. Olivier and J. Mos, Rodent models of aggressive behavior and serotonergic drugs, *Prog. Neuro-Psychopharmacol. Biol. Psychiatry 16*:847 (1992).
28. C. Sanchez, J. Arnt, J. Hyttel, and E.K. Moltzen, The role of serotonergic mechanisms in inhibition of isolation-induced aggression in male mice, *Psychopharmacology 110*:53 (1993).

29. S.M. White, R.F. Kucharik, and J.A. Moyer, Effects of serotonergic agents on isolation-induced aggression, *Pharmacol. Biochem. Behav. 39*:729 (1991).
30. C.H. Summers and N. Greenberg, Activation of central biogenic amines following aggressive interaction in male lizards, *Anolis Carolinensis, Brain Behav. Evol. 45*:339 (1995).
31. P. Marks, M. O'Brien, and G. Paxinos, 5,7-DHT-induced muricide: Inhibition as a result of exposure of rats to mice, *Brain Res. 135*:383 (1977).
32. M. Vergnes, C. Penot, E. Kempf, and G. Mack, Lesions selective des neurones serotoninergiques au raphe par la 5, 7-dihydroxytryptamine: Effets sur le comportement d'agression inter-specifique du rat, *Brain Res. 133*:167 (1977).
33. S.M. Korte, B. Buwalda, O. Meijer, E.R. De Kloet, and B. Bohus, Socially defeated male rats display a blunted adrenocortical response to a low dose of 8-OH-DPAT, *Eur. J. Pharmacol. 272*:45 (1995).
34. H.M. van Praag, J. Korf, and J. Puite, 5-Hydroxyindoleacetic acid levels in the cerebrospinal fluid of depressive patients treated with probenecid, *Nature. 225*:1259 (1970).
35. M. Asberg, L. Traskman, and P. Thoren, 5-HIAA in the cerebrospinal fluid: A biochemical suicide predictor? *Arch. Gen. Psychiatry 33*:1193 (1976).
36. C.M. Banki, G. Molnar, and M. Vojnik, Cerebrospinal fluid amine metabolites, tryptophan and clinical parameters in depression: Part 2. Psychopathological symptoms, *J. Affect. Disorder. 3*:91 (1981).
37. D. Lester, The concentration of neurotransmitter metabolites in the cerebrospinal fluid of suicidal individuals: A metaanalysis, *Pharmacopsychiatry 28*:45 (1995).
38. J.J. Lopez-Ibor, S.-R. Jeronimo, and J.C. Perez de los Cobos, Biological correlations of suicide and aggressivity in major depressions (with melancholia) : 5-Hydroxyindoleacetic acid and cortisol in cerebral spinal fluid, dexamethasone suppression test and therapeutic response to 5-hydroxytryptophan. *Neuropsychobiology 14*:67 (1985).
39. M.L. Rao, P. Braunig, and A. Papassotiropoulos, Autoaggressive behavior is closely related to serotonin availability in schizoaffective disorder, *Pharmacopsychiatry 27*:202 (1994).
40. H.M. van Praag, Depression, suicide and the metabolism of serotonin in the brain, *J. Affect. Disorder. 4*:275 (1982).
41. G.L. Brown, F.K. Goodwin, J. Ballenger, P.F. Goyer, and L.F. Major, Aggression in humans correlates with cerebrospinal fluid amine metabolites, *Psychiatry Res. 1*:131 (1979).
42. L. Oreland, A. Wiberg, M. Asberg, L. Traskman, L. Sjostrand, P. Thoren, L. Bertilsson, and G. Tybring, Platelet MAO activity and monoamine metabolites in cerebrospinal fluid in depressed and suicidal patients and in healthy controls, *Psychiatry Res. 4*:21 (1981).
43. L. Traskman, M. Asberg, L. Bertilsson, and L. Sjostrand, Monoamine metabolites in CSF and suicidal behavior, *Arch. Gen. Psychiatry 38*:631 (1981).
44. M. Virkkunen, J. De Jong, F.K. Goodwin, and M. Linnoila, Relationship of psychobiological variables to recidivism in violent offenders and impulsive fire-setters: A follow-up study, *Arch. Gen. Psychiatry 46*:600 (1989).
45. P.T. Ninan, D.P. van Kammen, M. Scheinin, M. Linnoila, W.E. Bunney, and F.K.

Goodwin, CSF 5-hydroxyindoleacetic acid levels in suicidal schizophrenic patients, *Am. J. Psychiatry 141*:566 (1984).
46. H.M. van Praag, CSF 5-HIAA and suicide in non-depressed schizophrenics, *Lancet 2*:977 (1983).
47. G.L. Brown, M.H. Ebert, P.F. Goyer, D.C. Jimerson, W.J. Klein, W.E. Bunney, and F.K. Goodwin FK, Aggression, suicide and serotonin—Relationships to CSF amine metabolites, *Am. J. Psychiatry 139*:741 (1982).
48. B. Bioulac, M. Benezech, B. Renaud, B. Noel, and D. Roche, Serotonergic functions in the 47, XYY syndrome, *Biol. Psychiatry 15*:917 (1980).
49. E. Rydin, D. Schalling, and M. Asberg, Rorschach ratings in depressed and suicidal patients with low levels of 5-hydroxyindoleacetic acid in cerebrospinal fluid, *Psychiatry Res. 7*:229 (1982).
50. L. Lidberg, M. Asberg, and U.B. Sundqvuist-Stensman, 5-hydroxyindoleacetic acid in attempted suicides who have killed their children, *Lancet 2*:928 (1984).
51. L. Lidberg, J.R. Tuck, M. Asberg, G.P. Scalia-Tomba, and L. Bertilsson, Homicide, suicide and CSF 5-HIAA, *Acta Psychiatr. Scand. 71*:230 (1985).
52. M.J.P. Kreusi, J.L. Rapoport, S. Hamburger, E. Hibbs, W.Z. Potter, M. Lenane, and G.L. Brown, CSF monoamine metabolites, aggression and impulsivity in disruptive behavior disorders of children and adolescents. *Arch. Gen. Psychiatry 47*:419 (1990).
53. F.X. Castellanos, J. Elia, M.J.P. Kreusi, C.S. Gulotta, I.N. Mefford, W.Z. Potter, G.F. Ritchie, and J.L. Rapoport, Cerebrospinal fluid monoamine metabolites in boys with attention-deficit hyperactivity disorder, *Psychiatry Res. 52*:305 (1994).
54. A. Roy, B. Adinoff, and M. Linnoila, Acting out hostility in normal volunteers: Negative correlation with levels of 5-HIAA in cerebrospinal fluid, *Psychiatry Res. 24*:187 (1988).
55. M. Linnoila, M. Virkkunen, M. Scheinin, A. Nuutila, R. Rimon, and F.K. Goodwin, Low cerebrospinal fluid 5-hydroxyindoleacetic acid concentration differentiates impulsive from non-impulsive violent behavior. *Life Sci. 33*:2609 (1983).
56. M. Linnoila and M. Virkkunen, Aggression, suicidality, and serotonin, *J. Clin. Psychiatry 53*:46 (1992).
57. M. Virkkunen, J. De Johng, J. Bartko, and M. Linnoila, Psychobiological concomitants of history of suicide attempts among violent offenders and impulsive fire setters, *Arch. Gen. Psychiatry 46*:604 (1989).
58. M. Virkkunen, A. Nuutila, F.K. Goodwin, and M. Linnoila, Cerebrospinal fluid monamine metabolite levels in male arsonists, *Arch. Gen. Psychiatry 44*:241 (1987).
59. M. Virkkunen, R. Rawlings, R. Tokola, R.E. Poland, A. Guidotti, C. Nemeroff, G. Bissette, K. Kalogeras, S.L. Karonen, and M. Linnoila, CSF biochemistries, glucose metabolism, and diurnal activity rhythms in alcoholic, violent offenders, fire setters, and healthy volunteers, *Arch. Gen. Psychiatry 51*:20 (1994).
60. A. Apter, R. Plutchik, S. Sevy, M.L. Korn, S.L. Brown, and H.M. van Praag, Defense mechanisms in risk of suicide and risk of violence, *Am. J. Psychiatry 146*:1027 (1989).
61. A. Apter, H.M. van Praag, R. Plutchik, S. Sevy, M.L. Korn, and S.L. Brown, In-

terrelations among anxiety, aggression, impulsivity, and mood: A serotonergically linked cluster? *Psychiatry Res. 32*:191 (1990).
62. A. Apter, M. Kotler, S. Sevy, R. Plutchik, S.L. Brown, H. Foster, M. Hillbrand, M.L. Korn, and H.M. van Praag, Correlates of risk of suicide in violent and nonviolent psychiatric patients, *Am. J. Psychiat. 148*:883 (1991).
63. S.L. Brown and H.M. van Praag, *The Role of Serotonin in the Psychiatric Disorders*, Brunner/Mazel, New York, 1991.
64. R. Plutchik, H.M. van Praag, and H.R. Conte, Suicide and violence risk in psychiatric patients, *Biol. Psychiatry 20*:761 (1985).
65. C. Morand, S.N. Young, and F.R. Ervin, Clinical response of aggressive schizophrenics to oral tryptophan, *Biol. Psychiatry 18*:575 (1983).
66. J. Volavka, M. Crowner, D. Brizer, A. Convit, H.M. van Praag, and R.F. Suckow, Tryptophan treatment of aggressive psychiatric inpatients, *Biol. Psychiatry 28*:728 (1990).
67. S.E. Smith, R.O. Pihl, S.N. Young, and F.R. Ervin, Elevation and reduction of plasma tryptophan and their effects on aggression and perceptual sensitivity in normal males, *Aggress. Behav. 12*:393 (1986).
68. R.O. Pihl, S.N. Young, P. Harden, S. Plotnick, B. Chamberlain, and F.R. Ervin, Acute effect of altered tryptophan levels and alcohol on aggression in normal human males, *Psychopharmacology 119*:353 (1995).
69. R.M. Salomon, C.M. Mazure, P.L. Delgado, P. Mendia, and D.S. Charney, Serotonin function in aggression: The effect of acute plasma tryptophan depletion in aggressive patients, *Biol. Psychiatry 35*:570 (1994).
70. M. Candito, F. Askenazy, M. Myquel, P. Chambon, and G. Darcourt, Tryptophanemia and tyrosinemia in adolescents with impulsive behavior, *Int. Clin. Psychopharmacol. 8*:129 (1993).
71. M. O'Neil, N. Page, W.N. Adkins, and B. Eichelman, Tryptophan-trazodone treatment of aggressive behavior, *Lancet 2*:859 (1986).
72. B. Olivier, J. Mos, and D. Rasmussen, Behavioural pharmacology of the serenic, eltoprazine, *Rev. Drug Metab. Drug Inter. 8*:31 (1990).
73. R.D. Porsolt, Report on the Third International I.T.E.M.-LABO Symposium on Strategies in Psychopharmacology: Serotonin: Animal models and clinical targets, *Pharmacopsychiatry 26*:20 (1993).
74. S.M. Stahl, The human platelet, *Arch. Gen. Psychiatry 34*:509 (1977).
75. P. Braunig, M.L. Rao, and R. Fimmers, Blood serotonin levels in suicidal schizophrenic patients, *Acta Psychiatr. Scand. 79*:186 (1989).
76. J.J. Mann, P.A. McBride, G.M. Anderson, and T.A. Mieczkowski, Platelet and whole blood serotonin content in depressed patients: Correlations with acute and lifetime psychopathology. *Biol. Psychiatry 32*:243 (1992).
77. S.R. Pliszka, G.A. Rogeness, P. Renner, J. Sherman, and T. Broussard, Plasma neurochemistry in juvenile offenders. *J. Am. Acad. Child Adolesc. Psychiatry 27*:588 (1988).
78. L.J. Siever and R.L. Trestman, The serotonin system and aggressive personality disorder, *Int. Clin. Psychopharmacol. 8*:33 (1993).

79. L. Lidberg, I. Modin, and L. Oreland, Platelet monoamine oxidase and psychopathy, *Psychiatry Res. 16*:22 (1985).
80. D. Schalling, M. Asberg, and G. Adman, Markers for vulnerability to psychopathology: Temperament traits associated with platelet MAO activity, *Acta Psychiatr. Scand. 76*:172 (1987).
81. M.S. Briley, R. Raisman, and S.Z. Langer, Human platelets possess high-affinity binding sites for 3H-imipramine, *Eur. J. Pharmacol. 58*:347 (1979).
82. Y. Sarne, J. Mandel, M.H. Goncalves, S. Brook, M. Gafni, A. Elizur, Inipramine binding to blood platelets and aggressive behavior in offenders, schizophrenics and normal volunteers, *Neuropsychobiology 31*:120 (1995).
83. M.F. Muldoon, S.B. Manuck, and K.A. Matthews. Lowering cholesterol concentrations and mortality: a quantitative review of primary prevention trials, *Br. Med J. 301*:309 (1990).
84. M.F. Muldoon, S.B. Manuck, and K.A. Matthews, Does cholesterol lowering increase non-illness-related mortality? *Arch. Intern. Med. 151*:1453 (1991).
85. J.M. Santiago and J.E. Galen, Cholesterol and violent behavior, *Arch. Intern. Med. 154*:1317 (1994).
86. M. Virkkunen, Serum cholesterol in antisocial personality, *Neuropsychobiology 10*:65 (1983).
87. M. Virkkunen, Lipid research clinics primary prevention trial results, *J.A.M.A. 253*:635 (1985).
88. J. Pekkanen, A. Nissinen, S. Punsar, and M.J. Karvonen, Serum cholesterol and risk of accidental or violent death in a 25-year follow-up: Finnish cohorts of the Seven Countries Study, *Arch. Intern. Med. 149*:1589 (1989).
89. D.K. Wysowski and T.P. Gross, Deaths due to accidents and violence in two recent trials of cholesterol-lowering drugs, *Arch. Intern. Med. 150*:2169 (1990).
90. C.D. McGee and C.E. Greenwood, Effects of dietary fatty acid composition on macronutrient selection and synaptosomal fatty acid composition in rats, *J. Nutr. 119*:1561 (1989).
91. M.F. Muldoon, J.R. Kaplan, S.B. Manuck, and J.J. Mann, Effects of a low-fat diet on brain serotonergic responsivity in cynomolgus monkeys, *Biol. Psychiatry 31*:739 (1992).
92. J.R. Kaplan, C.A. Shiveli, B. Fontenot, T.M. Morgan, S.M. Howell, S.B. Manuck, M.F. Muldoon, and J.J. Mann, Demonstration of an association among dietary cholesterol, central serotonergic activity, and social behavior in monkeys, *Psychosom. Med. 56*:479 (1994).
93. J.A. Golier, P.M. Marzuk, A.C. Leon, C. Weiner, and K. Tardiff, Low serum cholesterol level and attempted suicide, *Am. J. Psychiatry 152*:419 (1995).
94. D.L. Murphy, E.A. Mueller, N.A. Garrick, and C.S. Aulakh, Use of sertonergic agents in the clinical assessment of central serotonin function, *J. Clin. Psychiatry 47*:9 (1986).
95. S.L. Brown, S. Wetzler, and H.M. van Praag, Serotonin receptor dysfunction and violence, Unpublished manuscript, Albert Einstein College of Medicine, New York, 1993.

96. L.D. van der Kar, Neurendocrine aspects of the serotonergic hypothesis of depression, *Neurosci. Biobehav. Rev. 13*:237 (1989).
97. H.Y. Meltzer, R. Perline, B.J. Tricou, M.T. Lowy, and A. Robertson, Effect of 5-hydroxyptryptophan on serum cortisol levels in major affective disorders: II. Relation to suicide, psychosis, and depressive symptoms, *Arch. Gen. Psychiatry 41*:379 (1984).
98. A. Quattrone, G. Tedeschi, and F. Aguglia, Prolactin secretion in man: A useful tool to evaluate the activity of drugs on central 5-hydroxytryptaminergic neurones: Studies with fenfluramine, *Br. J. Clin. Pharmacol. 16*:471 (1983).
99. C. Barbieri, V. Magnoni, and W.G. Rauhe, Effect of fenfluramine on prolactin secretion in obese patients: Evidence for serotonergic regulation of prolactin in man, *Clin. Endocrinol. 19*:705 (1983).
100. D.A. Lewis and B.M. Sherman, Serotonergic regulation of prolactin and growth hormone secretion in man, *Acta Endocrinol. 110*:152 (1985).
101. D.H. Fishbein, D. Lozovsky, and J.H. Jaffe, Impulsivity, aggression and neuroendocrine responses to serotonergic stimulation in substance abusers, *Biol. Psychiatry 25*:1049 (1989).
102. G. Gerra, G. Fertonani, P. Tagliavini, A. Zaimovic, R. Delsignore, D. Maestri, P. Avanzini, R. Caccavari, and F. Brambilla, Serotonin function in detoxified heroin abusers: Prolactin and cortisol responses to fenfluramine challenge, *Psychiatry Res. 58*:153 (1995).
103. E.F. Coccaro, L.J. Siever, H.M. Klar, G. Maurer, K. Cochrane, T.B. Cooper, R.C. Mohs, and K.L. Davis, Serotonergic studies in patients with affective and personality disorders: Correlates with suicidal and impulsive aggressive behavior, *Arch. Gen. Psychiatry 46*:587 (1989).
104. V. O'Keane, E. Moloney, H. O'Neill, A. O'Connor, C. Smith, and T.G. Dinan, Blunted prolactin responses to D-fenfluramine in sociopathy, *Br. J. Psychiatry 160*:643 (1992).
105. L.J. Siever, D.A. Murphy, and S. Slater, Plasma prolactin changes following fenfluramine in depressed patients compared to controls: An evaluation of central serotonergic responsivity in depression, *Life Sci. 34*:1029 (1984).
106. D.M. Stoff, A.P. Pasatiempo, J. Yeung, T.B. Cooper, W.H. Bridger, and H. Rabinovich, Neuroendocrine responses to challenge with DL-fenfluramine and aggression in disruptive behavior disorders of children and adolescents, *Psychiatry Res. 231*:480 (1992).
107. F.G. Moeller, J.L. Steinberg, F. Petty, M. Fulton, D.R. Cherek, G. Kramer, and D.L. Garver, Serotonin and impulsive/aggressive behavior in cocaine dependent subjects, *Prog. Neuro-Psychopharmacol. Biol. Psychiatry 18*:1027 (1994).
108. E.F. Coccaro, Impulsive aggressive and central serotonergic system function in humans: an example of a dimensional brain behavior relationship, *Int. Clin. Psychopharmacol. 7*:3 (1992).
109. H.M. van Praag, R.S. Kahn, G.M. Asnis, S. Wetzler, S.L. Brown, A. Bleich, and M.L. Korn, Denosologization of biological psychiatry or the specificity of 5-HT disturbances in psychiatric disorders, *J. Affect. Disord. 13*:1 (1987).
110. M.A. Sills, B.A. Wolfe, and A. Frazer, Determination of selective and nonselec-

tive compounds for the 5-HT1A and 5-HT1B receptor subtypes in rat frontal cortex, *J. Pharmacol. Exp. Ther. 231*:480 (1984).
111. G.J. Kilpatrick, B.J. Jones, and M.B. Tyers, Identification and distribution of 5-HT3 receptors in rat brain using radioligand binding, *Nature, 330*:746 (1987).
112. J. Tuomisto and A. Manisto, Neurotransmitter regulation of anterior pituitary hormones, *Pharmacol. Rev. 37*:249 (1985).
113. A. Hamik and S.J. Peroutka, 1-(m-Chlorophenyl) piperazine (mCPP) interactions with neurotransmitter receptors in human brain, *Biol. Psychiatry 25*:569 (1989).
114. R. Invernizzi, S. Cotecchia, A. Deblaise, A. DeBlasi, T. Mennini, R. Pataccini, and R. Samanin, Effects of MCPP on receptor binding and brain metabolism of monoamines in rats, *Neurochem. Int. 3*:239 (1981).
115. R.W. Fuller, H.D. Snoddy, N.R. Mason, and J.E. Owen, Disposition and pharmacological effects of MCPP, *Neuropharmacology 20*:155 (1981).
116. A. Quattrone, G. Schettini, L. Annunziato, and G. Di Renzo, Pharmacological evidence of supersensitivity of central serotonergic receptors involved in the control of prolactin secretion, *Eur. J. Pharmacol. 76*:9 (1981).
117. J.A. Aloi, T.R. Insel, E.A. Mueller, and D.L. Murphy DL, Neuroendocrine and behavioral effects of m-chlorophenylpiperazine administration in rhesus monkeys, *Life Sci. 34*:1325 (1984).
118. R.S. Kahn, S. Wetzler, G.M. Asnis, R.F. Suckow, and H.M. van Praag, The effects of *m*-chlorophenylpiperazine in normal subjects: A dose response study, *Psychopharmacology 100*:339 (1990).
119. E.A. Mueller, D.L. Murphy, and T. Sunderland, Further studies of the putative serotonin agonist, MCPP: Evidence for a serotonin receptor mediated mechanism of action in humans, *Psychopharmacology 89*:388 (1986).
120. C.S. Aulak, R.M. Cohen, J.L. Hill, D.L. Murphy, and J. Zohar, Long-term imipramine treatment enhances locomotor and food intake suppressant effects of MCPP in rats, *Br. J. Pharmacol. 91*:747 (1987).
121. R. Samanin, T. Mennini, A. Ferraris, C. Bendotti, and F. Borsini, Hyper- and hyposensitivity of central serotonin receptors: (3H)serotonin binding and functional studies in the rat, *Brain Res. 189*:449 (1980).
122. H.B. Moss, J.K. Yao, and G.L. Panzak, Serotonergic responsivity and behavioral dimensions in antisocial personality disorder with substance abuse. *Biol. Psychiatry 28*:325 (1990).
123. T.R. Insel, Neurobiology of obsessive-compulsive disorder: A review, *Int. Clin. Psychopharmacol. 7*(1):31 (1992).
124. J. Zohar, T.R. Insel, R.C. Zohar-Zadouch, J.L. Hill, and D.L. Murphy, Serotonergic responsivity in obsessive-compulsive disorder: Effects of chronic clomipramine treatment, *Arch. Gen. Psychiatry 45*:167 (1988).
125. J.J. Lopez-Ibor, Serotonin and psychiatric disorders, *Int. Clin. Psychopharmacol. 7*:5 (1992).
126. S. Wetzler, R.S. Kahn, G.M. Asnis, M. Korn, and H.M. van Praag, Serotonin receptor sensitivity and aggression, *Psychiatry Res. 37*:271 (1991).
127. J.M. Stolk, R.L. Conner, S. Levine, and J.D. Barchas, Brain norepinephrine metabolism and shock-induced fighting behavior in rats: Differential effects of shock

and fighting on the neurochemical response to a common footshock stimulus, *J. Pharmacol. Exp. Ther. 190*:193 (1974).
128. D.J. Reis, The relationship between brain norepinephrine and aggressive behavior, *Res. Pub. Assoc. for Res. Nerv. Ment. Dis. 50*:266 (1972).
129. B. Eichelman and J.D. Barchas, Facilitated shock-induced aggression following antidepressant medication in the rat, *Pharmacol. Biochem. Behav. 3*:601 (1975).
130. K. Matsumoto, K. Ojima, and H. Watanabe, Noradrenergic denervation attenuates desipramine enhancement of aggressive behavior in isolated mice, *Pharmacol. Biochem. Behav. 50*:481 (1995).
131. B. Eichelman, N.B. Thoa, and J. Perez-Cruet, Alkali metal cations: Effects on aggression and adrenal enzymes, *Pharmacol. Biochem. Behav. 1*:121 (1973).
132. J.M. Stolk, W.J. Nowack, J.D. Barchas, and S.R. Platman, Brain norepinephrine: Enhanced turnover after rubidium treatment, *Science. 168*:501 (1970).
133. M.H. Sheard, The role of drugs affecting catecholamines on shock-elicited fighting in rats, *Catecholamines: Basic and Clinical Frontiers* (E. Usdin, ed.), Pergamon Press, New York, 1979, pp. 1690–1692.
134. L.R. Hegstrand and B. Eichelman, Increased shock-induced fighting with supersensitive B-adrenergic receptors, *Pharm. Biochem. Behav. 19*:313 (1983).
135. M.L. Leavitt, S.C. Yudofsky, J.C. Maroon, E.J. Riley, and M.B. Bavitz, Effect of intraventricular nadolol infusion on shockinduced aggression in 6-hydroxydopamine-treated rats, *J. Neuropsychiatry 1*:167 (1989).
136. B. Eichelman, Neurochemical and psychopharmacologic aspects of aggressive behavior, *Annu. Rev. Med. 41*:149 (1990).
137. G. Aston-Jones and F.E. Bloom, Norepinephrine-containing locus coeruleus neurons in behaving rats exhibit pronounced responses to non-noxious environmental stimuli, *J. Neurosci. 1*:887 (1991).
138. D.E. Redmond Jr, M.M. Katz, J.W. Maas, A. Swann, R. Casper, and J.M. Davis, Cerebrospinal fluid amine metabolites, *Arch. Gen. Psychiatry 43*:938 (1986).
139. G. Edman, M. Asberg, S. Levander, and D. Schalling, Skin conductance habituation and cerebrospinal fluid 5-hydroxyindoleacetic acid in suicidal patients, *Arch. Gen. Psychiatry 43*:586 (1986).
140. D. Lester, Biochemical correlates of suicidal behavior in arsonists. *Psychol. Rep. 64*:258 (1989).
141. A. Roy, P. Ninan, A Mazonson, D. Pickar, D. Van Kammen, M. Linnoila, and S.M. Paul, CSF monoamine metabolites in chronic schizophrenic patients who attempt suicide, *Psychol. Med. 15*:335 (1985).
142. J.D. Higley, P.T. Mehlman, D.M. Taub, S.B. Higley, S.J. Suomi, M. Linnoila, and J. Vickers, Cerebrospinal fluid monoamine and adrenal correlates of aggression in free-ranging rhesus monkeys, *Arch. Gen. Psychiatry 49*:436 (1992).
143. K.A. Miczek and P. Donat, Brain 5-HT system and inhibition of aggressive behavior, *Behavioral Pharmacology of 5-HT* (T. Archer, P. Bevan, and A. Cools, eds.), Lawrence Erlbaum, Hillsdale, NJ, 1990, pp. 117–144.
144. R.W. Cowdry, and D.L. Gardner, Pharmacotherapy of borderline personality disorder, *Arch. Gen. Psychiatry 45*:111 (1988).

145. L.A. Gottschalk, G.C. Gleser, and H.W. Wylie Jr, Effects of imipramine on anxiety and hostility levels, *Psychopharmacologia (Berlin) 7*:303 (1965).
146. D. Rampling, Aggression: A paradoxical response to tricyclic antidepressants, *Am. J. Psychiatry 135*:117 (1978).
147. P.H. Soloff, A. George, R.S. Nathan, P.M. Schulz, and J.M. Perel, Paradoxical effects of amitriptyline on borderline patients, *Am. J. Psychiatry 143*:1603 (1986).
148. F.A. Elliott, Propranolol for the control of belligerent behavior following acute brain damage, *Ann. Neurol. 1*:489 (1977).
149. J. Ratey, P. Sorgi, G.A. O'Driscoll, S. Sands, M.L. Daehler, J.R. Fletcher, W. Kadish, G. Spruiell, S. Polakoff, K.J. Lindem, J.R. Bemporad, L. Richardson, and B. Rosenfeld, Nadolol to treat aggression and psychiatric symptomatology in chronic psychiatric inpatients: A double-blind, placebo-controlled study, *J. Clin. Psychiatry 53*:41 (1992).
150. J.M. Silver, and S.C. Yudofsky, Propranolol in the treatment of chronically hospitalized violent patients, *Biological Psychiatry* (C. Shagass, R.C. Josiassen, W.H. Bridger, K.J. Weiss, D. Stoff, and G.M. Simpson, eds.), Elsevier Science Publishing Co., Amsterdam, 1986, pp. 174–176.
151. P.J. Sorgi, J.J. Ratey, and s. Polakoff, B-adrenergic blockers for the control of aggressive behaviors in patients with chronic schizophrenia, *Am. J. Psychiatry 143*:775 (1986).
152. E. Eichelman, Neurochemical and psychopharmacologic aspects of aggressive behavior, *Psychopharmacology: The Third Generation of Progress* (H.Y. Meltzer, ed.), Raven Press, New York, 1987, pp. 697–704.
153. M.H. Sheard, J.L. Marini, C.I. Bridges, and E. Wagner, The effect of lithium on impulsive aggressive behavior in man, *Am. J. Psychiatry 133*:1409 (1976).
154. F. Brambilla, M. Lampertico, A.E. Panerai, L. Sali, F. Salerno, and E.E. Muller, Effect of clonidine on the secretion of anterior pituitary hormones in heroin addicts and normal volunteers, *Psychiatr. Res. 13*:295 (1984).
155. K.S. Estes, J.W. Simpkins, and S.P. Kalra, Resumption with clonidine of pulsative LH release following acute norepinephrine depletion in ovarectomized rats, *Neuroendocrinology 35*:56 (1982).
156. E.E. Muller, G. Nistico, and U. Scapagnini, *Brain Neurotransmitters and Anterior Pituitary Function*, Academic Press, New York, 1978.
157. E. Eriksson, S. Eden, and K. Modigh, Up- and down-regulation of central postsynaptic alpha-2-receptors reflected in the growth hormone response to clonidine in reserpine pretreated rats, *Psychopharmacology 77*:327 (1982).
158. J.R. McWilliam and B.S. Meldrum, Noradrenergic regulation of growth hormone secretion in the baboon. *Endocrinology 112*:254 (1983).
159. E.F. Coccaro, T. Lawrence, R. Trestman, S. Gabriel, H.M. Klar, and L.J. Siever, Growth hormone responses to intravenous clonidine challenge correlate with behavioral irritability in psychiatric patients and healthy volunteers, *Psychiatry Res. 39*:129 (1991).
160. M.A. Geyer, and D.S. Segal, Shock-induced aggression: Opposite effects of intraventricularly infused dopamine and norepinephrine, *Behav. Biol. 10*:99 (1974).
161. A.J.J.C. Lammers, and J. Van Rossum, Bizarre social behaviour in rats induced

by a combination of a peripheral decarboxylase inhibitor and DOPA. *Eur. J. Pharmacol. 5*:103 (1968).

162. K.P. Datla, A.P. Sen, and S.K. Bhattacharya, Dopaminergic modulation of footshock induced aggression in paired rats, *Indian J. Exp. Biol. 30*:587 (1992).
163. K.A. Miczek, Differential antagonism of d-amphetamine effects on motor activity and agonistic behavior in mice, *Neurosci. Abstr. 7*:343 (1981).
164. K.A. Miczek, E. Weerts, M. Haney, and J. Tidey, Neurobiological mechanisms controlling aggression: Preclinical developments for pharmacotherapeutic interventions, *Neurosci. Biobehav. Rev. 18*:97 (1994).
165. C.M. Banki, M. Arato, Z. Papp, and M. Kurcz, Biochemical markers in suicidal patients: Investigations with cerebrospinal fluid amine metabolites and neuroendocrine tests, *J. Affect. Disord. 6*:341 (1984).
166. C.M. Banki, M. Arato, and C. Kilts, Aminergic studies and cerebrospinal fluid cations in suicide, *Ann. N.Y. Acad. Sci. 487*:221 (1986).
167. C.J. Earley and B.E. Leonard, The effect of testosterone and cyproterone acetate on the concentration of gamma-aminobutyric acid in brain areas of aggressive and non-aggressive mice, *Pharmacol Biochm. Behav. 6*:409 (1977).
168. P. Mandel, G. Mack, and E. Kempf, Molecular aspects of a model of aggressive behavior, *Interactions Between Putative Neurotransmitters in the Brain* (J.F. Pujol and R. Samanin, eds.), Raven Press, New York, 1968, pp. 285–303.
169. S. Puglisi-Allegra and P. Mandel, Effects of sodium dipropyl-acetate, muscimol hydrobromide and nipecotic acid amide on isolation-induced aggressive behavior in mice, *Psychopharmacology 70*:287 (1980).
170. S. Puglisi-Allegra, S. Simler, E. Kempf, and P. Mandel, Involvement of the GABAergic system on shock-induced aggressive behavior in two strains of mice, *Pharmacol. Biochem. Behav. 14*:13 (1981).
171. J.P. Da Vanzo and M. Sydow, Inhibition of isolation-induced aggressive behavior with GABA-transaminase inhibitors, *Psychopharmacology 62*:23 (1979).
172. K.A. Fox, J.R. Tuckosh, and A.A. Wilcox, Increased aggression among grouped male mice fed chlordiazepoxide, *Eur. J. Pharmacol. 5*:119 (1970).
173. K.A. Miczek, Alcohol and aggressive behavior in rats: Interaction with benzodiazepines, *Soc. Neurosci. Abstr. 11*:1290 (1985).
174. J. Mos, B. Olivier, and A.M. Van der Poel, Modulatory actions of benzodiazepine receptor ligans on agonistic behaviour, *Physiol. Behav. 41*:265 (1987).
175. C.L. Azcarate, Minor tranquilizers in the treatment of aggression, *J. Nerv. Ment. Dis. 160*:100 (1975).
176. A. DiMascio, The effects of benzodiazepines on aggression: Reduced or increased? *Psychopharamcologia 30*:95 (1973).
177. R.J. Rodgers and A.J. Waters, Benzodiazepines and their antagonists: A pharmacoethological analysis with particular reference to effects on "aggression," *Neurosci. Biobehav. Rev. 9*:21 (1985).
178. E.B. Gordon, Tranquilizers causing aggression, *Br. Med. J. 2*:36 (1975).
179. K. Rickels and R.W. Downing, Chlordiazepoxide and hostility in anxious outpatients, *Am. J. Psychiatry 131*:442 (1974).

180. R.J. Rodgers and K. Brown, Amygdaloid function in the central cholinergic mediation of shock-induced aggression in the rat, *Aggress. Behav.* *2*:131 (1976).
181. A. Siegel and K. Schubert, Neurotransmitters regulating feline aggressive behavior, *Rev. Neurosci.* *6*:47 (1995).
182. G.K. Hodge and L.L. Butcher, Catecholamine correlates of isolation-induced aggression in mice, *Eur. J. Pharmacol.* *31*:81 (1975).
183. E.F. Coccaro, R.J. Kavoussi, and J.C. Lesser JC, Self- and other-directed human aggression: The role of the central serotonergic system, *Int. Clin. Psychopharmacol.* *6*(suppl):70 (1992).
184. E. Hollander, D.J. Stein, C.M. Decaria, L. Cohen, M. Islam, and M. Frenkel, Disorders related to OCD neurobiology, *Clin. Neuropharmacol.* *15*(suppl 1):259A (1992).
185. M.R. Spoont, Modulatory role of serotonin in neural information processing: Implications for human psychopathology, *Psychol. Bull.* *112*:330 (1992).
186. D.W. Costain and A.R. Green, B-adrenoceptor antagonists inhibit the behavioural responses of rats to increased brain 5-hydroxytryptamine, *Br. J. Pharmacol.* *64*:193 (1978).
187. M. Weinstock, C. Weiss, and S. Gitter, Blockade of 5-hydroxytryptamine receptors in the central nervous system by B-adrenoceptor antagonists, *Neuropharmacology* *16*:273 (1977).
188. A.R. Green, and D.G. Grahame-Smith, The role of brain dopamine in the hyperactivity syndrome produced by increased 5-hydroxy-tryptamine synthesis in rats, *Neuropharmacology* *13*:949 (1974).
189. M. Virkkunen, and M. Linnoila, Brain serotonin, type II alcoholism and impulsive violence, *J. Stud. Alcohol* *11*:163 (1993).
190. M. Virkkunen, D. Goldman, D.A. Nielsen, and M. Linnoila, Low brain serotonin turnover rate (low CSF 5-HIAA) and impulsive violence, *J. Psychiatry Neurosci.* *20*:271 (1995).
191. F. Saudou, D.A. Amara, A. Dierich, M. LeMeur, S. Ramboz, L. Segu, M.C. Buhot, and R. Hen, Enhanced aggressive behavior in mice lacking 5-HT1B receptor, *Science* *265*:1875 (1994).
192. P.L. Roubertoux, M. Carlier, G. Degrelle, M.C. Haas-Dupertuis, J. Phillips, and R. Moutier, Co-segregation of intermale aggression with the pseudoautosomal region of the Y chromosome in mice, *Genetics* *136*:225 (1994).
193. H.G. Brunner M.R. Nelen, P. van Zandvoort, N.G.G.M. Abeling, A.H. van Gennip, E.C. Wolters, M.A. Kuiper, H.H. Ropers, and B.A. van Oost, X-linked borderline mental retardation with prominant behavioral disturbance: Phenotype, genetic localization, and evidence for disturbed monoamine metabolism, *Am. J. Hum. Genet.* *52*:1032 (1993).
194. O. Cases, I. Seif, J. Grimsby, P. Gaspar, K. Chen, S. Pournin, U. Muller, M. Aguet, C. Babinet, J.C. Shih, and E. De Maeyer, Aggressive behavior and altered amounts of brain serotonin and norepinephrine in mice lacking MAOA, *Science* *268*:1763 (1995).

4

Neurological and Medical Diseases and Violence

Karen E. Anderson and Jonathan M. Silver
Columbia University College of Physicians and Surgeons, New York, New York

I. INTRODUCTION

Explosive and violent behavior has long been associated with focal brain lesions as well as with diffuse damage to the central nervous system (CNS). Among patients who suffer brain injury, irritability and aggressiveness are a major source of disability to themselves and of stress to their families. This aggressive behavior often has typical characteristics, which contrast to the violent acts of individuals with personality disorders (Table 1).

Studies of aggression often vary greatly in the reported frequency of this behavior in various populations. Several factors may influence these findings. Definitions may differ as to requirements of frequency or severity for inclusion in criteria of aggression. Some studied separate self-injurious behavior from aggression. Also, in studies of aggression, cutoff rates vary for inclusion of behavior such as damage to property or injury to others. In addition, there are different rates of aggression for inpatient and outpatient populations.

In this chapter, we discuss common neurological and medical etiologies of aggressive behavior. When possible, we focus on studies that use standardized rating scales and well-defined samples. However, some of these disorders are uncommon, and in these instances, case studies are the chief source of information.

Table 1 Characteristic Features of Organic Aggression Syndrome

Reactive:	Triggered by modest or trivial stimuli
Nonreflective:	Usually does not involve premeditation or planning
Nonpurposeful:	Aggressive serves no obvious long-term aims or goals
Explosive:	Buildup is *not* gradual
Periodic:	Brief outbursts of rage and aggression punctuated by long periods of relative calm
Ego-dystonic:	After outbursts, patients are upset, concerned, embarrassed as opposed to blaming others or justifying behavior

Source: Reprinted from Yudofsky SC, Silver JM, Hales RE: Pharmacologic management of aggression in the elderly. *J. Clin. Psychiatry* 51(10,suppl):22 (1990). Copyright 1990, Physicians Postgraduate Press. Used with permission.

II. DEMENTIA

Behavioral disturbances are common in individuals with dementia. Up to 70 to 90% of patients with Alzheimer's disease have some form of emotional or behavioral problem (1–3). Rabins and coworkers' (4) survey of family and primary caregivers found that the most serious problem was aggressive behavior. Families are able to tolerate forgetfulness in their relative, it is more difficult to manage the sudden episodes of anger.

Aggressive behavior is one of the main factors leading to the placement of a demented person in a nursing home. Haupt and Kurtz (5) studied 66 outpatients who had Alzheimer's disease with mild to moderate dementia. Patients were examined twice over a 12-month interval. One-third of the patients were admitted to nursing homes during these 12 months. Of the seven variables that could be used to predict nursing home placement, aggression was the fifth most powerful. O'Donnell and coworkers (6) also found that aggression was an important factor leading to institutionalization. They studied 143 outpatients with dementia due to various causes, including Alzheimer's disease, multi-infarct dementia, and Parkinson's disease. Most patients were suffering from moderate to severe impairment of activities of daily living (ADLs). Incontinence and aggression were found to have a significant interaction in predicting institutionalization. After 1 year, 8% of patients who were neither incontinent nor aggressive were institutionalized. In the same year, 12% of patients who were either incontinent or aggressive were institutionalized. However, 62% of patients who were both incontinent and aggressive had been institutionalized. The authors conclude that either of these two disorders may be tolerated individually by caregivers, but that the combination of incontinence and aggression becomes overwhelming to them.

Hamel and others (7) studied predictors of aggression in patients and the reaction of caregivers to aggression in demented outpatients. They studied 213 demented patients and their caregivers. Demented patients were moderately impaired according to the Hierarchic Dementia Scale (8). Ryden's Aggression Scale was used to assess patients' behavioral disturbances (9,10). Aggression was reported in 57.2% of patients, with verbal aggression as the most common form, occurring in 51% of cases. Physical aggression, including threatening gestures, was reported in 34.1% of patients. Aggression most often occurred in a situation in which a patient was instructed to "do something." A history of aggressive personality traits predicted aggression in patients with dementia. This finding is in agreement with earlier studies by Ryden (10), Morrant and Ablog (11), and Post (12). However, the level of cognitive deterioration did not predict aggression, as we found earlier by Ryden (10). Troubled premorbid relationship between patient and caregiver also predicted aggressive behavior. Aggression was also noted by caregivers as influencing whether they would decide to institutionalize patients, although other factors, such as medical illness, were also important.

In a study of agitation and cognitive impairment in nursing home residents, Cohen-Mansfield (13) studied 408 residents of a large suburban nursing home. Agitation was rated using the Cohen-Mansfield Agitation Inventory (14). Dementia was assessed using the Brief Cognitive Rating Scale (15) in a modified version. Impairment of ADLs and cognitive impairment were associated with increased aggression. Aggressive behavior was associated with the individual being a married man, having poor current social interactions, to being more likely to fall, and to exhibiting more aggressive behavior before admission to the nursing home.

Patel and Hope (16) monitored levels of aggressive behavior in 90 inpatients at a long-stay psychogeriatric unit. Dementia was the primary diagnosis in 71% of patients. Prevalence of aggressive behavior was rated in each patient over a 3-day period. During this period, 45% of the patients in the study were rated as having been aggressive. When severity of aggression was examined, 11% were moderately aggressive and 4% were severely aggressive. The remainder were rated as mildly aggressive. Most types of aggressive behavior were observed at least once over a 3-day period in over 10% of subjects. Verbal aggression was the most common and sexually offensive behavior was the least commonly observed aggressive behavior. When patients were compared as to diagnosis and incidence of aggression, those with dementia had a significantly higher level of aggression. Most of the aggressive behavior was directed at staff and often occurred consistently around morning assistance with ADLs.

A. Aggression in Specific Dementing Illnesses

Several predictors of aggressive and violent behavior have been found in Alzheimer's disease. Devanand and others (17) looked at behavioral disturbances in 106 outpatients with probable Alzheimer's disease, using the Behavioral Syndromes Scale for Dementia. Aggression and agitation, as measured by this scale, were associated with greater functional impairment, but did not correlate with severity of cognitive decline. Deutsch and Bylsma (18) found that psychotic symptoms were a predictor of aggressive behavior in Alzheimer's patients. Charts of 181 clinic patients with probable Alzheimer's disease were reviewed. Patients were rated using a modified version of the Present State Examination (19) and the Scale of Psychosis in Alzheimer's Disease (20). Delusions and misidentifications (e.g., inability to recognize themselves in a mirror or believing that someone else was living in the house) were both associated with an aggressive episode in approximately 90% of cases. The prevalence of delusions and misindentifications was significantly higher in the physically aggressive group. Occurrence of hallucinations approached significance in the aggressive patients. Lopez and coworkers (21) found in a study of 17 Alzheimer's patients that those with delusions and hallucinations had a significantly higher incidence of aggressive behavior than those who did not have any psychotic symptoms. Aggression and hostility were associated with more rapid cognitive decline. In a recent multicenter study of 235 outpatients with Alzheimer's disease, Devanand and others (22) found physical aggression to be an uncommon symptom of Alzheimer's disease, persisting in only 2.8% of the sample for over 2 years. However, if physical aggression was reported at one visit, there was an over 50% probability that it would be reported by a caretaker at the next visit. The authors conclude that physical aggression may become a more persistent problem at later stages of Alzheimer's disease, since the patients became more demented as the study progressed.

Imaging studies have revealed correlations among structural and functional deficits and aggression. Burns and others (23) studied 178 patients with Alzheimer's disease. A correlation was found between atrophy of the temporal lobes on computed tomography and aggression. Wandering and aggression together were significantly associated with cognitive impairment. A positron emission tomography (PET) study by Sultzer and coworkers (24) of 21 Alzheimer's patients (16 outpatients, 5 inpatients) found that agitation/disinhibition, as rated on the Neurobehavioral Rating Scale (25), was correlated with frontal and temporal hypometabolism. Agitation/disinhibition was significantly correlated with global hypometabolism.

Behavioral disturbances in a subcortical dementia (Huntington's disease) and a cortical dementia (Alzheimer's disease) were compared in another study (26). Aggression was assessed using the Overt Aggression Scale (27). A total of 31 patients with Alzheimer's disease and 26 with Huntington's were studied. While apathy scores did not differ for the two groups, the Huntington's patients were significantly more aggressive than the Alzheimer's group, with 59% of the Huntington's group meeting the cutoff score for aggression, while only 32% of the Alzheimer's group met the criteria. Individual aggressive outbursts were also more severe in the Huntington's group. There was no interrelation between apathy, aggression, or irritability. The authors suggest that damage to deep subcortical structures such as the hypothalamus and limbic system may result in behavioral dyscontrol of aggression.

Victoroff and colleagues (28) performed a neuropathological investigation of individuals with Alzheimer's disease to determine correlates of agitation and physical aggression. For those patients with Alzheimer's disease who had "histories of unequivocal interpersonal violence," there was preservation of the pigmented substantia nigra neurons. This may be associated with relatively greater influence of dopamine. Changes in multiple neurotransmitter systems, including serotonin and norepinephrine, may play a role in the development of aggressive behavior in patients with Alzheimer's (29).

III. TRAUMATIC BRAIN INJURY

Aggression and agitation commonly occur after traumatic brain injury (TBI) (30). These behaviors, which occur during the acute stages of recovery from brain injury, can endanger the safety of patients and their caregivers. In the acute phase after brain injury, patients often experience a period of agitation and confusion that may last from days to months. Brooke and others (31) suggest that agitation usually appears in the first 2 weeks of hospitalization and resolves within 2 weeks. Restlessness may appear after 2 months and may persist for 4 to 6 weeks. Subsequently, patients may develop low frustration tolerance and explosive behavior that can be set off by minimal provocation or occur without warning. These episodes range in severity from irritability to outbursts that result in damage to property or assaults on others. In severe cases, affected individuals cannot remain in the community or with their families and are often referred to long-term psychiatric or neurobehavioral facilities (Table 2).

In the acute recovery period, 35 to 96% of patients are reported to have exhibited agitated behavior (32,33). After the acute recovery phase, irritability or bad temper is common. In a survey of individuals with TBI who were in skilled nursing facilities in Connecticut, Wolf and colleagues (34) found that agitation was present in 45% of 140 patients. There has only been one prospective study of the occurrence of agitation and restlessness that has been monitored by an objective rating instrument, the Overt Aggression Scale (31). These authors found that out of 100 patients with severe TBI (Glascow Coma Scale score less than 8, more than 1 hour of coma, and greater than 1 week of hospitalization), only 11 patients exhibited agitated behavior. Only 3 patients manifested these behaviors for more than 1 week. However, 35 patients were observed to be restless but not agitated. In follow-up periods ranging from 1 to 15 years after injury,

Table 2 Prevalence of Aggression After Traumatic Brain Injury

Authors	Severity	*N*	Follow-up	Irritability or temper	Agitation
Acute					
Levin and Grossman, 1978	All	62	Acute	–	35%
Rao et al., 1985	Severe	26	Acute	–	96%
Brooke et al., 1992	Severe	100	Acute	35% restless	11%
	Chronic				
Rao et al., 1985	Severe	–	Rehabilitation	–	42%
McKinlay et al., 1981	Severe	55	1 year	71%	67%
Brooks et al., 1986 (same pts as McKinlay)	Severe	42	5 years	64%	64%
Oddy et al., 1985	Severe	44	7 years	43%	31%
Thomsen, 1984	Severe	40	2–5 years	38%	–
Thomsen, 1984	Severe	–	10–15 years	48%	–
Van Zomeren and Van den Berg, 1985	Severe	57	2 years	39%	–
Levin et al., 1979	Severe	27	1 year	37%	–
McMill and Glucksman, 1987 (16% orthopedic controls)	Moderate	24	–	64%	–
Schoenhuber et al., 1978	Mild	–	1 year	54%	–
Dikmen et al., 1986	Mild	20	1 month and 1 year	70%	40% (control: 45% irrit, 30% temper NS)
Rutherford et al., 1979	Mild	131	1 year	5%	–

Source: From Silver JM and Yudofsky SC, *Aggressive Disorders, in Neuropsychiatry of Traumatic Brain Injury*, APPI, 1994.

these behaviors occur in 31 to 71% of patients who experienced severe TBI. Studies of mild TBI have evaluated patients for much briefer periods of time; 1-year estimates from these studies range from 5 to 70%. Carlsson and colleagues (35) examined the relationship between the number of traumatic brain injuries associated with loss of consciousness (LOC) and various symptoms and demonstrated that irritability increases with subsequent injuries. Of those men who did not have head injuries with LOC, 21% reported irritability, while 31% of men with one injury with LOC and 33% of men with two or more injuries with LOC admitted to this symptom ($p = 0.0001$).

IV. CONGENITAL BRAIN DISORDERS AND DEVELOPMENTAL DISORDERS

People with intellectual deficiencies who engage in aggression toward others or self-injurious behavior are more likely to require intensive supervision and management (36,37). Aside from the severity of intellectual impairment, aggression is the most important reason why patients are institutionalized (38). The mounting costs of caring for such individuals makes improved understanding of such behavior a crucial concern.

A. Inpatient Populations

Several recent studies have reviewed rates of aggressive behavior among institutionalized people with intellectual disabilities. Linaker (39) compared 57 people in an institution who had shown violence in the preceding year with 57 people in the same institution who had now shown violence. The groups were matched for age, sex, and level of retardation. The aggressive residents had significantly more resources allocated to them and more space available per client on the wards. Communication skills and ability to care for themselves did not differ between the two groups. Neuroleptic drugs were given in a higher percent in the assaultive group, and a higher level of psychopathology was found in this group. The number of patients with specific organic brain disorders such as Down's syndrome or infantile autism did not differ significantly except that Down's syndrome tended to be more common in the control group.

Ghaziuddin and Ghaziuddin (40) studied violent behavior in intellectually impaired persons over 1 year at a 100-bed unit at a university hospital. Of the 106 patients admitted to the unit during the study, 35% were involved in 145 violent incidents. Twelve patients who had associated psychiatric diagnoses were responsible for 86% of the incidents. Fourteen of the aggressive patients had a seizure disorder.

Sigafoos and others (41) studied a population of 2412 people with intellectual disability in Queensland, Australia. Of the sample, 48% were severely to profoundly mentally retarded, while 24% were moderately impaired and 9.6% were mildly impaired. Most individuals (59%) were male, and 16% of this population lived in institutions. Aggressive behavior was rated by a questionnaire given to those who cared for the patients. Of the group living in institutions, 35% exhibited aggressive behavior. Of those living in group homes, 17% were aggressive. For the entire sample, hitting others with a closed or open hand was the most common aggressive behavior (68%), followed by pushing others (64%). Three or more forms of aggressive behavior were displayed by 80% of those who were violent (e.g., hitting others, kicking, verbal abuse, pinching others). Persons who were identified as aggressive had more profound levels of retardation and lower verbal abilities. Self-injurious behavior was less common than aggression toward others.

B. Outpatients

Bouras and Drummond (42) conducted a study in a community setting in Southeast London, England, of 318 (190 men, 128 women) with intellectual deficiencies who were referred to the psychiatry division of a mental handicap service. Most patients (54.4%) had mild mental handicap; 28.6% had moderate and 17% had severe mental handicap. The Behavior Problems Rating Scale was used to assess aggression. Almost one-third of the patients demonstrated aggression toward others, and 13.2% engaged in self-injurious behavior. Those people with severe intellectual impairment were more severely and frequently aggressive.

In the study noted above by Sigafoos and coworkers (41), aggressive behavior occurred in 17% of those in group homes and 3% of those in community-based facilities. Davidson (43) studied 199 individuals who were referred to an outpatient crisis intervention program over a 2½-year period. All people in the study had IQs below 70, concomitant adaptive behavior deficits, and at least one severe behavior disorder, and all had behavioral problems that were severe enough to threaten their ability to stay in an outpatient community setting. In this cohort, 59% were male. One-half lived with family members, 22% in community residences, and 9% in intermediate community-based facilities for intellectually disabled persons. The remainder of those studied were either in family care or living independently or semi-independently. Intake evaluations, historical data from agency records, and medical records were reviewed as a source of data on aggressive behavior. After the cohort was sorted by presence or absence of primary referral involving explosive or assaultive behavior toward property or other individuals, 131 individuals were classified as aggressive at the time of the study. This study found that aggressive and nonaggressive patients had similar neurological histories and medical status. Central nervous system disorders, including seizures, were seen with a similar prevalence in both groups. The authors concluded that current aggressive behavior was best predicted by past aggressive behavior when found in males with lower cognitive functioning who might have been previously institutionalized.

C. Developmental Disabilities and Concomitant Psychiatric Diagnosis

Rojahn and others (44) conducted an extensive study of the relationship between psychiatric disorders and behavioral problems in developmental disabilities. Statewide data bases from clinical service agencies for those with intellectual disability were examined in New York (n = 45,683 patients) and California (n = 89,419 patients). The Clinical Developmental Evaluation Report was used in the California group, while the Developmental Disabilities Information Survey was used in New York. In New York, 5.4% of this population had one or more psychiatric diagnoses, and 41.4% of all patients had severe behavior problems, including aggression. In California, 3.9% had at least one psychiatric diagnosis and 21.1% had sever behvior problems. The difference in rates of behavioral problems is attributed to the differing methods of reporting problem behavior used in the two states. The California sample had a much larger number of children than the New York sample. Also, in the California group, approximately 70% of the sample fell into the mild/moderate range, while only 54% fell into this range in New York. There was a low association between psychiatric diagnosis and aggressive behavior. The strongest associations for both states' samples were found between aggression and property destruction and between aggression and self-injurious behavior. The authors speculate that the low correlation between behavioral problems and psychiatric diagnoses may be partly due to the fact that patients with behavioral problems are referred to behavior specialists, who are less likely to diagnose psychiatric disorders. Conversely, more isolated patients may more often be referred to a psychiatrist for evaluation and diagnosis.

Bouras and Drummond (42), when evaluating patients in a community setting, noted that those with more severe mental handicaps tended to have more behavioral problems while those with higher abilities more often had a psychiatric diagnosis. While in those with more mental capability, psychiatric diagnoses will probably look the same as they do in the general population, in people with severe intellectual disabilities, a psychiatric diagnosis may present a behavioral problem and be diagnosed as such.

In a study of whether diagnosis of depression specifically correlates with increased aggression, Reiss and Rojahn (45) evaluated 528 adults, adolescents, and children with intellectual disabilities. All subjects in the study were rated using either the Reiss Screen for Maladaptive Behavior or the Reiss Scales for Children's Dual Diagnosis. Patients who met criteria for depression on one of these subscales had an associated fourfold increase in probability of an aggressive behavior. Consistent with the above findings, studies of prison inmates with intellectual disabilities suggest that they have a higher incidence of offenses such as fighting and destruction of property as compared with inmates without documented intellectual deficiencies (46,47).

V. EPILEPSY

Epilepsy has long been felt to be a cause of or at least a contributor to acts of violence. Echoing a common though untested belief of his day, Maudsley noted in 1873 (48) that "Whenever a murder has been committed suddenly, without premeditation, without malice, without motive, openly and in a way quite different from the way in which murders are commonly done, we ought to look carefully for epilepsy . . . ." There has been substantial use of the "epilepsy defense"—such persons claim that they are not guilty of certain crimes, usually violent in nature, because they were seizing or in a period of confusion following a seizure (i.e., "postictal confusion"). Going back as far as 1889, Treiman (49) found 75 cases in the United States, reviewed by state or federal courts, in which the "epilepsy defense" was used by offenders charged with the commission of violent crimes ranging from rape to murder. However, the defense was successful in only one case.

Estimates of interictal aggressive acts have varied from 5 to 50% among individuals with epilepsy (50–52). There are several possible explanations for this variability. Many studies of "general populations" of epileptics are performed at large teaching hospitals, where the patients who are referred are likely to have more severe disorders than those seen in a general population of people with epilepsy. Aggressive behavior can result from structural lesions that cause seizures. Medications used to treat epilepsy can alter mood and behavior. Lastly, many reports of violent behavior in persons with epilepsy are anecdotal and do not rely on standardized rating scales.

In analyzing the occurrence of aggressive behavior in individuals with epilepsy, it is important to note when the behavior occurred. Aggressive acts can be ictal (during a seizure), postictal (immediately after a seizure), or interictal (in the period between seizures).

A. Ictal Aggression

Ictal aggression occurs most often during attempts to assist or restrain a patient during a seizure (49). Resistive violence has also been observed in animal seizure models. Ictal aggression is rarely directed. Delgado-Escueta and colleagues (53) reported that on video-electroencephalographic (EEG) recordings of ictal behavior in 5400 patients, only 19 showed aggression. Only 1 of these 19 demonstrated actual aggression directed toward another person. The others yelled loudly, spat, or destroyed property.

B. Postictal Aggression

Postictal aggression involves violent acts that occur when a patient is still confused following a seizure. Postictal aggression is most commonly seen following a general tonic-clonic seizure and occurs less often following a complex partial seizure. Attempts at restraint are the most typical cause of aggression during this time. Postictal psychosis is another likely cause of aggression that occurs during this period, especially if the patient is experiencing frightening hallucinations or paranoia (54).

C. Interictal Aggression

The occurrence of aggressive behavior between seizures is more controversial than ictal or postictal aggression in that there is no direct relationship between the aggression and the seizure event. Most epileptologists agree that the majority of patients with epilepsy are psychologically normal between seizures. It is unclear whether a small subset of persons with epilepsy behave differently between seizures asa result of brain alterations caused by the ictal events. Devinsky and coworkers used the Buss-Durkee Hostility Inventory (54) to study 61 adult patients with epilepsy (46 patients with temporal lobe epilepsy, 15 with absence epilepsy) and compared this group with 17 neurologically and medically normal controls. This study found no pattern of aggressive or hostile behavior among persons with epilepsy. These data are in agreement with earlier studies that did not demonstrate an increase in aggressive behavior among persons with epilepsy (55). Mendez (56) examined 44 patients with epilepsy who were referred for psychiatric evaluation because of violence. They concluded that interictal violence was associated more with underlying psychopathology, such as schizophrenia or mental retardation, than with seizure activity.

D. Temporal Lobe Pathology

While studies that examine general populations of individuals with epilepsy do not find a significant correlation with aggressive behavior, there is a large body of literature linking the interictal behavior of individuals with temporal lobe epilepsy to aggression. This may be due to the association of the "limbic lobe" with emotion and aggression. Patients with temporal lobe epilepsy may exhibit emotional lability, impairment of impulse control, and suspiciousness (57). The study by Devinsky and others (54) did find increased suspiciousness in patients with left temporal lobe epilepsy and increased assaultive behavior in persons with bilateral temporal lobe epilepsy.

Herzberg and Fenwick (58) retrospectively reviewed the records of 31 subjects admitted to the Maudsley Hospital from 1974 to 1983 with temporal lobe epilepsy. Fourteen of the subjects were identified as aggressive, based on chart case notes, while the others were classified as nonaggressive. The charts were then rated for certain patient characteristics. It was found that male sex, early seizure onset, and a history of long-standing behavioral problems were associated with aggression. Aggression was not associated with history of psychosis. The authors note that patients seen at Madusley tend to be particularly disabled, both physically and socially. On the 5-point Gunn and Robertson forensic scale (59), most subjects rated as aggressive were minimally aggressive.

Devinsky (60) reviewed five cases of aggression in temporal lobe epilepsy. These patients' symptoms were quite variable, including paranoia, auditory hallucinations to kill others, violent thoughts, fights with others, and threats to kill authority figures. One female patient held a knife to her former psychotherapist's neck for 3 hours and then left to slash her own wrists. She later brought the therapist some of her own blood in a container as an apology. Devinsky suggests that a chronic alteration of the limbic system takes place, which allows emotional events to trigger aggression at a much lower threshold.

Tonkonogy (61) performed an imaging study in 23 inpatients with diagnoses of organic mental syndromes. Of the 23 patients, 14 had violent behavior observed by staff. Five of the violent patients had localized lesions in the anteroinferior temporal lobe on magnetic resonance imaging (MRI) or computed tomography (CT). However, while four of these patients had epileptic activity on the EEG, only one met criteria for temporal lobe epilepsy. The other three had generalized seizures. The author proposes that anterior temporal structures may regulate release of violent behaviors—i.e., the amygdala in one hemisphere may inhibit violent behaviors originating in the amygdala of the other hemisphere.

Stenves (62), in reviewing several large older studies of aggression in temporal lobe epilepsy, concluded that people with temporal lobe epilepsy are not, as a group, more violent than those with other forms of epilepsy. Damage or dysfunction in the limbic area, and not temporal lobe epilepsy per se, was the significant factor in predisposing to violent behavior (63). Therefore, these studies suggest that temporal lobe epilepsy may be related to aggression as a result of pathological abnormalities or dysfunction of the temporal lobe.

VI. ENCEPHALITIS

The influence of viral and other forms of encephalitis on behavior first came to notice during the pandemic of encephalitis lethargica during World War I. Also known as Von Economo's encephalitis, the illness was noted to produce a plethora of psychiatric symptoms, including behavioral changes such as aggression, in previously normal persons. Other forms of encephalitis, most notably herpes encephalitis, are now also known to result in aggressive behavior.

A. Encephalitis Lethargica

Encephalitis lethargica was first described in detail by Constantine von Economo in 1917 (64). The agent that causes encephalitis lethargica has not yet been isolated. Besides producing physical symptoms of an acute central nervous system infection, encephalitis lethargica can at times progress to coma or death. Survivors were sometimes afflicted with parkinsonism or with bizarre behavioral disturbances. Some survivors, who were mostly adolescents, suffered pseudopsychopathic states. In a review of early work on the illness, Hoening (65) notes that children who had been normal because uninhibited, damaging property and attacking strangers in the street. Few neurological abnormalities were seen in these cases. Sporadic cases of encephalitis lethargica are still seen throughout the world. Honig describes a patient hospitalized in the early 1980s, after what was presumably a viral illness, who had postencephalitis parkinsonism. The patient "was withdrawn, appeared depressed, was noncompliant with medications, and was occasionally agitated and combative, throwing things and kicking, hitting, and biting staff" (65). The patient, was also suicidal and, despite his severe disabilities, made several attempts to throw himself over a balcony. Later in his hospitalization, the patient became psychotic. His physical condition continued to deteriorate, and he often had choking attacks.

B. Herpes Simplex Encephalitis

The herpes simplex virus (HSV-1) can produce a severe form of encephalitis. It is probably the most common cause of nonepidemic encephalitis in temperate zones (66). Mortality rates are as high as 70%. However, with new antiviral treatments, many patients are living longer. These people often have severe neurological sequelae, including profound behavioral disturbances. For unclear reasons, the herpesvirus tends to destroy the temporal lobes specifically. This can produce a Klüver-Bucy syndrome, in which patients are hyperoral, hypersexual, and may have an abnormal desire to explore objects (hypermetamorphosis) (67,68).

While Klüver-Bucy syndrome generally produces passive behavior, some patients with temporal lobe damage due to encephalitis are aggressive (69). Probably because of the low incidence of herpes simplex encephalitis, the literature on aggressive behavior consists only of case reports. Greer and coworkers (70) describe a 14-year-old patient with bilateral damage to the temporal lobes (right worse than left as visualized on CT scan) due to herpes simplex viral encephalitis. The encephalitis was initially diagnosed when the patient was in second grade. Along with severe intellectual deficits, the patient also had severe, uncontrollable motor activity, including aggressive and self-injurious behavior. He eventually required placement in a residential facility because of his violent behavior. During formal testing, the patient was noted to be particularly aggressive when questioned directly. At one point, he lunged at and tried to choke the tester.

Greenwood and others (69) describe four patients with herpes simplex encephalitis who exhibited aggressive behavior. The patients all exhibited some bizarre eating and chewing behaviors, mostly related to nonfood items such as bedding or feces. None were hypersexual or sexually inappropriate. All patients looked emotionless and had few facial expressions, but with questioning, three of the four patients flew into unpredictable rages. Greenwood notes that the patient who was the most unpredictably and violently aggressive was also the one with the least memory loss from the encephalitis. When in control, he could sit and play simple board games with staff. Yet when he became angered, he would throw food and feces, shout at staff, and swear. Greenwood suggests that since aggression does not occur in Klüver-Bucy monkeys, the aggression in some patients with herpes simplex encephalitis may be due to only partial involvement of limbic areas in these cases, while patients with a classical Klüver-Bucy syndrome have complete involvement of both temporal lobes.

C. Other Forms of Encephalitis

Since herpes simplex encephalitis is the only encephalitis known to localize to a particular brain area; it is the only encephalitis in which neuropsychiatric symptoms may be predictable. Other types of encephalitis produce more diffuse central nervous system damage. Himmelhoch and coworkers (68) report on eight cases of subacute encephalitis of various etiologies that cause numerous behavioral syndromes in patients, including marked aggression. The following are a few specific case reports.

1. Acquired Immune Deficiency Syndrome (AIDS) Encephalitis

AIDS causes numerous behavioral deficits, including dementia. Another common behavioral disturbance associated with agitated behavior in AIDS patients is AIDS-related mania. Patients can display symptoms seen in typical mania, including irritability and psychosis (71). AIDS encephalitis has been reported to cause depression and psychotic symptoms in some patients (72,73). Beresford and others (74) report on a patient with AIDS encephalitis who had severe "acting out," which was initially felt to be sociopathy. Among other things, the patient threatened his father with a knife. He was paranoid and uncooperative with interviews, although no overt hallucinations or delusions are reported. At autopsy, the patient was diagnosed with acute encephalitis felt to be secondary to AIDS.

2. Limbic Encephalitis

Paraneoplastic syndromes, a remote effect of malignancy and generally felt to be autoimmune in nature, are the most common cause of limbic encephalitis. Newman and coworkers (75) describe a 76-year-old man who was admitted to a psychiatric service following his brother's death. He was confused and had memory problems. His behavior deteriorated while he was in the hospital, such that he could not care for himself and was frequently aggressive toward staff. The patient died a few months after initial presentation. He was found to have an oat-cell carcinoma in his lung and a renal-cell carcinoma. Examination of the brain showed damage to the limbic system.

Khan and Wiesser (76) report on a 24-year-old patient who initially presented with complex partial seizures. The patient had worsening behavioral problems, including aggression, which the patient felt was out of character, and memory problems. A diagnosis of limbic encephalitis was made, and the behavioral disturbances were felt to be due to the temporal lobe seizures. The etiology of the limbic encephalitis was unclear in this case. Some improvement in the behavioral problems was seen with control of the seizures.

VII. MOVEMENT DISORDERS

Movement disorders often present with behavioral changes. Increased irritability and angry outbursts are reported in many movement disorders. Psychotic symptoms, which exacerbate underlying aggression, are also seen.

A. Gilles de la Tourette Syndrome

Gilles de la Tourette syndrome is a condition in which patients display both verbal and motor tics. These tics change over time in localization and presentation. Patients with Tourette's may display coprolalia (obscene speech) and copropraxia (obscene gestures). Numerous authors have cited behavioral problems as part of the clinical picture in some cases of Tourette's syndrome. Indeed, Tourette himself mentioned behavioral problems in his original description of the syndrome (77).

While obsessions, compulsions, and disorders related to attention-deficit hyperactivity disorder are generally the most commonly described psychiatric symptoms in Tourette's (78,79), aggressive outbursts have also been described. Robertson and others (80) studied the correlation between motor symptoms and behavioral disorders in 90 Tourette's patients. They found that 28 patients had been physically aggressive toward people (most typically family members), animals, or objects. Aggressive behavior was significantly associated with symptoms of being forced to touch and with copropraxia. There was no significant association between aggression and age of onset, personal or family history of psychiatric illness, EEG or neurological abnormalities, medication, distribution of tics, hyperactivity, or difficulty in concentration or attention as a child. Coprolalia was associated with a number of aggression subscales in the Hostility and Direction of Hostility Questionnaire (HDHQ) (81). Enchophenomena were associated with significantly high scores on the sum hostility scale of the HDHQ.

B. Wilson's Disease

Wilson's disease, or hepatolenticular degeneration, is an autosomal recessive disorder involving dysregulation of copper metabolism by the liver. Psychiatric symptoms in Wilson's disease were recognized as early as 1912 by Samuel Alexander Kinnier Wilson in his description of the disorder (82). Neurological, renal, and hepatic abnormalities are the usual findings in the disease. Kayser-Fleischer rings can often be seen on fundoscopic examination. All symptoms are caused by abnormal deposition of copper in organ systems. In a study of 42 patients with Wilson's disease, Akil and others (83) noted that 24 of the patients had psychiatric symptoms as the presenting complaint. Personality changes, seen in 17 patients, were the most common presenting psychiatric complaint. Some of these personality changes caused aggressive behavior. Family members would describe the patient as having more "temper" than usual or yelling and throwing things when angry. Psychosis, which could contribute to aggression, was the presenting complaint in two patients.

Dening and Berrios (84) assessed multiple neuropsychiatric symptoms in 195 patients with Wilson's disease. Aggression was present in 17 patients. They noted a robust association between incongruous behavior, aggression, and personality change and certain neurological symptoms such as dysarthria, dysphagia, drooling, and rigidity.

C. Huntington's Disease

Huntington's disease is an autosomally dominant disorder that can present with choreiform movements and/or psychiatric symptoms. Caine and Shoulson (81) studied a group of 17 patients with Huntington's disease, most of whom were referred for study because of behavioral problems. Those patients that were severely demented or were unable to provide informed consent were excluded from the study. The Schedule for Affective Disorders and Schizophrenia (85) was used for assessment. Two patients fulfilled criteria for intermittent explosive syndrome.

Burns and coworkers (86), using the Overt Aggression Scale (27) to assess 26 patients with Huntington's disease, found that 59% of the patients scored significantly on the aggression scale. Aggression and irritability were not correlated with apathy or with each other.

D. Parkinson's Disease

While aggression may not be a common manifestation of Parkinson's disease per se, it may develop as a result of treatment with dopaminergic medications (87).

VIII. MEDICATIONS AND DRUGS

Drug effects and side effects can result in disinhibition or irritability. In any individual with brain dysfunction, there is increased susceptibility to adverse behavioral effects of medication. By far the most common drug associated with aggression is alcohol, during both intoxication and withdrawal. Stimulating drugs such as cocaine and amphetamines, as well as stimulating antidepressants, may produce agitation. Antipsychotic medications often increase agitation through anticholinergic side effects, and agitation and irritability usually accompany severe akathisia. Many other drugs may produce confusional states, especially anticholinergic medications that cause agitated delirium. Other drugs that may produce aggressive behavior include steroids (prednisone, cortisone, and the anabolic steroids; see Ref. 88 for review), analgesics (opiates and other narcotics; Ref. 89), and anxiolytics (barbiturates and benzodiazepines; Ref. 90).

IX. BRAIN TUMORS

Aggression secondary to intracerebral malignancy has long been a part of the differential diagnosis considered by psychiatrists. It is, however, rare for violent behavior to manifest itself as the first symptom of a brain tumor. We believe that the more frequent use of brain imaging techniques has resulted in earlier detection of tumors, resulting in less frequent behavioral presentation. There have, to this date, been few studies of central nervous system malignancies as a cause of aggressive behavior. Remington and Rubert (91) reviewed records of one psychiatric hospital and looked at records of patients with discharge diagnoses of "psychosis due to brain tumor"; they found only 34 cases (0.2%) over a 30-year period. Among the "psychological" symptoms noted, 5 of the patients were reported to have "combative behavior." There is no comment on whether this was the presenting complaint.

Generally, behavioral symptoms attributed to brain tumors can be difficult to correlate with location, since tumor growth, especially when rapid, can cause widespread edema, bleeding, and large mass effects. Often, the patients present with lethargy as the predominant behavioral problem. There are a few case series, especially in the older literature, where attempts were made to correlate tumor location with manifestation of behavioral disturbance.

A. Limbic System Tumors

In a review of 18 cases of limbic system tumors, Malamud (92), found that 4 of the 9 patients with tumors in the temporal lobe had irritable, angry, or actual assaultive episodes during their clinical courses. Of 2 patients with cingulate tumors, 1 displayed aggressive behavior. Of 7 patients with tumors in the region of the third ventricle, 1 displayed aggressive behavior. While the tumors varied in histological type from glioblastoma to astrocytoma to colloid cyst, they were all relatively slow-growing, disrupting minaly limbic system structures, since they did not cause rapid shifts in intracranial pressure. Nearly all patients with temporal lobe or cingulate involvement were having psychomotor seizures. Thus, Malamud proposes that these patients' psychiatric symptoms may be related to the behavioral disturbances seen in temporal lobe epilepsy (reviewed above). He also suggests that the patients with tumors of the third ventricle may be comparable to those with hypothalamic tumors (discussed below). While thesc series of patients is too small to allow for generalizations about tumor type, it is striking that so many patients with limbic system tumors were aggressive, some to the point of assaultiveness toward family or staff.

B. Hypothalmic Tumors

Numerous studies with experimental animals have demonstrated that damage to the ventromedial hypothalmus can result in hyperphagia and occasionally rage. Reeves and Plum (93) describe a 20-year-old woman with a hypothalamic tumor who displayed episodes of extremely aggressive behavior during her 2-year illness. During formal testing, she "would hit, scratch and attempt to bite the examiner. Alternatively she was briefly pleasant and cooperative and occasionally even expressed regret for her unprovoked aggressiveness." She also had hyperphagia, with consequent morbid obesity, dementia, and auditory hallucinations. Function of the adrenal, gonadal, and thyroid systems were interrupted. On autopsy, a hamartoma was found at the base of the diencephalon. The bilateral ventromedial hypothalamus and the median eminence were destroyed. The tumor appeared to have caused little destruction anteriorly and laterally.

X. STROKE

Mood disorders following stroke have been reported in numerous case studies and reviews (94–97). Robinson's extensive studies on the relationship between lesion location and depression or mania (98–100) suggest that patients with left-hemisphere lesions are more likely to become depressed, while those with right-sided lesions are more likely to be unusually cheerful or even manic.

A. Poststroke Mania

Aggression can occur in poststroke mania, just as in primary mania. Robinson and others (98) compared lesion location in 17 patients with poststroke mania to the injured area in 31 poststroke patients with depression and 28 with no mood disorder after stroke. Patients with secondary mania were more likely to have lesions of the right hemisphere in areas connected to limbic areas than were patients in the other two groups. They were also more likely to have a family history of affective disorder. Aggressive behavior was not specifically addressed in this study.

Drake and coworkers (101) reports on two right-handed patients who exhibited secondary mania after ventral pontine lesions. Both patients exhibited aggressive behavior. The 52-year-old male patient with a right pontine lesion, who had premorbidly been a quiet person, had loud arguments with family during his manic state. At one point, he heard voices telling him to kill his family. He tried to fight the urge, but after a few days rushed at his family with a knife and wounded one of his children. The other patient, a 56-year-old man with a left ventral pontine lesion, who also had no premorbid history of aggression, engaged in fistfights while manic.

B. Catastrophic Reaction

Catastrophic reaction to stroke is a relatively rare mood disorder seen most commonly after left-hemispheric strokes, although it has also been described in other types of brain damage. It is often seen in individuals with aphasia. Patients may display anxiety, aggression, and extreme agitation. Some authors attribute this to frustration at not being able to communicate due to the aphasia.

Gianotti (102) conducted a study of behavioral and mood disorders in 160 patients with right- or left-sided hemispheric lesions. Both vascular and neoplastic lesions were included, although 53 of the 80 patients with left-hemispheric lesions and 58 of the 80 with right-hemispheric lesions had vascular lesions. Aggressive behavior was scored as irritation and expressions of anger toward the examiner. Actual physical violence is not mentioned. Eleven of 80 patients with left-hemispheric lesions and 8 of 80 patients with right-hemispheric lesions exhibited aggressive behavior. The author suggests that difficulty communicating and resulting frustration may be a particular cause of catastrophic reaction in these patients.

More recently, Teasell (103) reported on a patient with catastrophic reaction after a left-sided stroke involving the frontal, parietal, and subcortical areas. In addition to right hemiplegia, this 75-year-old man had deficits in both comprehension and expressive language. Comprehension returned to normal soon after the stroke, but the hemiplegia and expressive aphasia persisted with minimal improvement. While characterized as a peaceful person prior to this illness, the patient's poststroke course was characterized by outbursts of angry remarks and threatening gestures. He injured staff on several occasions and even attempted to bite staff members. He was verbally aggressive toward his wife. He expressed frustration with his physical disabilities. The authors note that the patient's aggressiveness did not improve as the demands placed on him by rehabilitation and other services were decreased.

XI. HYPOGLYCEMIA

A series of studies conducted by Virkunnen and colleagues in Finland examined biological correlates of aggression in a group of violent prisoners. One consistent finding has been that this group is prone to hypoglycemia and that they have an increase in irritability during these episodes. In one study (104), 33 successive male admissions to a psychiatric clinic in Helsinki, Finland, were studied. Of these men, 13 met criteria for antisocial personality and had exhibited violent behavior, often while using alcohol. Twenty of the patients had intermittent explosive disorder with violent tendencies. Patients who were retarded, had chromosomal abnormalities, or were psychotic were excluded. Of note, all violent offenders met DSM-III criteria for alcohol abuse. The patients were compared with a control group of men from the staff of the clinic matched for age and body weight. None of the control subjects reported alcohol or drug problems. Using a glucose tolerance test, Virkkunen et al. found that while both patient groups displayed greater hypoglycemia than controls, duration of hypoglycemia was longer in patients with antisocial personality disorder than in those with intermittent explosive disorder. The severity of the hypoglycemia was greater in those individuals with intermittent explosive disorder but their recovery from hypoglycemia was more rapid. Virkkunen and coworkers suggest that these results fit with the different clinical pictures of intermittent explosive disorder and antisocial personality disorder. Similar results were reported in an earlier study of 68 habitually violent male patients with either antisocial personality disorder or intermittent explosive disorder (105).

The main criticism of studies in violent populations is the confounding effect of alcohol. Since many of these patients have a history of extensive alcohol abuse, especially while perpetrating violent acts, it is unclear what contribution alcohol makes to the overall picture of violence (106). Other authors have questioned the usefulness of the oral glucose tolerance test as a measure of blood glucose levels in these circumstances and the differences in diet of patients compared with that of controls, which can be quite disparate for institutionalized persons (107). At this time, these results are not useful predictors of violent behavior in the general population.

XII. SLEEP DISORDERS

There have been a few reports of aggressive behavior during parasomnias, including violent attacks. Dyken and others (108) report on an elderly farmer who had a 10-year history of extremely vivid dreams, which often caused him to jump from his bed, at one point sustaining a subdural hemorrhage. The patient reported dreams in which cows chased him, causing him actually to run in his sleep. This disruptive behavior can also be directed toward others in a remarkably organized fashion. Mahowald and other workers (109) report on a 73-year-old man whose disturbing dreams caused him to grab or kick his wife. Formal sleep studies can help to determine the cause of this sleep-related behavior, including non-REM parasomnias, sleep-related seizures, REM behavior disorder, or psychogenic dissociative phenomena (110).

XIII. ENDOCRINE DISORDERS

Along with systemic effects, several endocrine disorders are known to produce behavioral symptoms and often have psychiatric symptomatology as the presenting complaint.

A. Thyroid Disorders

Hyperthyroid states can produce agitation and psychosis.

Thyrotoxicosis is caused by increased production of thyroid hormone by the thyroid gland, inflammation of the thyroid, or sources of thyroid hormone from outside the gland (i.e., exogenous thyroid hormone consumption or tumor production of thyroid hormone). Neuropsychiatric symptoms of thryotoxicosis include anxiety, insomnia, and intense dysphoria. Memory and concentration can be impaired. Psychosis is sometimes present, and this is when violence generally occurs, since patients may react dramatically to perceived threats or command hallucinations (111). When psychosis is seen, it may be a sign that the patient is progressing toward the more serious state of thyroid storm (112).

Two young women are described by Kutzer (113) as manifesting paranoid behavior due to undiagnosed thyroid conditions. Each was taken to see a psychiatrist after nonspecific violent acts toward family members. Both had severe hyperthyroidism, that caused an agitated, manic-like state with psychosis. The author postulates that this was due to metabolic encephalopathy.

Thryotoxicosis in children can present in numerous ways, including an ADHD-like picture, affective symptoms, and psychosis. Severe aggression is rarely reported in children with thyrotoxicosis. Fire setting and aggressive behavior is described by Bhatara and coworkers (114) in a 4-year-old boy with thryotoxicosis secondary to consumption of beef contaminated with bovine thyroid. Symptoms included bizarre behavior such as fecal smearing, stabbing of dolls, and hitting his mother. He was hospitalized after he attempted to set the house on fire several times. He also had weight loss, anxiety, and restlessness. The child's symptoms improved during hospitalization, while he was no longer eating contaminated beef. Thyroid tests, performed 3 days after admission, were normal. The authors believe that the child's thyroid hormone levels fell rapidly after admission to the hospital.

Hypothyroidism is usually primary; pituitary or hypothalamic disease causing hypothyroidism is rare. In psychiatric patients, lithium can cause hypothyroidism (115). Patients with hypothyroid conditions are usually characterized as depressed, apathetic, and lethargic. Elderly patients may look demented. However, there are case reports of agitation leading to violent behavior in persons with hypothyroidism. Approximately half of the patients with hypothyroidism will have some affective disturbance, and a small percentage of these will show signs of psychosis (116). Long-standing hypothyroidism can lead to myxedema. Patients with myxedema psychosis (or "myxedema madness," as this severe psychiatric disturbance in hypothyroid states was once termed) can become quite agitated (117,118).

Easson (118) describes a 31-year-old man who had a long history of thyroid disorder and behavioral problems. At age 17, he underwent a partial thyroidectomy for hyperthyroidism. He then took thyroid hormone replacement, stopping it sporadically at several points. At age 31, he stopped taking his thyroid replacement. During the 4 months after he stopped replacement, he felt tired and clumsy. He also became increasingly suspicious that people were ridiculing him. He began to hear voices commenting disparagingly on his sexual abilities. One day, he hit and killed a friend who was asleep, believing that the friend was sending him bad thoughts. He was arrested and sent to a forensic psychiatric unit. Tests showed severe hypothyroidism. One he received adequate thyroid replacement, the paranoia resolved and he had no further hallucinations. The patient was judged not guilty by reason of insanity and was sent to a forensic psychiatric hospital, although he was no longer psychiatrically ill at the time of trial.

B. Parathyroid Disorders

It has long been recognized that parathyroid disorders, and the resulting calcium abnormalities, can cause psychiatric symptoms. Since calcium is involved in neurotransmission, it is not surprising that hypercalcemia can have many psychiatric manifestations. Primary hyperparathyroidism can be caused by a tumor of the parathyroid or by parathyroid hyperplasia. The conditions usually causes depression, fatigue, and confusion (119,120). However, psychosis has been reported in rare cases and can lead to violent behavior. Brown (121) and coworkers describe a 68-year-old man with no prior psychiatric history who developed anxiety, confusion, and mild paranoia. He had hypercalcemia on laboratory testing and was treated with intravenous fluids. After increasing paranoia, during which time he thought his antihypertensives were poisonous, he woke early one morning and fatally shot his wife with a double-barreled shotgun and wounded a grandson who was trying to escape. He then called a local law enforcement center to report what he had done. He was able to give his correct name and address. He did not resist arrest and told his lawyer that he shot his family members because they were conspiring to kill him. He was found to have a parathyroid adenoma. Despite efforts by his lawyer to use an insanity defense, he was found guilty of both attacks and imprisoned. The authors note that while the behavioral disturbances seen in this case are extreme, the patient did follow a typical pattern of initial vague symptoms, which later progressed to psychiatric symptoms. Patients with hypercalcemia are also more likely than those with other endocrine disorders to display psychiatric symptoms with concomitant fully intact consciousness (112). There is some indication that patients with higher calcium levels are more likely to have psychotic symptoms (121,122).

Hypoparathyroidism can cause hypocalcemia. Hypoparathryoidism is usually associated with autoimmune disorders or other destruction of the parathyroid. Hypocalcemia has not been reported to cause violence. Patients with this disorder are often anxious and demented (112).

C. Cortisol Disorders

Patients with Cushing's syndrome due to adrenal tumors or adronocorticotropin hormone (ACTH)-secreting tumors have high levels of cortisol, which can cause metabolic encephalopathy and various psychiatric symptoms (113). Capenter and Gavin (123) report that psychotic symptoms can be precipitated by hypercortisolism. Older literature cites an example of homicidal psychosis afer exogenous ACTH use (124). Patients with Addison's disease, who have abnormally low cortisol levels, are generally depressed (123).

XIV. SEX HORMONES

A. Testosterone

"High testosterone levels" are often blamed for aggressive behavior in men, although the actual relationship between testosterone levels and violence is far from clear. There are several controlled studies of testosterone levels in serum, saliva, and spinal fluid, attempting to correlate these values with various measures of violence. For an extensive review of studies linking sex hormones and violence, see Volavka (125).

Several groups have examined testosterone levels in male prisoners who have committed violent acts, finding some correlation between elevated testosterone and aggression. Ehrenkranz and others (126) evaluated 12 offenders with chronic aggressive behavior in prison who continued to engage in fighting while incarcerated, 12 socially dominant prisoners who were incarcerated for nonviolent crimes such as theft, and 12 prisoners who were not violent or socially dominant. They found higher serum testosterone levels in the continuously violent group. The socially dominant group also had higher testosterone levels than the nondominant, nonaggressive group. None of the results of psychological rating scales of aggression correlated with testosterone levels. The authors suggest that higher anxiety levels in the socially dominant group, seen on the rating scales, help explain why there were able to keep their behavior more in check.

Rada and other workers (128) found higher serum testosterone levels in incarcerated rapists who used physical aggression against their victims as opposed to those who used only verbal threats or displayed a weapon but did not use it. Physically aggressive rapists also had higher testosterone levels than child molesters. Rapists as a group scored higher than controls on the Buss-Durkee Hostility Inventory (128). Individual test scores did not correlate with testosterone levels. The same group was unable to replicate these data in a later study (129) with similar groups of offenders.

In contrast, Kreuz and Rose (130) found no correlation between plasma testosterone and incidences of fighting and verbal aggression in prisoners. They studied 21 young prisoners (ages ranging from 19 to 32, with a mean age of 28), taking six plasma samples over a 2-week period. Testosterone levels did not correlate with current aggression as measured by the Buss-Durkee Hostility Inventory. Those prisoners with a more prominent history of violent crime in adolescence did have a higher level of testosterone than those without a significant early history of violence. The authors propose that high levels of testosterone may have a permissive effect on aggression early in life in some individuals who are more prone to commit crime in the first place. However, it is unclear whether high testosterone levels in adulthood correlate with increased testosterone early in life. Bain and others (131) also failed to find a significant difference in random serum testosterone levels between groups of offenders who had committed murder (n = 13), assault (n = 14) and 14 controls charged with property crimes.

More recently, Virkunnen and others (132) compared 43 impulsive and 15 nonimpulsive male alcoholic offenders with 21 normal, nonalcoholic volunteers. Testosterone levels in CSF were measured. It was found that these do not have the wide fluctuations that can be seen in serum and that they may provide a more steady-state picture of testosterone levels in the brain. The "impulsive" prisoners were divided into two groups, those with antisocial personality disorder (n = 17) and those with explosive personality disorder (n = 14). Those offenders with antisocial personality disorder had significantly higher testosterone levels than controls. Those with explosive personality disorder did not exhibit different testosterone levels from either group.

Saliva testosterone reflects testosterone levels more accurately than serum levels. Testosterone may also influence behavior in women. Dabbs and others (133) studied saliva testosterone levels in 84 female prisoners and 15 female college students. Of these offenders, 20 had committed violent crimes, including homicide and assault. Testosterone was higher in women who had committed an unprovoked crime but not in those women who had committed defensive violence (e.g., killing an abusive husband).

Testosterone may exert a modulatory effect in decreasing the threshold for violent crimes. However, most violent crime is not directly correlated with testosterone levels. Future studies using saliva or CSF testosterone may be more conclusive.

B. Premenstrual Dysphoric Disorder

Popular wisdom has linked the menstrual cycle to mood swings and unusual behavior since the early 1900s. However, there are few controlled studies that address the question of whether violence in women is linked to a certain phase or phases of the menstrual cycle.

The term *premenstrual syndrome*, which has been replaced by *premenstrual dysphoric disorder*, is used to describe a number of physical and or mood changes observed in a small percentage of women in association with their menstrual cycles. The psychiatric symptoms include tiredness, depression, and, in some women, irritability and anxiety (134). Some women experience hypoglycemia during the time prior to menses, and this has been postulated to account for increased irritability. However, work by Denicoff and others (135) has demonstrated that hypoglycemia is not related to symptoms of premenstrual dysphoric disorder.

Several studies have examined the relationship between stage of menstrual cycle and commission of a crime. D'Orban and Dalton (136) and Dalton (137) found that female prisoners committed crimes more often during premenstrual and menstrual stages of their cycles than at other times. However, this was true for both violent and nonviolent crimes. These studies, which rely on retrospective self-report by women, may be confounded by popular opinion, which may cause women to falsely recall that they were paramenstrual at the time a crime was committed, as an explanation or excuse for the behavior (138,139). There are no studies to date on women with premenstrual dysphoric disorder are more likely to commit crimes than women who do not meet criteria for this disorder.

Thus, the relationship between the menstrual cycle and aggression is unclear. Women who commit crimes may be more likely to do so during the premenstrual or menstrual phase of their cycle. However, these data may be influenced by suggestibility, in that women may retrospectively attribute their actions to a particular phase in their menstrual cycle. Some studies of prisoners may, as Volavka suggests in his review of the topic (125), simply imply that women are more likely to be apprehended if they commit a crime during the paramenstrual time of their cycle. He postulates that this could occur because depression or lethargy can reduce the motivation to escape arrest.

C. Prenatal Exposure to Exogenous Hormones

Prenatal exposure to androgens has occurred mainly when synthetic androgens were used to prevent abortion. It has been suggested that the exposure to androgens would masculinize females and could lead to higher levels of aggression. These cases are fortunately quite rare. Reinisch (140) studied 17 girls and 8 boys who were exposed to progestin in utero. Exposed children were compared with their same-sex siblings, who had not been exposed, using questionnaires about aggression. Both exposed boys and girls scored higher on the questions that predicted potential for aggression. However, no actual observation or whether the children displayed more aggression than their siblings was reported.

Prenatal diethylstilbestrol (DES) exposure was examined by Ehrhardt and others (141). Thirty adolescent and adult women who had been exposed were compared with 30 matched controls who had not been exposed. Questionnaires and interviews were given to patients and to their mothers. No increase in verbal or physical aggression was found in exposed females when compared with controls.

In summary, human studies on prenatal exposure to sex hormones do not provide conclusive evidence that exposure to androgens lead to an actual increase in violent behavior.

XV. NUTRITIONAL FACTORS

A. Vitamin Deficiencies

Vitamin deficiencies generally present with apathy as the foremost behavioral symptom. Pyridoxine (B_6) deficiency due to homocystinuria may cause psychosis. Folic acid deficiency in homocystinuria and hypomethioninemia may cause a schizophrenia-like syndrome (142).

There are a few case reports of dietary vitamin deficiencies causing agitation. Niacin deficiency can cause depression with psychotic features, including hallucinations and thought disorder. Patients with more severe psychotic symptoms may become agitated (143). As the disorder progresses, patients will become more demented and, ultimately, stuporous.

Zucker and others (144) report that B_{12} deficiency leading to pernicious anemia causes psychotic symptoms in 16% of patients. They also report that 30 to 80% of patients with pernicious anemia may have an organic brain syndrome including paranoia, violence, and depression. These symptoms all respond to correction of vitamin deficiencies. They note that psychiatric symptoms can be seen without neurological deficits or anemia.

B. Serum Cholesterol

In a review of nutritional factors and violence, Kanarek (107) discusses studies by Virkunnen and others suggesting that male offenders with antisocial personality disorder or intermittent explosive disorder who were habitually violent had lower cholesterol levels than those seen in other prisoners (145,146). The greatest differences were seen in those under 30 years of age. The authors propose that the lower cholesterol in violent offenders may be due to increased insulin secretion. However, as Kanarek notes, the studies did not control for variables such as alcohol consumption and dietary differences between the two groups. Muldoon (147) and others looked at causes of mortality in large groups of subjects who had specific interventions (diet changes or medications) to lower cholesterol. Cholesterol was reduced by 10% in treatment groups compared with controls. The risk of death from a violent cause, including suicide, was twice as great in treatment group, while their risk of death from coronary disease was lowered. In a long term follow-up study, Pekkanen and others (148) failed to replicate these findings. Thus, the association between cholesterol and violence remains unclear.

XVI. ELECTROLYTE IMBALANCE AND HYPOXIA

Electrolyte imbalance can precipitate delirium and confusional states. Patients may become acutely agitated and aggressive as a result of various electrolyte abnormalities. Sodium and calcium imbalanced are probably the most common abnormalities to cause agitation, since either state can result in disturbance of cell membrane equilibrium in the central nervous system (113,149,150).

Both acute cerebral hypoxia, a deficiency of oxygen in tissue, or hypoxemia (deficiency of oxygen in the blood, usually resulting from cardiac or pulmonary compromise) can also cause delirium. As with any delirious state, these patients may become combative. Patients with chronic cerebral anoxia may compensate for the condition at baseline but can become quite confused and aggressive if the anoxia is worsened by infection or other systemic illness (113). Numerous other medical conditions such as hypertensive encephalopathy, hypoglycemia, or intracranial bleeding can also cause delirium, occasionally with concomitant aggression (151).

XVII. TOXINS

Toxins will generally cause stupor and lethargy with acute intoxication. However, numerous toxins have been reported to cause irritability and even aggression in extreme cases, especially when exposure is gradual. As with the general medical illnesses discussed above, encephalopathy and psychosis are the main reasons for aggression. Chronic mercury exposure produces the best known neuropsychiatric side effects, leading to the expression "mad as a hatter," since mercury was formerly used in the manufacture of felt hats. Afflicted persons have mood lability and are shy, with decreased sleep and memory problems (152). Actual violence has not been reported. Organophosphates act by binding to acetincholinesterase and inactivating the enzyme. The immediate effect is accumulation of large amounts of acetylcholine in the synapse. Organophosphate toxicity, usually following pesticide use, commonly presents with neuropsychiatric symptoms (152). Aggression has been described in rare cases, including one incidence of a man and his pet cat who both became quite violent after organophosphate exposure in their home. The aggression resolved after the pesticides were discontinued (153).

Lead has been reported to cause mood disorders and irritability, among other neuropsychiatric symptoms, but aggression per se has not been reported (154). Adults are usually exposed to lead through occupational contact, while children commonly ingest lead paint. At highly toxic levels, lead intoxication causes encephalopathy, which is seen most commonly in children, since they absorb lead more readily. Encephalopathy can progress to psychosis (152). Chronic arsenic poisoning can also cause encephalopathy, and, in some case, psychotic symptoms (155). "Manganese madness" occurs most often in miners and processors of manganese. Besides parkinsonian symptoms, patients may have behavioral disturbances, including psychosis (156).

XVIII. CONCLUSION

Aggressive and violent behavior may result from many disorders of the central nervous system. These problems are common and constitute a major source of morbidity and mortality. Disruptive behavior is often the largest barrier to reintegration into the community for those with severe neurological illnesses.

Lesions that involve which the limbic lobes may be more frequently associated with aggression, but violent behavior is also seen with diffuse cortical disease. Patients with central nervous system disease may be violent in an unpredictable manner, but aggression often occurs when others attempt to restrain or assist a patient. This restrictive aggression is reported frequently in studies of demented patients, those with intellectual deficiency, and those with epilepsy who are postictal. Aggression is also seen as a result of severe medical illness, especially in individuals with chronic illness. Encephalopathy as a result of a medical condition can lead to agitation and aggression. Systemic medical illness can also cause psychosis, which may lead to violent behavior in response to paranoid ideation.

While aggression may appear to be unpredictable in these populations, patterns are evident in many forms of disruptive behavior. If a sudden change in behavior occurs, neurological or medical illness should be ruled out as a cause of the aggression. This may require a fairly extensive workup and consideration of uncommon conditions. Description and evaluation of aggression in the aggressive behavior is the first step toward treatment and prevention.

REFERENCES

1. B. Reisberg, J. Borenstein, S. Salbo, and S. H. Ferris, Behavioral symptoms in Alzheimer's disease: Phenomenology and treatment, *J Clin Psychiatry 48 (5 Suppl.)*: 9 (1987).
2. L. Teri, P. Rabins, P. Whitehouse, and B. Leonard, Management of behavior disturbance in Alzheimer's disease: Current knowledge and future directions, *Alzheimer Dis Assoc Disord 6*(2):77 (1992).
3. M.F. Weiner, L. Teri, and B.T. Williams, Psychological and behavioral management, *The Dementias: Diagnosis, Management, and Research*, 2d ed. (M. F. Weiner, ed.), American Psychiatric Press, 1996, pp. 139–173.
4. P.V. Rabins, N.L. Mace, and M.J. Lucas, The impact of dementia on the family, *J.A.M.A. 248*:333 (1982).
5. M. Haupt and A. Kurz, Predictors of nursing home placement in patients with Alzheimer's disease, *Int. J Geriat Psychiatry 8*:741 (1993).
6. B.F. O'Donnell, D.A. Drachman, H.J. Barnes, K.E. Peterson, J.M. Swearer, and R.A. Lew, Incontinence and troublesome behaviors predict institutionalization in dementia, *J Geriatr Psychiatry Neurol 5*:45 (1992).

7. M. Hamel, D. P. Gold, D. Andres, M. Reis, D. Dastoor, H. Grauer, and H. Bergman, Predictors and consequences of aggressive behavior by community-based dementia patients, *Gerontologist 30 (2)*:206 (1990).
8. D.P. Dastoor and M.G. Cole, Hierarchic Dementia Scale, *J Clin Exp Gerontol 5(3)*:219 (1983).
9. M. B. Ryden, Aggressive behavior in persons with dementia who live in the community, *Alzheimer Dis Assoc Disord 2(4)*:342 (1988).
10. M. Ryden, Aggressive behavior in cognitively impaired nursing home residents, paper presented at the Annual Scientific Meeting of the Gerontological Society of America, San Francisco, 1988.
11. J.C. Morrant and J.R. Ablog, The angry elderly patient: An approach to understanding, *Postgrad Med 74(6)*:93 (1983).
12. F. Post, Some problems arising from the study of mental patients over the age of sixty years, *J Ment Sci 90*:554 (1944).
13. J. Cohen-Mansfield, M.S. Marx, and A.S. Rosenthal, Dementia and agitation in nursing home residents: How are they related? *Psychol Aging* 5(1):3 (1990).
14. J. Cohen-Mansfield, Agitated behaviors in the elderly: II. Preliminary results in the cognitively deteriorated, *J Am Geriatr Soc 34*:722 (1986).
15. B. Reisberg and S.H. Ferris, A clinical rating scale for symptoms of psychosis in Alzheimer's disease, *Psychopharmacol Bull 21(1)*:101 (1985).
16. V. Patel and R.A. Hope, Aggressive behaviour in elderly psychiatric inpatients, *Acta Psychiatr Scand 85*:131 (1992).
17. D.P. Devanand, C.D. Brockington, B.J. Moody, R.P. Brown, R.M. Mayeux, J. Endicott, and H.S. Sackeim, Behavioral syndromes in Alzheimer's disease, *Int Psychogeriatr 4(2)*: 161 (1992).
18. L.H. Deutsch, F.W. Bylsma, B.W. Rovner, C.S. Steele, and M.F. Folstein, Psychosis and physical agitation in probable Alzheimer's disease, *American J Psychiatry 148(9)*:1159 (1991).
19. J.K. Wing, J.E. Cooper, and N. Sartorius, *The Measurement and Classification of Psychiatric Symptoms: An Instructional Manual for the PSE and CATEGO Programs*, New York, Cambridge University Press, 1974.
20. B. Reisberg and S.H. Ferris, A clinical rating scale for symptoms of psychosis in Alzheimer's disease, *Psychopharmacol Bull 21(1)*:101 (1985).
21. O.L. Lopez, J.T. Becker, R.P. Brenner, J. Rosen, O.I. Bajulaiye, and C.F. Reynolds, Alzheimer's disease with delusions and hallucinations: Neuropsychological and electroencephalographic correlates, *Neurology 41*:906 (1991).
22. D.P. Devanand, D.M. Jacobs, M. Tang, C. Del Castillo-Castaneda, M. Sano, K. Marder, K. Bell, F. W. Bylsma, J. Brandt, M. Albert, and Y. Stern. The course of psychopathologic features in mild to moderate Alzheimer's disease, *Arch Gen Psychiatry 54*:257 (1997).
23. A. Burns, R. Jacoby, and R. Levy, Psychiatric phenomena in Alzheimer's disease. IV: Disorders of Behaviour, *Br J Psychiatry 157*:86 (1990).
24. D.L. Sultzer, M.E. Mahler, M.A. Mandelkern, J.L. Cummings, W.G. Van Gorp, C.H. Hinkin, and M.A. Berisford, The relationship between psychiatric symptoms and regional cortical metabolism in Alzheimer's disease, *J Neuropsychiatry Clin Neurosci 7*:476 (1995).

25. H.S. Levin, W.M. High, and K.E. Goethe, The Neurobehavioral Rating Scale: Assessment of the behavioral sequelae of head injury by the clinician, *J. Neurol Neurosurg Psychiatry 50*:183 (1987).
26. A. Burns, S. Folstein, J. Brandt, and M. Folstein, Clinical assessment of irritability, aggression, and apathy in Huntington and Alzheimer disease, *J Nerv Ment Dis 178(1)*: 20 (1990).
27. S. C. Yudofsky, J. M. Silver, and W. Jackson, The Overt Aggression Scale for the objective rating of verbal and physical aggression, *Am J Psychiatry 143*:35 (1986).
28. J. Victoroff, C. Zarow, W.J. Mack, E. Hsu, and H.C. Chui, Physical aggression is associated with preservation of substantia nigra pars compact in Alzheimer disease, *Arch Neurol 53*:428 (1996).
29. M.M. Esiri, The basis for behavioural disturbances in dementia, *J Neurol Neurosurg Psychiatry 61*:127 (1996).
30. J.M. Silver and S.C. Yudofsky, Aggressive disorders, *Neuropsychiatry of Traumatic Brain Injury* (J.M. Silver, S. C. Yudofsky, and R. E. Hales, eds.), American Psychiatric Press, 1994, pp. 313–353.
31. M. M. Brooke, K. A. Questad, D. R. Patterson, and K.J. Bashak, Agitation and restlessness after closed head injury: A prospective study of 100 consecutive admissions, *Arch Phys Med Rehabil 73*:320 (1992).
32. N. Rao, H. M. Jellinek, and D. C. Woolston, Agitation in closed head injury: Haloperidol effects on rehabilitation outcome, *Arch Phys Med Rehabil 66*:30 (1985).
33. H. S. Levin and R. G. Grossman, Behavioral sequelae of closed head injury: A quantitative study, *Arch Neurol 35*:720 (1978).
34. A. P. Wolf, A. D. Gleckman, D. X. Cifu, and P. C. Ginsburg, The prevalence of agitation and brain injury in skilled nursing facilities: A survey, *Brain Injury 10(4)*:241 (1996).
35. G. S. Carlsson, K. Svardsudd, and L. Welin, Long term effects of head injuries sustained during life in three male populations, *J Neurosurg 67*:197 (1987).
36. B.K. Hill and R.H. Bruininks, Maladaptive behavior of mentally retarded individuals in residential facilities, *Am J Ment Defic 88*:380 (1984).
37. J.W. Jacobson, Problem behavior and psychiatric impairment within a developmentally disabled population: I. Behavior frequency, *Appl Res Ment Retard 3*:121 (1982).
38. W.I. Gardner and C.W. Moffatt, Aggressive behavior: Definition, assessment, treatment, *Int Rev Psychiatry 2(1)*:91 (1990).
39. O.M. Linaker, Assaultiveness among instutionalised adults with mental retardation, *Br J Psychiatry 164(1)*:62 (1994).
40. M. Ghaziuddin and N. Ghaziuddin, Violence against staff by mentally retarded inpatients, *Hosp Commun Psychiatry 43*:503 (1992).
41. J. Sigafoos, J. Elkins, M. Kerr and T. Attwood, A survey of aggressive behavior among a population of persons with intellectual disability in Queensland, *J Intell Disabil Res 38*:369 (1994).
42. N. Bouras and C. Drummond, Behaviour and psychiatric disorders of people with mental handicaps living in the community, *J Intell Disabil Res 36*:349 (1992).
43. P.W. Davidson, N.N. Cane, J.E. Sloane-Reeves, A. Van Speybroech, J. Segel, J.

Gutkin, L.E. Quijano, and B.M. Kramer, Characteristics of community-based individuals with mental retardation and aggressive behavioral disorders, *Am J Ment Retard 98*:704 (1994).
44. J. Rojahn, S.A. Bothwick-Duffy, and J.W. Jacobsen, The association between psychiatric diagnosis and severe behavior problems in mental retardation, *Ann Clin Psychiatry 5(3)*:163 (1993).
45. S. Reiss and J. Rojahn, Joint occurrence of depression and aggression in children and adults with mental retardation, *J Intellect Disabil Res 37*:287 (1993).
46. H.M. Boslow and A. Kandell, Psychiatric aspects of dangerous behavior: The retarded offender, *Am J Psychiatry 121*:646 (1965).
47. C. Smith, R.E. Schmid, L.R. Clark, and W.B. Crew, M. Nunnery, The mentally retarded inmate: Prison adjustment and implications for treatment, *J Offend Counsel 9*:8 (1988).
48. H. Maudsley, *Body and Mind*, Macmillan, London, 1873.
49. D.M. Treiman, Epilepsy and violence: Medical and legal issues, *Epilepsia 27 (Suppl. 2)*: S77 (1986).
50. S. Currie, K.W.G. Healthfield, R.A. Henson, and D.F. Scott, Clinical course and prognosis of temporal lobe epilepsy: A survey of 666 patients, *Brain 94*:173 (1971).
51. C. Ounstead, Aggression and epilepsy: Rage in children with temporal lobe epilepsy, *J Psychosom Res 13*:237 (1969).
52. E.A. Rodin, Psychomotor epilepsy and aggressive behavior, *Arch Gen Psychiatry 28*:210 (1973).
53. A.V. Delgado-Escueta, R.H. Mattson, L. King, E.S. Goldensohn, H. Spiegel, J. Madsen, P. Crandall, F. Dreifuss, and R. J. Porter, The nature of aggression during epileptic scizures, *N Engl J Med 305*:711 (1981).
54. O. Devinsky, D. Ronsaville, C. Cox, E. Witt, P. Fedio, and W.H. Theodore, Interictal aggression in epilepsy: The Buss-Durkee Hostility Inventory, *Epilepsia 35*:585 (1994).
55. B.P. Hermann and S. Whitman, Behavioral and personality correlates of epilepsy: A review, methodological critique, and conceptual model, *Psychol Bull 95*:451 (1984).
56. M. F. Mendez, R.C. Doss, and J.L. Taylor. Interictal violence in epilepsy: Relationship to behavior and seizure variables, *J Nerv Ment Dis 181*:566 (1993).
57. G. Garyfallos, N. Manos, and A. Adamopoulou, Psychopathology and personality characteristics of epileptic patients: Epilepsy, psychopathology and personality, *Acta Psychiatr Scand 78(1)*:87 (1988).
58. L.J. Herzberg and P. B. C. Fenwick, The aetiology of aggression in temporal lobe epilepsy, *Br J Psychiatry 153*:50 (1988).
59. J. Gunn and G. Robertson, Drawing a criminal profile, *Br J Criminol 16*:156 (1976).
60. O. Devinsky and D. Bear, Varieties of aggressive behavior in temporal lobe epilepsy, *Am J Psychiatry 141*:651 (1984).
61. J.M. Tonkonogy, Violence and temporal lobe lesion: Head CT and MRI data, *J Neuropsychiatry Clin Neurosci 3(2)*:189 (1991).
62. J.R. Stevens, Psychiatric aspects of epilepsy, *J Clin Psychiatry 49(4 Suppl)*:49 (1988).

63. J. R. Stevens and B. R. Herman, Temporal lobe epilepsy, psychopathology, and violence: The state of the evidence, *Neurology 31*:1127 (1981).
64. C. Von Economo, *Encephalitis Lethargica*, Oxford University Press, New York, 1931.
65. J. Hoening and S. Abbey, Von Economo's disease (encephalitis lethargica); Lessons for psychiatry, *Viruses, Immunity, and Mental Disorders* (E. Durstak, Z. J. Lipowski, and P. V. Morozov, eds.), Plenum Press, New York, 1987, pp. 423–439.
66. S. U. Ho and D. H. Harter, Editorial: Herpes simplex virus encephalitis, *J.A.M.A. 247*:337 (1982).
67. H.M. Friedman and N. Allen, Chronic effects of complete limbic lobe destruction in man, *Neurology (Minn) 19*:679 (1969).
68. J. Himmelhoch, J. Pincus, G. Tucker, and T. Detre. Sub-acute encephalitis: Behavioural and neurological aspects, *Br J Psychiatry 116*:531 (1970).
69. R. J. Greenwood, A. Bhala, and A. Gordon, J. Roberts, Behaviour disturbances during recovery from herpes simplex encephalitis, *J Neurol Neurosurg Psychiatry 46*:809 (1983).
70. M. Greer, M. Lyons-Crews, L. Mauldin, and F.R. Brown, A case study of the cognitive and behavioral deficits of temporal lobe damage in herpes simplex encephalitis, *J Autism Dev Disord 19(2)*:317 (1989).
71. C.G. Lyketsos, J. Schwartz, M. Fishman, and G. Treisman, AIDS mania, *J Neuropsychiatry Clin Neurosci 9*:277 (1997).
72. W. D. Snider, D. M. Simpson, S. Nielson, J.W.M. Gold, C.E. Metroka, and J. B. Posner, Neurological complications of acquired immune deficiency syndrome: Analysis of 50 patients, *Ann Neurol 14*:403 (1983).
73. H.G. Nurnberg, J. Prudic, M. Fiori, and E. P. Freedman, Psychopathology complicating acquired immune deficiency syndrome (AIDS), *Am J Psychiatry 141(1)*:95 (1984).
74. T. P. Beresford, F.C. Blow, and R. C. W. Hall, AIDS encephalitis mimicking alcohol dementia and depression, *Biol Psychiatry 21*:394 (1986).
75. N.J. Newman, I.R. Bell, and A.C. McKee, Paraneoplastic limbic encephalitis: Neuropsychiatric presentation, *Biol Psychiatry 27*:529 (1990).
76. N. Khan and H.G. Wieser, Limbic encephalitis: A case report, *Epilepsy Res 17*:175 (1994).
77. M. M. Robertson and D. Z. Reinstein, Convulsive tic disorder: Georges Gilles de la Tourette, Guinon and Grasset on the phenomenology and psychopathology of Gilles de la Tourette syndrome, *Behav Neurol 4*:29 (1991).
78. D. E. Comings and B. G. Comings, Tourette's syndrome and attention deficit disorder, *Tourette's Syndrome and Tic Disorders. Clinical Understanding and Treatment* (D. J. Cohen, R. D. Bruun, and J. F. Leckman, eds.), John Wiley & Sons, New York, 1988, pp. 119–135.
79. K. E. Towbin and M. A. Riddle, Attention deficit hyperactivity disorder, *Handbook of Tourette Syndrome and Related Tic and Disorders* (R. Kurlan, ed.), Marcel Dekker, New York, 1993, pp. 89–110.
80. M. M. Robertson, M. R. Trimble, and A. J. Lees, The psychopathology of Giles de la Tourette syndrome: A phenomenological analysis, *Br J Psychiatry 152*:383 (1988).

81. E.D. Caine and I. Shoulson, Psychiatric syndromes in Huntington's disease, *Am J Psychiatry 140*:728 (1983).
82. S.A.K. Wilson, Progressive lenticular degeneration: A familiar nervous disease associated with cirrhosis of the liver, *Brain 34*:295 (1912).
83. M. Akil, J. A. Schwartz, D. Dutchak, V. Yuzbasiyan-Gurkan, and G.J. Brewer, The psychiatric presentations of Wilson's disease, *J Neuropsychiatry Clin Neurosci 3*: 377 (1991).
84. T.R. Dening and G.E. Berrios, Wilson's disease: Psychiatric symptoms in 195 cases, *Arch Gen Psychiatry 46*:1126 (1989).
85. J. Endicott and R.L. Spitzer, A diagnostic interview: The Schedule for Affective Disorders and Schizophrenia, *Arch Gen Psychiatry 35*:837 (1978).
86. A. Burns, S. Folstein, J. Brandt, and M. Folstein, Clinical assessment of irritability, aggression, and apathy in Huntington and Alzheimer disease, *J Nerv Ment Dis 178(1)*:20 (1990).
87. P. J. Whitehouse, R. P. Friedland, and M. E. Strauss, Neuropsychiatric aspects of degenerative dementias associated with motor dysfunction, *American Psychiatric Press Textbook of Neuropsychiatry*, 2d ed. (S. C. Yudofsky and R. E. Hales, eds.), 1992, pp. 585–604.
88. H. G. Pope and D.L. Katz, Psychiatric and medical effects of anabolic-androgenic steroid use: A controlled study of 160 athletes, *Arch Gen Psychiatry 51*:375 (1994).
89. R. Spiga, D.R. Cherek, J.D. Roache, and K.A. Cowan, The effects of codeine on human aggressive responding, *Int Clin Psychopharmacol 5(3)*:195 (1990).
90. A. Bond and M.H. Lader, Differential effects of oxazepam and lorazepam on aggressive responding, *Psychopharmacology 95*:369 (1988).
91. F.B. Remington and S.L. Rubert, Why patients with brain tumors come to a psychiatric hospital, *Am J Psychiatry 119*:256 (1962).
92. N. Malamud, Psychiatric disorder with intracranial tumors of the limbic system, *Arch Neurol 17*:113 (1967).
93. A. G. Reeves and F. Plum, Hyperphagia, rage, and dementia accompanying a ventromedial hypothalamic neoplasm, *Arch Neurol 20*:616 (1969).
94. M.E. Drake, A. Pakalnis, and B. Phillips, Secondary mania after ventral pontine infarction, *J Neuropsychiatry Clin Neurosci 2*:322 (1990).
95. J.L. Cummings and M.F. Mendez, Secondary mania with focal cerebrovascular lesions, *Am J Psychiatry 141*:1084 (1984).
96. V. Chowdary and R. Abrams, Mania secondary to left and right hemisphere damage, *Am J Psychiatry 140*:1197 (1983).
97. L. B. Starr and K. L. Kubos, Mood changes in stroke patients: Relationship to lesion location, *Comp Psychiatry 24*:555 (1983).
98. R. G. Robinson, J.D. Boston, S.E. Starkstein, and T.R. Price, Comparison of mania and depression after brain injury: Causal factors, *Am J Psychiatry 145*:172 (1988).
99. R.G. Robinson, K.L. Kubos, L.B. Starr, K. Rao, and T.R. Price, Mood disorders in stroke patients: Importance of location of lesion, *Brain 107*:81 (1984).
100. S. E. Starkstein, R.G. Robinson, M.A. Honig, R. M. Parikh, J. Joselyn, and T.R. Price, Mood changes after right-hemisphere lesions, *Br J Psychiatry 155*:79 (1989).

101. M.E. Drake, A. Pakalnis, and B. Phillips, Secondary mania after ventral pontine infarction, *J Neuropsychiatry Clin Neurosci 2*:322 (1990).
102. G. Gainotti, Emotional behavior and hemispheric side of the lesion, *Cortex 8*:41 (1972).
103. R. Teasell, Catastrophic reaction after stroke: A case study, *Am J Phys Med Rehabil 72*:151 (1993).
104. M. Virkkunen, Insulin secretion during the glucose tolerance test among habitually violent and impulsive offenders, *Aggress Behav 12*:303 (1986).
105. M. Virkkunen, Reactive hypoglycemic tendency among habitually violent offenders: A further study by means of the glucose tolerance test, *Neuropsychobiology 8*:35 (1982).
106. S. C. Messer, T. L. Morris, and A. M. Gross, Hypoglycemia and psychopathology: A methodological review, *Clin Psychol Rev 10*:631 (1990).
107. R.B. Kanarek, Nutrition and violent behavior, *Understanding and preventing violence. Volume 2. Biobehavioral influences.* (A.J. Reiss, K.A. Miczek, and J.A. Roth, eds.), National Academy Press, 1994, pp. 515–539.
108. M. E. Dyken, D. C. Lin-Dyken, P. Seaba, and T. Yamada, Violent sleep-related behavior leading to subdural hemorrhage, *Arch Neurol (52)*:318 (1995).
109. M.W. Mahowald, S.R. Bundlie, T.D. Hurwitz, and C.H. Schenck, Sleep violence-Forensic science implications: Polygraphic and video documentation, *J Forens Sci 35*: 413 (1990).
110. Report of the American Academy of Neurology, Assessment, Techniques associated with the diagnosis and management of sleep disorders, *Neurology 42*:269 (1992).
111. A. L. Lazarus and R. Jaffe, Resolution of thyroid-induced schizophreniform disorder following subtotal thyroidectomy: Case report, *Gen Hosp Psychiatry. 8*:29 (1986).
112. M. B. Goldman, Neuropsychiatric features of endocrine disorders, *American Psychiatric Press Textbook of Neuropsychiatry*, American Psychiatric Press, 1992, pp. 519–540.
113. D. J. Kutzer, Psychobiological factors in violent behavior, *Violent Behavior. Vol. 1: Assessment and Intervention* (L. J. Hertzberg, G.F. Ostrum, and J.R. Field, eds.), PMA Publishing, 1990.
114. V. S. Bhatara, J. M. McMillin and M. Kummer, Aggressive behavior and fire-setting in a 4-year-old boy associated with ingestion of ground beef contaminated with bovine thyroid tissue: A case report and review of neuropsychiatric findings in pediatric thyrotoxicosis, *J Child Adolesc Psychopharmacol 5*:255 (1995).
115. V.R. Erhardt and M.B. Goldman, Drug-induced endocrine dysfunction, *Drug-Induced Dysfunction in Psychiatry: Diagnosis and Management* (M.S. Keshavan and J. Kennedy, eds.), Hemisphere Publications 295–310 (1991).
116. M.S. Bauer, M. Droba and P.C. Whybrow, Disorders of the thyroid and parathyroid, *Handbook of Clinical Psychoneuroendocrinology* (C. B. Nemeroff and P.T. Loosen, eds.), Guilford Press, New York, 1987, pp. 41–70.
117. M.N. Chalk, Psychosis in a 15 year old hypothyroid girl: myxoedematous madness? *Aust NZ J Psychiatry 25*:561 (1991).

118. W. M. Easson, Myxedema psychosis- Insanity defense in homicide, *J Clin Psychiatry 41*:316 (1980).
119. C. Joborn, J. Hetta, J. Rastad, H. Ågren, G. Åkerström, and S. Ljunghall, Psychiatric symptoms and cerebrospinal fluid monoamine metabolites in primary hyperparathyroidism, *Biol Psychiatry 23*:149 (1988).
120. S. J. McAllion and C. R. Paterson, Psychiatric morbidity in primary hyperparathyroidism, *Postgrad Med J 65*:628 (1989).
121. R. S. Brown, A. Fischman, and C. R. Showalter, Primary hyperparathyroidism, hypercalcemia, paranoid delusions, homicide, and attempted murder, *J Forensi Sci 32*:1460 (1987).
120. S. J. McAllion and C. R. Paterson, Psychiatric morbidity in primary hyperparathyroidism, *Postgrad Med J 65*:628 (1989).
121. R. S. Brown, A. Fischman, and C. R. Showalter, Primary hyperparathyroidism, hypercalcemia, paranoid delusions, homicide, and attempted murder, *J Forens Sci 32*:1460 (1987).
122. R. D. Alarcon and J. A. Franceschini, Hyperparathyroidism and paranoid psychosis: Case report and review of the literature, *Br J Psychiatry 145*:477 (1984).
123. W. T. Carpenter and P. H. Greun, Cortisol's effects on human mental functioning, *J Clin Psychopharmacol 2(2)*:91 (1982).
124. G. Train and G. Winkler, Homicidal psychosis while under ACTH, *Psychosomatics 3*:317 (1962).
125. J. Volavka, Neurochemistry of violence, *Neurobiology of Violence*, American Psychiatric Press, 1995, pp. 49–76.
126. J. Ehrenkranz, E. Bliss, and M. H. Sheard, Plasma testosterone: Correlation with aggressive behavior and social dominance in man, *Psychosomatic Medicine* 36:469 (1974).
127. R. T. Rada, D. R. Laws, and R. Kellner, Plasma testosterone levels in the rapist, *Psychosom Med 38*:257 (1976).
128. A.H. Buss and A. Durkee, An inventory for assessing different kinds of hostility, *J Consult Clin Psychol 21*:343 (1957).
129. R. T. Rada, R. Laws, R. Kellner, L. Stivastava, and G. Peake, Plasma androgens in violent and nonviolent sex offenders, *Bull Am Acad Psychiatry Law, 11(2)*:149 (1983).
130. L. E. Kreuz and R. M. Rose, Assessment of aggressive behavior and plasma testosterone in a young criminal population, *Psychosom Med 34*:321 (1972).
131. J. Bain, R. Langevin, R. Dickey, and M. Ben-Aron, Sex hormones in murderers and assaulters, *Behav Sci Law 5(1)*:95 (1987).
132. M. Virkunnen, R. Rawlings, R. Tokola, R.E. Poland, A. Guidotti, C. Nemeroff, G. Bissette, K. Kalogeras, S.L. Karonen, and M. Linnoila, CSF biochemistries, glucose metabolism, and diurnal activity rhythms in alcoholic, violent offenders, fire setters, and healthy volunteers, *Arch Gen Psychiatry 51(1)*:20 (1994).
133. J. M. Dabbs, R. B. Ruback, R. L. Frady, C.H. Hopper, and D. S. Sgoutas, Saliva testosterone and criminal violence among women, *Personality Indiv Diff 9(2)*:269 (1988).
134. American Psychiatric Association, *Diagnostic and Statistical Manual of Mental*

Disorders, 4th ed., Washington, DC: American Psychiatric Association, 1994, pp. 715–718.

135. K. D. Denicoff, C. Hoban, G. N. Grover, and D. R. Rubinow, Glucose tolerance testing in women with premenstrual syndrome, *Am J Psychiatry 147*:477 (1990).
136. P. T.d'Orban, J. Dalton, Violent crime and the menstrual cycle, *Psychol Med 10*:353 (1980).
137. K. Dalton, Menstruation and crime, *Br Med J 2*:1752 (1961).
138. D. N. Ruble, Premenstrual symptoms: A reinterpretation. *Science 197*:291 (1977).
139. M.B. Parlee, The premenstrual syndrome, *Psychol Bull 80*:454 (1973).
140. J. M. Reinisch, Prenatal exposure to synthetic progestins increases potential for aggression in humans, *Science 211*:1171 (1981).
141. A. A. Ehrhardt, H. F. L. Meyer-Bahlburg, L. R. Rosen, J. F. Feldman, N. P. Veridiano, E. J. Elkin, and B. S. McEwen, The development of gender-related behavior in females following prenatal exposure to diethylstilbestrol (DES), *Hormone Behav 23*:526 (1989).
142. R.D. Adams and M. Victor, Diseases of the nervous system due to nutritional deficiency, *Principles of Neurology*, 5th ed., McGraw-Hill, New York, 1993, pp. 850–876.
143. D.A. Bender, B Vitamins in the nervous system, *Neurochemi Int 6*:297 (1984).
144. K. Zucker, R.L. Livingston, R. Nakra, and P.J. Clayton, B12 deficiency and psychiatric disorders: Case reports and literature reviews. *Biol Psychiatry 16*:197 (1981).
145. M. Virkunnen, and H. Penttinen, Serum cholesterol in aggressive conduct disorder, *Biol Psychiatry 19*:435, (1984).
146. M. Virkunnen, Serum cholesterol levels in homicidal offenders, *Neuropsychobiology 10*:65 (1983).
147. M.F. Muldoon, S. B. Manuck, and K. A. Matthews, Lowering cholesterol concentrations and mortality: A quantitative review of primary prevention trials, *Br Med J 301*:309 (1990).
148. J. Pekkanen, A. Nissinen, S. Punsar, and M.J. Karvonen, Serum cholesterol and risk of accidental or violent death in a 25-year follow-up, *Arch Intern Med 149*:1589 (1989).
149. F. Plum and J.B. Posner, The diagnosis of stupor and coma, *Contemporary Neurology*, 3d ed., F.A. Davis Philadelphia, 1980.
150. P. Bannister, *Brain's Clinical Neurology*, 5th ed. Oxford University Press, New York, 1978.
151. M.G. Wise and G.T. Brandt, Delirium, *American Psychiatric Press Textbook of Neuropsychiatry*, American Psychiatric Press, 1992, pp. 291–310.
152. L. S. Gross and R. M. Nagy, Neuropsychiatric aspects of poisonous toxic disorders, *American Psychiatric Press Textbook of Neuropsychiatry*, American Psychiatric Press, 1992, pp. 541–561.
153. D. Bear, H. Rosenbaum, and R. Norman, Aggression in cat and human precipitated by a cholinesterase inhibitor, *Psychosomatics 27*:535 (1986).
154. R. S. Schottenfeld and M. R. Cullen, Organic affective illness associated with lead intoxication, *Am J Psychiatry 141*:1423 (1984).

155. W. L. Schoolmeester and D. R. White, Arsenic poisoning, *South Med J 73*:198 (1980).
156. C. Huang, N. Chu, C. Lu, C. Lu, J. Wang, J. Tsai, J. Tzeng, J. Tsai, E. C. Wolters, and D. B. Calne, Chronic manganese intoxication, *Arch Neurol 46*:1104 (1989).

5
Psychiatric Disorders and Violence

Leslie Citrome and Jan Volavka
New York University, New York and Nathan S. Kline Institute for Psychiatric Research, Orangeburg, New York

I. INTRODUCTION

The etiology of violent behavior in patients with psychiatric disorders is multifactorial: (a) comorbid substance abuse, dependence, and intoxication may facilitate violence; (b) the disease process itself may produce hallucinations and delusions that provoke violence, (c) poor impulse control because of neuropsychiatric deficits may facilitate the discharge of aggressive tendencies, (d) underlying character pathology such as antisocial personality traits may also influence the use of violent acts as a means to achieve certain goals, and (e) the ward or other environment may be chaotic, further encouraging maladaptive behaviors.

In addition to the differential diagnosis, the *pattern* of violent behavior may provide clues for management. Transient and the persistent violence may differ in their causes and treatments.

This chapter begins with an overview of the epidemiology of violence and mental disorders, followed by a review of several broad categories of psychiatric disorders with an emphasis on schizophrenia. Clinical vignettes preface each section. Also included is a discussion of whether or not pharmacotherapeutic interventions can lead to violent behavior.

II. OVERVIEW OF THE EPIDEMIOLOGY OF VIOLENCE AND MENTAL DISORDERS

Studies of relationships between mental disorders and violent behavior typically use one of two complementary approaches: a mental disorder can be seen as a risk factor for violent behavior or violent behavior can be seen as a risk factor for mental disorder (1). The first approach examines the prevalence of violent behavior among persons with mental disorders (in identified mental patients or in random community samples); the second examines the prevalence of mental disorder among persons exhibiting violent behavior (in identified criminal offenders or in random community samples).

A. Violent Behavior Among Persons with Mental Disorders

1. Community Samples

Self-reports of violent behavior were obtained in the Epidemiological Catchment Area (ECA) project. The primary purpose of the project was to estimate the prevalence of untreated psychiatric disorders in the population of the United States. To that end, structured diagnostic interviews were administered to over 20,000 persons residing in five areas of the United States, either in the community or in institutions (2).

In approximately 50% of this sample (i.e., approximately in 10,000 persons), data on violence were collected. The interviewers inquired about the following behaviors in the past year: use of a weapon in a fight, history of fighting, child beating, wife (or partner) beating, and physical fights while drinking. On the basis of this self-report, the subjects were dichotomously classified as either violent or nonviolent. A logistic regression model of predictors of violence was performed (3). The predictors included gender, age, socioeconomic status, marital status, and psychiatric diagnosis. The effect of psychiatric diagnosis on the probability of being violent was computed after the effects of the other predictors were accounted for statistically (i.e., the other predictors were used as covariates). The resulting probability estimates for various diagnoses are displayed in Table 1.

Table 1 shows that the probabilities of violent behavior in male and female patients with schizophrenia were, respectively, 5.3 and 5.9 times higher than in persons without any diagnosed mental disorder. The probabilities were also higher for patients diagnosed with affective disorder but not for those with anxiety disorder. Patients with a mental disorder and a comorbid substance-abuse disorder had the highest probabilities of all.

The results reported by Swanson et al. (3) were supported by a smaller epidemiological study comparing 385 psychiatric patients (current or former) living in a community with 365 other community residents who have never received psychiatric treatment (the number of subjects reported in this study varies slightly depending on the availability of data) (4,5). The self-reports of violent behaviors—hitting someone, fighting, and using a weapon—were,

Table 1 Violent Behavior, Gender, and Psychiatric Diagnosis

Current Year Psychiatric Diagnosis	Percent Probability of Violent Behavior		Adjusted Chi-Square	Statistical Significance
	Male	Female		
None	2.45	1.38	–	–
Anxiety disorder	2.91	1.79	0.42	n.s.
Affective disorder	8.41	5.70	10.57	$p < .0001$
Schizophrenia or schizoaffective	13.12	8.16	5.04	$p < .05$
Substance abuse	21.64	17.10	127.72	$p < .0001$
Mental disorder and substance abuse	22.29	17.43	61.87	$p < .0001$

Source: Adapted from Ref. 3.

respectively, 2.4, 1.7, and 3.6 times more frequent in the patients than in the nonpatients (5). Interestingly, these violent behaviors were specifically related to three psychiatric symptoms: feeling of domination by external force, thought insertion, and the feeling that others wished to harm one.

A study of an unselected Swedish birth cohort by Hodgins (6) supported and expanded the relationships reported by Swanson (3) and Link (4,5). The cohort consisted of 15,117 persons born in Stockholm in 1953. Among persons without mental disorder, the conviction rate for violent offenses was 5.7% in the men and 0.5% in the women. Men with major mental disorders were approximately four times more likely to have been convicted of violent offenses than men without any mental disorder, and women were approximately 27 times more likely to be convicted than women without mental disorder.

A larger unselected cohort comprising of 324,401 Danes born between January 1, 1944, and December 31, 1947, was followed up to the age of 43 years with respect to psychiatric admission and criminal proceedings as documented in national registries (7). Both men and women hospitalized at least once with major mental disorders (schizophrenia, manic-depressive psychosis, psychogenic psychosis, or other psychosis), mental retardation, antisocial personality disorder, drug-abuse disorders, alcohol-abuse disorders, and other mental disorders were more likely to have registered for at least one violent crime than persons with no history of psychiatric admissions. This was not the case for women diagnosed with organic disorders where there was no statistically significant increase in relative risk for violent crime. For the period 1978 to 1990, where computerized national police data were used in the analysis, men hospitalized with major mental disorders were approximately nine times more likely to have been convicted of at least one violent offense than men with no history of psychiatric hospitalizations. For women, this relative risk was approximately 4.5. A hierarchy of diagnoses was used, taking into account only one diagnosis per subject, with major mental disorders at the top of the hierarchy; thus comorbidity with alcohol or substance abuse was not evaluated.

These Scandinavian studies indicate that links between violent behavior in the community and major mental illness, demonstrated in the American studies, are not limited to the United States. However, generalizing the actual odds ratios to the United States may be inappropriate. The rates of violent crime committed by persons without mental disorders are much higher in the United States than in Scandinavia.

Thus, the results obtained in the American and Scandinavian populations indicate that major mental disorders elevate the risk for violent behavior. However, a causal relationship between the two phenomena (violence and psychosis) has not been established by these studies. A hypothesis stating that psychosis causes violence would be supported by a finding of clear temporal linkage between them; one would also test whether the patients are more violent when they are more psychotic.

That linkage was studied by interviewing 121 incarcerated psychotic forensic patients about the motives for the offenses committed while they were living in the community (8). Most of these patients were diagnosed with schizophrenia. The author estimated that 82% of their offenses (violent and nonviolent offenses combined) were attributable to their illness. Delusions were the driving force for violent offending among these patients. Thus, this study has established the time linkage between delusions and the offense that was lacking in the studies discussed above (3–5): the patients were delusional at the time when they committed their offenses.

Data from the ECA project and the other recent studies we discussed represent a major advance in the epidemiology of violent behavior in psychiatric disorders. However, they have certain weaknesses. One of these weaknesses is that violent behaviors (e.g., fighting) are presented as categorical variables (present or absent). Thus, recidivistically violent patients are lumped together with those who are violent just once. Frequency of violent behavior is an important variable. We return to this issue later.

2. Hospital Samples

a. Short-Term Hospitalization. Violent or threatening behavior is a frequent reason for the admission to a psychiatric inpatient facility, and that behavior may continue after the admission. The association between preadmission threats and postadmission violence is particularly strong among schizophrenic patients and did not reach statistical significance for patients with mania (9). During the first 24 hours after the admission to a psychiatric inpatient unit, 33 (13.0%) of 253 patients physically attacked another person (10). Manic patients were the most likely diagnostic group to be assaultive during the initial phase of hospitalization, with 12 out of 46 patients (26.1%) attacking another person. In contrast, 9 out of 87 (10.3%) diagnosed with schizophrenia, and 12 out of 120 (10%) diagnosed with a disorder other than schizophrenia or mania attacked another person during the same period. Another group reported that in the first 8 days after hospitalization, 25 of 289 schizophrenic or schizoaffective patients (8.7%) assaulted someone at least once (11).

b. Long-Term Hospitalization. A study of 5164 long-term patients indicated that 7% of them physically attacked another person at least once during a 3-month period (12). Assaultive patients were more likely than nonassaultive patients to have a primary diagnosis of nonparanoid schizophrenia, psychotic organic brain syndrome, mental retardation, or personality disorder. Mania was not reported on in this study.

This and similar studies do not distinguish between recidivistic and transient assaultiveness. But such distinction is important. Persistent (recidivistic) and transient violence may differ in their neurobiological underpinning, management, and social consequences (13–15). A 6-month study of 1552 inpatients with various diagnoses detected 576 violent incidents; a small group of recidivistic patients (5%) caused 53% of the incidents (16). The diagnosis of schizophrenia was slightly overrepresented among the male recidivists; personality and impulse disorder diagnoses were frequent among the male and female recidivists.

B. Mental Disorders Among Violent Criminal Offenders

Traditionally, frequency estimates of violent behavior relied heavily on *arrest records*. These records tend to show an increase of the arrest rates of mental patients in the United States over the past several decades. However, many problems complicate the interpretation of arrest data. If a suspect is apprehended, the police have considerable discretion in deciding whether to arrest and what to charge. The discretionary power to adopt alternatives to arrest is typically exercised when suspects are juvenile or when they appear ill (in which case they may be taken to a hospital emergency room rather than to the police station). Even if an arrest is made, the charge may not fully reflect the severity of the criminal behavior. Arrest statistics thus underestimate the "true" crime rate and provide a biased description of offender characteristics as well as of the type of criminal behaviors actually occurring. Therefore, it is not surprising that arrest record yield rather "soft" data. Controversies surrounding these data are reviewed elsewhere

(17). Rather than studying arrest data, one can focus on mental illness among prisoners. Severe mental illness has a much higher prevalence among prisoners than in the general population (18). Like the arrest data, prisoners' mental health statistics do not yield very specific information on the relationship between violent acts and mental illness.

Such information can be obtained by focusing research on offenders convicted of a specific violent crime. To maximize the data's validity, the crime that is selected for such research should be one that is not underreported and that has a high rate of clearance (i.e., the perpetrator is identified and arrested). Homicide meets these criteria.

Prevalence of mental illness was studied among persons who committed homicide in Finland during an 8 year period (19). The Finnish police solved 96.9% of all homicides during this period. Finnish courts of law ordered a comprehensive forensic psychiatric examination on 693 of the 994 offenders. Each subject was evaluated with a psychiatric examination, a battery of psychological tests, laboratory tests, and observation in a hospital normally lasting from 4 to 8 weeks. The 301 offenders not evaluated were considered not mentally disordered, but the authors noted that, on occasion, the Finnish courts of law consider that offenders with alcohol problems, antisocial personality disorder, anxiety disorders, or dysthymia do not need to be examined by this thorough forensic examination. Male homicide offenders were approximately eight times more likely to have schizophrenia (49.2% having paranoid schizophrenia), twelve times more likely to have antisocial personality disorder, and eleven times more likely to have alcoholism than men in the general population. Major depression increased the risk only slightly in men. There was no increased risk in mental retardation. Female homicide offenders were approximately 6.5 times more likely to have schizophrenia, 54 times more likely to have antisocial personality disorder, and 40 times more likely to have alcoholism than women in the general population.

If analogous studies were conducted in the United States, the risk for serious mental illness among homicide offenders would perhaps be lower than that in Finland. We assume that the easy availability of guns, violence associated with the illegal drugs traffic, and various racial and socioeconomic factors would be expected to reduce the relative importance of serious mental illness for homicide (and other violent crime) in the United States. Some data supporting this assumption have been published (20); cross-cultural studies of this type are very difficult to implement.

In summary, mental illness is associated with elevated prevalence of violent behavior, and violent crime is associated with elevated prevalence of mental illness.

III. SCHIZOPHRENIA AND OTHER PSYCHOTIC DISORDERS

A. Auditory Hallucinations and Paranoid Delusions

John is a 25-year-old white male with a history of two prior psychiatric hospitalizations for schizophrenia. He lives alone, is unemployed, and has few social contacts. He has missed his last two monthly appointments at the Community Mental Health Center, where he had been receiving injections of haloperidol decanoate, a depot neuroleptic, for the past 9 months. He was brought in by the police to the local community hospital after having assaulted a clerk at a nearby grocery store. John is currently exhibiting disorganized speech and is rambling about the CIA, FBI, and KGB conducting an investigation about him and that the grocery store clerk was a spy who was going to shoot him.

Patients with schizophrenia may present acutely with aggressive and violent behavior. This may be due to acute decompensation secondary to covert or overt noncompliance with psychotropic medication. Decompensation may also be due to a failure of the current medication regimen. The clinical features expected would be a worsening of psychotic symptoms and possibly command hallucinations, although the importance of the latter in violent behavior is in dispute (21–24). Studies report that from 24 to 44% of aggressive incidents committed by individuals with schizophrenia occur during an acute phase of the illness (21,25,26). Neuroleptic blood levels have been found to be inversely correlated with danger-related events in a group of recently hospitalized male schizophrenic patients (27).

A patient with paranoid schizophrenia with a delusional focus on interpersonal relationships may be sufficiently intact to actually plan and execute violent acts (28), but the presence of paranoid delusions in itself may not predict violence (29). This has been a focus in the prevention of violence in the workplace (30), where paranoid schizophrenia, delusional disorder, and paranoid personality disorder are considered. Those who make threats toward the president of the United States or other prominent American political figures are typically described as having chronic paranoid schizophrenia (31).

B. Comorbid Substance Abuse

Susan is a 30-year-old black female who has been hospitalized in the past at several local and state hospitals for schizophrenia. She usually presents with auditory hallucinations of a male voice commenting on her behavior. She also believes that her telephone is tapped and that her television is "reverse-broadcasting" her picture back to the television studio. She attends a local day-treatment program but lately has been seen at night with known drug dealers in the community. After several days of absence at the day-treatment program, the crisis service receives a call from the police precinct. Susan was witnessed by several people to have stabbed another woman but is telling the police that she was at her program. Susan later admitted to have smoked "crack" cocaine and becoming even more paranoid, although she vehemently denies that she actually stabbed anyone.

Some of the violent behavior occurring among schizophrenic patients is attributable to comorbidity with substance abuse (3,32). The relationship is illustrated by Table 1, which shows that substance abuse elevates the probability of violent behavior substantially more than schizophrenia alone. Schizophrenia and substance abuse disorders cooccur more frequently than expected by chance. Data from the ECA project, discussed earlier, indicate that 47% of all individuals with a lifetime diagnosis of schizophrenia have also met criteria for substance abuse or dependence (2).

Schizophrenia was found to elevate very significantly the risks for alcohol dependence as well as for drug dependence. Conversely, substance use disorders elevated the risk for schizophrenia. Aggressive and violent behavior in patients with schizophrenia can be precipitated by alcohol, cocaine, phencyclidine (PCP), or amphetamine intoxication (33). The importance of these findings is underscored by the reported increase in the prevalence estimates of comorbid substance abuse with schizophrenia over several decades (34). In 1993, illicit drugs were detected in urine samples of the majority of the arrested males in 23 U.S. cities (ranging from 54% in Omaha to 81% in Chicago) (35). Odds of violence are particularly elevated for schizophrenic or schizoaffective patients having a pattern of polysubstance abuse (36). Inpatients can also be abusing illicit substances, because access to drugs and alcohol, although difficult, is not impossible. Caffeine intoxication, water intoxication, antihistamine intoxication, and the ingestion of deodorants and aerosols have also been described in inpatients (37).

C. Neurological Impairment

Martin is a 50-year-old white male hospitalized continuously for the past 15 years at the State Psychiatric Center. For the last 6 years he has been housed on the special secure unit because of his history of unprovoked attacks on other patients. He shows no interest in his environment, does not participate in therapeutic groups, and has poor personal hygiene. Despite having emphysema, he does smoke cigarettes at every opportunity and is easily frustrated and irritated if his smoking is curtailed by staff. He has a history of auditory hallucinations and bizarre delusions in the past but is relatively uncommunicative now, and the current presence of hallucinations or delusions cannot be readily ascertained. He has been nonresponsive to several typical neuroleptic medications and is being considered for therapy with clozapine if only he would consent to the mandatory weekly blood testing. On his annual routine physical examinations, no physical signs of coarse brain disease were ever evident. When examined by the consultant from the local medical school, Martin showed subtle impairment on frontal motor tasks.

Central to the development of a differential diagnosis is the analysis of the pattern of violence. Factors such as whether aggressive episodes are singular or repetitive, regular or sporadic, and with low or high potential for actual injury will guide the clinician in formulating immediate management plans, a provisional diagnosis, and long-term strategy. Some patients are transiently violent when in a chaotic environment, others are persistently violent independent of the milieu (38). The persistently violent were found to be more likely to have neurological impairments as evidenced by impairments in stereognosis, graphesthesia, tandem walk and walking-associated movements, and selective impairment in visual-spatial functioning found on neuropsychological testing (14,39). In another study, lateralized abnormalities in EEGs were found in a group of persistently violent psychiatric inpatients, most of whom had schizophrenia (40). Organic brain dysfunction has been found in maximum-security forensic psychiatric patients (41). A Quantified Neurological Examination has been developed to assess subtle neurological dysfunction and has been demonstrated to differentiate violent from matched nonviolent psychiatric inpatients (42). It has also been related to the degree of violence and to poor treatment response (39). Brain computed tomography (CT) has been employed to compare violent and nonviolent schizophrenic inpatients (43), but the results of this pilot study did not demonstrate any significant differences other than a possible larger sylvian fissure for the violent group. A more detailed discussion regarding the neurology of aggression in general can be found elsewhere (44,45), as can a review of the psychobiology of the violent offender (46), and the neurobiology of violence (17).

In contrast to the persistently violent patient, those who were transiently violent were more likely to respond to a new structured environment (47). Environmental factors leading to increased aggressive behavior on a psychiatric ward include crowding (48) and possibly an overauthoritative attitude by nursing staff and underinvolvement of medical staff with ward activities (49). Time of day may be a factor with a peak problem period of 7 to 9 a.m. reported in one facility (50). It appears that the transiently violent are more responsive to typical neuroleptic medication and have less neurological impairment than the persistently violent patient (51).

Medical conditions such as newly developed brain tumors or metabolic disturbances may precipitate aggressive behavior in a patient not normally known to be violent.

D. Comorbid Antisocial Personality Disorder

> David is a 30-year-old white male recently rehospitalized for the third time, having expressed paranoid delusions that his landlord was plotting to kill him. On the hospital ward the staff noted that although David had no money when admitted, he had soon accumulated over $100. Other patients revealed that they had bought cigarettes from David and that one patient sold his portable radio to David for "$2 and a cigarette." When confronted by the staff, he denied any wrongdoing. He was later accused of punching another patient who David thought had informed on him. When the Incident Review Committee conducted an investigation, they located an old psychiatric assessment dating back to when David was 14 years old, when he was diagnosed as having a conduct disorder. David was noted to have been a bully who often initiated physical fights. He was once accused of forcing another child into sexual activity. He ran away from home several times and was often truant from school, starting at age 12. The Incident Review Committee also uncovered that David had several other hospital admissions under a different name and that most admissions were notable for irritability, aggressiveness, and stealing from other patients and staff.

Antisocial personality disorders may coexist with schizophrenia, and antisocial personality traits may be present even if the full disorder cannot be diagnosed. Data from the ECA study indicate that in males diagnosed with antisocial personality disorder, schizophrenia occurs at the rate that is seven times higher (and in the females, twelve time higher) than the expected rate (52). These strong cross-sectional associations between schizophrenia and antisocial personality disorder are consistent with the observation of frequent conduct problems in the premorbid history of schizophrenic patients (53). Violence secondary to the comorbidity of schizophrenia and antisocial personality disorder/traits may be evaluated by examining the context of the aggressive incident. Intimidation of patients and staff or material gain may be factors. For example, there may be some fighting over money, cigarettes, access to sexual partners, and attacks on caregivers who deny a patient's request or try to set limits to patients' behaviors (such as enforcing a smoking ban). Engagement in illegal activities, rule breaking, lying, and a lack of remorse are only a few of the criteria in the diagnosis of antisocial personality disorder in DSM-IV (54). These characteristics may be found in both inpatient and outpatients populations. Misdiagnosis of schizophrenia as antisocial personality disorder can occur, possibly missing an opportunity for treatment (55). Chronically psychotic patients can also make sociopathic adaptations to the environments imposed on them as a result of their illnesses, and this can distort the clinical picture, an example being the individual whose psychotic symptoms diminish when his welfare check is due to arrive (56).

IV. PERSONALITY DISORDERS AND IMPULSE CONTROL

A. Antisocial Personality Disorder (ASP)

> Brian is a 50-year-old white male currently incarcerated for armed robbery. As a child he was noted to be disruptive and cruel to animals; he also often played with matches. As an adolescent he would vandalize the property of others and was well known by the local police. He spent close to a year at a special Division for Youth facility after he was arrested for a burglary that had escalated into a robbery and during which the homeowner was stabbed. As an adult, Brian has spent a great deal of his time in various municipal lockups and county jails. He once served 6 years at the state prison after a conviction of manslaughter. Brian has never held a job for more than a few weeks at a time. He would often be dismissed after getting into a fight with his coworkers and supervisors. He has never shown remorse or regret.

Among the subtypes of personality disorder, ASP has the closest links to violence and is, in part, defined by acts of violence. In the DSM-IV (54), diagnostic criterion B calls for evidence of conduct disorder with onset before age 15. Of the 15 items defining conduct disorder, 7 involve physical aggression against people or animals: bullying, fighting, using weapons, physical cruelty to people or animals, robbing, forcing someone into sexual activity. Furthermore, "repeated physical fights or assaults" are listed as an optional item for the diagnostic criterion C (concerned with behavior after the age of 15).

The validity of the ASP definitions in the DSM-III and DSM-IIIR (which were closely related to the current DSM-IV definition) was supported by neurobiological studies (57). Nevertheless, these definitions of ASP have some disadvantages for violence research. Since only 7 of the 15 items defining conduct disorder in the DSM-IV involve physical aggression and since only 3 of the 15 criteria need to be met for the diagnosis of conduct disorder, Criterion B for ASP can be met without a history of violence, or it can be met exclusively (or partly) by items reflecting violence. Criterion C can be met with or without violence. Thus, without the individual items leading to the diagnosis (which are rarely published), the ASP diagnosis per se does not allow an inference about violence.

An answer to the question "Does ASP predict violent behavior?" thus depends on the items constituting the diagnosis in individual cases. Since the mix of items varies among subjects and studies, ASP-based results concerning violent behavior are difficult to replicate. Furthermore, the list of ASP diagnostic criteria contains many behaviors that are against the law. The criteria needed for the ASP diagnosis can be met without any history of illegal behavior, or they can be met exclusively (or partly) by items reflecting illegal behavior. The diagnosis of ASP per se does not allow any inference about illegal behavior. However, we can assume that offenders who meet the ASP criteria do so primarily for the same reasons that brought them to the attention of the criminal justice system. This reduces the utility of the ASP diagnosis in studies of prisoners and similar populations: a diagnostic procedure is not needed to determine that these subjects broke laws.

This problem was recognized in a study of mental disorders among jail detainees (58–60). The investigators addressed it by omitting from some of their analyses the responses to two questions "directly related to arrest and conviction history"; these questions were part of the diagnostic interview for the ASP (61). The omission affected the results very little.

Comorbidity of ASP with other disorders may affect the likelihood of violent behavior. ASP diagnosis was associated with violent crime among jail detainees, and the number of arrests for violent crime was further elevated among detainees who had substance abuse disorders cooccurring with ASP (58). Cooccurrence of schizophrenia and ASP was discussed earlier.

The term *psychopathy* was used loosely until Cleckley endowed it with specific content, a conceptual framework, and classic clinical descriptions (62). Hare developed a Psychopathy Checklist based on Cleckley's work (63–66). Unlike the current ASP criteria, the checklist focuses on personality traits and psychological processes rather than criminal behaviors (67,68). These traits and processes may be more difficult to define and ascertain than discrete criminal behaviors such as an arrest for driving while intoxicated. Several studies using either the checklist or its earlier version demonstrated that the psychopathy defined by these instruments was associated with violent crime (69). The instruments were typically used to classify offenders into two or three categories (psychopaths and nonpsychopaths, or psychopaths, mixed, and nonpsychopaths). Convictions of violent crime were more frequent among the psychopaths (85%) than the nonpsychopaths (54%). Very similar group differences were obtained for violent behavior observed in prison (69).

B. Borderline Personality Disorder

> Louise is a 24-year-old white female living with her well-to-do parents. She has just completed graduate studies in sociology and is seeking employment. The past 8 years have been punctuated by frequent but short hospital admissions, usually occurring after a breakup with a boyfriend, when she would mutilate herself by cutting her arms with a razor. Her interpersonal relationships would be marked by extremes of idealization and devaluation. She also had several periods of promiscuity and substance abuse. When angry, Louise would frequently throw a temper tantrum. This latter behavior would sometimes escalate into a physical fight. Her psychotherapist reports that Louise has been working on identity issues and her chronic feelings of emptiness.

Borderline personality disorder is defined in part by impulsiveness, recurrent anger with lack of control reflected by physical fights, and suicidal threats or behavior (54). Borderline (or antisocial) personality traits were found among men who physically abused women (70). A significant association between the presence of borderline symptomatology and recent use of physical violence inside and outside the hospital was found in a retrospective review of 4800 consecutive admissions to a hospital operated by the U.S. Department of Veterans Affairs (71).

Borderline behavioral features are linked to a central serotonin disturbance. Some important studies of the biological aspects of personality disorders are concerned with central serotonergic function. Among 17 patients meeting diagnostic criteria for various personality disorders, 8 with borderline personality disorder showed a particularly pronounced dysfunction of the central serotonergic system, and they may have largely accounted for the reported relationship between aggressive behavior and serotonergic dysfunction (72).

C. Impulse Control

Richard is a 35-year-old black male working in commercial construction as a mason. He is married with two children and has no history of drug or alcohol abuse. He describes "spells" or "attacks" in which he feels tense, followed by relief only after he has destroyed something nearby. This usually occurs during periods of stress, when pressure is placed on him at work to be more efficient. It has sometimes led to job loss, but his area of work is in such high demand that he never has trouble getting other employment Sometimes he strikes other people, and he has been arrested in the past. He has never actually been incarcerated and has always expressed remorse, regret, and embarrassment about his "losing control." Richard has never presented with clinically significant depression and has never expressed psychotic symptoms. He has no significant medical illnesses.

Impulse control is a concept of pivotal importance for the psychobiology of violence (73). It links criminologists' explanations of criminal propensity by inadequate "self-control" (74) or impaired "impulse control" (75) to the data on the role of serotonin in impulsive violence (76,77) and to the animal research on capacity to wait (delay response) (78). Inadequate impulse control may be a relatively permanent personality attribute (impulsiveness as a trait).

Barratt (79) describes three aspects of disinhibitory psychopathology that define, in part, syndromes or diagnostic categories. These aspects or subtraits were labeled as motor, cognitive, and "nonplanning" impulsiveness. Motor impulsiveness (physical activity without forethought) is a core symptom of attention-deficit hyperactivity disorder; furthermore, it is negatively related to a measure of central serotonergic activity in patients with personality disorders (72).

Cognitive impulsiveness involves rapid and careless decision making. Non-planning impulsiveness implies lack of concern for the future.

DSM-IV (54) has a special section on "Impulsive Control Disorders Not Elsewhere Classified." Intermittent explosive disorder has the following (abbreviated) diagnostic criteria:

> A. Several discrete episodes of loss of control of aggressive impulses resulting in serious assaultive acts or destruction of property. B. The degree of aggressiveness during episodes is out of proportion to precipitating stress. C. The episodes of loss of control are not better accounted for by antisocial or borderline personality disorders, psychosis, attention deficit/hyperactivity disorder, and are not due to the direct effects of a substance or a general medical condition (e.g., personality change due to head injury).

Many patients diagnosed in the 1960s and 1970s with "episodic dyscontrol syndrome" (80) or "explosive personality" (DSM-II), would now be diagnosed with "intermittent explosive disorder." Patients diagnosed with episodic dyscontrol syndrome have shown numerous signs of neuropsychiatric dysfunction (81–83). Such signs are probably also detectable by careful examination in many patients diagnosed with intermittent explosive disorder today. The signs may not be obvious to clinicians (who therefore use this residual diagnostic category). It is not clear whether any patients would retain the diagnosis of intermittent explosive disorder after the other disorders (which must be ruled out before this diagnosis can be made) are excluded by careful examination. Thus, the usefulness of intermittent explosive disorder as a diagnostic category is in doubt.

Offenders diagnosed (DSM-III) with explosive personality disorder were among the impulsive violent criminals reported to have low CSF 5-HIAA levels (84). Serotonergic dysfunction could be a neurobiological basis of explosive personality disorder. All subjects with explosive personality disorder, however, also had a diagnosis of borderline personality disorder, and their violent behavior occurred frequently under the influence of alcohol. It is uncertain how many of these subjects would meet the newly introduced (DSM-IV) diagnostic criterion C for intermittent explosive disorder.

A relationship between the childhood history of fire setting and adult violent crime (murder, assault, robbery, and rape) was reported among prisoners examined at a psychiatric forensic unit (85). Fire setting alone, as well as a combination of fire setting, enuresis, and cruelty to animals, was reported more frequently among prisoners charged with violent crimes than among the other prisoners. Twenty adult arsonists "who apparently did not set fire for economic gains" were compared with 20 habitually violent offenders and 10 normal controls (86). The arsonists had lower CSF levels of two monoamine metabolites (5-HIAA and MHPG) than the other groups and low glucose nadirs in the oral glucose tolerance test. Of the 20 arsonists, 19 were diagnosed (DSM-III) with borderline personality disorder and 17 with alcohol abuse; 18 set fires under the influence of alcohol. It is not clear whether the arsonists' primary impulse was to drink alcohol or to set fires. Impulsive features are shared by impulse control disorders, substance abuse disorders, eating disorders, and personality disorders (87).

V. MOOD DISORDERS

Helga is a 40-year-old single white female with a 15-year history of bipolar disorder. She has been noncompliant with her mood stabilizer, lithium carbonate, saying that it "slows her down" and "gives her tremors." For the past week she has been irritable and sleeping very little. She has been more talkative than usual and has been expressing thoughts of starting her own business selling gambling novelties across all the K-Mart stores in the United States. She has been sexually promiscuous, which ordinarily is out of character for her. Her sister brought her in to the local emergency room and told the triage nurse that her sister was having a manic episode and needed to be put back on her medication. Helga appears distracted and has no insight as to why she was brought to the hospital. She becomes enraged when the interviewing psychiatrist suggests hospitalization and strikes him the face with her pocketbook. She is then admitted on an emergency basis as an involuntary patient.

Using a sample of 1140 recently incarcerated male felons, evidence was found of a direct relationship between a lifetime diagnosis of dysthymia and an arrest or incarceration history for robbery as well as with multiple incidents of fighting since age 18 (88). The authors did not find as strong an association between manic symptoms and violence. In a sample of 20 inpatients with mania and 856 other diagnoses, assaultiveness was not present in the manic group even though agitation was seen more frequently when compared to all other diagnostic categories (89). In contrast, another investigator reported that manic patients were the most likely diagnostic group to be assaultive during the initial phase of hospitalization (10). In a psychiatric intensive care unit operated within a Veteran Administration Medical Center, the manic state was associated with violent behavior among 40 male psychiatric inpatients diagnosed with bipolar disorder (90).

The association between homicide and depression has also been reported on (91–93). Comorbidity with alcohol/substance abuse and/or personality disorders appears to be a prominent feature in these cases.

VI. ANXIETY DISORDERS

Charles is a 55-year-old black male who, while serving as a private in the Marines in Vietnam, witnesses the death of his entire squad in an ambush.

He remembers vividly how an explosive decapitated his best friend. Charles survived only because he was under the body of another solider and was left for dead. Upon return to his home in New York City he experienced recurrent and intrusive recollections of the events in Vietnam and was plagued with nightmares. He found that he had to avoid going to Chinatown because it made him very anxious. He was wary of all Orientals. Charles became a loner and felt detached from others. He had not expected to live to his present age and felt guilty about surviving when all his buddies had died. He engaged in risky behaviors, including intravenous drug abuse. He never married, finding himself unable to have loving feelings. Charles developed chronic sleep problems, difficulty concentrating, and significant irritability. He became involved in fights with strangers when they got in his way. It was during one of these chance encounters that he knocked his opponent into a concrete wall, causing his death. This led to Charles being incarcerated. In prison, he continues to be considered by the other inmates as disturbed and as someone to be avoided.

Posttraumatic stress disorder (PTSD) has been associated with anger, hostility, and violence, although the presence of comorbid conditions such as mood disorders and substance abuse disorders may be confounding. In a study of 27 Vietnam veteran outpatients with PTSD and 15 non-PTSD Vietnam combat veteran controls, PTSD subjects scored significantly higher than non-PTSD subjects on measures of hostility and violence (94). Excluded were subject candidates with a current diagnosis of organic mental, bipolar, schizophrenic, paranoid, delusional, or other psychotic disorder or with alcohol or other substance dependence or abuse within the preceding year. Comorbid disorders in the PTSD subjects included major depression, dysthymia, and other anxiety disorders as well as antisocial personality disorder. Analysis of covariance was done to control for the potentially confounding effects of group differences in psychiatric comorbidity, education, combat exposure, neurological soft signs, and past history of substance abuse or dependence. Results for the aggression measures remained statistically significant when adjusted for these covariates with only one exception for one of the scales (Hostility Inventory) with one of the covariates (education). Adjusted partial correlations indicated that there was a significant relationship between PTSD severity and aggression. This study may not be generalizable to females with PTSD or to persons with non-combat-related PTSD.

A nationally representative sample of 1200 male Vietnam veterans and the spouses or partners of 376 of these veterans were extensively interviewed using a structured set of questions (95). Elevated levels of violence were found in the homes of veterans with PTSD, both by the veteran and by his spouse or partner.

Panic disorder with aggressive thoughts and behaviors in association with panic symptoms has been reported in a series of three patients (96). The case descriptions hint at significant disturbances of mood, impulse control, and the presence of substance abuse and history of trauma.

VII. MENTAL RETARDATION

> Elizabeth is a 22-year-old black female with moderate mental retardation living in a group home with five other mentally retarded adults. She has a low frustration tolerance and has been difficult to manage. The group home's director has been asking for help from the psychiatric consultant and a trial of thioridazine was recommended. Despite the sedative effects of the thioridazine, Elizabeth remained intermittently agitated and, during one of these episodes, struck one of the attendants with a telephone, causing a laceration on his scalp. Elizabeth was then brought to the local hospital emergency room, where the group home's direct or demanded that she be admitted before "someone else gets hurt."

Aggressive behavior in the mentally retarded is a common clinical problem. In a survey of 2158 mentally handicapped patients institutionalized in Eastern Ontario, 920 (43%) were identified as problem cases, with roughly a third considered aggressive (97). In a study of psychoactive drug use in public and community residential facilities for mentally retarded persons in Missouri, out of a random sample of 466 subjects, 26% were described as having serious behavior problems (defined as clients who were considered dangerous to themselves or who frequently exhibited violent or destructive behavior) and 58% as having moderate behavior problems (defined as clients whose behaviors while not frequently being dangerous or destructive might disrupt or jeopardize residential or program placement) (98). Utilization of neuroleptic medication was common for these groups.

In an unselected Swedish birth cohort followed up to age 30 years (6), intellectually handicapped men were five times more likely to commit a violent offense than men with no disorder or handicap. Intellectually handicapped women were 25 times more likely to commit a violent offense. This contrasts with the major mental disorders (schizophrenia, major affective disorders, paranoid states, and other psychoses), were the increase in risk for committing a violent offense was 4 times for men and 27 times for women. Another birth cohort from Denmark, followed to age 43, provided similar findings, with the relative risk estimate of committing a violent crime being the same or higher for mental retardation as for the major mental disorders (7).

Grizenko (99) reported on 176 mentally retarded individuals from two facilities and nine group homes in Montreal. Age range was 11 to 58 years, with a mean of 25. Behavior was measured using a standardized 113-item questionnaire with several subscales describing degrees of hyperactivity, aggressivity, immaturity, uncommunicativeness, delinquency, anxiety, schizoid behavior, and somatization. Moderately retarded subjects presented with more severe behavior problems, including aggression, than the severely mentally retarded. The severity of the behavior disturbance did not vary with age.

A Norwegian study of assaultiveness among institutionalized adults with mental retardation also revealed an association between the degree of mental retardation and assaultive behavior (100). Fifty-seven patients with mental retardation who had shown assaultive behavior during the prior year were compared with an equal number of controls from the same institution matched on gender, age, and functional level. Aggressive behavior was more frequent among the moderately mentally retarded than in patients with profound mental retardation, possibly because of reduced mobility for some of the profoundly retarded patients. The assaultive group was younger than the comparison group, had more psychopathology, and consumed more psychotropic medications. There were no group differences found in level of vision, hearing impairment, personal hygiene, ability to feed, tendency to get lost outside the ward, ambulation ability, and communication skills. The assaultive group had more resources allocated to it, including better-educated personnel, access to single rooms, and greater living space.

Among mild to moderate mentally retarded persons, the cooccurrence of mental retardation and antisocial personality disorder has been described (101). In all six of the cases, violent crime was a predominant feature. The investigators caution that the development of antisocial personality disorder among the mentally retarded may not be rare and that recognition of this is important in order to prevent further violence.

VIII. DO PSYCHOTROPICS CAUSE VIOLENT BEHAVIOR?

Paradoxical reactions to benzodiazepines, as exhibited by hostility or violence, has been an area of concern (102,103), but the evidence is not convincing. Disinhibition with benzodiazepines is in any event uncommon (104) and even more unlikely to occur when given within the context of single or limited doses in a crisis situation (17).

Concomitant seizure disorder may complicate the clinical picture, in particular if neuroleptic therapy appears to worsen the condition. However, for patients with a history of seizure disorder, recent evidence suggests that interictal violence is associated more with psychopathology and mental retardation than with epileptiform activity or other seizure variables (105).

Adverse drug effects such as akathisia increases irritability and may serve as stimulus for striking out (106,107). High-dose haloperidol treatment of chronic schizophrenia (60 mg/day) has been associated with violence (108); akathisia might have been the mediating variable. It is possible that some of the antiaggressive effects of beta-adrenergic antagonists added to antipsychotics may actually be due to a reduction of akathisia (109).

Fluoxetine has been blamed for inducing murder or suicide and has been used as a legal defense and as a plaintiff's argument in seeking compensatory and punitive damages in a variety of court cases (110,111). In early 1990 there was a case report of six depressed patients free of recent serious suicidal ideation who developed intense and violent suicidal preoccupations after starting fluoxetine treatment (112). The authors recommended that fluoxetine be used cautiously. In another study, increased aggression was observed in a group of 19 adult, mentally retarded inpatients with epilepsy and a history of current or recent aggressive behavior (113). Each was concurrently taking other psychotropic medication and there was wide individual differences in fluoxetine drug response. The emergence of self-destructive behavior in six children and adolescents during fluoxetine treatment has also been reported (114). In these cases the subjects were being treated for obsessive-compulsive disorder and four of the six had major risk factors for self-destructive behavior. Given fluoxetine's pharmacological action as a specific serotonin reuptake inhibitor and the role that serotonergic imbalance or dysfunction may have in the genesis of aggressive behavior, one would have predicted the opposite effect (115). Indeed, there are studies utilizing fluoxetine as a therapeutic agent in the control of self-injurious behavior. One such study of 21 severely to profoundly mentally retarded persons with aggression and self-injurious behavior treated with fluoxetine on an open-label basis demonstrated a positive outcome for 19 of the subjects, with no worsening attributable to fluoxetine reported for the remaining 2 patients (116). In a preliminary medication trial with five refractory borderline patients, fluoxetine led to a decrease in impulsiveness (117,118). In a double-blind, placebo-controlled, 12-week clinical trial of fluoxetine in the treatment of impulsive aggressive behavior in personality disordered individuals without major depression, fluoxetine had significant antiaggressive effects independent of any antidepressant effects (119). In a postmarketing surveillance study of 1577 fluoxetine-treated and 1209 sertraline-treated patients, fluoxetine-treated patients reported a higher frequency of anger or aggression, but the relative risk reported was not statistically significant (120). A similar trend, not reaching statistical significance, was reported in a comparison of fluoxetine with trazodone using the same methodology (121). The Lilly Research Laboratories have published several metanalyses concluding that fluoxetine is not associated with increased suicidality in treatment for obsessive-compulsive disorder (122), increased suicidality during pharmacotherapy for depression (123), or increased aggression (124). Specifically, a relative risk analysis of 3992 subjects enrolled in several double-blind, placebo-controlled clinical trials across multiple indications (depression, obesity, bulimia nervosa, obsessive compulsive disorder, smoking cessation, and alcoholism) demonstrated a fourfold higher likelihood of an aggressive event for patients receiving placebo as opposed to fluoxetine.

A consequence of the fluoxetine controversy may be the reluctance of some patients to accept fluoxetine and for some physicians to prescribe it. This barrier to the use of fluoxetine is unfortunate, given that older antidepressant medications are usually not as well tolerated with regard to side effects and are more toxic in overdose. Mann and Kapur (125) remark that paradoxical suicidal ideation is not limited to any one psychiatric diagnosis or any specific type of antidepressant and may be more frequent in nonresponders, patients with unrecognized akathisia, and in those with a history of attempted suicide. They recommend that patients be warned that worsening of symptoms may occur regardless of what medication they may be taking and that the clinician be informed quickly if this should happen.

IX. CONCLUSIONS

Violent or threatening behavior is a frequent reason for the admission to a psychiatric inpatient facility, and that behavior may continue after the admission. For patients with schizophrenia, the association between preadmission threats and postadmission violence is impressive. Patients chronically hospitalized may also be aggressive. In both psychotic and nonpsychotic disorders, comorbidity with substance and alcohol abuse and personality disorders may further predispose a patient to exhibit violent behavior. The distinction between transient and recidivistic assaultiveness is important, since a small group of recidivistic patients may cause the majority of violent incidents. Mental retardation is an additional risk factor. Psychotropic medication may be a causative factor in some cases of patient violence, but the evidence for this is weak, and it is the lack of treatment or undertreatment of psychiatric disorders that most likely places patients at risk for violence.

REFERENCES

1. J. Monahan, Mental disorder and violent behavior: Perceptions and evidence, *Am. Psychol. 47*:511 (1992).
2. D.A. Regier, M.E. Farmer, D.S. Rae, B.Z. Locke, S.J. Keith, L.L. Judd, and F.K. Goodwin, Comorbidity of mental disorders with alcohol and other drug abuse: Results from the Epidemiologic Catchment Area (ECA) Study, *J.A.M.A. 264*:2511 (1990).
3. J.W. Swanson, Mental disorder, substance abuse, and community violence: An epidemiological approach, *Violence and Mental Disorder: Developments in Risk Assessment* (J. Monahan and H.J. Steadman, eds.), University of Chicago Press, Chicago, 1994, pp. 101–136.

4. B.G. Link, F.T. Cullin, and H. Andrews. The violent and illegal behavior of mental patients reconsidered, *Am. Sociol. Rev.* 57:275 (1992).
5. B.G. Link and A. Stueve, Psychotic symptoms and the violent/illegal behavior of mental patients compared to community controls, in *Violence and Mental Disorder: Developments in Risk Assessment* (J. Monahan and H.J. Steadman, eds.), University of Chicago Press, Chicago, 1994, pp. 137–159.
6. S. Hodgins, Mental disorder, intellectual deficiency, and crime: Evidence from a birth cohort, *Arch. Gen. Psychiatry 49*:476 (1992).
7. S. Hodgins, S.A. Mednick, P.A. Brennan, F. Schulsinger, and M. Engberg, Mental disorder and crime: Evidence from a Danish birth cohort, *Arch. Gen. Psychiatry 53*:489 (1996).
8. P.J. Taylor PJ: Motives for offending among violent and psychotic men, *Br. J. Psychiatry 147*:491 (1985).
9. D.E. McNiel and R.L. Binder, Relationship between preadmission threats and later violent behavior by acute psychiatric inpatients, *Hosp. Commun. Psychiatry 40*:605 (1989).
10. R.L. Binder and D.E. McNiel, Effects of diagnosis and context on dangerousness, *Am. J. Psychiatry 145*:728 (1988).
11. E.D. Tanke and J.A. Yesavage, Characteristics of assaultive patients who do and do not provide visible cues of potential violence, *Am. J. Psychiatry 142*:1409 (1985).
12. K. Tardiff and A. Sweillam, Assaultive behavior among chronic inpatients, *Am. J. Psychiatry 139*:212 (1982).
13. M.I. Krakowski and P. Czobor, Clinical symptoms, neurological impairment, and prediction of violence in psychiatric inpatients, *Hosp. Commun. Psychiatry 45*:700 (1994).
14. M. Krakowski, A. Convit, J. Jaeger, S. Lin, and J. Volavka, Inpatient violence: Trait and state, *J. Psychiat. Res. 23*:57 (1989).
15. M.I. Krakowski, J. Jaeger, and J. Volavka, Inpatient psychiatric violence: Its course and associated symptomatology. *Current Approaches to the Prediction of Violence* (D.A. Brizer and M.L. Crowner, eds.), Washington, DC, American Psychiatric Press, 1989, pp. 149–161.
16. A. Convit, D. Isay, D. Otis, and J. Volavka, Characteristics of repeatedly assaultive psychiatric inpatients, *Hosp. Commun. Psychiatry 41*:1112 (1990).
17. J. Volavka, *Neurobiology of Violence*, Washington, DC, American Psychiatric Press, 1995.
18. L.A. Teplin, The prevalence of severe mental disorder among male urban jail detainees: Comparison with the Epidemiologic Catchment Area Program, *Am. J. Public Health 80*:663 (1990).
19. M. Eronen, P. Hakola, and J. Tiihonen, Mental disorders and homicidal behavior in Finland, *Arch. Gen. Psychiatry 53*:497 (1996).
20. J. Coid, The epidemiology of abnormal homicide and murder followed by suicide, *Psychol. Med. 13*:855 (1983).
21. M.S. Humphreys, E.C. Johnstone, J.F. MacMillan, and P.J. Taylor, Dangerous

behavior preceding first admission for schizophrenia, *Br. J. Psychiatry 161*:501 (1992).
22. J. Junginger, Command hallucinations and the prediction of dangerousness, *Psychiatr. Serv. 46*:911 (1995).
23. D.E. McNiel, Hallucinations and violence, *Violence and Mental Disorders* (J. Monahan and H.J. Steadman, eds.), University of Chicago Press, Chicago, 1994, pp. 183–202.
24. R. Rogers, D. Nussbaum, and R. Gillis, Command hallucinations and criminality: A clinical quandary, *Bull. Am. Acad. Psychiatry Law 16*:251 (1988).
25. M.N. Beaudoin, S. Hodgins, and F. Lavoie, Homicide, schizophrenia and substance abuse or dependency, *Can. J. Psychiatry 38*:541 (1993).
26. M. Virkkunen, Observations on violence in schizophrenia, *Acta Psychiatr. Scand. 50*:145 (1974).
27. J.A. Yesavage, Inpatient violence and the schizophrenic patient: An inverse correlation between danger-related events and neuroleptic levels, *Biol. Psychiatry 17*:1331 (1982).
28. M. Krakowski, J. Volavka, and D. Brizer, Psychopathology and violence: A review of the literature, *Comp. Psychiatry 27(2)*:131 (1986).
29. A.L. Calcedo-Barba and A. Calcedo-Ordonez, Violence and paranoid schizophrenia, *Int. J. Law Psychiatry 17(3)*:253 (1994).
30. P.A. Boxer, Assessment of potential violence in the paranoid worker, *J. Occup. Med. 35(2)*:127 (1993).
31. D. Shore, C.R. Filson, and W.E. Johnson, Violent crime arrests and paranoid schizophrenia: The White House case studies, *Schizophr. Bull. 14(2)*:279 (1988).
32. P. Lindqvist and P. Allebeck, Schizophrenia and assaultive behaviour: the role of alcohol and drug abuse, *Acta Psychiatr. Scand. 82*:191 (1990).
33. J. Smith and S. Hucker, Schizophrenia and substance abuse, *Br. J. Psychiatry* 165:13 (1994).
34. B.J. Cuffel, Prevalence estimates of substance abuse in schizophrenia and their correlates, *J Nerv. Ment. Dis. 180*:589 (1992).
35. K. Maguire and A.L. Pastore (eds.), *Sourcebook of Criminal Justice Statistics 1994.* U.S. Department of Justice, Bureau of Justice Statistics, Washington, DC, 1995, p. 415.
36. B.J. Cuffel, M. Shumway, T.L. Chouljian, and T. Macdonald, A longitudinal study of substance abuse and community violence in schizophrenia, *J. Nerv. Ment. Dis. 182*:704 (1994).
37. A.B. Koczapski, B. Ledwidge, J. Paredes, C. Kogan, and J. Higenbottam, Multisubstance intoxication among schizophrenic inpatients: Reply to Hyde, *Schizophr. Bull. 16*:373 (1990).
38. M. Krakowski, P. Czobor, M.D. Carpenter, K. Nolan, J. Libiger, M. Kunz, H. Papezova, B.B. Parker, L. Schmader, and T. Abad, Violent crime in psychiatric patients: Relationship to frontal lobe impairment, *American Journal of Forensic Psychiatry 17(4)*:53 (1996).
39. M. Krakowski, A. Convit, J. Jaeger, S. Lin, and J. Volavka, Neurological impairment in violent schizophrenic inpatients, *Am. J. Psychiatry 146*:849 (1989).

40. A. Convit, P. Czobor, and J. Volavka, Lateralized abnormality in the EEG of persistently violent psychiatric inpatients, *Biol. Psychiatry 30*:363 (1991).
41. D.A. Martell, Estimating the prevalence of organic brain dysfunction in maximum-security forensic psychiatric patients, *J. Forens. Sci. 37*:878 (1992).
42. A. Convit, J. Jaeger, S.P. Lin, M. Meisner, and J. Volavka, Predicting assaultiveness in psychiatric inpatients: A pilot study, *Hosp. Commun. Psychiatry 39*:429 (1988).
43. A. Convit, R. Douyon, K. Yates, G. Smith, J. Volavka, P. Cozobor, J. de Asis, Vitrai, C. Evangelista, and L. Camus, Fronto-temporal abnormalities in violence, *Aggression and Violence: Genetic, Neurobiological and Bioscocial Perspective* (D. Stoff and R. Cairns, eds.), Lawrence Erlbaum, Hillsdale, NJ, 1996. In press.
44. W.A. Weiger and D.M. Bear, An approach to the neurology of aggression, *J. Psychiatr. Res. 22*:85 (1988).
45. B. Hamstra, Neurobiological substrates of violence: An overview for forensic clinicians, *J. Psychiatry Law 14*: 349 (1986)
46. J. Volavka, D. Martell, and A. Convit, Psychobiology of the violent offender, *J. Forens. Sci. 37*:237 (1992).
47. M. Krakowski, A. Convit, and J. Volavka, Patterns of inpatient assaultiveness: Effect of neurological impairment and deviant family environment on response to treatment, *Neuropsychiatry Neurophyschol. Behav. Neurol. 1*:21 (1988).
48. T. Palmstierna, B. Huitfeldt, and B. Wistedt, The relationship of crowding and aggressive behavior on a psychiatric intensive care unit, *Hosp. Commun. Psychiatry 42*:1237 (1991).
49. D.S. Brailsford and J. Stevenson, Factors related to violent and unpredictable behavior in psychiatric hospitals, *Nurs. Times 69*(suppl):9 (1973).
50. E. Fottrell, A study of violent behavior among patients in psychiatric hospitals, *Br. J. Psychiatry 136*:216 (1980).
51. J. Volavka and M. Krakowski, Schizophrenia and violence, *Psychol. Med. 19*:559 (1989).
52. L.N. Robins, J. Tipp, and T. Przybeck, Antisocial personality, *Psychiatric Disorders in America: The Epidemiologic Catchment Area Study* (L.N. Robins and D.A. Regier, eds.), The Free Press, New York, 1991, pp. 258–290.
53. L.N. Robins, *Deviant Children Grown Up: A Sociological and Psychiatric Study of Sociopathic Personality*, Baltimore, Williams & Wilkins, 1966, p. 240.
54. American Psychiatric Association, *Diagnostic and Statistical Manual of Mental Disorders*, 4th ed. American Psychiatric Association, Washington, DC, 1994.
55. S. Travin and B. Protter, Mad or bad? Some clinical considerations in the misdiagnosis of schizophrenia as antisocial personality disorder, *Am. J. Psychiatry 139*:1335 (1982).
56. M.P. Geller, Sociopathic adaptations in psychotic patients, *Hosp. Commun. Psychiatry 31*(2):108 (1980).
57. M. Virkkunen, R. Rawlings, R. Tokola, et al., CSF biochemistries, glucose metabolism, and diurnal activity rhythms in alcoholic, violent offenders, fire setters, and heathy volunteers, *Arch. Gen. Psychiatry 51*:20 (1994).

58. K. Abram, The effect of co-occurring disorders on criminal careers: interaction of antisocial personality, alcoholism, and drug disorders, *Int. J. Law Psychiatry 12*:133 (1989).
59. K.M. Abram and L.A. Teplin, Drug disorder, mental illness, and violence, *NIDA Res. Monogr. 103*:222 (1990).
60. K.M. Abram and L.A. Teplin, Co-occuring disorders among mentally ill jail detainees: Implications for public policy, *Am. Psychol. 46*:1036 (1991).
61. L.N. Robins, J.E. Helzer, J. Croughan et al., NIMH Diagnostic Interview Schedule: Version III (unpublished). National Institute of Mental Health, Division of Biometry and Epidemiology, Rockville, MD, 1981.
62. H. Cleckley, *The Mask of Sanity*, 5th ed. Mosby, St. Louis, 1976.
63. R.D. Hare, A research scale for the assessment of psychopathy in criminal populations. *Personal. Individ. Diff. 1*:111 (1980).
64. R.D. Hare, *The Hare Psychopathy Checklist—Revised*, Multi-Health Systems, Toronto, 1991.
65. S.D. Hart, R.D. Hare, and T.J. Harpur, The psychopathy checklist-revised (PCL-R): An overview for researchers and clinicians, *Advances in Psychological Assessment* (J.C. Rosen and P. McReynolds, eds.), Plenum Press, New York, 1992, pp. 103–130.
66. S.D. Hart, R.D. Hare, and A.E. Forth, Psychopathy as a risk marker for violence: Development and validation of a screening version of the revised psychopathy checklist, *Violence and Mental Disorder. Developments in Risk Assessment* (J. Monahan and H.J. Steadman, eds.) University of Chicago Press, Chicago, 1994, pp. 81–98.
67. R.D. Hare, S.D. Hart, and T.J. Harpur, Psychopathy and the DSM-IV criteria for antisocial personality disorder, *J. Abnorm. Psychol. 100*:391 (1991).
68. R.D. Hare, Psychopathy and antisocial personality disorder: A case of diagnostic confusion, *Psychiatric Times February*:39 (1996).
69. R.D. Hare and L.M. McPherson, Violent and aggressive behavior by criminal psychopaths, *Int. J. Law Psychiatry 7*:35 (1984).
70. L.T. Else, S.A. Wonderlich, W.W. Beatty, et al., Personality characteristics of men who physically abuse women, *Hosp. Commun. Psychiatry 44*:54 (1993).
71. S. Snyder, W.M. Pitts, and A.D. Pokorny, Selected behavioral features of patients with borderline personality traits, *Suicide Life-Threat. Behav. 16(1)*:28 (1986).
72. E.F. Coccaro, L.J. Siever, H.M. Klar, et al., Serotonergic studies in patients with affective and personality disorders, *Arch. Gen. Psychiatry 46*:587 (1989).
73. E.S. Barratt, Impulsiveness and aggression, *Violence and Mental Disorder: Developments in Risk Assessment* (J. Monahan and H.J. Steadman, eds.), University of Chicago Press, Chicago, 1994, pp. 61–79.
74. M.R. Gottfredson and T.A. Hirschi, *A General Theory of Crime*, Stanford University Press, Stanford, CA, 1990, pp. 87–94.
75. J.Q. Wilson and R.J. Herrnstein, *Crime and Human Nature*, 2nd ed. Simon & Schuster, New York, 1986, pp. 435–437.
76. M. Virkkunen and M. Linnoila, Serotonin and personality disorders with habitual violence and impulsivity, *Mental Disorder and Crime*, (S. Hodgins, ed.), Sage, Newbury Park, CA, 1993, pp. 227–243.

77. D.J. Stein, E. Hollander, and M.R. Libeowitz, Neurobiology of impulsivity and the impulse control disorders. *J. Neuropsychiatry Clin. Neurosci. 5*:9 (1993).
78. E. Soubrie and J.C. Bizot, Monoaminergic control of waiting capacity (impulsivity) in animals, *Violence and Suicidality: Perspectives in Clinical and Biological Research* (H.M. Van Praag, R. Plutchik, and A. Apter, eds.), Brunnzer/Mazel, New York, 1990, pp. 257–272.
79. E.S. Barratt, Impulsiveness subtraits: arousal and information processing, *Motivation, Emotion and Personality* (J.T. Spence and C.E. Izard, eds.), Elsevier North-Holland, Amsterdam, 1985, pp. 137–146.
80. R.R. Monroe, *Episodic Behavioral Disorders*. Harvard University Press, Cambridge, MA, 1970.
81. G. Bach-y-Rita, J.R. Lion, C.E. Clement, et al., Episodic dyscontrol: A study of 130 violent patients, *Am. J. Psychiatry 127*:1473 (1971).
82. G. Bach-y-Rita and A. Veno, Habitual violence: A profile of 62 men, *Am. J. Psychiatry 131*:1015 (1974).
83. R.R. Monroe, *Brain Dysfunction in Aggressive Criminals*. Lexington Books, DC Heath, Lexington, MA, 1978.
84. M. Linnoila, M. Virkkunen, M. Scheinin et al., Low cerebrospinal fluid 5-hydroxyindole acetic acid concentration differentiates impulsive from non-impulsive violent behavior, *Life Sci. 33*:2609 (1983).
85. D.S. Hellman and N. Blackman, Enuresis, firesetting and cruelty to animals: A triad predictive of adult crime, *American Journal of Psychiatry*:1431 (1966).
86. M. Virkkunen, A. Nuutila, F.K. Goodwin, et al., Cerebrospinal fluid monoamine metabolites in male arsonists, *Arch. Gen. Psychiatry 44*:241 (1987).
87. H. Lacey and C.D. Evans, The impulsivist: a multi-impulsive personality disorder, *Br. J. Addict. 81*:641 (1986).
88. J.J. Collins and S.L. Bailey, Relationship of mood disorders to violence, *J. Nerv. Ment. Dis. 178(1)*:44 (1990).
89. J.T. Craig, An epidemiologic study of problems associated with violence among psychiatric inpatients, *Am. J Psychiatry 139*:1262 (1982).
90. J.A. Yesavage, Bipolar illness: Correlates of dangerous inpatient behaviour, *Br. J. Psychiatry 143*:554 (1983).
91. A. Husain, D.E. Anasseril, and P.W. Harris, A study of young-age and mid-life homicidal women admitted to a psychiatric hospital for pre-trial evaluation, *Can. J. Psychiatry* 28:109 (1983).
92. M. Rosenbaum and B. Bennett, Homicide and depression, *Am. J. Psychiatry 143*:367 (1986).
93. D. Bourget and J.M.W. Bradford, Homicidal parents, *Can. J. Psychiatry 35*:233 (1990).
94. N.B. Lasko, T.V. Gurvits, A.A. Kuhne, S.P. Orr, and R.K. Pitman, Aggression and its correlates in Vietnam veterans with and without chronic posttraumatic stress disorder, *Comp. Psychiatry 35:*373 (1994).
95. B.K. Jordan, C.R. Marmar, J.A. Fairbank, W.E. Schlenger, R.A. Kukla, R.L. Hough, and D.S. Weiss, Problems in families of male Vietnam veterans with posttraumatic stress disorder, *J. Consult. Clin. Psychology 60*:916 (1992).

96. D.T. George, P. Anderson, D.J. Nutt, and M. Linnoila, Aggressive thoughts and behavior: Another symptom of panic disorder? *Acta Psychiatr. Scand. 79*:500 (1989).
97. J.B. Tu and J.T. Smith, The Eastern Ontario survey: A study of drug-treated psychiatric problems in the mentally handicapped, *Can. J. Psychiatry 28*:270 (1983).
98. J. Intagliata and C. Rinck, Psychoactive drug use in public and community residential facilities for mentally retarded persons, *Psychopharmacol. Bull. 21*:268 (1985).
99. N. Grizenko, H. Cvejic, S. Vida, and L. Sayegh, Behavior problems of the mentally retarded, *Can. J. Psychiatry 36:*712 (1991).
100. O.M. Linaker, Assaultiveness among institutionalised adults with mental retardation, *Br. J. Psychiatry 164*:62 (1994).
101. A.D. Hurley and R. Sovner, Six cases of patients with mental retardation who have antisocial personality disorder, *Psychiatr. Serv. 46*:828 (1995).
102. A. Bond and M. Lader, Benzodiazepines and aggression, *Psychopharmacology of Aggression* (M. Sandler, ed.) Raven Press, New York, 1979, pp. 173–182.
103. J.O. Cole and J.C. Kando, Adverse behavioral events reported in patients taking alprazolam and other benzodiazepines, *J. Clin. Psychiatry 54(10, suppl):49* (1993).
104. J.T. Dietch and R.K. Jennings, Aggressive dyscontrol in patients treated with benzodiazepines, *J. Clin. Psychiatry 49*:184 (1988).
105. M.F. Mendez, R.C. Doss, and J.L. Taylor, Interictal violence in epilepsy. *J. Nerv. Ment. Dis 181*:566 (1993).
106. W.A. Keckich, Neuroleptics: Violence as a manifestation of akathisia. *J.A.M.A. 240*:2185 (1978).
107. S.G. Siris, Three cases of akathisia and "acting out." *J. Clin. Psychiatry 46*:395 (1985).
108. J.N. Herrera, J.J. Sramek, J.F. Costa, et al., High potency neuroleptics and violence in schizophrenics. *J. Nerv. Ment. Dis. 176*:558 (1988).
109. J.F. Lipinski Jr., P.E. Keck Jr., S.L. McElroy, Beta-adrenergic antagonists in psychosis: Is improvement due to treatment of neuroleptic-induced akathisia? *J. Clin. Psychopharmacol. 8*:409 (1988).
110. T.M. Burton, Medical flap: Anti-depression drug of Eli Lilly loses sales after attack by sect. *Wall Street Journal*, Friday, April 19, 1991.
111. M.J. Grinfeld, Jury finds Prozac did not cause violence. *Psychiatric Times, February:33* (1995).
112. M.H. Teicher, C. Glod, and J.O. Cole, Emergence of intense suicidal preoccupation during fluoxetine treatment. *Am. J. Psychiatry 147*:207 (1990).
113. A. Troisi, E. Vicario, F. Nuccetelli, N. Ciani, and A. Pasini, Effects of fluoxetine on aggressive behavior of adult inpatients with mental retardation and epilepsy. *Pharmacopsychiatry 28*:73 (1995).
114. R.A. King, M.A. Riddle, P.B. Chappell, M.T. Hardin, G.M. Anderson, P. Lombroso, and L. Scahill, Emergence of self-destructive phenomena in children and adolescents during fluoxetine treatment. *J. Am. Acad. Child Adolesc. Psychiatry 30(2)*:179 (1991).
115. E.F. Coccaro, J.L. Astill, J.L. Herbert, and A.G. Schut, Fluoxetine treatment of

impulsive aggression in DSM-III-R personality disorder patients, *J. Clin. Psychopharmacol. 10*:373 (1990).

116. P.I. Markowitz, Effect of fluoxetine on self-injurious behavior in the developmentally disabled: A preliminary study, *J. Clin. Psychopharmacol.* 12:27 (1992).
117. J.R. Cornelius, P.H. Soloff, J.M. Perel, and R.F. Ulrich, Fluoxetine trial in borderline personality disorder, *Psychopharmacol. Bull. 26(1)*:151 (1990).
118. J.R. Cornelius, P.H. Soloff, J.M. Perel, and R.F. Ulrich, A preliminary trial of fluoxetine in refractory borderline patients, *J. Clin. Psychopharmacol. 11*:116 (1991).
119. E.F. Coccaro and R.J. Kavoussi, Fluoxetine and aggression in personality disorder. American Psychiatric Association 148th Annual Meeting New Research Program and Abstracts. May 23, 1995, NR170, p. 101.
120. S. Fisher, T.A. Kent, and S.G. Bryant, Postmarketing surveillance by patient selfmonitoring: Preliminary data for sertraline versus fluoxetine, *J. Clin. Psychiatry 56*:288 (1995).
121. S. Fisher, S.G. Bryant, and T.A. Kent, Postmarketing surveillance by patient selfmonitoring: Trazodone versus fluoxetine, *J. Clin. Psychopharmacol. 13*:235 (1993).
122. C.M. Beasley, J.H. Potvin, D.N. Masica, D.E. Wheadon, B.E. Dornseif, and L.A. Genduso, Fluoxetine: No association with suicidality in obsessive-compulsive disorder, *J. Affect. Dis. 24*:1 (1992).
123. G.D. Tollefson, A.H. Rampey, C.M. Beasley, G.G. Enas, and J.H. Potvin, Absence of a relationship between adverse events and suicidality during pharmacotherapy for depression, *J. Clin. Psychopharmacol. 14*:163 (1994).
124. J.H. Heilgenstein, C.M. Beasley, and J.H. Potvin, Fluoxetine not associated with increased aggression in controlled clinical trials, *Int. Clin. Psychopharmacol. 8*:280 (1993).
125. J.J. Mann and S. Kapur, The emergence of suicidal ideation and behavior during antidepressant pharmacotherapy, *Arch. Gen. Psychiatry 48*:1027 (1991).

6
Substance Abuse and Violence

Jan Volavka
New York University, New York and Nathan S. Kline Institute for Psychiatric Research, Orangeburg, New York

Kenneth Tardiff
Cornell University Medical College, New York, New York

I. INTRODUCTION

Alcohol and drugs can cause violence through their acute pharmacological effects in persons with no other psychiatric psychopathology. They can exacerbate the psychopathology found in other psychiatric disorders—for example, cocaine or other stimulants worsening agitation in mania or delusions in schizophrenia. There can be polysubstance abuse—for example, cocaine users frequently use alcohol and/or opiates to sooth the irritability of cocaine. Alcohol and some substances such as benzodiazepines and opiates are associated with withdrawal syndromes, which can present with agitation and violence. With acute violence, as seen in the emergency room, the violent patients may be intoxicated with alcohol, in a withdrawal state from alcohol, be intoxicated with one or more drugs, and/or be in withdrawal from some drugs. Heavy alcohol or drug abuse can cause changes in the brain that lead to chronic organic impairment characterized by dementia or other symptoms such as delusions, which, in turn, can be related to violent behavior. Thus, the effects of alcohol and drugs on violent behavior can be very complex.

II. ALCOHOL

Alcohol has been linked to violence through epidemiological, laboratory, and clinical studies. A recent study in Finland assessed 693 homicide offenders, representing a large majority of all homicide offenders in Finland during the study period (1). Most of the offenders were intoxicated at the time of the crime. Approximately 39% of the offenders received the diagnosis of alcoholism. The offenders were compared with the general population of Finland on several variables, including the diagnosis of alcoholism. The men with the diagnosis of alcoholism were approximately 12 times more likely to be convicted of homicide than men without that diagnosis. However, these Finnish findings cannot be directly applied to the United States. Organized crime, drug abuse, availability of guns, and many other cultural factors in the United States are much less important in Finland.

In any event, the rates of diagnosed alcoholism among violent offenders are considerably lower than the rates of drinking by the offender during or immediately prior to the commission of a violent crime. Those latter rates are generally above 50% (2). In the United States, it appears that while acute effects of alcohol are generally associated with incarceration for violent crime, the prevalence of alcohol use disorders is not (3,4). Most authors reporting links between alcohol use and violent crime have not controlled for cooccurring disorders. It is therefore possible that such links are mediated by a third variable such as antisocial personality disorder. Data supporting this possibility have been published (4). Alternatively, a subtype of alcohol abuse may be inherited jointly with antisocial personality disorder. Cloninger and his group (5) have demonstrated the existence of two types of alcohol abuse. Type 2 abusers frequently fight (and get arrested) under the influence of alcohol. This type of alcohol abuse is transmitted from fathers to sons and develops early in life. Patients with type 2 alcohol abuse show many features characteristic of antisocial personality disorder.

The extensive literature reviewed elsewhere (3) indicates that the assailants were under the influence of alcohol in more than 50% of assaults and homicides and that this percentage was lower for nonviolent criminal offenses. Furthermore, alcohol ingestion by the victims was a factor that precipitated assault and homicide. Association between acute effects of alcohol and violence was thus overwhelmingly supported by correlational studies. However, such studies do not directly address the causal relationships and mechanisms underlying that association. Studies of alcohol effects under controlled laboratory conditions are better suited to this purpose.

The mechanisms through which alcohol causes violence are complex and not completely known. One of the most common mechanisms discussed in the early literature is that of disinhibition (6). Alcohol is thought to release one from one's inhibitions, so that urges and behaviors that would be unacceptable in the sober state, in this case, violence, erupt despite one's personal and societal restraints against violence. Yet, the theory of disinhibition seems too nonspecific in terms of how alcohol affects the brain.

There have been studies that have explored how alcohol affects cognitive functions of the brain; these may elucidate how alcohol produces violence (7,8). Subjects were given varying doses of alcohol or a placebo and then evaluated with psychological tests. Alcohol produced impairment in tasks associated with the frontal lobes, such as assessment, planning, organization of behavior, ability to abstract, and impaired memory. Alcohol did not affect previously learned information but rather affected the ability to deal with threatening or new situations. This supports the theory that decreased functions of the frontal lobe due to intoxication may be responsible for violence when the individual is faced with provocation. In addition to impaired planning and other cognitive processes, communication skills may not be sufficient to allow the intoxicated individual to deal with the situation in a verbal rather than physical—i.e., violent—manner. In addition to violence due to decreased ability to deal with probative situations, cognitive impairment of the brain caused by alcohol may exaggerate provocation through misinterpretation of real events, such as perceiving an insult in a bar or in a marital discussion. The intoxicated individual may not appreciate the consequences of violence because of cognitive impairment.

The pharmacology of how alcohol produces impairment in the brain is not known. Most laboratory work with animals has focused on serotonin and the receptor for gamma-aminobutyric acid (GABA) (10). Serotonin but not GABA has been extensively studied in relation to human aggression. A study of male criminals in Finland found that impulsive violence was associated with low levels of serotonin metabolites in cerebrospinal fluid (11). More work on these and other neurotransmitters remains to be done.

The pharmacological effects of alcohol that produce violence must be seen in the context of environmental factors and psychological processes. The environment contains social cues that may provoke an intoxicated individual, such as the frustrations, disappointments, threats, fears, and provocations that occur in families and in society (12,13). Cognitive impairment from intoxication may lead to misinterpretation or exaggeration of these stressors. Furthermore, the use of alcohol may distance or isolate the individual from familial and social supports that help deal with these stressors. Drinking may interfere with work and otherwise limit financial resources to deal with these stressors. In the end, self-esteem is threatened and violence is a way to restore it, particularly for men. Last, the view in society that alcohol produces violence and other antisocial behaviors may be a self-fulfilling prophecy. Violence is an expected effect of alcohol; this allows the intoxicated individuals to transfer blame to the alcohol rather than accept the blame themselves.

Many of the laboratory studies done to assess the association of alcohol and aggression used college students or other "normal" subjects. Typical violent offenders differ from these subjects in a number of ways. Their educational achievement is generally lower; therefore they may have limited resources and outlets to express hostility verbally (rather than physically). Unlike college students, many violent offenders grew up in what was termed "a subculture of violence" (14). This background made them prone to violence because of the established pattern of such behavior in their community. Thus violent offenders may be more likely than college students to expect elevations of aggressiveness after drinking. Furthermore, violent offenders may differ from college students in other areas of functioning besides the aggressive behavior and such differences may facilitate that behavior. For example, violent offenders frequently meet the criteria for psychopathy (15) or antisocial personality disorder (16).

Above and beyond personality disorders, many violent offenders show signs of neuropsychiatric impairment resulting from various types of brain damage (e.g., head injuries). Brain damage is an important intervening variable between drinking and violence, since it changes the organism's response to alcohol (17). The relationship between the dose of alcohol and the person's response may be changed quantitatively and qualitatively. *Alcohol intolerance* may be described as a largely quantitative change: the sequence of intoxicated behaviors proceeds as usual from initial excitement to sleep, but the dose of alcohol required to elicit the effect is reduced. This intolerance can be expressed quantitatively as a shift of the dose-response curve to the left.

Furthermore, certain qualitative features of the alcohol effect may be altered. Violent offenders reported more frequently than the controls that alcohol ingestion made them feel paranoid and inferior (18). These offenders also tended to show more neuropsychiatric impairment on a test battery than the controls (18). Such feelings may conceivably account for some instances of violence under the influence of alcohol. Deviant alcohol effects were also reported in persons whose brain function was impaired due to a combination of factors which may act in an additive or interactive fashion. Thus schizophrenics who also abuse drugs may be particularly likely to become assaultive under the influence of alcohol (19).

These results were based on self-reports of alcohol effects and alcohol doses were not controlled (18,19). Perhaps the violent individuals drank more than others, and the differing effects on mood and assaultiveness were due to a higher dose of alcohol. Nevertheless, it appears that neuropsychiatric impairments predispose to a qualitatively different, maladaptive response to alcohol. The nature of such impairments and the disorders responsible for them remain unclear. Alcohol is sometimes associated with aggressive behavior that is incongruous with the personality of the drinker, inappropriate to the situation, and apparently independent of the dose of alcohol ingested. Pathological intoxication (also known as *idiosyncratic intoxication*) may represent an extreme example of this effect. This category is controversial. Although it had been listed in previous DSM editions, DSM-IV (16) omits it because of lack of supporting evidence. However, pathological intoxication is an important concept in the forensic literature.

In this condition, assaultive or other maladaptive behavior which is atypical of the person when not drinking occurs shortly after a small amount of alcohol. Amnesia for such behaviors is frequently reported. The definitions of the "small amount" varied slightly as the criteria developed. Early criteria stipulated a "minimal alcohol intake" (DSM-I and DSM-II); this was changed to an "amount of alcohol insufficient to induce intoxication in most people" (DSM–III and DSM-III-R). Unfortunately, the change has not helped. The questions have just become more difficult to answer: Who are the "most people"? What is their age, gender, and race? Some European textbooks state that small amounts of alcohol are "frequently" sufficient to elicit pathological intoxication (20–22). Predisposing factors for idiosyncratic intoxication include brain damage due mostly to trauma or encephalitis; other factors include unusual fatigue or debilitating physical illness.

Behavioral manifestations of pathological intoxication start and stop rather suddenly, the behavior is incongruous with the patient's personality and with the situation, and amnesia is frequent. These clinical features make it similar to temporal lobe epilepsy (partial complex seizures). A syndrome indistinguishable from idiosyncratic intoxication may apparently be elicited by alcohol in epileptics, particularly in patients with temporal lobe epilepsy.

Alcohol use increases the likelihood of seizures in epileptic patients. It is well known that seizures may be elicited as a part of the alcohol withdrawal syndrome. Recent evidence suggests that alcohol may increase the risk of seizures in epileptic patients more directly, without any withdrawal (23). Short of clinical seizures, epileptogenic effect of alcohol may be manifested by an electroencephalographic (EEG) "activation," i.e., the induction of EEG abnormalities not apparent before the administration of alcohol or an enhancement of preexisting EEG abnormalities. For all these reasons, epileptics are advised not to drink, but some do anyway. Although there is no evidence that epilepsy in general leads to violent behavior, it appears that violent behavior with amnesia may be elicited in epileptics by relatively small doses of alcohol. Such behavior has never been demonstrated in epileptics after experimental alcohol administration under controlled conditions; however, EEG activation by approximately 60 to 90 mL of alcohol by mouth was demonstrated in a series of patients with posttraumatic epilepsy who had a history of episodes of violence after alcohol (24). It is important to note that the patients did not show any aggressive behavior during these EEG activation tests. Attempts at EEG activation by intravenous alcohol in 10 patients with a clinical history of pathological intoxication (some of whom had epilepsy) have failed (25).

However, another author has elicited behavioral changes similar to those described by others in pathological intoxication (26). Subjects were selected for this study because of their history of violent or psychotic behavior while under the influence of alcohol. Presumably they were not epileptic. They were given intravenously relatively large amounts of alcohol (100 to 300 mL), and 11 of the 22 subjects developed "inappropriate rage". The blood alcohol level (BAL) in two of the subjects (measured around the time of their violent reaction) were respectively 117 and 210 mg/dL. (In order to put these results into context, we note that drivers with a BAL of 100 mg/dL and above are legally considered intoxicated in most jurisdictions.) The EEG effects of alcohol observed in this study were diagnostically nonspecific and were not related to violent behavior. Most of the subjects in this study were alcohol abusers and some were alcohol-dependent. Maletzky argued that the diagnostic criterion stipulating a small amount of alcohol needed to elicit pathological intoxication (see above) makes little sense in patients who have an increased tolerance due to antecedent chronic use or abuse of alcohol (26).

Pathological intoxication is an important forensic concept, since it offers "perhaps the only genuine exculpating condition linked to acute drug use" (27). The defense may claim that the defendant's action was caused not by simple drunkenness but by an unusual reaction to alcohol that was due to an underlying brain disease. Numerous objections have been raised against this argument, but a critical analysis of these objections suggests that pathological intoxication provides "a potentially significant defense in many serious cases" (28).

Thus idiosyncratic reactions to alcohol remain controversial from the standpoint of psychiatry, neurology, clinical pharmacology, electroencephalography, and the law. Everybody is confused. Pathological (or idiosyncratic) intoxication is a concept that has eluded a clear and generally accepted definition. Its very existence has been doubted (28,29). In spite of all the confusion, it is clear that links between epilepsy, alcohol, amnesia, and violence do exist. However, one should keep in mind that alcoholic blackouts are frequent and that they occur in patients without any evidence of seizure disorder.

In summary, it appears that interactions between various types of underlying neuropsychiatric impairments and the acute effects of alcohol account for a proportion of alcohol-associated violence. Such an interaction has been proposed (18) but not tested. This presents an interesting opportunity for future research.

III. CRIME AND THE EFFECTS OF DRUGS

In 1991, illicit drugs were detected in urine samples of 59% of male arrestees in 24 U.S. cities (30). Of the male arrestees charged with robbery 65% tested positive; of those charged with assault, 48% tested positive. Cocaine and marijuana were the drugs most frequently detected. Cocaine was detected in the urine of male arrestees at rates ranging from 14% in Omaha to 62% in Manhattan (New York City) (30). The detection rates for marijuana were generally lower. Some of these positive-testing persons were arrested for possession or sale of drugs, having committed no other crime. In the United States, however, drug violations account for less than 10% of offenses charged (30). Taken together, these data suggest that illicit drug use may increase the likelihood of committing crimes above and beyond drug violations. However, these correlational observations do not prove a causal relationship between drugs and crime. Such information is difficult to interpret without urine samples from persons in the same community who were *not* arrested. Such control samples would be needed, since acute drug effects may increase the likelihood of arrest of those who commit crimes and since comparable persons in the same community who do not commit crimes (other than drug possession) may be using drugs at rates similar to those of the arrestees. The need for control samples is illustrated by self-reports of recent (within preceding 30 days) drug use among young adults in the United States. Marijuana was used by 13.3% and cocaine by 1.8% of the respondents (30).

Evidence for linkage between drug abuse and crime varies depending on the drug. The most persuasive data on linkage exist for opioids. This is not due primarily to specific pharmacological effects of opioids on aggression. The availability of evidence is rather due to the long history and relatively high prevalence of opioid abuse in the United States and the history of funding for research in this area. One of the major achievements of the methadone treatment programs in the 1970s was a dramatic reduction in the arrest rates of their clients. The arrest charges were not specified in the major follow-up reports (31,32), but the decline in arrest rates was so great that one can perhaps assume a reduction of arrests for violent crime in patients currently in methadone treatment (in addition to the obvious reduction of arrests for drug possession). The arrest rate returned to the original (pretreatment) high levels in patients who dropped out of the methadone programs (31).

A research group (33) interviewed 132 opioid addicts about their drug use and criminal activity. The interviews covered a period of 15 years (average). During that time, the subjects experienced periods of "addiction" and "nonaddiction." A period of opioid addiction was defined as a "period of one month or more while at large in the community during which the subject illicitly used opiates 4 or more days a week." This definition, albeit idiosyncratic, yielded data on long-term fluctuations of opioid intake; such fluctuations are generally related to changes in severity of substance use disorders.

Self-reported criminal activity was higher during the addiction than during the nonaddiction periods. Furthermore, there was a long-term trend for the criminal activity (including violent crime) to decrease after a peak occurring during the first period of addiction.

These results emphasized the importance of close temporal relationships between the level of drug use and crime. Most crime is committed during periods when the offender is using maximal amounts of drugs. This finding may explain why a diagnosis of drug-use disorder (lifetime or current) did not account for significant proportions of variance of criminal activity (34). Diagnosis misses important information on temporal fluctuations of the amount of drugs used. Similar data stressing the importance of temporal relationship of drinking to crime (rather than the diagnosis of alcohol abuse or dependence) were mentioned in the preceding section on alcohol.

The data discussed so far suggest a relationship between drug abuse and crime, including violent crime. In regard to the nature of that relationship, Goldstein classifies drug-related violence into three types: psychopharmacological, economically compulsive, and systemic (35). Psychopharmacological mechanisms elicit violence directly; they involve intoxication or drug withdrawal. Economic compulsive violent crime is committed by drug-dependent individuals in order to obtain money to purchase drugs. Some of these individuals are driven to criminal violence by withdrawal symptoms. These cases blur the difference between the psychopharmacological and the economic-compulsive types of violent behavior. Systemic violence is intrinsic to involvement with illicit drugs. Typical examples include territorial fights among dealers, elimination of informers, and punishment for selling adulterated drugs or for unpaid debts. Systemic violence may be committed under the influence of drugs, which again somewhat blurs the distinction between the psychopharmacological and other types of violence.

Each of these three types of drug-related violence affects the drug users and distributors (as aggressors or victims) as well as innocent people not involved with drugs who are victimized intentionally (e.g., in a robbery) or unintentionally (e.g., hit by stray bullets in gun battles). The relative importance of the three types of drug-related violence was explored by interviewing a sample of methadone maintenance treatment clients and untreated controls (36). The interviews were concerned with violent events occurring over a sample period of time. Slightly more than 50% of all violent events reported by these subjects were drug-related. Within this drug-related subset, psychopharmacological and systemic violence occurred with similar frequencies, whereas economic compulsive violence (mostly related to cocaine) was less frequent.

A subsequent report by this group (37) indicated that the proportions of psychopharmacological, economic-compulsive, and systemic drug-related violent events depended on race and gender of the participants. The involvement of white males tended to be classified as psychopharmacological, whereas African-American males were relatively more involved in the systemic subtype of violence. Psychopharmacological subtype predominated among females irrespective of their racial/ethnic identification. There is clinical and epidemiological evidence that cocaine use among young women may increase the risk of being victims of violence as they trade sex for cocaine (38–40). On the other hand, young men who use cocaine and alcohol are frequently killed with guns on the streets during disputes around drug dealing (41).

IV. PSYCHOPHARMACOLOGICAL EFFECTS AND VIOLENCE

A. Psychostimulants

Psychostimulants most frequently involved in violence are cocaine and amphetamine. Effects of stimulants on aggression in animals have been extensively studied. These effects are variable, depending on the animal species, the individual's experience with aggression, the dose of the drug (low doses may elicit aggression, high doses may have opposite effect), and the animal's social position in a group (dominant or subordinate individuals in primate groups).

Cocaine is used as either the hydrochloride salt or the free base. Free base can be prepared from the hydrochloride by individual users. Since the mid-1980s, preprocessed free base (crack) has become available on the streets of U.S. cities. Most users take the hydrochloride powder intranasally or dissolve it in water and inject intravenously. Crack is volatile at temperatures above 90°C, which makes it more suitable for smoking.

Immediately after the intravenous administration or the inhalation of smoked cocaine, the user experiences an extremely pleasurable feeling (a "rush") that lasts for a few minutes. This is followed by feelings of anxiety, depression (a "crash"), and intense craving for more cocaine. The effects of intranasal administration are less intense and delayed (due to slower absorption). Intranasal or intravenous administration of single doses of cocaine to normal subjects under experimental conditions did not result in any obvious hostility or aggression (42). However, patients treated for cocaine addiction did report increased anger and overt violent behavior among the acute effects of cocaine (43–45). These effects were reported to be more often expressed after smoking or intravenous injection than after nasal insufflation, but these differences were possibly confounded by cultural or personality factors that were not controlled in this study. Smoking crack is more prevalent among African Americans, whereas intranasal use is preferred by whites.

The craving during a crash may lead to an immediate additional administration of cocaine, and the cycle is repeated until the drug supply is exhausted or the user becomes too incapacitated to continue. This type of binge use results in high cumulative doses, which may elicit an intoxication or a delirium. Most of the violent behavior elicited by the pharmacological effects of cocaine apparently occurs during these states. Other symptoms of intoxication or delirium include auditory, visual, and tactile hallucinations, paranoid and other delusions, irritability, confusion, and psychomotor agitation (sometimes extreme). Violent behavior in patients presenting with cocaine intoxication was observed in hospital emergency rooms and other treatment settings (46–51), although this finding is not always confirmed (52). Violence was more pronounced in patients reporting higher levels of cocaine usage in the preceding month (50), in patients presenting with psychotic symptoms (51), and in patients who smoked crack or used cocaine intravenously (compared with intranasal users) (53). This relation between route of administration and violence may be mediated by cocaine dose: intranasal users may be taking lower doses, and the cocaine dose they take is less efficiently absorbed. Cocaine plasma level curves after intravenous administration and smoking are very similar (54).

Symptoms of intoxication or delirium typically disappear within 2 days after the last dose of cocaine. However, a delusional syndrome may linger for a week or more after the last dose. This syndrome is characterized by persecutory delusions, which may elicit violence against misperceived "enemies." The emergency room reports (48–50) do not contain sufficient clinical details to separate the delusional syndrome from the more acute manifestations (intoxication and delirium).

Violence may be elicited by cocaine alone. However, in addition to cocaine, alcohol and heroin are frequently used to counter the irritability and other unpleasant effects of cocaine. These substances may contribute to the violent behaviors observed. This hypothesis was tested in three groups of patients: those with cocaine and alcohol abuse, alcohol abuse only, and cocaine abuse only. The alcohol and cocaine abuse group had a higher likelihood of homicidal ideation and plans than the alcohol-only and the cocaine-only groups (55). A review of the literature concluded that the use of alcohol and cocaine involves a greater risk of violence than the use of these substances separately (56).

Amphetamine may cause intoxication, delirium, or a delusional disorder; these conditions are clinically indistinguishable from those produced by cocaine (see above). Paranoid delusions may result in assault (57) or homicide (58). The mechanism of amphetamine effects on aggression is unclear, but observations in subjects withdrawn from opioids suggest that opioid peptides may play a modulatory role in these amphetamine effects (59).

B. Phencyclidine

Pencyclidine (PCP) may be smoked or taken orally, intranasally, or intravenously. Intoxication is manifested by belligerence, assaultiveness, ataxia, dysarthria, muscle rigidity, seizures, and hyperacusis. PCP delirium may last longer than that caused by cocaine (because of a slower clearance of PCP); otherwise it is clinically similar. PCP delusional disorder is similar to that elicited by cocaine (see above). Early descriptions of PCP-related violence relied largely on self-reports (60,61), which were not quite clear about the time elapsed between the last PCP dose and the violent act. Furthermore, some of the subjects reported using other drugs and alcohol in addition to PCP. Inpatients detoxifying from PCP were not especially assaultive (62). Yet another study found that 64% of patients with PCP intoxication presenting to an emergency room were combative or agitated (63). History of PCP abuse given by male schizophrenic inpatients predicted their assaultiveness in the hospital (19,64). This finding might have been caused by cooccurring (but undiagnosed) personality disorders in the PCP users. Alternatively, schizophrenic patients may be especially vulnerable to some long-term PCP effects which perhaps facilitate violence.

C. Cannabis

Cannabis preparations (marijuana and hashish) have been associated with violence in folk tales for centuries (65). However, evidence linking cannabis to violence has been scarce. In animals, cannabis extracts and its principal active component, delta-9-tetrahydrocannabinol (THC), reduced aggressive behavior and increased flight and submission under most conditions (66). THC tended to suppress aggression in healthy human volunteers in the experimental paradigm described above for testing alcohol effects (67). A survey of adolescent delinquents indicated that cannabis was used for calming effect and that it decreased assaultiveness (68). Numerous experiments studying the acute and chronic effects of cannabis in American (69) and Green (70) users were conducted without any emergence of hostility or violence. The administration of marijuana or hashish seemed to make the subjects more friendly. There is some anecdotal evidence that cannabis preparations may elicit violence in persons with various preexisting mental disorders (65). However, evidence suggests that cannabis preparations may be associated with violence only under exceptional conditions in predisposed persons.

D. Opioids

Opioids generally suppress aggressive behavior in animals (66). This suppression is nonspecific. Other behaviors are suppressed as well by the overall sedative effect. However, when withdrawal from opioids occurs while other animals are present, aggressive or defensive behavior is displayed by rodents and rhesus monkeys (66).

In pain-free humans, short-term effects of morphine include mental clouding, sedation (but sometimes excitation), and euphoria (but sometimes dysphoria). The effects of heroin (diacetylmorphine) are similar to morphine. Heroin penetrates the blood-brain barrier faster than morphine; accordingly, its central effects have an earlier onset. Heroin is quickly metabolized to morphine. In persons dependent on opioids, the euphoria that follows an intravenous administration of heroin has two phases. The first phase (the "rush") is an intensive orgasm-like experience that usually lasts for several minutes after the injection. The second phase, lasting several hours, is experienced as a peaceful, pleasant, and sleepy period. Ex-abusers who were administered moderate doses of heroin under experimental conditions (71) have become friendly and "mellow" rather than displaying any aggressive reaction.

In general, clinical observations suggest that opioids have short-term pacifying effects. Methadone was used to treat rage in a schizophrenic patient (72). Potential merits of opioids as antiaggressive treatment were considered (73), but ethical and practical considerations have precluded any systematic tests of opioid treatment for aggression.

Withdrawal from opioids elevates aggressive behavior in animals under various experimental conditions. The evidence for this effect in humans is based on clinical observations rather than on controlled experiments. Dysphoria, irritability, and increased hostility were reported in humans (74). There are anecdotal reports of violent behavior elicited by withdrawal from opioids—e.g., prostitutes in opioid withdrawal attacking and robbing their clients rather than just tricking them out of their money using more common nonviolent means (35).

E. Anabolic Steroids

Anabolic steroids have been illegally misused by athletes and body builders to enhance muscle growth, strength, and performance. Increased irritability and aggressiveness were recently recognized as unintended side effects of this practice in a series of published case reports (75–79). The reports describe young male athletes who had not demonstrated any aggressive behavior or other psychopathology until they started medicating themselves with various steroids, sometimes at high doses, in order to improve their performance or their size. After several weeks or months of self-medication, the men became irritable and combative, committing violent crimes that included homicide, assault, and robbery. Their irritability and violent outbursts disappeared within several months after steroid discontinuation.

A controlled study compared 88 athletes who were using steroids with 68 nonusers (80). The users showed a higher frequency of mood disorders that were sometimes associated with aggressive behavior. Although the effects of anabolic steroids on aggressive behavior was demonstrated in individual cases of athletes, the contribution of this factor to the population rates of violent crime is not likely to be very high. Interviews of 133 consecutive male convicts in a forensic facility has revealed two cases of apparent steroid-induced crimes (81).

Neuropsychiatric effects of anabolic steroids were assessed in two studies of normal male volunteers (82). Various mood changes were observed, including increases of violent feelings, hostility, and impulsivity. These changes would be consistent with reports of violent behavior in naturalistic settings.

In general, the literature on anabolic steroids and violence shows various methodological problems. These include the retrospective, uncontrolled nature of the observations, the failure to characterize the subjects in terms of their psychiatric history and personality, and the lack of information on the coadministration of other drugs. Furthermore, some of the perpetrators of violent crimes might have provided distorted information on steroid use to present the unintended behavioral effects of the steroids as a mitigating circumstance. Nevertheless, these cases share a pattern of aggressiveness appearing during the use of steroids and disappearing after their discontinuation; this commonality makes the syndrome credible.

F. Benzodiazepines

There have been a few reports of benzodiazepines being associated with "paradoxical rage" attacks (83,84). One clinical study found that patients with borderline personality were more likely than those on placebos to have dyscontrol on alprazolam (85). A review of case reports, experimental studies, and incident reports found that loss of control and violence with benzodiazepines is very infrequent (86).

V. POLYSUBSTANCE ABUSE

To simplify the presentation, the relationships between violence and substances of abuse were discussed separately for each substance. In reality, however, *polysubstance abuse* is very common. Substances may be taken simultaneously, even in the same injection (such as the "speedball" combination of cocaine and heroin). Alcohol is frequently combined with drugs of abuse during the same occasion, or it may be used on separate occasions. Polysubstance use may result from a deliberate decision on the part of the user or from a drug supplier's decision to mix several substances together. These mixtures are then sold to users on the streets under various names that do not necessarily imply their true composition. No Food and Drug Administration regulations on product labeling protect these consumers. Users do not necessarily know that they are using more than one drug. The combinations of substances result in multiple interactions, and very little is known about the effects of these interactions on aggression in animals or on violence in humans.

VI. OCCURRENCE WITH OTHER DISORDERS

Coocurrence of substance abuse and other mental disorders is very frequent. The contribution of such cooccurring disorders to violent behavior is discussed in Chapter 5. Cooccurrence of substance abuse and antisocial personality disorder is particularly important in assessing the contribution of alcohol and drugs to violent behavior. Alcohol abuse or dependence may be related to crime (including violent crime) primarily via the antisocial personality disorder (4). Substance abuse and other psychiatric disorders were studied in relation to violent behavior in the community within the framework of the Epidemiologic Catchment Area survey (87). Substance abuse was associated with an elevated level of self-reported violence, as was schizophrenia. Mood disorders and anxiety disorders alone appeared unrelated to violence. However, a substantial elevation of violence was seen in respondents whose substance abuse cooccurred with either a mood disorder or an anxiety disorder. In general, the risk for violent behavior increased with the number of the respondent's psychiatric diagnoses. Only Axis I diagnoses (DSM-III) were reported in this study; personality disorders remained unexplored (87).

In a follow-up study of discharged schizophrenic patients in Sweden, it was noted that violent crime was linked to cooccurring substance abuse (88). Violent behavior among (sober) hospitalized schizophrenics was related to self-reported history of assaultive or "loud" behavior under the influence of alcohol or drugs (19). The effects of alcohol in the neuropsychiatrically impaired patients were described above.

In summary, studies of prisoners, hospital patients, and community samples suggest that the effects of alcohol and drugs on violence are codetermined by the mental disorders of the user. The evidence for interaction between substance abuse, violence, and antisocial personality appears convincing. Similar interaction data for schizophrenia and other disorders are emerging. Such interactions among cooccurring disorders and violence have to be addressed in future research, prevention, and treatment efforts.

VII. SUMMARY AND CONCLUSIONS

There are no substances that specifically promote (or inhibit) violent behavior through their pharmacological effects. The direction and the size of these effects depend on the dose, user's personality and experience with the substance, and social setting (including the availability and behavior of potential victims). The effects of alcohol and drugs on aggression are extremely complex, and it appears that many mechanisms are involved.

REFERENCES

1. M. Eronen, P. Hakola, and J. Tiihonen, Mental disorders and homicidal behavior in Finland, *Arch. Gen. Psychiatry 53*:497 (1996).
2. D. Murdoch, R.O. Pihl, and D. Ross, Alcohol and crimes of violence: Present issues, *Int. J. Addict. 25*:1065 (1990).
3. J. J. Collins and W.E. Schlenger, Acute and chronic effects of alcohol use on violence, *J. Stud. Alcohol 49*:516 (1988).
4. K. Abram, The effect of co-occurring disorders on criminal careers: Interaction of antisocial personality, alcoholism, and drug disorders, *Int. J. Law Psychiatry 12*:133 (1989).
5. C. R. Cloninger, M. Bohman, and S. Sigvardsson, Inheritance of alcohol abuse: Cross-fostering analysis of adopted men, *Arch. Gen. Psychiatry 38*:861 (1981).
6. S.P. Taylor and K.E. Leonard, Alcohol and human aggression, *Aggression: Theoretical and Empirical Reviews*, Vol. 2, (R.G. Green and E.I. Donnerstein, eds.), Academic Press, New York, 1983, pp. 77–101.
7. J.B. Peterson and R.O. Pihl, Information processing, neuropsychological function, and the inherited predisposition to alcohol, *Neuropsychol. Rev. 1*:343 (1990).
8. J.B. Peterson, J. Rolhfleisch, P.D. Zelazo, and R.O. Pihl, Acute intoxication and cognitive functioning, *J. Stud. Alcohol 51*:114 (1990).
9. B.J. Bushman, Effects of alcohol on human aggression: Validity of proposed explanation, *Recent Dev Alcohol 13*:227 (1997).
10. K.A. Miczek, E.M. Weerts, and J.F. De Bold, Alcohol, aggression, and violence: Biobehavioral determinants in alcohol and interpersonal violence: *Fostering Multidisciplinary Perspective* (S.E. Martin, ed.), Research Monograph No. 24, National Institutes of Health (Pub No 93-3496), Rockville, MD, 1993, pp. 83–119.
11. M. Virkkunen and M. Linnoila, Serotonin in early onset, male alcoholics with violent behaviour, *Ann. Med. 22*:327 (1990).
12. J. Fagan, Intoxication and aggression, *Drugs and Crime* (M. Tonry and J. Wilson eds.), University of Chicago Press, Chicago, 1990, pp. 241–320.
13. T.A. Ito, N. Miller, and V.E. Pollock, Alcohol and aggression: A meta-analysis on the moderating effects of inhibitory cues, triggering events and self-focused attention, *Psychol. Bull. 120*:60 (1996).
14. M.E. Wolfgang and F. Ferracuti, *The Subculture of Violence*, Tavistock, London, 1967.
15. R.D. Hare and L.M. McPherson, Violent and aggressive behavior by criminal psychopaths, *Int. J. Law Psychiatry 7*:35 (1984).
16. American Psychiatric Association, *Diagnostic and Statistical Manual of Mental Disorders*, 4th ed., American Psychiatric Association, Washington, DC, 1994.
17. S. Finger and D.G. Stein, *Brain Damage and Recovery*, Academic Press, New York, 1982.
18. R. Langevin, M. Ben-Aron, G. Wortzman, R. Dickey, and L. Handy, Brain damage, diagnosis, and substance abuse among violent offenders, *Behav. Sci. Law 5*:77 (1987).

19. J.A. Yesavage and V. Zarcone, History of drug abuse and dangerous behavior in inpatient schizophrenics, *J. Clin. Psychiatry 44*:259 (1983).
20. R. Tolle, *Psychiatrie*, 8th ed., Springer-Verlag, Berlin, Heidelberg, 1988.
21. G. Huber, *Psychiatrie*, 4th ed., Schattauer, Stuttgart, 1987.
22. M. Dufek, *Forensic Psychiatry for Lawyers and Physicians*, Orbis, Praha, 1975 (in Czech).
23. S.K. Ng, W.A. Hauser, J.C. Brust and M. Susser, Alcohol consumption and withdrawal in new-onset seizures, *N. Engl. J. Med. 319*:666 (1988).
24. A.A. Marinacci and K.O. Von Hagen, Alcohol and temporal lobe dysfunction: Some of its psychomotor equivalents, *Behav. Neuropsychiatry 3*:2 (1972).
25. G. Bach-y-Rita, J.R. Lion, and F.R. Ervin, Pathological intoxication: Clinical and electroencephalographic studies, *Am. J. Psychiatry 127*:698 (1970).
26. B.M. Maletzky, The diagnosis of pathological intoxication, *J. Stud. Alcohol 37*:1215 (1976).
27. C. Mitchell, Intoxication, criminality, and responsibility, *Int. J. Law Psychiatry 13*:1 (1990).
28. L.P. Tiffany and M. Tiffany, Nosologic objections to the criminal defense of pathological intoxication: What do the doubters doubt? *Int. J. Law Psychiatry 13*:49 (1990).
29. J.G. Small, Psychiatric disorders and EEG, *Electroencephalography, Basic Principles, Clinical Applications and Related Fields* (E. Niedermeyer and F. Lopes da Silva, eds.), Baltimore, Urban & Schwarzenberg, 1987, pp. 528–529.
30. K. Maguire, A.L. Pastore, and T.J. Flanagan (eds.), *Sourcebook of Criminal Justice Statistics, 1992*, U.S. Department of Justicc, Bureau of Justice Statistics, Washington, DC, 1993.
31. F. R. Gearing and M.D. Schweitzer, An epidemiologic evaluation of long-term methadone maintenance treatment for heroin addiction, *Am. J. Epidemiol. 100*:101 (1974).
32. V.P. Dole and H. Joseph, Long-term outcome of patients treated with methadone maintenance, *Ann. N.Y. Acad. Sci. 311*:181 (1978).
33. T.E. Hanlon, D.N. Nurco, T.W. Kinlock, and K.R. Duszynski, Trends in criminal activity and drug use over an addiction career, *Am. J. Drug Alcohol Abuse 16*:223 (1990).
34. K.M. Abram and L.A. Teplin, Drug disorder, mental illness, and violence, *NIDA Res. Monogr. 103*:222 (1990).
35. P.J. Goldstein, The drugs/violence nexus: A tripartite conceptual framework, *J. Drug Issues* 493 (1985).
36. B.J. Spunt, P.J. Goldstein, P.A. Bellucci, and T. Miller, Drug relationships in violence among methadone maintenance treatment clients, *Adv. Alcohol Subst. Abuse 9*:81 (1990).
37. B.J. Spunt, P.J. Goldstein, P.A. Bellucci, and T. Miller, Race/ethnicity and gender differences in the drugs-violence relationship, *J. Psychoact. Drugs 22*:293 (1990).
38. K. Tardiff, P.M. Marzuk, A.C. Leon, C.S. Hirsch, M. Stajic, L. Portera, and N. Hartwell, Homicide in New York City: cocaine use and firearms, *J.A.M.A. 272*:43 (1994).

39. J.A. Inciardi, D. Lockwood, and A.E. Pottieger, *Women and Crack Cocaine*, Macmillan, New York (1993).
40. C.P. Dukarm, R.S. Byrd, P. Auinger, and M. Weizman, Illicit substance use, gender, and risk of violent behavior among adolescents. *Arch. Pediatr. Adolesc. Med. 150*:797 (1996).
41. K. Tardiff, P.M. Marzuk, A.C. Leon, C.S. Hirsch, M. Stajic, L. Portera, and N. Hartwell, A profile of homicides on the streets and in the homes in New York City, *Public Health Rep.110*:13 (1995).
42. R.B. Resnick, R.S. Kestenbaum, and L.K. Schwartz, Acute systemic effects of cocaine in man: A controlled study by intranasal and intravenous routes, *Science 195*:696 (1977).
43. A.J. Giannini, N.S. Miller, R.H. Loiselle, and C.E. Turner, Cocaine-associated violence and relationship to route of administration, *J. Subst. Abuse Treat. 10*:67 (1993).
44. R.A. McCormick and M. Smith, Aggression and hostility in substance abusers: The relationship to abuse patterns, coping style, and relapse triggers, *Addict. Behav. (England) 20*:555 (1995).
45. F.G. Moeller, J.L. Steinberg, F. Petty, M. Fulton, D.R. Cherek, G. Kramer, and D.L. Garver, Serotonin and impulsive/aggressive behavior in cocaine dependent subjects, *Prog. Neuropsychopharmacol. Biol. Psychiatry (England) 18*:1027 (1994).
46. D.H. Lowenstein, S.M. Massa, M.C. Rowbotham, S.D. Collins, H.E. McKinney, and R.P. Simon, Acute neurologic and psychiatric complications associated with cocaine abuse, *Am. J. Med. 83*:841 (1987).
47. R. Mendoza and B.L. Miller, Neuropsychiatric disorders associated with cocaine use, *Hosp. Commun. Psychiatry 43*:677 (1992).
48. W.G. Honer, G. Gerwirtz, and M. Turey, Psychosis and violence in cocaine smokers (letter), *Lancet 2*:451 (1987).
49. S.L. Brody, Violence associated with acute cocaine use in patients admitted to a medical emergency department, *NIDA Res. Monogr. 103*:44 (1990).
50. K.J. Brower, F.C. Blow, and T.P. Beresford, Forms of cocaine and psychiatric symptoms (letter), *Lancet 1*:50 (1988).
51. T.C. Manschreck, J.A. Laughery, C.C. Weisstein, D. Allen, B. Humbelstone, M. Neville, H. Podlewski, and N. Mitra, Characteristics of freebase cocaine psychosis, *Yale J. Biol. Med. 61*:115 (1988).
52. D. Dhossche and J. Rubinstein, Drug detection in a suburban psychiatric emergency room, *Ann. Clin. Psychiatry 8*:59 (1996).
53. K.J. Brower, R. Hierholzer, and E. Maddahian, Recent trends in cocaine abuse in a VA psychiatric population, *Hosp. Commun. Psychiatry 37*:1229 (1986).
54. C.E. Johanson and M.W. Fischman, The pharmacology of cocaine related to its abuse, *Pharmacol. Rev. 41*:3 (1989).
55. I.M. Salloum, D.C. Daley, J.R. Cornelius, L. Kirisci, and M.E. Thase, Disproportionate lethality in psychiatric patients with concurrent alcohol and cocaine abuse, *Am. J. Psychiatry 153*:953 (1996).
56. M.E. Denison, A. Paredes, and J.B. Booth, Alcohol and cocaine interactions and aggressive behaviors, *Recent Dev. Alcohol (United States) 13*:283 (1997).

57. B.M. Angrist and S. Gershon, Amphetamine abuse in New York City—1966 to 1968, *Semin. Psychiatry 1*:195 (1969).
58. E.H. Ellinwood, Assault and homicide associated with amphetamine abuse, *Am. J. Psychiatry 127*:1170 (1971).
59. K.A. Miczek and J.W. Tidey, Amphetamines: aggressive and social behavior, *NIDA Res. Monogr. 94*:68 (1989).
60. M.A. Fauman and B.J. Fauman, Violence associated with phencyclidine abuse, *Am. J. Psychiatry 136*:1584 (1979).
61. M.A. Fauman MA and B.J. Fauman, Chronic phencyclidine (PCP) abuse: A psychiatric perspective—Part I: General aspects and violence (proceedings), *Psychopharmacol. Bull. 16*:70 (1980).
62. A.M. Khajawall, T.B. Erickson, G.M. Simpson, Chronic phencyclidine abuse and physical assault, *Am. J. Psychiatry 139*:1604 (1982).
63. D.N. Bailey, Phencyclidine abuse, clinical findings and concentrations in biological fluids after nonfatal intoxication, *Am. J. Clin. Pathol. (United States) 72*:795 (1979).
64. A. Convit, Z.C. Nemes, and J. Volavka, History of phencyclidine use and repeated assaults in newly admitted young schizophrenic men, *Am. J. Psychiatry 145*:1176 (1988).
65. E.L. Abel, The relationship between cannabis and violence: A review, *Psychol. Bull. 84*:193 (1977).
66. K.A. Miczek, The psychopharmacology of aggression, *Handbook of Psychopharmacology*, Vol. 19 (L.L. Iversen, S.D. Iversen, and S.H. Snyder, eds.), Plenum Press, New York, 1987, pp. 230–231.
67. S.P. Taylor, R.M. Vardaris, A.B. Rawtich, C.B. Gammon, J.W. Cranston, and A.I. Lubetkin, The effects of alcohol and delta-9-tetrahydrocannabinol on human physical aggression, *Aggress. Behav. 2*:153 (1976).
68. J.R. Tinklenberg, W.T. Roth, B.S. Kopell, and P. Murphy, Cannabis and alcohol effects on assaultiveness in adolescent delinquents, *Ann. N.Y. Acad. Sci. 282*:85 (1976).
69. J. Volavka, R. Dornbush, S. Feldstein, G. Clare, A. Zaks, M. Fink, and A.M. Freedman, marijuana, EEG and behavior, *Ann. N.Y. Acad. Sci. 191*:206 (1971).
70. M. Fink, Study of long-term hashish users in Greece: Summary and discussion, *Hashish: Studies of Long-Term Use* (C. Stefanis, R. Dornbush, and M. Fink, eds.), New York, Raven Press, 1977; pp. 151–158.
71. J. Volavka, R. Levine, S. Feldstein, and M. Fink, Short-term effects of heroin in man, *Arch. Gen. Psychiatry 30*:677 (1974).
72. G.H. Berken, M.M. Stone, and S.K. Stone, Methadone in schizophrenic rage: A case study, *Am. J. Psychiatry 135*:248 (1978).
73. K. Verebey, J. Volavka, and D. Clouet, Endorphins in psychiatry: An overview and a hypothesis, *Arch. Gen. Psychiatry 35*:877 (1978).
74. J.R. Tinklenberg and R.C. Stillman, Drug use and violence, *Violence and the Struggle for Existence*, (D.N. Daniels, M.F. Gilula, and F.M. Ochberg, eds.) Boston, Little, Brown and Company, 1970, pp. 327–365.
75. P.Y.L. Choi, A.C. Parrott, D. Cowan, High dose anabolic steroids in strength athletes: Effects upon hostility and aggression, *J. Psychopharmacol. 3*:102 (1989).

76. H.G. Jr. Pope and D.L. Katz, Homicide and near-homicide by anabolic steroid users, *J. Clin. Psychiatry 51*:28 (1990).
77. J.T. Dalby, Brief anabolic steroid use and sustained behavioral reaction (letter), *Am. J. Psychiatry 149*:271 (1992).
78. H.B. Moss and G.L. Panzak, Steroid use and aggression (letter), *Am. J. Psychiatry 149*:1616 (1992).
79. H.M. Schulte, M.J. Hall, and M. Boyer, Domestic violence associated with anabolic steroid abuse (letter), *Am. J. Psychiatry 150*:348 (1993).
80. H.G. Pope Jr. and D.L. Katz, Psychiatric and medical effects of anabolic-androgenic steroid use: A controlled study of 160 athletes, *Arch. Gen. Psychiatry 51*:375 (1994).
81. H.G. Jr. Pope, E.M. Kouri, K.F. Powell, C. Campbell, and D.L. Katz, Anabolic-androgenic steroid use among 133 prisoners, *Compr. Psychiatry 37*:322 (1996).
82. T. Su, M. Pagliaro, P.J. Schmidt, D. Pickar, O. Wolkowitz, and D.R. Rubinow, Neuropsychiatric effects of anabolic steroids in male normal volunteers, *J.A.M.A. 269*:2760 (1993).
83. A. Bond and M. Lader, Benzodiazepines and aggression, *Psychopharmacology of Aggression*, (M. Sandler, ed.), Raven Press, New York, 1979, pp. 173–182.
84. J.O. Cole and J.C. Kando, Adverse behavioral events in patients taking alprazolam and other benzodiazepines, *J. Clin. Psychiatry 54:*49 (1993).
85. D.C. Gardner and R.W. Cowdry, Alprazolam-induced dyscontrol in borderline personality disorder, *Am. J. Psychiatry 142*:98 (1985).
86. J.T. Dietch and R.K. Jennings, Aggressive dyscontrol in patients treated with benzodiazepines, *J. Clin. Psychiatry 49*:184 (1988).
87. J.W. Swanson, C.E. Holzer, V.K. Ganju, and R.T. Jono, Violence and psychiatric disorder in the community: Evidence from the Epidemiologic Catchment Area surveys, *Hosp. Commun. Psychiatry 41*:761 (1990).
88. H. Petursson and G.H. Gudjonsson, Psychiatric aspects of homicide, *Acta Psychiatr. Scand. 64*:363 (1981).

7
Evaluation of Violent Patients

William H. Reid
University of Texas Health Science Center, San Antonio, Texas

I. INTRODUCTION

This chapter focuses on evaluation of adults known to have been violent, many of whom are at significant risk for future violence. Many of the people discussed are *patients*. Others are more accurately described as *evaluees*, since no doctor-patient relationship exists. In this chapter, the term *patient* may refer to either. Although the chapter provides a number of *guidelines* for evaluation and risk assessment, one should not consider these to be standards, mandates, or requirements for any specific clinical or medicolegal situation.

Violence is common. Virtually everyone can be broadly described as "violent" at one time or another. Some definitions include suicidal behavior and/or physically insignificant acts such as verbal aggression, brief threats, or minor agitation. This chapter refers primarily to violence associated with significant physical or property damage, separate from self-destructive activity identified—directly or indirectly—with mental illness.

Most mental illness does not give rise to violence. Although violence is not uncommonly indirectly related to substance abuse or a mental disorder (or both), mental illness itself contributes only 2 or 3% to the overall base rate of significant violence in the United States. Nevertheless, some disorders deserve special attention, and some subgroups of the population are at more risk than others (e.g., patients' families).

The chapter blends two different kinds of evaluation: *evaluation of the violent patient* and *assessment of violence potential*. In the first, one may be trying to understand the cause of a person's violence in order to diagnose, manage, or treat it; trying to understand the source or pattern of existing violence also implies attempts to predict the likelihood of future violence. In the second, one is attempting to assess risk potential. We address this pair of concepts by considering only those patients or evaluees for whom there is already a history of violence or for whom reasonable clinicians would consider violence in a treatment or discharge plan.

It is not feasible to launch exhaustive evaluations for all patients. Before applying the principles discussed here, the clinician should consider individual need and the context of the evaluation and evaluation request. Rather than discuss a protocol or algorithm for each of countless clinical presentations, Several general considerations have been chosen.

A. Allocating Necessary Time and Resources

There are many constraints on clinicians in busy practices, managed-care settings, public clinics and hospitals, and the like. One often hears that there is insufficient time or other resources to do a complete workup. This author takes the simplistic stance that the appropriate expenditure and duration for evaluation of a violent or potentially violent patient is *whatever time and resources are required to address adequately the questions asked and to complete an evaluation acceptable to a knowledgeable professional for the purpose requested.*

It is critical that the physician in charge of admission, diagnostic, treatment, and discharge decisions be able to distinguish real from "practical" or "implied" constraints on the evaluation and that he or she understand clearly that it is the managing physician who is responsible for its quality. One is often asked to evaluate, make clinical (and safety) decisions, treat, and eliminate psychiatric problems within far less time than most clinicians believe optimal. The important thing is that one not misunderstand the difference between real constraints and those other obstacles which should not stand in the way of the doctor's responsibility to self and patient.

Once the patient has been accepted for evaluation and significant violence is a clinical or safety issue, time and money must become far less important. Limitations on admission, hospital stay, use of consultations or diagnostic procedures, etc., should not go unquestioned unless the physician is convinced that those limitations pose no reasonable threat to the accuracy and the reliability of the evaluation. If the doctor believes he or she is forced to limit the evaluation for nonclinical reasons (e.g., lack of insurance coverage, hospital policy, on length of stay), then this belief—and a request to the appropriate authority for permission to proceed—should be documented in the medical record at once, not just after the final decision has been made.

B. Purpose and Expectations

When violent behavior is the reason for referral, the clinician may first determine whether or not it represents a *psychiatric* problem. Violent individuals may be referred for psychiatric evaluation for a number of reasons not directly related to a probability of mental disorder, such as criminal recidivism, frustrated correctional personnel, family hopes that the doctor will find a "diagnosis" to explain bad behavior, legal proceedings, or presumed malingering.

One must be concerned with the expectations of the patient, family, and referral source. Is this to be a first-pass screening for common psychiatric or neurological syndromes or an exhaustive search for explanations of violent behavior? Are resources scant, or is there ample opportunity and funding for sophisticated staff and technology? Will the findings be used for major decisions involving the patient's health or liberty or simply to clarify his or her condition? Do the family and referral source expect some magically complete answer, or do they understand the limitations of our knowledge and abilities?

Regardless of the answers to these questions, the comments and recommendations herein should not be construed as providing any "standard" for evaluation in individual cases and contexts.

II. PATIENT EVALUATION

A. The Evaluation Process

An ordinary psychiatric history, interview, and mental status examination is very useful for finding and clarifying clinical mental illness. In some cases, it leads to diagnoses and treatments that directly address violent behavior. However, there are a number of differences when the purpose is to evaluate violence per se.

1. Corroborating Information

First, the clinician must obtain as much separate and corroborating information about the patient's history and current behavior as possible. This is necessary in part because of the possibility that the patient will lie in the interview; however, other sources of information may be inaccurate as well. Parents may play down their offspring's violence; spouses, police officers, or correctional personnel may have reason not to tell the truth. In addition, while laypersons' observations of specific behaviors may be generally accurate, these individuals cannot be expected to notice every clinical nuance that may be significant to the psychiatrist, and their memories are often fallible. The need for corroboration is further illustrated by studies of violence and mental illness in which neighborhood and family corroboration efforts revealed significant recent and past violent behavior that was not discovered in careful admission interviews and record reviews.

In this era of diagnostic and treatment teams, too much fragmentation of the workup can be a bad thing. In taking history from family, for example, much may be missed if the person interviewing them is not both highly qualified in the topic at hand (comprehensive evaluation of violence, in this case) *and* familiar enough with the case to ask patient-specific questions and follow patient-specific leads in the conversation. In most cases, family and other corroborating sources should be contacted by the primary evaluating clinician, either initially or to follow up interviews by another professional.

2. Multiple Observations

When comprehensive understanding of the patient is the goal, he or she should be observed or interviewed on more than one occasion and often by more than one person. Serial office interviews, for example, reveal more than a single session, allowing the patient to become familiar with the setting, decreasing some defenses, increasing opportunities to remember important things, and offering a chance to see the patient in different parts of his or her daily life.

Just as multiple interviews and observations are useful, multiple observers add to the validity and reliability of the evaluation. In inpatient settings, there are usually professional and direct-care staff who observe and document their findings. They offer more than one viewpoint and varying opportunities to see patients as they present to different kinds of staff at different times of the day. Each staff person should be trained in observation, documentation, and interpretation to the extent appropriate for his or her role in the evaluation.

"Multiple observers" may also refer to the use of several different forms of observation and interpretation. Structured and unstructured interviews yield different, complementary kinds of data. Reports from ordinary interactions such as dining, medication administration, or social outings—as well as from special settings such as jails or courts—are helpful. Psychological testing and other forms of consultation (see below) increase the number of "windows" through which the evaluator or clinical team can view the patient/evaluee.

3. Protection During the Evaluation

The evaluator(s) and others who may come into contact with the patient should be appropriately warned and cautious. Many patients do not require extraordinary protective measures; however, the possibility of assault or flight by the patient should be assessed and the results documented. One must not ignore other patients, nonclinical staff, and visitors in this consideration, since they will not have worked with the evaluation team or read the patient's chart. Physical control, containment, and/or close monitoring of potentially violent patients, while often unpleasant, may be the best way to protect those in his or her environment until it becomes clear that there is little or no danger.

Seclusion, restraint, and other control procedures are unfortunately often misunderstood by laypersons, hospital regulators, policymakers, and even some clinicians. While procedures for patient control are not to be used for punishment or mere staff convenience, there are several circumstances in which they are clearly indicated for safety, other legitimate clinical reasons, patient comfort, or all three.

Indications for patient control, whether seclusion, some level of restraint, sedating medication, or some broader restriction such as close observation or a locked ward, are more varied than one might think. Safety of the patient and others is a major consideration; however, violence per se is not the sole clinical indication for, for example, seclusion or restraint. They may also be employed when the patient is a serious threat to property, the unit milieu, or the treatment program; to decrease sensory stimulation (often necessary on chaotic "psychiatric intensive care" units); preventively, when the patient's behavior or other symptoms suggest that violence is imminent or when part of the evaluation process is likely to precipitate violence (e.g., when attempting to replicate alcohol idiosyncratic reactions); as part of a behavior therapy (e.g., "contingent restraint") program; or when requested by the patient (e.g., to decrease anxiety, "calm down," or when the patient believes that he or she is about to become violent).

The concept of "least restrictive *clinically appropriate* alternative" is an important part of the modern institutional lexicon. Critics of patient control policies often note that adequate numbers of trained staff can decrease the need for seclusion, restraint, sedating medication, and locked doors. The experienced clinician will note, however, that there are many different situations in which some sort of control is indicated, and not all are best managed with additional personnel, no matter how well trained. For example, the patient may respond better to limited restraint (e.g., waist ties that allow movement on the ward but prevent swinging of the arms or grabbing others) than to continuous, expensive one-to-one monitoring.

Different individual procedures may be more or less restrictive, depending on the situation. Suicide is difficult to predict among violent patients, whether or not they have expressed self-destructive thoughts. For such patients, restraint may be safer than seclusion unless the room is safe and carefully monitored. For the patient who responds poorly to isolation and sensory deprivation, seclusion may be the worst alternative. Properly designed ambulatory restraints allow many violent patients to participate in the ward milieu and social interaction. On the other hand, some patients are extremely intolerant of four- or five-point restraint, experiencing panic even when an attendant is present. Chemical sedation, particularly a sedative neuroleptic, is sometimes considered the most humane form of restraint; however, it also offers potential for side effects, sensory deprivation and isolation, as well as a loss of control which is global rather than targeting the violence.

4. Examiner Safety

The interview setting should be comfortable and nonthreatening, with sufficient privacy for the examination but not enough to isolate the evaluator or place him or her in danger. Both the facility and the examining clinician (or team) should be aware of personal safety principles from the outset. In correctional settings, the staff are usually aware of security needs and can easily remain visible and/or able to recognize and respond to danger (but out of earshot for private conversation).

Sometimes, however, clinicians may be asked if they want to talk with a prisoner in his cell or be shown to a remote examining room, as if a psychologist or psychiatrist could recognize assault potential and magically prevent it. In some psychiatric facilities, unfortunately, single clinicians examine patients late at night, in remote parts of an institution or mental health center. When faced with such a situation, or any situation in which one may feel unsafe, it is important to request appropriate safeguards and not to proceed until they are provided. *The evaluator should not tolerate being placed in isolation or other jeopardy with a potentially violent patient.* Many clinicians, because of inexperience, denial, reticence, or misplaced embarrassment, do not adequately consider their own safety needs. *Estimates of danger to the examiner should not be left to intuition.*

When using a clinical examining room or one's own office, one should be aware of the contents *vis à vis* this special patient population and evaluation purpose. Ordinary office items that could be used as weapons should be identified and removed if necessary. Exit routes should be clear. Emergency notification equipment, appropriate for some settings, should be easily reachable and in working order. Procedures for using alarms, "panic buttons," safety response teams, aggressive behavior management techniques, etc., should be well practiced. One may consider removing personal items, particularly those that identify one's family, address, telephone number, etc., from the room. In many cases, clothing or jewelry that might be used quickly to injure the examiner (e.g., a necktie or necklace) should be removed as well. One must remember that the violence evaluation process is not a routine clinical discussion or therapy session.

B. Notice and Documentation

This chapter does not offer a specific format for documenting the evaluation; however, there are a few violence-relevant special issues that may be overlooked by even experienced clinicians. Some of these are particularly applicable to risk-assessment evaluations, which may be done either within or outside a routine treatment relationship (e.g., for commitment or other court procedure, special discharge panel, parole board, or certain employment consultations).

The patient/evaluee should be notified of the evaluator's duties and allegiances before any interview. The purpose of the session and limitations on confidentiality should be clear. If the patient is not able to understand, the interview and other parts of the personal assessment can usually proceed as long as appropriate attention is paid to the patient's rights against self-incrimination as relevant to the particular setting and purpose at hand. Note that in many cases the person's *consent* is not required for the interview or evaluation; however, he or she may decline to participate (which should be noted and considered in one's eventual conclusions).

The extent to which the patient's rights must be balanced with the rights of potential victims is sometimes a complex legal, ethical, and philosophical issue. The patient/evaluee may want to avoid the evaluation or may not be able to understand its purpose and consequences. Each evaluation type and setting is different in this regard, some giving the evaluator *carte blanche* and others severely limiting access even to relevant clinical information. Speaking broadly, this author places considerable emphasis on protecting others from serious damage or injury; however, the evaluator should be aware of his or her own legal and ethical circumstances with respect to patients' rights issues and consult a knowledgeable attorney, colleague, or other reference as necessary.

In some cases, data may be gathered outside the personal interview and physical examination without regard to evaluee cooperation. Much of the history may be obtained without disturbing the issue of confidentiality, and background information may sometimes be obtained from anyone willing to provide it. The absence of a clinician-patient relationship may be helpful in this regard, since the evaluator may thus not have any duty of confidentiality to the evaluee. Even when a clinician-patient relationship exists, the patient may be told at the outset (e.g., on hospital admission or at the beginning of therapy) that when the issue of significant danger to others is raised, individual privilege will be weighed against the need to protect potential victims. In this chapter we are not speaking of warning or protecting per se, but *this author recommends that questions of patient privilege not be allowed to interfere with good-faith efforts to obtain information that is reasonably necessary to protect others from significant harm.*

If the patient refuses to authorize release of information, two techniques of gathering outside information may be helpful in cases involving a clinician-patient relationship. Both rely on one or more of the patient's relatives or friends already being aware that he or she is a patient; that is, this particular fact would not be a confidential matter for those persons. In such a case, there should be no legal or ethical consequence to asking them about the nonconsenting patient *provided that they are not given further information about him or her.* Such a "one-way" conversation, in which the clinician asks for information but does not discuss (or informally hint about) the patient's care or condition, can be very helpful. Further, since the same family member or friend is not constrained by legal or professional issues of confidentiality, one may ask him or her to question other sources of important information (e.g., relatives, employers, coworkers, friends) whom the doctor cannot contact without authorization. The information obtained will be secondhand but may be much better than none at all.

It is important to document these "legalistic" parts of the evaluation procedure, just as one documents the clinical items. A brief note that prior to personal interview the patient/evaluee has been told the purpose, confidentiality limitations, examiner allegiance, and possible consequences of the interview—and that he or she understands the information—is usually sufficient. In some cases, written notice (not a "consent") may be provided (see the Appendix at the end of this chapter). Other items that are useful to include in the examination note or report include the referral source, evaluator's role (if any) in contemplated legal or administrative proceedings, the specific purpose of the interview, a detailed description of the setting, and sources of corroborating information. One may also provide estimates of the reliability of the information obtained and the patient's/evaluee's ability to participate (e.g., fluency in English, presence of psychosis or mental retardation), and a note about his or her understanding of the examination process.

C. Preliminary Assessment

Tardiff (1) has recommended that evaluation of the violent patient begin with an "instant differential diagnosis" in order to set the initial examination procedure and assess needs for immediate control or treatment. Such a gross differentiation, into three general categories, may or may not relate directly to the violence or its cause and should not be an end in itself; however, it adds helpful structure to the initial phase of the evaluation process.

Patients with *"organic" mental disorders* (including substance-related syndromes) are often unable to provide clinical or historical data themselves and respond poorly to verbal efforts at control. If controlling violence during the evaluation is necessary, neuroleptics and other drugs that further cloud the cognitive picture should generally be avoided in favor of treatment of the underlying general medical disorder or substance abuse. When this is contraindicated or impossible, humane physical restraint should be used as necessary to allow the evaluation to proceed safely. Patients with *psychotic disorders* not caused by a general medical problem or a substance (e.g., schizophrenic, manic, or other delusional patients), who are acutely violent or agitated, are usually best treated with rapid pharmacologic relief of their psychoses. Those with *nonpsychotic, nonorganic disorders* (e.g., severe personality disorders, nonpsychotic depression, or impulse-control disorders) can often be evaluated without medication, seclusion, or restraint; however, safeguards for patient and staff should be considered. Treatment of psychiatric symptoms (e.g., depression) can usually proceed during the violence workup.

D. Historical Information

The following have been found useful in at least some studies and settings involving violence. Note that this should not be considered an exhaustive list, nor is everything here relevant to every evaluation. Context and individual situation are important. Different historical items may or may not be important to different types of violence. Finally, one should not forget that the history should not be limited to information from the patient; corroboration is critical.

1. Violence History

Understanding the characteristics of past violence, attempts, plans, thoughts, and fantasies is arguably the most important part of the evaluation. The vast variety of form, level, and context of violence demands that each case be considered individually, not generically. Once there is detailed understanding, the behavior may fit a pattern that contributes to diagnosis, treatment, or risk assessment. Each negative or, especially, positive finding should trigger follow-up questions consistent with the particular case. While an organized approach is recommended, strict assessment protocols and algorithms may not be flexible enough for a truly individualized evaluation.

Type, onset, duration, course, and frequency should be explored. Type of violence is critical. Is there one kind in the history or are there several? When, where, and how did it or they begin? Was the behavior relatively constant over time, regular, sporadic, or isolated? Has it increased, decreased, fluctuated, or remained about the same in frequency and severity? When was the last episode? Does it continue during hospitalization or evaluation? It is important not to forget vehicular violence, relevant verbal threats and aggression, and other significant aggression not always traditionally considered to be "violence."

Inquiring about superlatives is useful in many evaluations. What is the *most* anger the person has ever experienced? What is the *worst* outburst in the history? The *worst* injury to another person? The *worst* property damage? How often has that level of violence occurred? When and under what specific circumstances? What happened afterward?

Additional exploration of the violent behavior should consider associated *events, setting, illness, substance use or abuse, people* (e.g., groups, accomplices, onlookers), and *relationship* (real or symbolic) *to the victim(s)*. In directed violence, is the choice of victim logical or foreseeable? In seemingly indirect or random violence, is there any discernible pattern?

Is the violence *affective* or *predatory*? This is, does it appear to be a response to autonomic stimulation such as global threat or "fight-or-flight" (as when a cat responds to a large, barking dog), or is it careful and planned (as when the same cat slowly stalks a bird).[2] Is it *purposeful* or *random*? *controlled* or *explosive*? Does it involve obvious alterations of mood, affect, though process, reality testing, memory, cognition, or consciousness? Is the violence incidental to a crime or does it represent the crime itself? Is there *remorse* afterward? Confusion? Dissociation? Apathy? Is the perpetrator willing to recognize and/or accept *responsibility* for the violence? Able to appreciate the *consequences*? Does he or she believe that the violence is/was worth later consequences such as arrest or self-injury?

Another set of inquiries may address *response to past treatment* and management techniques. Has the patient sought treatment voluntarily? Has he or she complied with treatment programs? What worked and what did not? What has changed in the patient's life or environment, if anything, that might change one's view toward current and future violence, treatment, or risk-management decisions?

2. Psychiatric History

A number of cohort and retrospective studies of severe Axis I and II disorders over at least two decades have shown that, broadly speaking, persons with mental illness have significantly increased risk of violence and violent crime as compared with matched populations without mental illness (2–5).[3] This general association with violence is easily misunderstood. First, only a few diagnoses contribute very much to increases over general population rates. In most disorders and situations (but not all), factors other than illness per se contribute most of the risk. Even when the mental illness is a critical factor, as in some paranoid or postpartum psychosis, the phase of illness, severity of symptoms, and symp-

---

[2]Thanks to Dr. Phil Resnick for this example.

[3]Note that the statistical importance of the association between Axis I mental illness and violence to the overall incidence of violent acts in a society is related to the base rate of violence in the population being studied. Thus many studies of severely ill patients from relatively low-violence Scandinavia and Switzerland show a manyfold increase compared to the non-mentally-ill population, whereas in countries with higher violence rates, the contribution of mental illness is relatively smaller. Although studies in the former societies may help highlight the effect of the mental illness per se, by lessening variance from the base rate, the relationship is complicated by other factors, such as social expectations regarding violence, which may be felt by the mentally ill more or less than by the general population.

tom content (e.g., form of delusion or hallucination) are important considerations (5,6).

Thus, although one should consider those diagnoses that are inherently, commonly, or infrequently associated with violence (Table 1), attribution of causation or risk is a more complex matter. Any association may be partial or incidental and is likely to be related to factors outside the diagnosis itself (e.g., active substance abuse, treatment compliance, physical setting, provocation, victim characteristics). One must remember that *violence is a generic, "final common pathway" phenomenon, usually the result of multiple factors coming together at a particular time and place.*

The paragraphs below offer several examples of clinical considerations. They are not intended to be a comprehensive list of psychiatric illness factors in violence, nor are they relevant to every evaluation.

Chronically psychotic patients charged with lethal and potentially lethal violence appear to have a higher incidence of delusions about specific victims and/or targets and delusions about significant others being replaced by imposters (*Capgras syndrome*) than do those charged with property crimes. They also have higher intelligence and more family members who were victims of lethal violence (7). Silva et al. (8) recently reviewed 82 cases of *delusional misidentification.* Paranoid delusions are often more subtle than other schizophreniform characteristics and may be hidden from other people. Paranoia is more often associated with organized, predatory violence than are more disorganized forms of psychosis. Misidentification and Capgras syndrome are both associated with more violence than ordinary paranoia and should be documented if found. In other forms of schizophrenia, violence may arise from delusions or hallucinations as well as from other factors.

Command hallucinations are not always an ominous sign. The clinician should try to determine several characteristics of the commands before deciding whether or not they suggest imminent danger. For example, is the voice a familiar one? Familiar voices (except for God or Satan) are more likely to be associated with commands eventually being carried out. Is the command a violent one or something benign? Benign commands are more likely to be carried out and do not necessarily predict the presence of violent ones. What is the patient's perceived penalty for *not* carrying out the command? The belief that he or she can save the world by killing someone is an ominous thought indeed; the feeling that some unbearable tension will be relieved is also worrisome. On the other hand, if the patient is accustomed to resisting the commands without ill effects, the risk of violence is much lower.

Modestin and Ammann (5) found a fivefold higher lifetime prevalence of violent crimes, three times the drug abuse, and 2 1/2 times more property crimes, in Swiss *schizophrenic* men ($n = 282$) than in highly matched controls from the general population. Stage of illness (schizophreniform, acute, chronic) contrib-

Table 1 DSM-IV Diagnoses and Conditions Which May Be Associated with Some Form of Violent Behavior*

Those listing violence as an essential diagnostic feature:

Conduct disorder
Intermittent explosive disorder
Pyromania
Sexual sadism
Child or adult physical abuse

Those with which some level of violence is frequently associated:

Oppositional defiant disorder
Disruptive behavior disorder
Delirium
Dementia
Substance-related disorders involving alcohol, amphetamines/stimulants, cocaine, hallucinogens, inhalants/"sniffing", opiates, phencyclidine, and similar substances
Schizophrenia/other psychotic disorders with paranoid, disorganized, catatonic-excited, delusional, shared, post-partum, and substance-induced psychotic syndromes, and those due to general medical conditions
Substance-induced mood disorder
Post-partum mood disorder with psychotic features (and other post-partum psychoses)
Pedophilia
Sexual sadism
Child or adult sexual abuse
Adjustment disorder with disturbance of conduct
Paranoid personality
Antisocial personality
Borderline personality
Adult or child/adolescent antisocial behavior

Those for which violence is less frequent but may be considered:

Attention-deficit hyperactivity disorder, adolescent or adult
Substance-related disorders other than above
Mental disorders due to a general medical condition other than above
Psychotic disorders other than above (including delusional depression)
Bipolar disorder, manic, and rapid-cycling
Posttraumatic stress disorder
Dissociative identity disorder
Schizotypal personality
Narcissistic personality
Neuroleptic-induced akathisia
Relational problems
Noncompliance with treatment

Table 1 Continued

Those for which violence is a potential but infrequent feature:

Mental retardation
Depressive disorders other than above (particularly post-partum syndromes)
Bipolar disorders other than above
Panic disorders
Acute stress disorder
Obsessive-compulsive disorder
Substance-induced anxiety disorder
Dissociative disorders other than above
Other paraphilias
Gender identity disorder
Parasomnias
Other impulse control disorders
Personality disorders other than above
Medication effects other than above
Borderline intellectual functioning
Age-related cognitive decline
Acculturation problem

*Not including solely self-destructive violence. Note caveats in the text about relying solely on diagnosis to explain causation or assess risk. For most disorders and conditions listed, the violence may be clinically related (e.g., violent response to a paranoid delusion), peripherally related (e.g., mentally retarded persons encouraged by others to commit crimes, opioid addicts using violence to procure drugs), or both.

uted to the variance. Studies from the same authors indicate that, with some exceptions, other psychiatric diagnosis per se contributes little to risk of criminality in their Swiss population. Substance abuse, separate from other demographic factors, accounts for much of this variance (9). In Finland, which has a very low base rate of homicide, the risk of committing murder was about 10 times greater for schizophrenic patients of both genders than it was for the general population. Schizophrenia without alcoholism increased the risk about 7 times; schizophrenia with *coexisting alcoholism* increased it more than 17 times (3). *Antisocial personality* was associated with an even greater increase in "odds ratio," especially for women (up to 50 times). Affective disorders, anxiety disorders, dysthymia, and mental retardation did not measurably increase the likelihood of homicide (2).

Grossman et al. (10) found that state hospital patients with *schizoaffective disorder* were more likely to have been convicted of a violent crime than those with other schizophreniform and mood disorders. Presence of *psychosis, paranoia*, and *substance abuse* increased past risk. In some studies, *affective disor-*

der patients show a peak in aggressiveness during spring and winter (11). Aggressive activity among schizophrenics appears unrelated to time of year per se.

Patients with chronic psychosis can be violent for reasons other than their psychosis. They must often live in violence-prone locations, are sometimes involved with drug abuse, and often become depressed and frustrated with their disability.

Borderline personality traits are proportionately overrepresented among murderers. In some studies, decreasing stability of relationships and affect is linearly associated with increasing violence (12). The presence of *coexisting antisocial personality* increases indices of criminality (e.g., earlier age of onset, more convictions) in major mental disorder compared to either diagnosis alone; however, at least one study found no increase in violence per se (13).

Spouse abuse has a number of psychiatric correlates but is not apparently associated with major mental illness. Dinwiddie (14) found that wife batterers had significant increases in lifetime alcoholism, antisocial personality, and depression but not other disorders. Early adolescent violence was not a differentiating factor. Dutton (15) found that male perpetrators of spouse abuse were more likely than controls to have symptoms of *posttraumatic stress disorder (PTSD)* on the MCMI-II (Millon Clinical Multiaxial Inventory); however, these findings are colored by the fact that many of the men had characteristics of antisocial personality as well, and the MCMI is poorly validated for such applications.

Violent impulse control disorders such as *intermittent explosive disorder* usually have a better prognosis than characterologic violence (such as that found in borderline or antisocial personality). The remorse such patients usually feel, and their greater sensitivity to consequences of violence (e.g., marriage problems), increase treatment motivation and compliance.

3. General Medical History

Medical history, particularly regarding neurological and endocrine (including menstrual) conditions, toxins, and medication reactions, must not be omitted. A great many medical syndromes have occasionally been associated with severe violence [cf., exceptional cases of killing during a postictal confusional state or sleep-related phenomenon (16) or arising from depression or irritability related to chronic illness (17)]. This does not mean that such illnesses or confusional states are always significant risk factors, however. When signs of a general medical condition are found in the violence evaluation, potential association with the violence should be explored.

Neurological abnormality is a fairly consistent differentiating factor among psychiatric patients with persistent, transient, and little or no violence (18). After substance abuse, brain damage is the single most common organic contributor to violent behavior. As with mental illness, however, the association is complex and far from ubiquitous. Set and setting continue to be important for most patients. The nature and severity of the violence is so varied that general assumptions should be discouraged. For example, one may say that some level of "violence" is frequently seen in Alzheimer's disease, with or without organic psychosis (19). Alzheimer's patients are rarely directly dangerous to others, however, although their confusion or forgetfulness may indirectly cause fires or other hazards.

It is usually easy to uncover current or past symptoms of central nervous system (CNS) irritability, affective instability, dyscontrol episodes, dementia, and other suggestions of brain damage. Poor judgment, impulsivity, or lack of insight are less specific features of organicity but also increase the probability of violence. When these are present in violent patients, careful workup may reveal a focal neurological abnormality or more diffuse dysfunction. When the problem is diffuse and/or not directly treatable (e.g., from inhalant abuse or trauma), response to intervention is correspondingly poorer.

It is difficult to generalize about the relationship of behavior after brain damage to preexisting behavior. In some cases, the brain dysfunction weakens higher functions and impulse control; in others, the patient becomes more docile and "flat" (but may nevertheless be prone to act without adequately considering the consequences).

Post-ictal violence is usually related to confused states but may also be due to encephalomalacia from extended convulsions or *status epilepticus*. Violence during partial complex seizures is rare, often without purpose, and rarely serious. Violence during post-seizure encephalopathy is more subtle but does occur.

Overall rates of violence generally increase with decreased intelligence down to an IQ of roughly 70. Some clinicians are reluctant to recognize antisocial syndromes in persons with mental retardation; however, when there is violent behavior, particularly with predatory behavior and lack of remorse, such diagnoses should be made (20). Patients with severe CNS dysfunction or very low IQ have a decreased probability of directed violence and, in most cases, of violence in general.

The relationship of neurological abnormality to violent behavior is often complicated by past and continuing substance abuse, which, in turn, complicates behavioral management (2). Since the source of the CNS abnormality is often some sort of reckless or antisocial behavior before injury (e.g., driving while intoxicated or other risk taking), careful comparison of past and present is important to understanding the role of the brain damage.

4. Social History

A detailed social history should include the setting in which violence has occurred and may suggest a specific pattern or syndrome. One should incorporate questions and follow-up about all kinds of violence, including reckless driving and other automobile incidents, verbal altercations, fights (whether or not started by the patient), and sports violence. This part of the history may be more comprehensive than the "psychiatric" portion with regard to clarifying the phenomenology of violent behavior and describing three levels of concern: violent thoughts, plans, and behaviors.

In trying to rate the seriousness of plans and behaviors, one should be alert for evidence that these could or would have been serious if not somehow interrupted. For example, if clear plans to kill a spouse are serendipitously discovered in a patient's diary without other violent behavior, they should be considered ominous. If a person on his way to kill a superior at work is distracted by something else, the behavior should be considered an "attempt" for purposes of the evaluation. *Psychiatric evaluation of violent patients should not be confused with criminal investigations or trials. It is quite appropriate to consider information that might not be allowed in a legal proceeding.*

Work and interpersonal relationships provide important psychosocial information. Family, marital, friend, and work relationships should be addressed and their characteristics and stability noted. It goes without saying that marital and family relationships should be examined for domestic violence.

Changes in work or relationships (especially those associated with past violent behavior) should be explored. Real or psychodynamic loss (or threatened loss) is particularly associated with violence in susceptible individuals, in part because of commonly related issues of shame, humiliation, self-image, narcissism, helplessness, dependency, and/or retribution. Details of divorce, separation, child custody, job loss, school failure, and even property damage may be helpful in both assessing risk and building a foundation for diagnosis and treatment. Although a general threat of job loss—for example, from company downsizing—may cause psychiatric symptoms, at least one study has found no increased violence in persons not actually laid off (22).

Legal or criminal history is often minimized by patients/evaluees. The examiner should ask specific and detailed questions about misdemeanor and felony arrests and charges, driving offenses, substance-related offenses, divorces and domestic disputes, and civil matters (e.g., lawsuits). Patients who say they were never "convicted" should be asked about times they were detained or arrested. Those who describe a "misunderstanding" with the law or a "couple of days in jail" should be pressed for details and the history corroborated when feasible. Many patients, particularly those with antisocial, narcissistic, paranoid, or hysteroid characteristics, are unreliable in their descriptions of past antisocial behavior, criminal charges, and other legal entanglements.

Cultural issues may also be important. For example, several authors note that love-obsessional or erotomanic violence is often associated with men brought up in sexually repressive cultures who misunderstand or overinterpret relatively benign communications from American women. Words or behavior considered merely social in the United States or Canada, such as accepting a date or a good-night kiss, may be misconstrued as connoting a deeper relationship. When the woman does not continue the misperceived commitment, a seed of obsession or paranoia may be planted in which the man feels slighted, cuckolded, or otherwise humiliated. (With regard to either men or women, there is danger to persons who come between the perpetrator and the love object, as well as a danger *to* the love object.) The role of mental illness in such violent clashes of cultures varies. In addition, culturally based forms of violence, such as *amok*, if recognized, may help the North American clinician understand otherwise baffling behavior (23).

Military experience offers a unique opportunity for extensive information about a significant portion of the patient's life. Military records are usually easy to obtain and offer a fairly objective view of a person's overall work behavior, disciplinary problems, and ability to interact with others. In addition, the military history can provide information about weapons training and use, combat experience, responses to severe (sometimes life-threatening) stress, and similar topics. It is useful to know the extent to which the patient retains combat skills and/or attitudes.

Being a victim of violence appears to increase the likelihood of violence among female criminals. Lake (24) studied 83 inmates and found that assault by husbands and partners and early physical abuse was associated with earlier entry into crime and more diverse criminal activity. Note that although women have measurably less serious violence in the general population, gender is not a differentiating factor in risk of violence among psychiatric patients in either the hospital or the community (25).

5. Substance History

The extraordinary association of substance abuse with violence makes a careful substance history critical to any evaluation. Substance-abuse disorders alone are linked to various forms of violence. Intoxication increases risk of irritability or violence (e.g., with amphetamines, phencyclidine, some anabolic steroids); decreases judgment, inhibitions, or impulse control (alcohol, cocaine, others); and/or alters sensorium or perception (barbiturates, hallucinogens, others). Other associations between substance use and violence include those related to idiosyncratic reactions (e.g., to alcohol and some benzodiazepines), withdrawal, brain damage (especially inhalants), the substance-abusing environment, drug-seeking behavior, and illegal activity.

The combination of substance abuse with other psychiatric diagnoses (sometimes markedly) increases the probability of violence and is an important factor in treatment planning. Such dual diagnosis adds direct risk from intoxication or substance dependence, compromises already tenuous social and emotional conditions, threatens treatment compliance, and complicates diagnosis.

6. Developmental History

Birth or early childhood trauma, attachment problems, neglect, abandonment, family violence, physical (but in some studies not sexual) abuse, parental loss, parental violence or criminality, delayed developmental milestones, childhood attention and hyperactivity disorders, conduct disorders, cruelty, other antisocial behavior, and school problems are all positively correlated with later violence. *None is pathognomonic for adult violence, however, and it is inappropriate to imply a causative or one-to-one relationship in most cases.*

7. Family History

Family history should determine the structure of the nuclear and extended families and then search for violence, criminality, certain psychiatric illnesses, substance abuse, and suicide. Specific details of each, particularly violence and criminality, should be sought, along with any direct effects on the patient (such as parental abuse, neglect, abandonment, or modeling during development). Sibling characteristics, especially for twins, are particularly important. Paternal criminality is among the best documented correlates of adult antisocial behavior. It is important to be sure that all "family" are encompassed, including second-degree relatives and any unrelated persons who were consistent parts of the developmental environment.

E. Psychological Tests and Behavioral Analysis

1. Tests and Rating Scales

Anger, hostility, and aggression scales on general tests such as the Brief Psychiatric Rating Scale (BPRS), Positive and Negative Symptom Scale (PANSS), or Hopkins Symptom Checklist (SCL-90) tend not be very useful for assessing violence per se but may help clarify general psychopathology. The Nurses' Observation Scale for Inpatient Evaluation (NOSIE) is a common inpatient observation instrument but contains little concerning primary presentations of aggression or violence.

There are few comprehensive diagnostic scales for aggression. Most are designed for observations in inpatient settings and so suffer from a lack of context outside the hospital or institution. All have limitations, and the reader should become familiar with each before relying on its results. Self-report instruments such as the Buss-Durkee Inventory tend not to be very valid and are questionably useful when the patient has an important stake in the outcome (e.g., to avoid incarceration or to be discharged from hospital).

Bech and Mak (26) describe several scales for measuring aggressive behavior, particularly in the context of assessing target symptoms and response to treatment. Many are briefly summarized below. Unfortunately, they are limited to settings in which patients can be observed directly, and validation is often limited.

The Carolina Nosology of Destructive Behaviors (CNBD) (27) has codes and axes for different forms of aggressive behavior. It is "promising" but has not been well validated to date (26). The Scale for Assessment of Agitated and Aggressive Behavior (SAAB) was developed for violent adolescents (28). The Overt Aggression Scale (OAS), developed for children and adults, is described as moderately valid and has recently been modified to address some earlier shortcomings (29). The Social Dysfunction and Aggression Scale (its SDAS-9 items focus on outwardly directed violence) is quite brief but may be useful for both generalized and specific aggressive episodes (30,31). Validation has largely been in patients with personality disorders and psychotic and mood disorders. The Staff Observation Aggression Scale (SOAS) was developed for elderly patients (32). The Rating Scale for Aggression in the Elderly (RAGE) is oriented toward hospital or nursing home geriatric patients, often with dementias (33).

General psychometrics may reveal generic correlates of violence, such as certain kinds of emotional conflict, reality testing, impulsivity, depression, low intelligence, and/or frustration intolerance. Although helpful in clarifying diagnosis, they are often not very useful for assessing risk of violence or ascertaining its primary cause.

Neuropsychological testing is a valuable noninvasive tool for assessing actual brain function. In experienced hands, it can provide clues to both primary behavioral abnormality and organic brain substrate that may predispose the patient to aberrance (e.g., out of frustration with CNS deficits, inability to form alternative behaviors, or inability to recognize or respond to cues in various environments and situations).

Baseline or interim outcome information in chronically institutionalized persons is often best assessed with comprehensive *behavior analysis*. Long-term inhabitants of institutions—such as some people with mental retardation, incapacitating developmental disabilities, chronic severe psychoses, and dementias as well as some criminals—may be best understood using individualized, highly detailed observations through which behavior can be scrutinized for diagnosis, tracked for changes or improvement, and reliably compared with earlier levels after management or treatment techniques. Behavior analysis is most useful in controlled settings in which the interventions and environment can be either held constant or shaped for extended periods. Its usefulness in community settings is much more limited.

F. Psychiatric Interview and Examination

It is not possible to describe interview techniques for every violent or potentially violent patient. Traditional interview and mental status examination principles apply to some extent, with special attention to therapist protection, completeness, the probability that the patient will not be completely truthful, and examiner agency (discussed below).

G. Diagnostic Procedures and Laboratory Tests

Although other consultations may also be indicated, neurological and endocrinological examinations are most likely to be helpful in violence evaluations. Genetic workup is occasionally useful as well. When comprehensive evaluation is indicated, the patient should receive complete psychiatric and physical examinations with blood and urine screening (including drug screens for outpatients and new admissions).

Blake et al. (34) found that 20 of 31 convicted or accused murderers showed frontal dysfunction on careful neurological examination. Temporal symptoms were present in 9 and 20 qualified for a neurological diagnosis (including 9 with borderline intelligence or mental retardation). All subjects had abnormal neuropsychological testing, and 8 of 20 who received electroencephalography (EEG) had some abnormality (usually bilateral spikes and slowing, common in studies of very violent men). Magnetic resonance imaging (MRI) or computed tomography (CT) often showed brain atrophy or other white matter changes. Paranoia, "misunderstood social situations," and protracted past physical abuse were very common. MRI offers more information than CT scanning. Wong et al. (35) found similar temporal EEG tracings in violent British maximum security patients as well as abnormal temporal lobe structure (overall decreased size and/or dilated temporal horns of the ventricles), both greatly overrepresented in the highly violent group. In a small study of patients on a violent behavior unit, Convit et al. (36) found a significant relationship between violent psychiatric patients and lateralized frontotemporal EEG abnormality. Electroencephalography is more productive if nasopharyngeal leads and activating techniques are used.

Cerebrospinal fluid 5-hydroxy indoleacetic acid (5-HIAA) in 10 violent schizophrenics was identical to that in 10 matched nonviolent schizophrenics studied by Kunz et al. (37). In a much larger Scandinavian study (n = 114), Virkkunen et al. (38) found increased family histories of paternal violence and alcoholism in male alcoholic violent offenders and firesetters with low CSF 5-HIAA and homovanillic acid (HVA). Low plasma cholesterol, which has been reported as both positively and negatively associated with various forms of violence and hostility (39), was linked to family history of paternal alcoholism but not violence. After 4.5 years of follow-up, further violence and firesetting was predicted by low CSF 5-HIAA and 3-methoxy 4-hydroxyphenylglycol (MHPG) concentrations as well as by early paternal absence.

A few years earlier, Virkkunen's group found that impulsive offenders with alcoholism and antisocial personality disorder had lower CSF 5-HIAA and corticotropin and higher CSF testosterone than nonimpulsive and nonalcoholic controls. Those with intermittent explosive disorder had a very low blood glucose after glucose challenge. Low CSF 5-HIAA concentration was primarily associated with impulsivity and high CSF testosterone concentration with aggressiveness or interpersonal violence (40). Moderately low cholesterol was statistically linked to male aggression in a study of inpatients by Hillbrand et al. (41). No study thus far has implied any clinical usefulness of the above lipid findings.

III. RISK ASSESSMENT

A. Risk Factors

It is useful to point out the difference between "prediction of violence" and "assessment of risk." The presence of a "risk factor" does not necessarily imply significant risk increase, singular significance (as contrasted with incremental and contextual significance), prediction of future violence, prediction of a particular form or severity of violence, or applicability to persons outside the group being discussed. For example, a recent study of violent psychiatric emergency department patients found that commonly described demographic "risk factors" (young age, male sex, past history of violence) did not differentiate them from an equal number of nondangerous patients (42).

Everyone has "risk factors"; many people with very little propensity for violence have many risk factors; and most people with many risk factors do not become significantly violent. This disclaimer is intended to stop naive clinicians—and nonclinicians such as judges and attorneys—from using risk factors and decision algorithms in a simplistic way, either to predict future behavior or to criticize unfairly decisions made by psychiatrists and others on the treatment team. Risk assessment provides a probabilistic context within which individualized treatment, violence prevention plans, etc., can be considered as necessary. "Prediction," on the other hand, is the much more difficult task of forecasting a specific outcome for a specific patient.

B. Context

Evaluation of violence potential must be seen as *context-sensitive*. It is inappropriate to expect *more* workup than the clinical situation requires for reasonable diagnosis and probable safety (e.g., in pre-discharge or pre-pass screening when there is little reason to expect violence), just as it is inappropriate to expect *less* than is necessary when there is cause to expect problems (e.g., in some forensic settings or when behavior, symptoms, or diagnosis should suggest caution). Some violence evaluations are done in emergency departments to assess need for admission; others relate to approving the patient/evaluee for some level of activity (e.g., a pass, discharge, return to work, visitation with children). Still others are part of an extensive workup to try to understand a pattern or disorder and arrive at a definitive diagnosis. The recommended evaluation process thus depends on the context in which patient/evaluee and clinician find themselves. The primary requirement for the clinician is thoughtful consideration of that context, the clinical question asked, and, in many cases, potential risk.

Note the phrase *thoughtful consideration* in the last sentence. The psychiatrist or other responsible person(s), reasonably aware of the patient's background *vis á vis* the current setting and situation, should conduct an evaluation that is consistent with the present clinical and social context. In some cases, this requires only brief consideration with little or no documentation. In others, extensive review, corroboration of history, examination, testing, consultation with other professionals, referral to intensive evaluation settings, and/or physical control of the patient/evaluee may be necessary. Most situations require something between the two extremes. There is no universal standard for violence evaluations, only reasonable actions that fit the current patient in his or her current situation.

C. Purpose vs. Patient Need

Clinicians sometimes forget that assessment of violence risk should not focus primarily on the patient's needs but on danger to others. In spite of the professional ethic of beneficence toward patients, investigations centered on the safety or protection of others are necessarily different from (but may overlap with) those whose main purpose is diagnosis or treatment. Some of the differences are subtle (e.g., accurate diagnosis and effective treatment of the patient can clarify and decrease danger to others); others are not (e.g., efforts to minimize workplace violence regardless of the patient's diagnosis or treatment needs). In most settings, both purposes can be considered in some proportion consistent with patient need and risk of serious harm.

D. Agency: "Patient" vs. "Evaluee"

In a broad sense, we are all asked to protect potential victims of predictable violence. Some psychiatrists and psychologists, however, assess potential violence for courts, prisons, law enforcement organizations, other government agencies, or even private employers. Although this may seem unusual for a profession that generally denies its ability to predict violence, it is nevertheless proper—and often important—that we participate in the process when we can contribute to it.

In most clinical settings, the doctor has a *fiduciary* relationship with the patient; that is, the doctor has agreed to perform certain services *in the patient's interest*. In others, however, it is important to define one's professional relationship (or *agency*) in a different way.

When the evaluator assumes some of the patient's care (or makes decisions about care), a clinician-patient relationship probably exists. If the evaluator is solely a tool for the primary clinician's evaluation, then there may not be a clinician-patient relationship (depending, for example, on whether the patient was examined in person, seen or treated by someone under the supervision of the evaluator, or evaluated solely through record review). Consultants retained specifically for some legal or administrative purpose (such as presentencing evaluation, independent pre-release parole review, or employment-related examination) are agents of the employer, state, attorney, etc., and should inform the patient/evaluee of such.

The presence or absence of a clinician-patient relationship is not merely a legal or liability issue; it determines where the primary interests of the evaluation lie. If one is the patient's "doctor," then one must act in the patient's interest unless or until there is a measurable potential for serious danger to others (at which time the patient's interest must be balanced in some appropriate way with those of potential victims). Without a doctor-patient relationship, one's duty is to be objective about risk regardless of any effect on the evaluee.

E. Who Sets the Standards for Evaluation?

It is a truism that when patient violence occurs, the most recent evaluation will be brought into question and may be the center of inquiry or litigation. As stated above, there is no generic "standard" for evaluations of violence potential, nor should one be broadly applied. Clinicians and lawyers may look to textbooks and scholarly articles, but the principles of context and consideration just mentioned should guide their interpretations.

Nevertheless, guidelines, and sometimes "standards," do exist in some settings. Citizens exhort their legislators to pass laws ensuring that murderers and pedophiles will not be released from prisons or hospitals unless they are 100% safe. Risk managers and hospital lawyers seek "safe harbor" guidelines which, if not completely reliable, will at least meet some legal test of reasonableness. These fears and demands meet clinicians in arenas such as malpractice risk, forensic hospital release standards, and commitment laws. More subtle but nonetheless influential pressures may be felt from the media and third-party payers.

It is important that clinicians, especially those physicians who control decisions about admission, treatment, and discharge, champion procedures that are clinically and behaviorally reasonable and within the bounds of safety; they should not give up their defense of what is clinically right in favor of bureaucratic or political "correctness." We must obey the law and at times help protect our communities but also use what special knowledge we have in the service of both individual and society. When necessary, we can advocate for what we believe is right, and work toward that which appropriately balances public safety with clinical need.

A wise Oriental philosopher once said that "Perfect is the enemy of good." Violence evaluation should be aimed at maximizing return and minimizing danger in a particular context, with resources commensurate with the case at hand. Although the *goal* may be to locate all risk and prevent any violence, complete success is not a reasonable *objective*, any more than completely eradicating hunger is a reasonable objective for food banks and soup kitchens.

The clinician's responsibility for future violence is tied largely to his or her awareness of the elements of an appropriate evaluation, to the pursuit of the relevant elements of the evaluation, and to good-faith attention to the results of the evaluation. Although it is uncomfortable to have one's *judgments* prove wrong, especially if the outcome is tragic, it is far worse to have used an imprudent or inappropriate *process* in coming to those judgments.

F. Site of the Evaluation

Almost all violence evaluations are done in clinical settings, and a large portion of the remainder are done in correctional environments. Patients/evaluees are rarely examined in "natural" settings or in the settings in which violence has occurred. This makes it doubly important to be aware of the possibility that evaluation in a hospital or jail will miss important information about the set and setting of past or future violence.

The first step in correcting this problem is to be aware of it. Its potential effects on accuracy and reliability should be acknowledged and documented, then efforts may be made to overcome those effects. Complete, corroborated history is the cornerstone of the process.

In a few cases, it may be possible to reproduce the setting in which violence has occurred. Usually, this takes place in the form of off-ward passes in which the patient's feelings and behavior are monitored. Role-playing, fantasy, hypnosis, and even biological challenge (e.g., with small amounts of alcohol in suspected alcohol idiosyncratic syndromes) may also be employed. Nevertheless, it is usually impossible to reproduce the complex combination of location, surroundings, participants, and physical and emotional condition.

The patients' interest in the outcome of the evaluation should be considered, since his or her motivations and expectations are not usually the same as those of an ordinary patient. Sometimes a pass or discharge from the hospital is at stake. Recommendations regarding legal responsibility for violent acts, child custody, or incarceration are also common outcome topics. The patient may thus be only marginally cooperative in the evaluation process. In some cases, the patient is genuinely disturbed by his or her violent behavior and outwardly strives to understand and change it; however, one still must allow for unconscious resistances to diagnosis and treatment.

Principles of safety also apply when one is considering an outpatient evaluation or trial placement: one must think about safety before proceeding. Psychiatrists who are accustomed to striving for short hospital stays and extensive community treatment opportunities, particularly when driven by cost considerations, should be certain their decisions place safety higher than cost priorities and may wish to support their decisions with a subspecialist's second opinion and extra documentation.

For most patients, the most critical point in evaluating the patient's ability to function without violence outside the hospital is not, as some would say, the point of discharge, nor is it the point of giving unaccompanied passes in the community. The most critical decision point in this regard is the first unaccompanied pass off the locked ward. While on the ward, the patient has little opportunity to be violent and particularly no opportunity to recreate the setting and victim environment that existed when he or she was violent outside the institution. One should be very cautious when allowing a nonpsychotic, non-organically disordered patient, especially, to leave the ward unaccompanied for the first time, since he or she may have planned to escape the facility or may respond to an impulse to escape when given the new opportunity to do so. *The fact that the off-ward pass may be for a short time or may have a therapeutic purpose, such as to attend a program, should not obscure the additional fact that the patient's behavior is now governed solely by his or her internal controls.*

APPENDIX: Sample Document
Understanding Your Forensic Psychiatry Evaluation

I, ______, understand that I am seeing Dr. ______ for psychiatric evaluation. The purpose of my evaluation is legal or administrative, not treatment or treatment-related diagnosis. This means, in part, that Dr. ______ is not "my doctor"; I do not have a "doctor-patient" relationship with Dr. ______, and this evaluation does not create one.

I understand that the things that I discuss with Dr. ______ are not confidential in the same way that a "doctor-patient" interview might be. For example, Dr. ______ may write a report for some other person or organization entitled to information about my evaluation. He may also be asked to testify in court or at a hearing about the things I discuss in the evaluation. Nevertheless, I understand that I should try to cooperate in the interview as best I can, and be honest and straightforward in my answers.

A copy of this statement will be given to me to keep, and I may ask questions of Dr. ______ at any time during the interview. If I have questions later, they should be referred to my primary doctor or my attorney.

__________________________ Date ____________

__________________________ Date ____________

Witness

REFERENCES

1. K. Tardiff, Violence, *American Psychiatric Press Textbook of Psychiatry*, 2d ed. (R.E. Hales, S.C. Yudofsky, and J.A. Talbott, eds.), American Psychiatric Press, Washington, DC, 1994.
2. M. Eronen, P. Hakola, and J. Tiihonen, Mental disorders and homicidal behavior in Finland, *Arch. Gen. Psychiatry 53*:497 (1996).
3. Eronen M, Tiihonen J, Hakola P: Schizophrenia and homicidal behavior, *Schizophr. Bull. 22(1)*:83 (1996).
4. S. Hodgins, S.A. Mednick, B.A. Brennan, F. Schulsinger, and M. Engberg, Mental disorder and crime: Evidence from a Danish birth cohort, *Arch. Gen Psychiatry 53*:489 (1996).
5. J. Modestin and Ammann, Mental disorder and criminality: Male schizophrenia. *Schizophr. Bull. 22(1)*:69 (1996).
6. J. Junginger, Psychosis and violence: The case for a content analysis of psychotic experience, *Schizophr. Bull. 22(1)*:91 (1996).
7. P.G. Nestor, J. Haycock, S. Doiron, J. Kelly, and D. Kelly, Lethal violence and psychosis: A clinical profile, *Bull. Am. Acad. Psychiatry Law 23*:331 (1995).
8. J.A. Silva, G.B. Leong, R. Weinstock, K.K. Sharma, and R.L. Klein, Delusional misidentification syndromes and dangerousness, *Psychopathology 27(3–5)*:215 (1994).
9. J. Modestin and R. Ammann, Mental disorders and criminal behaviour, *Br. J. Psychiatry 166*:667 (1995).
10. L.S. Grossman, T.W. Haywood, J.L. Cavanaugh, J.M. Davis, and D.A. Lewis, State psychiatric hospital patients with past arrests for violent crimes, *Psychiatr. Serv. 46*:790 (1995).

11. M. Fux, M. Weiss, and D. Elhadad, Aggressive behaviour as a cause of psychiatric admission: A comparison between schizophrenic and affective disorder patients, *Med. Law 14(3–4)*:293 (1995).
12. A. Raine, Features of borderline personality and violence, *J. Clin. Psychol. 49*:277 (1993).
13. S. Hodgins and G. Cote, Major mental disorder and antisocial personality disorder: A criminal combination, *Bull. Am. Acad. Psychiatry Law 21*:155 (1993).
14. S.H. Dinwiddie, Psychiatric disorders among wife batterers, *Compr. Psychiatry 33*:411 (1992).
15. D.G. Dutton, Trauma symptoms and PTSD-like profiles in perpetrators of intimate abuse, *J. Trauma Stress 8*:299 (1995).
16. E.A. Nofzinger and R.M. Wettstein, Homicidal behavior and sleep apnea: A case report and medicolegal discussion, *Sleep 18*:776 (1995).
17. M. Ghahramani and V. Gooriah, Chronic fatigue syndrome associated with a psychotic state resulting in multiple murders, *Bull. Am. Acad. Psychiatry Law 23*:613 (1995).
18. M.I. Krakowski, A. Convit, J. Jaeger, S. Lin, and J. Volavka, Inpatient violence: Trait and state, *J. Psychiatr. Res. 23(1)*:57 (1989).
19. D. Aarsland, J.L. Cummings, G. Yenner and B. Miller, Relationship of aggressive behavior to other neuropsychiatric symptoms in patients with Alzheimer's disease, *Am. J. Psychiatry 153*:243 (1996).
20. A.D. Hurley and R. Sovner, Six cases of patients with mental retardation who have antisocial personality disorder, *Psychiatr. Serv. 46*:828 (1995).
21. J.S. Kreutzer, J.H. Marwitz, and A.D. Witol, Interrelationships between crime, substance abuse, and aggressive behaviours among persons with traumatic brain injury. *Brain. Inj.* (*Engl.*) *9*:757 (1995).
22. R. Catalano, D. Dooley, R.W. Novaco, G. Wilson, and R. Hough, Using ECA survey data to examine the effect of job layoffs on violent behavior. *Hosp. Commun. Psychiatry 44*:874 (1993).
23. Y. Kon, Amok, *Br. J. Psychiatry 165*:685 (1994).
24. E.S. Lake, An exploration of the violent victim experiences of female offenders, *Violence Vict. 8(1)*:41 (1993).
25. C.E. Newhill, E.P., Mulvey, and C.W. Lidz, Characteristics of violence in the community by female patients seen in a psychiatric emergency service, *Psychiatr. Serv. 46*:785 (1995).
26. P. Bech and M. Mak, Measurements of impulsivity and aggression, *Impulsivity and Aggression*, (E. Hollander and D. Stein, eds.), John Wiley & Sons, Chichester, England, 1995.
27. B. Eichelman and A. Hartwig, The Carolina Nosology of Destructive Behaviors (CNBD), *J. Neuropsychiatry 2*:288 (1990).
28. D.A. Brizer, A. Convit, M. Krakowski, and J. Volavka, A rating scale for reporting violence on psychiatric wards, *Hosp. Commun. Psychiatry 38*:769 (1987).
29. J.M. Silver and S.C. Yudofsky, The Overt Aggression Scale: Overview and guiding principles, *J. Neuropsychiatry 3(suppl.)*:23 (1991).
30. P. Bech, *Rating Scales for Psychopathology, Health Status, and Quality of Life: A*

Compendium on Documentation in Accordance with the DSM-III-R and WHO Systems, Springer-Verlag, Berlin, 1993.
31. ERAG, Social Dysfunction and Aggression Scale (SDAS-21) in generalized aggression and in aggressive attacks: A validity and reliability study, *Int. J. Meth. Psychiatr. Res. 59*:420 (1992).
32. T. Palmstierna and B. Wistedt, Staff Observation Aggression Scale (SOAS): Presentation and evaluation, *Acta Psychiatr. Scand. 76*:657 (1987).
33. V. Patel and R. Hope, A rating scale for aggressive behaviour in the elderly: The RAGE, *Psychol. Med. 22*:211 (1992).
34. P.Y. Blake, J.H. Pincus, and C. Buckner, Neurologic abnormalities in murderers, *Neurology 45*:1641 (1995).
35. M.T. Wong, J. Lumsden, G.W. Fenton, and P.B. Fenwick, Electroencephalography, computed tomography and violence ratings of male patients in a maximum-security mental hospital, *Acta Psychiatr. Scand. 90(2)*:97 (1994).
36. A. Convit, P. Czobor, and J. Volavka, Lateralized abnormality in the EEG of persistently violent psychiatric inpatients, *Biol. Psychiatry 30*:363 (1991).
37. M. Kunz, J. Sikora, M. Krakowski, A. Convit, T.B. Cooper, and J. Volavka, Serotonin in violent patients with schizophrenia, *Psychiatry Res. 59(1–2)*:161 (1995).
38. M. Virkkunen, M. Eggert, R. Rawlings, and M.A. Linnoila, Prospective follow-up study of alcoholic violent offenders and firesetters, *Arch. Gen. Psychiatry 53*:523 (1996).
39. D.S. Freedman, T. Byers, D.H. Barrett, N.E. Stroup, E. Eaker, and H. Monroe-Blum, Plasma lipid levels and psychologic characteristics in men, *Am. J. Epidemiol. 141*:507 (1995).
40. M. Virkkunen, R. Rawlings, R. Tokola, R.E. Poland, A. Guidotti, C. Nemeroff, G. Bissette, K. Kalogeras, S.L. Karonen, and M. Linnoila, CSF biochemistries, glucose metabolism, and diurnal activity rhythms in alcoholic, violent offenders, fire setters, and healthy volunteers, *Arch. Gen. Psychiatry 51*:20 (1994).
41. M. Hillbrand, R.T. Spitz, and H.G. Foster, Serum cholesterol and aggression in hospitalized male forensic patients, *J. Behav. Med. 18(1)*:33 (1995).
42. J.C. Beck, K.A. White, and B. Gage, Emergency psychiatric assessment of violence, *Am. J. Psychiatry 148*:1562 (1991).

8
Prediction of Violence

Kenneth Tardiff
Cornell University Medical College, New York, New York

I. INTRODUCTION

This chapter presents practical clinical guidelines on the evaluation of patients to determine a patient's potential for violence toward others. The word *patient* in the first sentence is a key word in this chapter and book since it delineates the responsibility of the physician or other clinicians for the prediction, prevention, and control of violence in our society. There are many types of violence in our society that are beyond the expertise of medicine, psychology, nursing, social work, and other health care disciplines. These include violence associated with economically motivated crimes such as robbery or violence that is part of the business of selling and buying illicit drugs, as in territorial disputes and retaliation. As discussed in Chapter 16, the duty of the physician and other clinicians to protect potential victims from violence by patients rests on the special relation that exists between the clinician and the potentially violent patient. This special relation exists when patients are in the custody of our hospitals and other health care institutions and when they are outpatients in treatment.

Clinicians must make predictions about the risk of violence by patients many times each day, whether they realize it or not. The psychiatrist who is evaluating a new patient for the first time in a clinic, a private office, or an emergency department does it. Nurses and psychiatrists on an inpatient unit do it as they determine level of supervision for a patient and whether a patient should be given a pass or discharged from the hospital. Social workers do it as they investigate the possibility of child abuse. The purpose of these predictions is to determine whether the patient poses a danger of physical violence in the near future and, if so, what should be done to protect others from violence by the patient. This may be hospitalizing the patient, increasing levels of supervision, changing medication or other treatments, keeping the patient in the hospital on a closed unit, or taking potential targets of violence, such as dependent children, out of the home.

II. STUDIES OF RISK OF VIOLENCE BY PATIENTS

Studies prior to 1981 found that psychiatrists and psychologists were not accurate in making predictions as to whether a patient will be violent over several years (1). Since then, studies have shown that mental health professionals have improved to the point that their predictions of violence are better than one would expect by chance alone (2–5).

Studies on risk factors for violence done in the 1980s and 1990s filled the literature. They may account for the increased accuracy in the prediction of violence by psychiatrists and other mental health professionals. These studies looked at violent behavior in large clinical populations of psychiatric patients. Tardiff and Sweillam studied thousands of patients to determine which factors were related to violence in the community prior to admission to public hospitals (6). Similar studies of violence by psychiatric patients just prior to admission to psychiatric hospitals followed, with similar findings (7–11).

These studies found that from 10 to 20% of patients were violent toward other persons in the month prior to admission to psychiatric hospitals. Patients with increased frequency of violence were those diagnosed as being schizophrenic or manic or having alcohol- or substance-abuse disorders and certain personality disorders, particularly antisocial or borderline types. Younger and male patients were usually more likely to have been violent that older or female patients.

There have been studies of violence by patients while in psychiatric hospitals. These have found lower rates, from 3 to 9%, than studies of violence before hospitalization (12–17). One study found a higher rate, but the percentage of patients who were violent varied greatly across units (18). Other studies, including those of patients hospitalized in Australia, Britain, Canada, Ireland, Sweden, Denmark, and the United States, found rates of inpatient violence in the range of 25 to 50% (19–24). Some studies looked at inpatient violence for the first 3 days and first week of hospitalization and found that 13 to 16% of patients were violent (25,26).

Studies differed as to which types of patients posed increased risks of violence in psychiatric hospitals. Many studies have found that younger patients have an increased risk of inpatient violence (12,13,16,17,19,22,23). Other studies have not found differences in the frequency of inpatient violence with regard to age (14,15,18,27). Most studies have not found differences in the frequency of inpatient violence among men and women (13–16,18,19,23). Some studies have found higher rates of inpatient violence for male patients as compared with female patients (17,27). Other studies have found that female patients had higher rates of inpatient violence than male patients (12,22).

A fairly consistent finding across studies is the increased risk of inpatient violence among schizophrenic patients (12–15,17,19,21,23,24,26). In addition to schizophrenia, patients with psychotic organic disorders also pose an increased risk of inpatient violence (13,26,27). Patients with alcohol- and/or drug-abuse problems in the absence of other psychiatric disorders have been found by some studies to have an increased risk of inpatient violence (22,27). One study found that patients with personality disorders and those with bipolar disorder had a greater likelihood of inpatient violence that did patients with schizophrenia or other disorders (18).

There have been studies of violence among patients living in the community. An earlier study by this author of patients presenting to outpatient clinics found that 3% had recently attacked persons (28). Patients who were more likely to have been violent were those with personality disorders, not schizophrenia. A recent study by this author of patients discharged from a psychiatric hospital found a similar pattern—that 3% of these patients attacked other persons within 2 weeks of discharge and that the patients with increased likelihood of violence were those with personality disorders, not schizophrenia or other Axis I disorders (29). Among those patients who had attacked someone before and after hospitalization, the targets of the attacks were the same for 70% of the patients.

Several studies have followed patients discharged from inpatient settings for longer periods of time and have reached different conclusions as to which patients in the community pose an increased risk of violence. These studies have been done in the United States, Great Britain, and Sweden (30–32). When patients are followed for longer periods of time after discharge, Axis I pathology, particulary psychosis, is related to increased risk of violence. There is evidence that comorbidity of major mental disorders, such as schizophrenia, with substance abuse greatly increases the risk of violence by persons living in the community (33,34).

III. CLINICAL GUIDELINES FOR PREDICTION OF VIOLENCE

Based on these studies and the clinical experience on which they rest, a number of authors have developed clinical guidelines for deciding whether a patient poses a significant risk of violence in the near future (3,35–38). These guidelines are rather consistent in describing what information should be collected in the evaluation of a patient to determine the potential for violence.

The model proposed in this paper represents that consensus, but it has not been empirically tested for accuracy. On the other hand, this model has been successfully used by the author as a standard in a number of malpractice suits involving violence by patients. The model includes information that the clinician should collect so as to make a decision about a patient's potential for violence in the near future, i.e., the next few days or a week at most. Beyond a week, there is the opportunity for intervening factors to change the state of the patient and the environment that existed at time the evaluation of violence potential was done. These intervening factors can include noncompliance with medication, resumption of drinking or substance use, threats of divorce by a spouse, and other stressors.

A. Sources of Information

The essential components of this model for the short-term prediction of violence rely on information collected from the interview with the patient, but other sources of information must be sought. These include past records from treatment, police records, and other records. It is essential that the clinician speak or attempt to speak to the family, therapist, police, and others who may have knowledge of the patient.

In the routine evaluation of patients, a screening question such as "Have you ever lost your temper?" should be asked. If the answer is yes, the clinician proceeds to inquire about the specifics of past violent behavior and ideation. Some patients, such as those with paranoid delusions, may be reluctant to divulge thoughts of violence, so the clinician must listen carefully and follow up on any hints of violence that may surface during the interview. If there are thoughts of violence or even threats, the degree of formulation of the ideas or threats of violence must be assessed.

B. Degree of Formulation

A well-formulated or detailed plan should raise concern about the risk of violence posed by a patient. This includes details about where, when, and how the patient will attack the victim as well as knowledge about the potential victim's personal life, such as daily schedules and home address. For example, vague thoughts of "getting even" are not as serious, all other things being equal, as specific thoughts of how and when the patient plans to attack someone.

C. Intent

If a patient has thoughts of harming someone, it is important to assess his or her *intent* to harm the person. The mere fact that thoughts of violence arise in a patient's mind may not be sufficient to warrant action by the clinician. For example, a young schizophrenic woman told her therapist that she had fleeting thoughts and images of killing her sister's newborn baby. She was very upset about these thoughts and it was clear that they were not delusional. She was judged not to be risk of violence and has not harmed the baby since.

D. Availability of Victims

The availability of a potential victim is important. This refers to daily vulnerability of the victim as well as geographic distance between the patient and potential victim. For example, a potential victim living in an apartment with a doorman is generally safer than one living in a house in the suburbs. Geography plays a part in the assessment of risk of violence to a potential victim. For example, a schizophrenic patient threatening his father who lives on the opposite coast is less of a danger than a schizophrenic patient who is threatening his father who is living in the patient's household.

E. Weapons

Availability of a weapon is a major factor in whether violence will occur and in the lethality of the violence. The patient should be asked, if there is a concern about violence as well as suicide, if there is a gun in the household, whether he or she has other access to other guns, or how he or she would go about buying a gun.

F. History of Violence and Other Impulsive Behaviors

A history of violence or other impulsive behaviors by the patient is a major factor in the assessment of potential for violence. Past violence predicts future violence. Episodes of past violence—for example, the most recent episode—must be dissected in a detailed, concrete manner by the clinician. This includes details of the time and place of the violence, who was present, who said what to whom, what the patient saw, what the patient remembers, what family members or staff remember, why the patient was violent (e.g., delusions versus anger), and what could have been done to avoid the violent confrontation. Often there is a pattern of escalation of violence, whether it involves the dynamics of a couple interacting in domestic violence or the schizophrenic patient on the inpatient unit escalating as interactions with other patients become too intense.

The "past history" of violence should be treated as any other medical symptom. This includes the date of onset, frequency, place (targets), and severity. Severity is measured by degree of injury to the victim(s) from pushing, to punching, to causing injuries such as bruises, to causing injuries such as broken bones, lacerations, internal injuries, or even death. Severity and frequency may be measured by the Overt Aggression Scale (39). The past history of violence should include the presence of other clinical phenoma, such as disorientation, amnesia, and guilt after the violent episode. Last, past history of violence should include prior evaluations—for example, psychological testing or imaging—and treatment, as well as hospitalization, medications, and response to treatment.

G. Psychosis and Schizophrenia

Psychosis increases potential for violent behavior if the patient has thoughts of violence. Schizophrenia is the disorder most frequently found where there is psychosis and violence. Schizophrenic patients can be violent because of delusions, particularly paranoid delusions. These patients are violent because they believe others are attempting to harm them or have harmed them (40–42). They regard violence as justified, as in self-defense or retaliation. Frequently, the theme of the delusion associated with violence persists throughout the course of the illness, as in the case of a schizophrenic woman who was admitted to the hospital on numerous occasions. From her first admission in college, she had a delusion that involved people poisoning her. As would be expected, she was violent against her parents at home and other patients in the hospital around mealtimes. Hallucinations, particularly auditory hallucinations, can be associated with violence by schizophrenic patients (43,44). These may be command auditory hallucinations telling the patient to kill others or harm themselves.

H. Other Aspects of Schizophrenia

It is important to recognize that schizophrenic patients can be violent for reasons other than psychosis per se. Violence by schizophrenic patients may be due to comorbid alcohol or substance abuse (33,34). Violence due to alcohol and substance abuse is discussed later in this chapter. There may be a superimposed insult to the brain that results in a low threshold for violence. These insults may include any of the organic disorders discussed later in this chapter, ranging from substance abuse, to head trauma, to AIDS, and to other neurological and systemic medical disorders. Mentally retarded schizophrenic patients may resort to violence in response to frustration due either to demands from family or staff or to the inability to verbalize needs and conflicts.

Comorbid antisocial or borderline personality disorders increase the potential for violence (34,45). Violence can be manipulative, used by these patients to control or to express anger, and not being related to the schizophrenic disorder itself. For example, a paranoid schizophrenic patient with antisocial personality who was no longer psychotic deliberately punched a nurse in the face upon being told that his weekend pass was rescinded.

I. Delusional Disorder

Delusional disorder can be associated with violent behavior, especially the paranoid and jealous types. Patients with paranoid delusional disorder harbor grudges against those whom they believe have wronged them. For example, a patient who believed that his activities were being monitored by the CIA harbored ideas of putting a bomb in the offices of a telephone company that he suspected was collaborating with the CIA. Patients with delusional disorders of the jealous type are known to retaliate violently against their spouses or the suspected third persons in illicit affairs.

J. Mania

Patients experiencing a manic episode can be violent because of psychosis and/or gross disorganization of thoughts and/or behavior (46,47). Targets of violence are often random in these cases. Manic patients who are more intact are often violent when they feel restricted or when limits are being set by staff. For example, a middle-aged woman who was manic attacked a female psychiatric resident in the emergency department as the resident told the patient that she would be admitted involuntarily to the hospital. Later, when the patient, who had been stabilized, was interviewed, she apologized for the attack but commented that she felt trapped. She said that "when you're manic, you want to be free, to shop, to move around, everything."

K. Personality Disorders

Some personality disorders, namely the antisocial and borderline types, increase the risk of violence (48–51). The patient with antisocial personality is violent in a vicious, "macho" way in order to seek revenge or bolster his image. Frequently the victim is a stranger or someone known to the patient in a superficial manner. Characteristically, the patient with antisocial personality shows no remorse after the attack and, instead, regrets that more injury was not inflicted on the victim, who he believes deserved it. Although this type of patient may appear glib and/or attractive, the clinician can expect violence if the patient's self-esteem or macho image is threatened.

Patients with borderline personality are violent in several contexts. Violence can be a manifestation of affective instability or manipulation and as such can be unpredictable. On the other hand, violence is predictable when the patient with borderline personality is or feels that he or she has been rejected or abandoned. This rejection may come from a lover, as in the case of Alex in the film *Fatal Attraction*, or from a therapist in the context of termination of treatment.

Patients with paranoid personality frequently threaten violence, since they often feel persecuted and/or discriminated against because of race, gender, or some other personal attribute. This often leads to arguments with people in their lives. They have thoughts or even plans of violence but do not usually act on their violent thoughts. However, if violence occurs, it can be catastrophic, as in the case of mass murder. For example, a man who was fired from a large company revealed to his outpatient therapist that he had a list of employees of the company—from human resource staff to high executives—and that he planned to kill them if he lost his lawsuit aimed at winning back his disability benefits and/or his old job. The crisis involved the possibility of loss of his apartment, which he described as the "bunker" in his fight against the company. An ad hoc meeting was held with the therapist, the present author, and a representative from legal affairs from our hospital. The decision was made to involve his sister so as to obtain financial resources to enable the patient to keep his apartment. This plan was successful, and the group decided that he did not pose an immediate danger to his former employer. No violence occurred for over a year.

L. Posttraumatic Stress Disorder

Patients with posttraumatic stress disorder (PTSD) can become violent, particularly when the original stressor was related to violence (52,53). In some cases, the violence may be due to the use of alcohol associated with PTSD; however, it may also be related to trigger phenoma. For example, a man developed PTSD while serving in Vietnam. With counseling, he became able to control episodes of anxiety. One day he was arrested wrongly by the police. After spending a humiliating night in jail, he was released. His former symptoms of PTSD recurred and hospitalization was necessary to deal with his rage attacks against people and objects, particularly when he read about or saw stories of police brutality in the news.

M. Alcohol Use and Substance Abuse

Alcohol has been found to increase the risk of violence in a number of ways. It is thought to release inhibitions, so that urges and behaviors that would be unacceptable in a sober state—in this case, violence—erupt despite the individual's personal and societal restraints against violence (54–56). Alcohol produces impairment in tasks associated with the frontal lobes, such as assessment, planning, and organization of behavior as well as ability to abstract and to remember. The intoxicated individual's communication skills may not be sufficient to allow him or her to deal with the situation in a verbal rather than a physical manner. Cognitive impairment of the brain caused by alcohol may exaggerate provocation through misinterpretation of real events, such as perceiving an insult in an encounter at a bar or in a marital conflict. The intoxicated individual may not appreciate the consequences of violence because of his or her cognitive impairment.

Cocaine produces violent behavior, usually during severe intoxication and/or delirium (57–60). Symptoms of intoxication include auditory, visual, and tactile hallucinations; paranoid and other delusions; irritability, confusion, and psychomotor agitation. Symptoms of intoxication or delirium typically disappear within 2 days after the last dose of cocaine. However, a delusional syndrome may linger for a week or more after the last dose. This syndrome is characterized by persecutory delusions that may elicit violence. Violence may also be elicited by cocaine alone. However, in addition to cocaine, alcohol and heroin are frequently used to counter the irritability and other unpleasant effects of cocaine. These substances may contribute to the violent behaviors observed (61,62).

Amphetamine may cause intoxication, delirium, or a delusional disorder; these conditions are clinically indistinguishable from those produced by cocaine, discussed above. Paranoid delusions may result in assault or homicide (63,64).

Phencyclidine may be smoked or taken orally, intranasally, or intravenously. Intoxication is manifest by belligerence, assaultiveness, ataxia, dysarthria, muscle rigidity, seizures, and hyperacusis. Phencyclidine delirium may last longer than that caused by cocaine; otherwise it is clinically similar (65–67).

Anabolic steroids have been used by athletes and body-builders to enhance muscle growth, strengths, and performance. Increased irritability and aggressiveness may occur as side effects of these drugs (68–70). Male athletes have demonstrated aggressive behavior and other psychopathology after taking steroids, sometimes at high doses. After several weeks or months of self-medication, the men became irritable and combative, committing violent crimes that included homicide, assault, and robbery. Their irritability and violent outbursts disappeared within several months after steroid discontinuation.

Polysubstance abuse is very common. Substances may be taken simultaneously, even in the same injection (such as the "speedball" combination of cocaine and heroin). Alcohol is frequently combined with drugs of abuse on the same occasion, or it may be used on separate occasions. Polysubstance use may result from a deliberate decision on the part of the user or from a drug supplier's decision to mix several substances together. The user does not necessarily know that he or she is using more than one drug. The combinations of substances result in multiple interactions.

N. Organicity

Organicity increases the risk of violence. Central nervous system disorders that have been associated with violent behavior include traumatic brain injuries, intracranial infections (such as encephalitis and postencephalitic syndrome), tumors, seizures (especially postictally), cerebrovascular disorder, Huntington's disease, Alzheimer's disease, Wilson's disease, multiple sclerosis, and normal-pressure hydrocephalus (71–79). Systemic disorders that can produce violence include metabolic disorders, electrolyte imbalances, hypoxia, uremia, Cushing's disease, vitamin deficiencies (e.g., pernicious anemia), systemic infections, systemic lupus erythematosus, porphyria, and toxins (80–87).

O. Background of the Patient

The sociocultural background of the patient must be taken into consideration as one tries to determine whether he or she poses a risk of violence. Violence is an accepted way of expressing oneself in some segments of society, usually characterized by poverty and lack of education. Although this environment may be more prevalent for African Americans and Latinos in inner-city areas, lack of legitimate means of attaining one's needs and the need to appear tough, rather than ethnicity, is important in these cases. A patient from this background who talks of violence will probably be violent and can be expected to have problems with aggression within an institution. For example, an African-American adolescent was admitted to a university hospital inpatient unit where the staff and other patients were predominantly white. The adolescent was frequently in physical fights for no apparent reason—for example, over selecting a television program in the lounge or while playing in the gym. When these episodes were explored, it became apparent that he saw the actions of other patients as disrespectful or demeaning to him, and he responded violently in the same way he would be expected to do in his neighborhood.

P. Compliance with Treatment

Compliance with treatment is a factor in determining a patient's risk of violence. This involves regular attendance for treatment sessions and compliance with medication and other treatments. Blood levels of medications assist the clinician in monitoring compliance with medication. Contact with the patient's family also helps in monitoring compliance with medication. Schizophrenic patients with a history of violence related to psychosis are best managed with haloperidol given as a depot drug or fluphenazine so as to assure compliance with medication.

IV. THREATS OF VIOLENCE TOWARD CLINICIANS

Patients can threaten the clinician in a number of different ways, from the impulsive, emotional outburst; the calm, serious statement; the joking, flippant manner; or through vague innuendos. Threats can be made face to face, on an answering machine, or by letter. All threats of violence must be taken seriously by the clinician, who should not deny the existence or seriousness of a threat. Often the clinician can confront the patient and clarify the meaning of the threat. If it is resolved, then therapy can proceed. If there is uncertainty or the clinician feels that the threat may be serious, it should be discussed with a supervisor, colleagues, and family so as to assess the risk of harm and to develop a plan to deal with it.

One possibility is a meeting consisting of representatives of various parts of the organization such as security, legal affairs, administration, employee health, human affairs, the director of clinical services, and a psychiatric consultant familiar with violence. This group will benefit from the various perspectives in terms of evaluating different options, from the legal to the therapeutic, in responding to the threat.

In evaluating the risk of violence, information along the lines discussed above must be obtained. This may involve meeting with the patient in a safe setting or obtaining information from other staff, patients, records, or by other means. This situation is particularly problematic where threats by telephone or mail are anonymous.

If the risk of violence is significant, a plan of action must be put in place. This includes security measures, restraining orders, and other means of preventing access to the intended victim. The mental state of the threatener must be assessed so as to determine whether there are grounds for involuntary hospitalization. It is helpful to use the institution as a buffer between the threatening patient and the victim; for example, "it is the policy of the hospital to not tolerate threats of violence to other staff and patients, therefore the hospital intends to . . . etc." This hopefully will deflect or at least not intensify the wrath of the threatener as the plan or action is implemented.

Anonymous threats are difficult to respond to and are frightening. Correspondence should be kept, preferably in a plastic bag, for further investigation. Telephone threats should be documented in terms of exactly what was said, whether the threatener had an accent or other speech characteristic, whether there were background noises, and so on. If possible the clinician might attempt to engage the threatener in a nonconfrontational manner so as to obtain further information as to his or her identity and further details of the threat so as to determine the risk of violence.

V. MALPRACTICE CASES

The author has had the opportunity to serve as an expert witness in a number of cases where prediction of violence was an issue. In one case, a patient killed his boss as they were laying carpet on a job. The author served as an expert for the defense. The patient had been seen on a regular basis in the medication clinic of a Veterans Administration Hospital for over a decade after a medical discharge from the U.S. Army following hospitalization for a psychotic episode. His diagnosis was paranoid schizophrenia. He continued to have a delusion that he was a spy for the United States. There was no history of violence on his part. The psychiatric resident in the medication clinic regularly noted that he was "not homicidal" despite his delusional thoughts. He complained about taking haloperidol but was compliant in taking another antipsychotic medication. He denied any ideas of violence and, in fact, his diaries mentioned no ideas of his employer being a spy or any thoughts of violence toward him. Summary judgment was in favor of the defendant, since there was no foreseeable victim.

Another case involved a young schizophrenic man, where the author served as an expert for the plaintiff—the victim of violence in this instance. The patient was in treatment with a private psychiatrist in the community. The patient attacked his father, with whom he lived, with a baseball bat. The psychiatrist did not recognize that the patient was delusional, in that the patient believed that his father was conspiring with the police to have him arrested and jailed. In the psychiatrist's records there was no evidence of the assessment of violence or suicide potential despite evidence that he knew of the attack on the father. When the psychiatrist did start to suspect that the patient was delusional, he started the patient on depo-haloperidol instead of hospitalizing him or using oral haloperidol. The case was settled for the plaintiff.

Another case where the author served as an expert for the plaintiff involved a young male schizophrenic with antisocial personality who was a patient in a medical unit in a state hospital. He was on the medical unit because he had broken his leg and its condition required monitoring. On the medical unit were a number of elderly demented patients with medical problems. The young schizophrenic patient had a history of violence toward persons in a particularly vicious manner outside the hospital. In the hospital, he made comments such as "I think these people need a date with the coroner" a number of times. Despite this, the man remained on the unit. One day an elderly woman was found bludgeoned to death with severe bloody skull fractures. It could not be proven that the young schizophrenic patient had killer her, but a foot rest of his wheelchair was found hidden under the mattress of a patient who resided in a room adjacent to his room. The communal bathroom was soaked as if someone had recently washed something vigorously. The case was decided by a jury in favor of the plaintiff. The staff and hospital should have predicted that the patient would attack someone on the medical unit because of his history of violence and statements about killing elderly people.

VI. SUMMARY OF PREDICTION OF VIOLENCE

The assessment of violence potential for the short term (i.e., within days or a week) is analogous to the assessment for suicide potential. The clinician must consider the following: subtle questioning of the patient if violence is not mentioned; how well planned the threat of violence is; available means of inflicting injury; past history of violence and impulsive behavior with attention to frequency, degree of past injuries to others and self, toward whom, and under what circumstances; alcohol and drug use; presence of other organic mental disorders; presence of schizophrenia, mania, or other psychosis; presence of certain personality and impulse control disorders; and noncompliance with treatment in the past.

All of these factors are weighed in the final assessment of whether the patient poses a significant risk to others, so that some action is necessary on the part of the evaluator. Action may include hospitalizing the patient or warning the intended victim and/or the police. All of the data determining the decision as to whether the patient is or is not a risk for violence must be documented in writing. The thinking process through which the decision was made should be evident in the written documentation. Reassessment of violence potential should be made at short intervals (e.g., from visit to visit or every few days) if the patient is to continue to be treated outside of the hospital or other institution.

REFERENCES

1. J. Monahan, The Clinical Prediction of Violent Behavior, National Institute of Mental Health, Rockville, MD, 1981.
2. C.W. Lidz, E.P. Mulvey, and W. Gardner, The accuracy of predictions of violence to others, *J.A.M.A. 269*:1007 (1993).
3. J. Monahan and H. Steadman (eds.), *Violence and Mental Disorder: Developments in Risk Assessment*, University of Chicago Press, Chicago, 1994.
4. D. Mossman, Assessing predictions of violence: Being accurate about accuracy. *IJ. Consult. Clin. Psychol. 62*:783 (1994).
5. R. Otto, The prediction of dangerous behavior: A review and analysis of "second generation" research, *Forens. Rep. 5*:103 (1992).
6. K. Tardiff and A. Sweillam, Assault, suicide and mental illness, *Arch. Gen. Psychiatry 37*:164 (1980).
7. T.J. Craig, An epidemiologic study of problems associated with violence among psychiatric inpatients. *Am. J. Psychiatry 139*:1262 (1982).
8. A.M. Rossi, M. Jacobs, M. Moteleone, et al., Violent or fear-inducing behavior associated with hospital admission, *Hosp. Commun. Psychiatry 36*:643 (1985).
9. D.E. McNeil and R.L. Binder, Predictors of violence in civilly committed acute psychiatric patients, *Am. J. Psychiatry 145*:965 (1988).

10. K. Tardiff, Characteristics of assaultive patients in private hospitals, *Am. J. Psychiatry 141*:1232 (1984).
11. K. Tardiff, P.M. Marzuk, A.C. Leon, L. Porter, and C. Weiner, Violence by patients admitted to a private psychiatric hospital, *Am. J. Psychiatry 154*:88 (1997).
12. E. Fottrell, A study of violent behavior among patients in psychiatric hospitals, *Br. J. Psychiatry* 216 (1980).
13. K. Tardiff and A. Sweillam, Assaultive behavior among chronic inpatients, *Am. J. Psychiatry* 212 (1982).
14. J. Edwards, D. Jones, and W. Reid, Physical assaults in a psychiatric unit of a general hospital, *Am. J. Psychiatry 145*:1568 (1988).
15. P. Noble and S. Roger, Violence by psychiatric inpatients, *Br. J. Psychiatry 155*:384 (1989).
16. W.D. Walker and R.P. Caplan, Assaultive behavior in acute psychiatric wards and its relationship to violence in the community: A comparison of two health districts, *Med. Sci. Law 33*:299 (1993).
17. M. Pearson, E. Wilmot, and M. Padi, A study of violent behavior among inpatients in a psychiatric hospital, *Br. J. Psychiatry 149*:232 (1986).
18. R.J. Miller, K. Zadolinnyj, R.F. Hafner, and M. Phil, Profiles and predictors of assaultiveness for different psychiatric ward populations, *Am. J. Psychiatry 150*:1368 (1993).
19. D.V. James, N.A. Findberg, A.K. Shah, and R.G. Priest, An increase in violence on an acute psychiatric ward: A study of associated factors, *Br. J. Psychiatry 156*:846 (1990).
20. A.K. Shah, Violence on an acute ward, *Br. J. Psychiatry 160*:571 (1992).
21. A.F. Cooper and J.D. Mendonca, A prospective study of patient assaults on nurses in a provincial psychiatric hospital in Canada, *Acta Psychiatr. Scand.* 163 (1991).
22. T. Palmstierna and B. Wistedt, Staff observation aggression scale, SOAS: Presentation and evaluation, *Acta Psychiatr. Scand. 76*:657 (1987).
23. C. Karson and L.B. Bigalow, Violent behavior in schizophrenic inpatients, *J. Nerv. Ment. Dis. 175*:161 (1987).
24. S. Benjaminsen, K. Gotzsche-Larsen, B. Norrie, L. Harder, and A. Luxhoi, Patient violence in a psychiatric hospital in Denmark: Rate of violence and relation to diagnosis, *Nordic J. Psychiatry* 233 (1996).
25. T.K. Greenfield, D.E. McNeil, and R.L. Binder, Violent behavior and length of psychiatric hospitalization, *Hosp. Commun. Psychiatry 40*:809 (1989).
26. D.E. McNeil and R.L. Binder, Correlates of accuracy in the assessment of psychiatric inpatients' risk of violence, *Am. J. Psychiatry 152*:901 (1995).
27. S.R. Kay, F. Wolkenfeld, and L.M. Murrill, Profiles of aggression among psychiatric patients: II. Covariates and profiles. *J. Nerv. Ment. Dis. 176*:547 (1988).
28. K. Tardiff and H.W. Koenigsberg, Assaultive behavior among psychiatric outpatients, *Am. J. Psychiatry 142*:960 (1985).
29. K. Tardiff, P.M. Marzuk, A.C. Leon, and L. Portera, A prospective study of violence by psychiatric patients after hospital discharge, *Psychiatr Serv 48*:678 (1997).
30. B.G. Link, F.T. Cullen, and H. Andres, The violent and illegal behavior of mental patients reconsidered. *Am. Soc. Rev. 57*:275 (1992).

31. P.J. Taylor, Schizophrenia and crime: Distinctive patterns and associations, *Mental Disorder and Crime* (S. Hodgins, ed.), Sage, Newbury Park, CA, 1993.
32. S. Hodgins, Mental disorder, intellectual deficiency, and crime: Evidence from a birth cohort, *Arch. Gen. Psychiatry 49*:476 (1992).
33. P. Lindqvist and P. Allebeck, Schizophrenia and assaultive behavior: The role of alcohol and drug abuse. *Acta Psychiatr. Scand. 82*:191 (1990).
34. J.W. Swanson, C.E. Holzer, V.K. Ganju, and R.T. Jono, Violence and psychiatric disorder in the community: Evidence from the epidemiologic catchment area survey. *Hosp. Commun. Psychiatry 41*:761 (1990).
35. D.A. Brizer and M.L. Crowner (eds), *Current Approaches to the Prediction of Violence*, American Psychiatric Press, Washington, DC, 1989.
36. E.P. Mulvey and C.W. Lidz, Conditional prediction: A model for research on dangerousness to others in a new era, *Int. J. Law Psychiatry 18*:129 (1995).
37. K. Tardiff, *Assessment and Management of Violent Patients*, 2d ed., American Psychiatric Press, Washington, DC, 1996.
38. T. Sensky et al., *Assessment and Clinical Management of Risk of Harm to Other People*, Council Report CRS3, Royal College of Psychiatrists, London, 1996.
39. S.C. Yudofsky, J.M. Silver, W. Jackson, et al., The Overt Aggression Scale: An operationalized rating scale for verbal and physical aggression, *Am. J. Psychiatry 143*:35 (1986).
40. M. Krakowski, J. Volavka, and D. Brizer, Psychopathology and violence: A review of the literature, *Compr. Psychiatry 27*:131 (1986).
41. M.S. Humpreys, E.C. Johnstone, J.F. MacMillan, and P.J. Taylor, Dangerous behavior preceding first admission for schizophrenia, *Br. J. Psychiatry 161*:501 (1992).
42. D. Shore, C.R. Filson, and W.E. Johnson, Violent crime arrests and paranoid schizophrenia: The White House case studies, *Schizophr. Bull. 14*:279 (1988).
43. J. Junginger, Psychosis and violence: The case for a content analysis of the psychotic experience, *Schizophr. Bull. 22*:91 (1996).
44. J. Junginger Command hallucinations and the prediction of dangerousness, *Psychiatr. Serv., 47*:430 (1996).
45. M.P. Geller, Sociopathic adaptation by psychotic patients, *Hosp Commun. Psychiatry 31*:108 (1980).
46. R.L. Binder and D.E. McNiel, Effects of diagnosis and context on dangerousness, *Am. J. Psychiatry 145*:728 (1988).
47. J.A. Yesavage, Bipolar illness: Correlates of dangerous inpatient behavior, *Br. J. Psychiatry 143*:554 (1983).
48. K. Abram, The effect of co-occurring disorder on criminal careers: Interaction of antisocial personality, alcoholism and drug disorders, *Int. J. Law Psychiatry 12*:133 (1989).
49. K. Abram and L.A. Teplin, Co-occurring disorders among mentally ill jail detainees: Implications for public policy, *Am. Psychol. 46*:1036 (1991).
50. R.D. Hare and L.M. McPherson, Violent and aggressive behavior by criminal psychopaths, *Int. J. Law Psychiatry 7*:35 (1984).
51. L.T. Else, S.A. Wonderlich, and W.W. Beatty, Personality characteristics of men who physically abuse women, *Hosp. Commun. Psychiatry 44*:54 (1993).

52. B.K. Jordan, C.R. Marmar, J.A. Fairbank, W.E. Schlenger, R.A. Kulka, R.L. Hough, and D.S. Weiss, Problems in families of male Vietnam veterans with posttraumatic stress disorder, *J. Consult. Clin. Psychol. 60*:916 (1992).
53. N.B. Lasko, T.V. Gurvits, A.A. Kuhne, S.P. Orr, and R.K. Pitman, Aggression and its correlates in Vietnam veterans with and without chronic posttraumatic stress disorder, *Compr. Psychiatry 35*:373 (1994).
54. J.J. Collins and W.E. Schlenger, Acute and chronic effects of alcohol use on violence, *J. Stud. Alcohol 49*:516–521 (1988).
55. S.P. Taylor and K.E. Leonard, Alcohol and human aggression *Aggression: Theoretical and Empirical Reviews*, Vol. 2, (R.G. Green and E.I. Donnerstein, eds.), Academic Press, New York, 1983, pp. 77–101.
56. B.J. Bushman, Effects of alcohol on human aggression: Validity of proposed explanation, *Recent Dev. Alcohol 13*:227 (1997).
57. A.J. Giannini, N.S. Miller, R.H. Loiselle, and C.E. Turner, Cocaine-associated violence and relationship to route of administration, *J. Subst. Abuse Treat. 10*:67 (1993).
58. R.A. McCormick and M. Smith, Aggression and hostility in substance abusers: The relationship to abuse patterns, coping style, and relapse trigger. *Addict. Behav. (England) 20*:555 (1995).
59. D.H. Lowenstein, S.M. Massa, M.C. Rowbotham, S.D. Collins, H.E. McKinney, and R.P. Simon, Acute neurologic and psychiatric complications associated with cocaine abuse. *Am. J. Med. 83*:841 (1987).
60. R. Mendoza and B.L. Miller, Neuropsychiatric disorders associated with cocaine use, *Hosp. Commun. Psychiatry 43*:677 (1992).
61. I.M. Salloum, D.C. Daley, J.R. Cornelius, L. Kirisci, and M.E. Thase, Disproportionate lethality in psychiatric patients with concurrent alcohol and cocaine abuse, *Am. J. Psychiatry 153*:953 (1996).
62. M.E. Denison, A. Paredes, and J.B. Booth, Alcohol and cocaine interactions and aggressive behaviors, *Recent Dev. Alcohol 13*:283 (1997).
63. E.H. Ellinwood, Assault and homicide associated with amphetamine abuse, *Am. J. Psychiatry 127*:1170 (1971).
64. K.A. Miczek and J.W. Tidey, Amphetamines: Aggressive and social behavior, *N.I.D.A Res. Monogr. 94*:68 (1989).
65. M.A. Fauman and B.J. Fauman, Violence associated with phencyclidine abuse. *Am. J. Psychiatry 136*:1584 (1979).
66. A.M. Khajawall, T.B. Erickson, and G.M. Simpson, Chronic phencyclidine abuse and physical assault. *Am. J. Psychiatry 139*:1604 (1982).
67. A. Convit, Z.C. Nemes, and J. Volavka, History of phencyclidine use and repeated assaults in newly admitted young schizophrenic men, *Am. J. Psychiatry 145*:1176 (1988).
68. P.Y.L. Choi, A.C. Parrott, and D. Cowan, High dose anabolic steroids in strength athletes: Effects upon hostility and aggression, *J. Psychopharmacol. 3*:102 (1989).
69. H.G. Pope Jr. and D.L. Katz, Homicide and near-homicide by anabolic steroid users, *J. Clin. Psychiatry 51*:28 (1990).
70. H.G. Pope Jr. and D.L. Katz, Psychiatric and medical effects of anabolic-androgenic steroid use: A controlled study of 160 athletes, *Arch. Gen. Psychiatry 51*:375 (1994).

71. N. Molamud, Psychiatric disorder with intracranial tumors of the limbic system, *Arch. Neurol. 17*:113 (1967).
72. R.J. Greenwood, A. Bhalla, A. Gordon, and J. Roberts, Behavioral disturbances during recovery form herpes simplex encephalitis, *J. Neurol. Neurosurg. Psychiatry 46*:809 (1983).
73. H.G. Nurnberg, J. Prudic, M. Fiori, and P. Freedman, Psychopathology complicating acquired immune deficiency syndrome (AIDS). *Am. J. Psychiatry 141*:95 (1984).
74. A. Burns, S. Folstein, Brandt, and M. Folstein, Clinical assessment or irritability, aggression and apathy in Huntington and Alzheimer disease, *J. Nerv. Ment. Dis. 178*:20 (1990).
75. M. Akil, A. Schwartz, D. Dutchok, V. Yuzbasiyan-Gurkan, and G.J. Brewer, The psychiatric presentations of Wilson's disease, *J. Neuropsychiatr. Clin Neurosci. 3*:377 (1991).
76. L. Teri, P. Rabins, P. Whitehouse, and B. Leonard, Management of behavioral disturbance in Alzheimer's disease: Current knowledge and future directions, *Alzheimer Dis. Assoc. Dis. 6*:77 (1992).
77. K.J. Bashak, Agitation and restlessness after closed head injury: A prospective study of 100 consecutive admissions, *Arch. Phys. Med. Rehab. 73*:320 (1992).
78. Teasell R. Catastrophic reaction after stroke: A case study, *Am. J. Phys. Med. Rehab. 72*:151 (1993).
79. O. Devinsky, D. Ronsaville, C. Cox, E. Witt, P. Fedio, and W.H. Theodore, Interictal aggression in epilepsy, *Epilepsia 35*:585 (1994).
80. W.M. Easson, Myxedema psychosis insanity defense in homicide, *J. Clin. Psychiatry 41*:316 (1980).
81. K. Zucker, R.L. Livingston, R. Nakra, and P.J. Clayton PJ. B_{12} deficiency and psychiatric disorders: case reports and literature reviews, *Biol Psychiatry 16*:197 (1981).
82. R.S. Schottenfeld and M.R. Cullen, Organic affective illness with lead intoxication, *Am. J. Psychiatry 141*:1423 (1984).
83. D. Bear, R. Rosenbaum, and R. Norman, Aggression in cats and humans precipitated by a cholinesterase inhibitor, *Psychosomatics 27*:535 (1986).
84. M. Virkkunen, Insulin secretion during the glucose tolerance test among habitually violent and impulsive offenders, *Aggress. Behav. 12*:303 (1986).
85. R.S. Brown, A. Fischman, and C.R. Showatter, Primary hyperparathyroidism, hypercalcemia, paranoid delusions, homicide and attempted murder, *J. Forens. Sci. 32*:1460 (1987).
86. C. Huang, N. Chu, C. Lu, J. Lu, J. Wang, J. Tsoi, J. Tzeng, J. Tsoi, C. Wolters, and D.B. Caine, Chronic Manganese intoxication, *Arch. Neurol. 46*:1104 (1989).
87. J. Volavka, *Neurobiology of Violence*, American Psychiatric Press, Washington, DC, 1995.

9
Clinician Safety

William R. Dubin
AmeriChoice Behavioral Healthcare and Jefferson Medical College, Philadelphia, Pennsylvania

I. INTRODUCTION

The practice of medicine symbolizes compassion, healing, and charity. The fact that a clinician can be the target of violence by a patient is an inconceivable thought to most caregivers. Yet clinicians are at significant risk for being assaulted. The American Psychiatric Association recognized the importance of this issue and established the Task Force on Clinician Safety to study the issue of violence against psychiatrists and make proposals to facilitate clinician safety (1). The American College of Emergency Physicians (2) and the American Nurses Association (3) have also addressed this issue. Despite the increased attention to this problem, clinicians are still reluctant to proactively develop and implement strategies for their own safety. This chapter reviews the incidence of assaults against clinicians and presents strategies to improve clinician safety. Strategies for the management of threats and interpersonal confrontations are reviewed, including approaches to managing patients with weapons. Issues of office and hospital safety are reviewed as they relate to clinician safety.

II. INCIDENCE OF VIOLENCE AGAINST CLINICIANS

A. Assaults Against Clinicians

Published studies on nonfatal assaults against psychiatrists have reported an incidence that varies from 3½ to over 40% of respondents who reported being assaulted, with most studies reporting an assault rate of 40% (4–9). Faulkner and coworkers (10) categorized 227 assaults against 150 psychiatrists as follows: 11%

resulted in serious or moderate physical harm requiring medical treatment, and 38% resulted in mild physical harm that did not require treatment. The remainder of the assaults had a potential for harm—i.e., chair thrown, gun brandished.

Violence against psychiatric residents is high and ranges from 28 to 48% of respondents who report being assaulted (11–14). Three studies found a high incidence of repeat assaults. Chaimowitz and Moscovitch (15) found that 31% of the residents were assaulted twice and 8% were assaulted three or more times. Other studies found that 10 to 12% of residents were assaulted more than once (13,16). The highest rates of assaults against residents appeared to be in the emergency room (12–14).

Among nonpsychiatric physicians, Reid and Kang (8) found that 3.3% of family practitioners in their study were assaulted, compared with 3.2% of psychiatrists. In a university school of medicine, Milstein (16) queried 177 medicine residents and found that, of the 70 respondents (60%), 16% were assaulted once and 6% were assaulted more than once. Perhaps the most dramatic case of violence in the past few years was the incident at the Los Angeles County–University of Southern California Medical Center in which a heavily armed patient wounded three doctors and held two women hostage for several hours before freeing them unharmed (17).

Statistics regarding the homicide rate within the medical profession do not exist. There are no statistics available within either the American Medical Association or American Psychiatric Association regarding death by homicide. Most fatal assaults are reported as case reports, clinical anecdotes, or newspaper reports (18–32). A review of many of these cases suggests that failure to understand safety issues may have helped contribute to the physicians' death.

B. Assaults Against Nurses

Of all clinical staff, nurses experience the greatest number of assaults (33). This appears to be a function of the amount of time spent in direct patient care and the involvement in various types of limit-setting activities, including the containment of violence (34–37). The types of injuries sustained range from minor bruises and scratches to severe sprains, lacerations, fractures, and head trauma, with head injury being the most common (34–37).

C. Assaults Against Therapists and Mental Health Workers

Studies of assaults against social workers and psychologists are virtually nonexistent. One study queried 184 Cincinnati mental health workers in the disciplines of psychiatry, psychology, and social work and found that 7% of 27 psychologist respondents and 20% of 20 social worker respondents reported being assaulted by patients (4). Bernstein (38) surveyed a group of psychiatrists (n = 171), psychologists (n = 252), clinical social workers (n = 244), and marriage, family, and child counselors (n = 404). Of the 988 surveyed therapists, 46% (453) responded to the questionnaire. The results of this survey were not broken down by discipline. Of all respondents, 14.22% indicated that they had been assaulted and 35.5% indicated they had been threatened by patients. Psychiatrists were threatened and attacked more frequently than other therapists. Hillen (39) reported that over 50% of the 600 psychologists attending the British Psychological Society's annual meeting had been physically attacked by a patient and 9 out of 10 felt threatened at some time. None of the attacks resulted in serious injury.

D. The True Incidence of Assaults and Injury

Despite the increasing number of reports on violence, the true incidence of assault is still unknown. Studies have repeatedly documented the underreporting of assaults. The rate of underreporting in these studies has ranged from 1.5 to 5 times the actual number of incidents (40–43). Similarly, the actual number and severity of injuries sustained in an assault have also been underreported. Problems include a uniform definition of assault and injury, inaccuracy of reporting, and suppression of reporting (44–47). Methodological issues concerning the descriptions of assaults and the threshold for reporting (i.e., only "sufficiently severe" assaults warrant inclusion) have further hindered the accurate reporting of assaults. Lanza and Campbell (41) and Lion et al. (40) have noted that staff can become inured to the problem of violence, which leads to the mentality that being assaulted is part of the job. The matter of guilt as it impedes the reporting of aggressive events has also been described (40). Staff may fear that the administration will criticize their handling of a violent event. Lanza and Campbell (41) have further discussed the bureaucratic problems of reporting assaults.

E. The Role of Weapons in Assaults

The role of weapons in assaults against clinicians is gaining increasing attention. Hatti and colleagues (7) found that guns were used in 24% of the attacks against psychiatrists and knives in 11%. These weapons were used exclusively in outpatient settings. Attacks against psychiatrists on inpatient units were more likely to involve fists, chairs, tables, and ashtrays. Dubin and coworkers (48) reported that of 91 psychiatrists, who reported an assault in an outpatient setting, 17 had been threatened with a gun, 15 with a knife, and 59 had been assaulted with thrown objects or by physical attack. Faulkner et al. (10) found that weapons used during assaults included the following: hand or foot (72%), an object such as an ashtray or chair (23%), a gun (3%), or a knife (2%).

The incidence of weapons brought into the emergency department by patients has generated concern. Thompson et al. reported that 6 months of screening for weapons at Henry Ford Hospital yielded 33 handguns, 1324 knives, 97 Mace-type sprays, and many other items that could be used as weapons (49). Other studies of violence in the emergency department have reported frequent occurrences of verbal threats, physical violence, threats with weapons, and hostage incidents at knife point (50,51).

Between 4 and 8% of patients seen in psychiatric emergency services have been reported to have weapons (52–54). These included knives, razor blades, heavy chains, a meat cleaver, and Mace. The increasing risk of violence has led several emergency and outpatient departments to install metal detectors or weapon screening procedures (49,55,56).

III. CLINICIAN SAFETY

A. Threat Management

An important issue in clinician safety is threat management. Unfortunately, there is a paucity of research in this area. There are no data detailing the clinical context in which most threats occur or of the outcome of threats. Threats can take many forms. They can be verbal or written, be made by phone, or relayed by a third party. Patients can threaten the clinician in an impulsive, emotional outburst; by a clam, serious statement; by a joking, flippant manner; or through vague innuendoes (57). Threats can be in the form of property damage, visits to a therapist's home, or loitering around a therapist's office on days when the patient has no appointment (58). The sending of love letters, pornographic materials, or vacation pictures can also represent threats (58). Threats can also take the form of veiled comments showing that a patient is involved in the clinician's personal life (59). Such comments might include the knowledge of the clinician's car or home address or the names of the clinician's children (59). These statements are made as a way of showing interest in the clinician but are usually out of proportion to the therapeutic relationship (59).

Threats to clinicians can occur in a variety of settings. These include clinical settings such as the emergency department, inpatient unit, outpatient clinic, or private office. Threats to clinicians can also occur in custody hearings, disability evaluations and hearings, forensic evaluations and hearings, competency hearings, from spouses of patients, and in nonpsychiatric medical settings.

Threats are often a way for a patient to gain control of others by manipulation (59). Maier (59) notes that when patients make manipulative comments, they are often of a nature that the clinician is not encouraged to share them with his or her peers. For instance, a patient may ask a female clinician if she is pregnant or has her period. He may tell a male clinician that he looks hung over or makes some comment about his sexual identity. The interplay between positive comments and personal judgments can provide for effective manipulation, resulting in the clinician's behavior becoming predictable and used by the patient at some future time. In this process, the patient establishes a secret relationship with the clinician, binding the clinician to the patient, governing the clinician's conduct, and distorting his or her judgment (59). Sharing the secret with a colleague is the first step in managing this process.

A written threat must be preserved with a minimal disruption of the physical evidence. Envelopes and all packaging materials must be saved and exposed to minimal handling, preferably with cotton gloves touching extreme edges and storing in a plastic bag (60). Telephone threats that are on tape should be saved. Under no circumstances should the tape be erased. If a threat is by telephone or in person, an attempt should be made to reconstruct the conversation verbatim and to immediately record as much detail as possible (60).

Recently, Brown et al. (61) have begun to address this issue systematically by interviewing psychiatrists who were threatened by patients. The investigators followed the threatened psychiatrist until the threat situation was resolved. In a preliminary study of 19 threat situations, the authors found that threats could be divided into two types. *Situational* threats occurred when a psychiatrist was acting as an administrator, usually on an inpatient unit or emergency department. The psychiatrist had frustrated the patient's wish by denying a request—e.g., to go out on a pass or to get more medication. The patient threatened the psychiatrist, a code was called, the patient was restrained or escorted from the hospital, and the threat situation ended with no psychiatrist being injured.

A *transference* threat occurred in the context of ongoing therapy. The threats were often insidious and in several instances were ongoing for many years. While no psychiatrist who were the targets of transference threats were physically injured, the threats were very disruptive, both to the psychiatrist and to his or her family.

Transference threats were often tolerated by the treating psychiatrist, who initially viewed the threat as an issue to be resolved in therapy. The threat situation often continued for many months before the psychiatrist recognized the inherent danger. Rather than diluting the transference by disengaging from the patient, many therapists intensified the transference by increasing the frequency of treatment sessions. Therapists often have difficulty disengaging from a patient. Such situations may be compared to the problem of marital separation when two parties are locked in a pathological relationship (62). By the time the treating psychiatrist sought consultation from a colleague he or she was so enmeshed in the patient's distorted or psychotic transference that the resolution of the threat situation was complicated if not impossible.

Psychiatrists must pay close attention to any changes in either transference or countertransference feelings as they arise in the therapy situation. Any changes in behavior or affect, by either the therapist or the patient, should alert the clinician to a potential change in the therapeutic relationship. Such behavior might include patient requests for more therapy sessions, frequent phone calls or messages on the answering machine, notes or gifts between sessions, increased and frequent flattery, or increased anger, hostility, or withdrawal. Therapists who treat more primitive character disorders or paranoid or psychotic patients run a certain risk as closeness develops (62). This is a risk that must be continuously assessed and dealt with. Often, subtle actions, such as the patient moving back his or her chair, defensive posturing, or tardiness late in the course of therapy should alert a clinician to a problem in the transference (62). In such situations, reviewing the case with a colleague is a prudent first step toward understanding the change in the therapeutic relationship, assessing whether a threat exists, and, if so, the risk of the threat. Similarly, a clinician should also monitor his or her countertransference. Feelings of increasing attraction, dread, anxiety, or anger toward a patient might signal the beginning of a distorted transference.

When a threat is made, a clinician should act decisively and immediately. Threats are messages and require comment (62). To ignore them is to indicate that the clinician is indifferent to suffering and does not care. Direct confrontation is often useful when a clinician is threatened. Comments such as "You're scaring me with your threat" or "Why do you have to go around scaring me and others with your threats? Is this the only way that you can relate to people, to be scary?" are often effective (62). If there is any alliance with the patient, interpretive statements such as "Why do you go around threatening and alienating people?" or "Do you have any positive feeling about our therapy?" can facilitate understanding and resolution of the threat (62).

The therapist may try to clarify the meaning of the threat, but the patient's failure to respond to reasonable interventions and continued threats are considerations for termination of therapy. Rather than intensifying the transference by continuing to engage the patient in therapy, the therapist should focus on diluting the transference by establishing distance and separation from the patient. For clinicians who work in institutional settings, this can be done by involving the chief clinical administrator. The administration should notify the patient that he or she is aware of the threat situation and that it will not be tolerated. Furthermore, the patient should be informed that the threatened clinician will not accept phone calls or letters or have any further interaction with the patient. The administrator should offer to help the patient find another therapist should he or she wish to continue therapy. Legal assistance should also be concomitantly obtained. The hospital legal staff should unambiguously convey to the patient that threatening a staff clinician is behavior that will not be tolerated and that he or she will be prosecuted if the threats continue. For psychiatrists in private practice, involving the district attorney is more effective than obtaining help from the family lawyer. Threats must be dealt with decisively and without ambivalence.

Another useful strategy in developing a response to a threat is to meet with departmental representatives from security, legal affairs, administration, employee health, human affairs, the director clinical services, and a psychiatric consultant familiar with violence management techniques (57). This group can provide various perspectives on evaluating different options, from legal to therapeutic, in responding to threats (57).

When threats persist despite the interventions discussed, additional steps should be considered. If the patient is told not to return to the therapist's office, security guards or doormen should be alerted not to allow the patient entrance and to notify the therapist if the patient tries to enter the building. A description of the patient should be given to the security staff. If security staff or doormen are not available, the local police precinct should be notified immediately if the patient is seen on the premises. While the threat is ongoing, the therapist should alter his or her schedule and not leave the office at night alone or come in early in the morning alone. The therapist should park near the office and in as public a location as possible. The therapist should avoid parking in isolated, dark areas with little traffic where there are places for a patient to hide. In severe, ongoing threats, the therapist should consider varying his or her routines and travel routes. While this can be disruptive to the therapist's life, it also increases his or her safety.

B. Facilitating Clinician Safety

The most effective strategy for enhancing clinician safety is to anticipate potential aggression. In Chapter 8, Tardiff has suggested that there are certain clinical, psychological, and historical variables that increase a patient's potential for violence. These include a past history of violence; agitation, anger, or disorganized behavior; poor compliance with treatment; a detailed plan or threat of violence; available means for inflicting injury, such as ownership of a weapon; presence of an organic disorder; presence of psychotic psychopathology, especially delusions or command hallucinations; presence of alcohol or drug use; and belonging to a demographic group with an increased prevalence of violence: the young, male, lower socioeconomic group. While there is no specific combination or number of these risk factors that can predict violence, their presence alerts the clinician that the patient poses a risk for violence. The clinician who is aware of these risk factors has the opportunity to develop treatment strategies to minimize the potential for violence. For instance, a clinician may change the site of

Table 1 Physical Defense

• Stand sideways, not facing patient
• Have arms ready for defense
• Deflect kicks with the legs
• Use office objects as shield for sharp weapons
• Use mattress as shield for sharp objects on inpatient units
• Use force against patient's thumb if grabbed
• Control patient's hand if hair is grabbed
• Tuck chin rapidly if a choke hold is attempted by the patient

Source: Adapted from Ref. 57.

treatment—e.g., from a private, secluded office to an outpatient clinic or emergency department setting. Appointments can be scheduled for the middle of the day, when numerous staff are present, as opposed to early morning or late evening. Sessions may be scheduled so that other staff are immediately available in the vicinity of the office or in the interview room during the appointment. For high-risk patients, the clinician may chose to leave the office door open during the interview, with staff or security present. Anticipation of violence leads to preventive treatment planning and can significantly enhance safety.

A risk assessment also begins to neutralize the potent psychological defense of denial in the clinician. Denial leads clinicians to minimize or ignore threats to their own safety despite the clinical evidence that the patient is escalating toward an aggressive event. By establishing the potential for violence through a risk assessment during the initial evaluation, a clinician can develop a treatment plan that incorporates safety issues before a patient displays threatening behavior.

A major issue in fostering safety is for the clinician to appreciate and adhere to the dynamics of violence. Succinctly stated, a patient is at risk for aggressive behavior when he or she feel helpless, impotent, or humiliated. A clinician who encounters a threatening or potentially violent patient should avoid becoming verbally or physically aggressive toward the patient. Psychiatrists who respond to threatening patients with physical or verbal aggression are significantly more likely to be injured or to have property destroyed than those who acknowledge their fear but also express a desire to help the patient (48). The strategy of a nonthreatening offer to provide help is reassuring to the patient and is the centerpiece for intervention with a potentially violent patient.

Aggression rarely occurs suddenly and unexpectedly. Usually there is a prodromal syndrome consisting of increasing tension and anxiety, increased verbal stridency and abuse, and increased motor activity usually characterized by pacing behavior. Intervention using talk-down strategies during this period of escalation will frequently avert violent behavior. In such an escalating situation, the clinician must be sure that the patient can hear and respond. A patient who is under the influence of alcohol is not a good candidate for talk-down techniques. By using a soft, assertive voice and short sentences, the clinician rapidly determine if the patient if paying attention (59). The clinician should talk down a patient by agreeing with him or her and not arguing. It is important not to respond to the content of the patient's speech. The patient should be overdosed with agreement (59).

The key to deescalating a potentially violent patient is affect management. Patients who are affectively aroused will need to ventilate their history and the clinician should not overly intrude into the interview (63). Often the patient who is overwhelmed with an angry affect intimidates the clinician, who responds with logical and rational explanations. This type of intervention only inflames the patient. Affect management involves acknowledging the patient's affect, validating the affect when appropriate, and encouraging the patient to talk about his or her feelings. For instance, the clinician might say, "I can see how angry this makes you. If I were given medication against my will I would be as angry as you are. Let's talk more about your feelings." Phrases such as "ventilate," "talking it out," "getting it off your chest," or "catharsis" are colloquialisms that refer to the process of allowing a person to discharge his or her affect. Addressing the affect serves several purposes. It teaches the patient to reduce his or her internal state of tension by verbalizing his or her feelings and that it is not necessary to hit someone or destroy furniture in order to feel better. Giving the patient the opportunity to ventilate his or her affect often defuses escalating emotions and averts a more violent confrontation.

An emotionally distraught patient requires an active response form the clinician. Active eye contact and body language that signal attentiveness and connectedness to the patient will reduce the probability that the patient will need to explode or attack to get his or her point across (63). Eichelman (63) has described interventions that are effective in the management of aggression. The use of active listening techniques, such as paraphrasing to the patient in brief, encapsulated form the content of his or her statements, helps to show that the clinician understands what the patient is experiencing. It is important to be honest and precise in responding to patients. Dishonesty may set the clinician up for either retribution or a tenuous therapeutic relationship. Eichelman (63) further recommends that in all situations the clinician keep a proper physical distance from the patient. It has been demonstrated that assaultive patients have a larger body buffer zone, and a rule of thumb would be to keep two quick steps or at least an arm's length away from the patient. If the patient is standing, the clinician should stand. If the patient is sitting, the clinician should also sit and not stand over the patient during the interview. If the patient is pacing, the clinician can model for the patient by walking with the patient, but at a much slower pace.

Clinicians frequently react to escalating or agitated behavior with punitive threats, in the belief that they are setting limits that will deter aggression. A threatening intervention, however, is contrary to the dynamics of violence, as it evokes feeling of impotence or humiliation in the patient and increases the risk of violence. Limit setting can be therapeutic and avert violent behavior. Too often, however, this is done in a provocative manner. According to Green and colleagues (64), the basic philosophy behind limit setting is to contain and counteract maladaptive behavior that interferes with therapy and threatens the clinician's safety. These authors have described the important elements of limit setting (64). Effective limit setting involves clear identification of the specific behaviors that need to be altered and precise articulation of the consequences that will follow if the inappropriate behavior persists. If the therapist lacks clarity in his or her thinking or communications to the patient concerning inappropriate behavior, the intervention may confuse and disorganize the patient. Whenever possible, interpretive or confrontational interventions should precede the imposition of limits, because this affords the patient greater flexibility in exercising his or her own autonomy and discretion.

An ultimatum that certain interventions—e.g., restraints, injections, loss of privileges—will ensue if certain behaviors do not cease is contrary to the dynamic of violence. Successful limit setting is most effective when the following sequence is carried out (64):

The patient is told of the behavior that is unacceptable.
The patient is told why the behavior is unacceptable.
The patient is offered several alternative treatment interventions.

For example, the clinician can say to the patient, "You cannot yell, curse or threaten other patients in the day room. They are afraid of you and they think that you will harm them. Therefore, you can either go to your room and listen to the radio until you feel calmer, or we can walk to the seclusion room and I will give you some medication." When a patient is offered options, he or she will usually accept the preferred option. Each time the patient is given a choice, he or she will pause and cognitively consider the options. Each pause decreases the amount of energy behind the anger and, as the process continues, the patient will slowly gain self-control (59). Offering only one choice invites the patient to argue and negotiate, which leads to further escalation and frequently culminates in an assault against the clinician or restraint of the patient.

Thackrey (65) describes several important clinical caveats regarding limit setting. Alternatives regarding both expected and prohibited behaviors must be stated concretely and in terms of actions that can be performed immediately. Whenever possible, directives or alternatives should be expressed in positive terms ("Do this," which describes acceptable behavior) rather than negative terms ("Don't do that," which describes no acceptable alternatives). The best limits are absolute rather than relative (such as, "Don't bang on the windows," rather than

"Don't bang on the windows so hard"). An essential part of limit setting is for the clinician to determine if the patient is capable of responding. In general, the greater the degree of cognitive impairment, the less able the patient is to understand or respond to limit setting. In these instances and depending on the location of the threat, the clinician should call for help or leave the interview office immediately if no one else is available to assist in the management of the patient.

When interviewing patients who have been violent or who have the potential for violence, the clinician should remove his or her glasses if possible (57). Neckties should be removed or tucked in and jewelry such as necklaces and earrings should be removed (57).

The clinician should leave when a situation seems totally uncontrollable (66). Before leaving, the clinician should consider what must be done to escape and what is the nearest safe place. The clinician should not run as a panic reaction but should leave as a positive action (66). The clinician should run toward a place of safety and not just away from danger. Once beginning the escape, the clinician should not hesitate or stop until he or she is free and clear. While running, one should consider where to run, how far it is, and what is the best way there (66). If it will help, one should take off one's shoes to make running easier (66).

Training and practice are essential if a clinician is to develop the necessary skills to manage aggressive patients. Unfortunately, psychiatrists receive limited training in the management of aggression during their residency. Hospital staff often have limited training as well. As a result, when aggressive incidents occur, there is often no agreed upon management philosophy and strategy. The lack of a uniform strategy can lead to mismanagement of aggressive events and to staff injury. Clinicians and staff should have ongoing training to enhance and maintain their skill level. Treatment teams should review all aggressive events in order to develop a cohesive philosophy of aggression management, so that agreed upon intervention strategies are employed simultaneously by all staff.

C. The Armed Patient

If a patient appears in a treatment setting with a weapon, as few staff as possible should be exposed to the risk of injury (57). Staff should retreat to an office. If trapped, the clinician should acknowledge the obvious—"I see you have a gun" (57). He or she should be calm and not become counteraggressive or threatening. The clinician should encourage the patient to talk during the initial phases and should repeat the patient's concerns. The firearm is almost invariably an expression of feelings of inadequacy and fear. The clinicians should try to speak to the underlying psychological issues (65). It is important to identify areas where the patient's viewpoint is correct rather than initially trying to demonstrate the areas where the patient's viewpoint is wrong. The alliance can be enhanced if the clinician can identify similarities between himself or herself and the patient.

If a short time passes during which the patient does not fire the gun, the likelihood of its eventual use is diminished. Initially, however, the clinician should comply with whatever demand the patient may make and take special care to avoid upsetting the patient further. There should be no attempt to take the weapon from the patient. One may suggest that the patient put the weapon down gently (57) but not reach for the gun or tell the patient to drop the gun, since it might then discharge (57).

D. Physical Defense by the Clinician

Generally, the clinician should avoid aggressive physical confrontation with the patient. Such a confrontation increases the risk of harm to the clinician. However, there are certain physical maneuvers that are helpful in managing attacks by patients. These are summarized in Table 1. A more detailed description of defensive maneuvers can be found elsewhere (57,65,66).

IV. OFFICE AND INSTITUTIONAL SAFETY

A. Office Safety

The most problematic situation is that of the individual clinician who practices alone. Office safety requires planning and persistence, and clinicians should be cognizant of safety issues. Ideally, the clinician's office should have two doors, one into the reception room and another locked door leading into the actual treatment room. This second door should have a peephole so that the clinician will be able to see who is in the outer office. In an ideal situation, the clinician may wish to have two entrances to his or her office so that, if a threatening patient comes into the reception area, there is another exit from the office.

If the clinician does not have a receptionist, he or she should consider a panic alarm or buzzer system to notify either building security or police in the event of a visit by a threatening or aggressive patient. Clinicians who practice alone should be cautious about the type of patients that they will evaluate and treat, especially in the evening or early morning. One strategy might be to initially interview all first-time and unknown patients in a more secure setting such as an outpatient department, crisis service, or emergency department. At a minimum, all new patients should have at least a 15- or 20-minute interview on the phone, which would include a risk assessment for violence.

Another controversial issue is whether the clinician should keep Mace or some other weapon in the office as a means of protection. Unfortunately, there is no literature to guide the clinician. Clinicians have reported that when they have had mace or other weapons in their office, they often forgot that they had the weapon when a patient became violent (48). Unless a clinician is highly skilled in the use of a weapon, there is considerable risk that the weapon could be used by the patient against the clinician. Preferably, clinicians should consider implementing most of the above strategies as opposed to keeping weapons in the office.

B. Office Safety in the Clinic Setting

Institutional outpatient sites should be constructed so that there is a physical and personal buffer for the clinician. Offices in outpatient clinics should have panic buttons and/or an organized strategy to notify a receptionist, other staff, or even the police of a threatening situation. A protocol should be developed to train office staff to recognize patients who may pose the risk of violence. Strategies should be put in place so that the office staff can notify the clinical staff or, if necessary, the police without alarming the patient when he or she begins to make escalating threats or presents at the office in a threatening manner. For instance, a simple code such as "Dr. Smith, can you see Mr. Jones *immediately*?" may be a signal that Mr. Jones is demonstrating behavior that suggests the risk of violence. This nonthreatening phone call then allows the clinician to implement other strategies, such as calling the police or mobilizing other clinic staff to help contain the patient.

A different code should be developed to alert staff that an armed patient is in the waiting area. Such an alarm should be simple and not threatening: e.g., "Is room 22 available?" Direct alarm systems to the police should also be considered, especially for the situation in which a patient has a weapon or is suspected of having a weapon. Such a system should be inconspicuous so as not to alert the patient that an alarm is being sounded.

Certain architectural features can further enhance safety. An office should be decorated in a manner that is consistent with the type of patient the clinician is treating. If the clinician is treating patients with a history of aggression or psychotic patients or if he or she frequently evaluates new patients, specific office safety issues should be considered. Safe offices should have heavy pieces of furniture that cannot be lifted or used as weapons. Offices, especially in emergency departments or inpatient units, should not contain hard, sharp objects such as small ashtrays, art work, lamps, or other decorations that could be thrown or used as weapons. All office doors should swing out into a hall and not into an office. This prevents a patient from blocking the therapist's egress by leaning against the door.

C. Safety in the Hospital

In emergency departments, interview rooms should be large enough that physical restraint can be implemented if necessary (63). Space for five staff members must be available as well as floor or gurney space making it possible to place an individual in a prone or supine position (63).

To further enhance safety, nursing stations should be constructed to provide a maximum view of the unit. Shatterproof Plexiglas should be employed in the windows of the nursing station if it is partially enclosed and in the windows of seclusion rooms (63). Closed-circuit television or convex mirrors should be used for blind spots on units (63). Dangerous furniture should be minimized, and heavy ashtrays or chairs that could be thrown should be replaced. Units with a high frequency of assault can also use individual portable alarm systems that can be carried by staff (63). A more detailed discussion of architecture and safety can be found elsewhere (63,67).

A controversial issue is whether to install metal detectors. The documented increase in violence in emergency departments coupled with the uncontrolled public access to an emergency department has led this author to conclude that, in a health care setting, an emergency department should have metal detectors to enhance clinician safety. Metal detectors can be effective while being nondisruptive to patient care. Consideration should also be given to the use of metal detectors in outpatients clinics, especially in high-crime areas or programs that treat patients who may be at a higher risk for violence. If metal detectors are employed, it is also important for the facility to develop protocols for managing patients and visitors when weapons are detected and for disarming a patient.

Another controversial issue is whether police should be allowed to carry their weapons into an emergency department. This author is aware of several situations in which patients have taken a police officer's gun and killed the officer or another patient. The safest strategy is to have all officers leave their guns in a secure area before going into patient areas in the hospital.

V. CONCLUSION

Clinicians can significantly enhance their safety by adhering to basic principles of safety. However, denial often leads clinicians to minimize the risk, and, as a result, they may take no steps to enhance their own security. In order to enhance safety, however, protocols must be developed, discussed repeatedly, and rehearsed; also, safety systems must be reviewed periodically and checked to assure that they are in working order. Immediate and rapid consultation with colleagues when threatening situations develop further helps to reduce the risk of violence. Optimal clinical safety not only enhances the security of the clinician but helps to facilitate effective treatment.

REFERENCES

1. W.R. Dubin and J.R. Lion, eds. *Task Force Report #33: Clinician Safety*, American Psychiatric Association, Washington, DC, 1992.
2. American College of Emergency Physicians, *Emergency Department Violence: Prevention and Management*, Dallas, 1988.
3. M.L. Lanza, The multiple costs of patient assault, *Creating a Secure Workplace: Effective Policies and Practices in Health Care* (J.R. Lion, W.R. Dubin, and D.E. Futrell, eds.) American Hospital Publishing, Chicago, 1996, p. 25.
4. R. M. Whitman, B. B. Armao, and O.B. Dent, Assault on the therapist, *Am. J. Psychiatry 133*:426 (1976).
5. D.J. Madden, J. R. Lion, and M.W. Penna, Assaults on psychiatrists by patients, *Am. J. Psychiatry 133*:422 (1976).
6. K. Tardiff, and W.L. Maurice, The care of violent patients by psychiatrists: A tale of two cities, *Can. Psychiatr. Assoc. J. 22*:83 (1977).
7. S. Hatti, W.R. Dubin, and K.J. Weiss, A study of the circumstances surrounding patient assaults on psychiatrists, *Hosp. Commun. Psychiatry 33*:660 (1982).
8. W.H. Reid and J.S. Kang. Serious assaults by outpatients or former patients, *Am. J. Psychother. 40*:594 (1986).
9. H. Carmel and M. Hunter, Psychiatrists injured by patient attacks, *Bull. Am. Acad. Psychiatry Law 19*:309 (1991).
10. L.R. Faulkner, N.R. Grimm, B. H. McFarland, et al., Threats and assaults against psychiatrists, *Bull. Am. Acad. Psychiatry Law 18*:37 (1990).
11. I. Ruben, G. Wolkon, and J. Yamamoto, Physical attacks on psychiatric residents by patients, *J. Nerv. Ment. Dis. 168*:243 (1980).
12. G.E. Gray, Assaults by patients against residents at a public psychiatric hospital, *Acad. Psychiatry 13*:81 (1989).
13. D.L. Fink, B. Shoyer, and W.R. Dubin, A study of assaults against psychiatric residents, *Acad. Psychiatry 15*:94 (1991).
14. M. Fireman, J.D. Bloom, and L.R. Faulkner, Violence toward psychiatric residents, presented at the 143rd Annual Meeting of the American Psychiatric Association, New York City, May 15, 1990.
15. G.A. Chaimowitz and A. Moscovitch, Patient assaults against psychiatric residents: The Canadian experience, *Can. J. Psychiatry 36*:107 (1991).
16. V. Milstein, Patient assaults on residents, *Indiana Med. 80*:753 (1987).
17. M. White, Gunman shoots three in emergency room, *Philadelphia Inquirer*, February 9, 1993.
18. W. R. Dubin, Assaults with weapons, *Patient Violence and the Clinician* (B.S. Eichelman and A. C. Hartwig, eds.) American Psychiatric Press, Washington, DC, 1995, p. 53.
19. W. R. Dubin and J.R. Lion, Violence against the medical profession, *Creating a*

Secure Workplace: Effective Policies and Practices in Health Care (J.R. Lion, W.R. Dubin, and D. E. Futrell, eds.), American Hospital Publishing, Chicago, 1996, p. 3.
20. L.V. Annis, H.A. McClaren, and C. A. Baker, Who kills us? Case study of a clinician's murderer, *Violence in the Medical Care Setting: A Survival Guide* (J.T. Turner, ed.), Aspen Publications, Rockville, MD., 1984, p. 19.
21. L.V. Annis and C. A. Baker, A psychiatrist's murder in a mental hospital, *Hosp. Commun. Psychiatry 37*:505 (1986).
22. B. Bowers, When a psychiatrist is murdered, *Psychiatric News*, January 15, 1982.
23. American Medical Association, MD recovers from office shooting, *A.M.A. News*, November 21, 1986.
24. K. Clarke and P. Windsor, Motive arises in shooting, *Ann Arbor News*, June, 27, 1992.
25. Assaults on doctors (editorial), *Br. Med. J. 6122*:1229 (1978).
26. J. Kron, Appointment, *Allure*, February 1994, p. 102.
27. R. Minter, Gunman kills one at Augusta hospital, *Atlanta Constitution*, October 9, 1991.
28. Funeral services for slain doctor, *New York Times*, February 10, 1987.
29. J. Perrone, Deadly disputes. *American Medical News*, January 13, 1992.
30. E. Revitch, Patients who kill their physician, *J. Med. Soc. N.J. 76*:429 (1979).
31. W.R. Wineke, Man shoots doctor, self; both dead. *State Journal*, Madison, WI, February 1, 1983.
32. W.R. Wineke, UW doctor and patient die of heart wounds, The *State Journal*, Madison, WI, February 2, 1983.
33. S.L. Lusk, Violence in the workplace, *J. Am. Assoc. Hosp. Nurses 40*:212 (1992).
34. H. Carmel and M. Hunter, Staff injuries from inpatient violence, *Hosp Commun. Psychiatry 40*:41 (1989).
35. M.L. Lanza, The reactions of nursing staff to physical assault by a patient, *Hosp. Commun. Psychiatry 34*:44 (1983).
36. M.L. Lanza, Reactions of nurses to a patient assault vignette, *West. J. Nurs. Res., 10*:45 (1988).
37. M. L. Lanza and H. Kayne, Staff and environmental characteristics related to patient assault, *Issues Ment. Health Nurs. 12*:253 (1991).
38. H. A. Bernstein, Survey of threats and assaults directed toward psychotherapists, *Am. J. Psychother. 35*:542 (1981).
39. S. Hillen, U.K. study: Half of therapists attacked, *APA Monitor* 22:22 (1991).
40. J. R. Lion, W. Synder, and G.L. Merrill, Underreporting of assaults on staff in a state hospital, *Hosp. Commun. Psychiatry 32*:497 (1981).
41. M.L. Lanza and D. Campbell, Patient assault: A comparison study of reporting methods, *J. Nurs. Care Qual. 5*:60 (1991).
42. A. Convit, D. Isay, R. Gadioma, et al., Underreporting of physical assaults in schizophrenic inpatients, *J. Nerv. Ment. Dis. 176*:504 (1988).
43. D.A. Brizer, A Convit, M. Krakowski et al., A rating scale for reporting violence on psychiatric wards, *Hosp. Commun. Psychiatry 38*:769 (1987).
44. M. Pearson, E. Wilmot, and M. Padi, A study of violent behavior among in-patients in a psychiatric hospital, *Br. J. Psychiatry 142*:232 (1986).

45. M.L. Lanza, Factors relevant to patient assault, *Issues Ment. Health Nurs. 9*:239 (1988).
46. J. Monahan, The prediction of violent behavior: Toward a second generation of theory and policy, *Am. J. Psychiatry 141*:10 (1984).
47. H. Carmel and M. Hunter, Staff injuries from patient attack: Five years' data. *Bull. Am. Acad. Psychiatry Law 21*:485 (1993).
48. W.R. Dubin, S.J. Wilson, and C. Mercer, Assaults against psychiatrists in outpatient settings, *J. Clin. Psychiatry 49*:338 (1988).
49. B.M. Thompson, J. Nunn, I, Kramer, et al., Disarming the department: Weapon screening and improved security to create a safer emergency department environment, *Ann Emerg Med 17*:419 (1988).
50. G.A. Pane, A.M. Winiarski, and K.A. Salness, Aggression directed toward emergency department staff at a university teaching hospital, *Ann. Emerg. Med. 20*:283 (1991).
51. F.W. Lavoie, G.L. Carter, D.F. Danzi, et al., Emergency department violence in the United States teaching hospitals, *Ann. Emerg. Med. 17*:1127 (1988).
52. A.A. Anderson, A.Y. Ghali, and R.K. Bansil, Weapon carrying among patients in a psychiatric emergency room, *Hosp. Commun. Psychiatry 40*:8456 (1989).
53. M.R. Privitera, M.O. Springer, and R.A. Perlmutter, To search or not to search: Is there a clinical profile of a patient harboring a weapon? *Gen. Hosp. Psychiatry 8*:442 (1986).
54. D.E. McNeil and R.L. Binder, Patients who bring weapons to the psychiatric emergency room, *J Clin Psychiatry 48*:230 (1987).
55. S. Eth, G.B. Leong, Weapon screening (letter). *Hosp. Commun. Psychiatry 38*:203 (1987).
56. W. McKillop, Weapon screening (letter), *Hosp. Commun. Psychiatry 38*:203 (1987)
57. K. Tardiff, Clinician safety, *Assessment and Management of Violent Patients*, 2d ed., American Psychiatric Press, Washington, DC, 1996, p. 19.
58. P.L. Jenkins, Harassment, *Hazards of Psychiatric Practice*, Year Book Medical Publishers, Chicago, 1989, p. 14.
59. G.J. Maier, Managing threatening behavior: The role of talk down and talk up, *J. Psychosoc. Nurs. 34*:25 (1996).
60. P.E. Dietz, Defenses against dangerous people when arrest and commitment fail, *Review of Clinical Psychiatry and the Law*, Vol. 1 (R.I. Simon, ed.), American Psychiatric Press, Washington, Dc, 1990, p. 205.
61. G.P. Brown, W.R. Dubin, J.R. Lion, et al., A preliminary classification of threats against clinicians, *Bull. Am. Acad. Psychiatry Law 24*:367 (1996).
62. J.R. Lion, Verbal threats against clinicians, *Patient Violence and the Clinician* (B.S. Eichelman and A.C. Hartwig, eds.) American Psychiatric Press, Washington, DC, 1995, p. 43.
63. B.S. Eichelman, Strategies for clinician safety, *Patient Violence and the Clinician* (B.S. Eichelman and A.C. Hartwig, eds.) American Psychiatric Press, Washington, DC, 1995, p. 139.
64. S.A. Green, R. L. Goldberg, D.M. Goldstein, et al., The art of limit setting, *Limit Setting in Clinical Practice* (S.A. Green, R.L. Goldberg, D.M. Goldstein, et al., eds.), American Psychiatric Press, Washington, DC, 1988, p. 1.

65. M. Thackrey, Psychological intervention techniques, *Therapeutics for Aggression*, Human Sciences Press, New York, 1987, p. 42.
66. V. Bowie, *Coping with Violence*, Karabuni Press, Sydney, Australia, 1989.
67. D. J. Allison and R. T. Matthews, Facility design and security, *Creating a Secure Workplace: Effective Policies and Practices in Health Care* (J.R. Lion, W.R. Dubin, and D.E. Futrell), American Hospital Publishing, Chicago, 1996, p. 235.

10
Acute Management of Violent Patients

Kenneth Tardiff
Cornell University Medical College, New York, New York

I. INTRODUCTION

There are a number of psychiatric disorders that are associated with violence. Since time is of the essence in an emergency, the clinician must decide immediately which of the three types of violent patients he or she faces so as to manage violence effectively with verbal means, restraint, seclusion, and/or medication.

II. THREE TYPES OF VIOLENT PATIENTS

A. The Psychotic Patient

The first type of violent patient is the *psychotic patient.* Violence with psychotic patients will probably not respond to verbal means of deescalation and attempts to appeal to rational thinking on the part of the patient. Medication with or without restraint and seclusion will probably be necessary. Psychosis and violence are often associated with schizophrenia (1,2). Schizophrenic patients can be violent as the result of delusions, particularly paranoid delusions (3,4). They believe people are trying to harm them or are spying on them, and they retaliate with violence. Hallucinations, particularly command hallucinations, may account for the violence as the psychotic patient hears voices telling him or her to attack someone (5).

Schizophrenic patients can be violent for reasons not related to psychosis per se. This includes general disorganization, lack of impulse control, or akathisia, as they are restless and bump into other patients, thus provoking fights. Schizophrenics may have comorbid conditions that cause the violence, such as alcohol or substance abuse, antisocial or borderline personality, or neurological impairment (6–8).

Other psychiatric disorders, such as mania and depression, can involve psychosis and violence (9,10). Manics are characteristically violent when they feel trapped or restricted, while psychotic depressed patients are violent as the result of delusions of guilt and/or paranoid delusions.

B. The Organic Patient

The second type of violent patient is the *organic patient* with a neurological or medical disorder (11). Such a patient may or may not be psychotic. As in the case of the first type of patient, this second type will probably not respond to verbal intervention. Restraint and/or medication will probably be necessary. The patient may be organic due to intoxication with alcohol or drugs such as cocaine, hallucinogens, amphetamines, or other drugs. A number of primary diseases of the brain can be associated with violence, such as infections, head trauma, toxins, dementias, and other deteriorative diseases of the brain. Organicity may come from other impacts on the brain, such as hypoxia, electrolyte imbalances, diseases of the thyroid, liver, kidney, and other organs, systemic infections, and other medical diseases.

C. The Nonpsychotic, Nonorganic Patient

The third type of violent patient is *Nonpsychotic, Nonorganic patient.* Verbal attempts to deescalate violence can be successful with these patients, who have personality disorders or other disorders with problems of impulse control (12–14). Patients with antisocial personality are violent and have no sense of guilt associated with their violence. They believe that the victim deserved the attack. Patients with borderline personality are violent in response to rejection or perceived rejection and because of their unstable, chaotic character structure. Patients without personality disorders who have poor impulse control and are violent usually feel guilty about their violence. Thus they have the best prognosis in terms of responding to verbal intervention and deescalation.

III. SAFETY

Violence among psychiatric patients can erupt unexpectedly in any clinical setting: in the emergency department, the inpatient unit, or even the outpatient clinic. If verbal deescalation is successful, further discussion with the patient is indicated. The ideal situation is that of being alone with the patient in a closed room; however, this may not always be advisable for safety reasons. Safety is the most important factor in managing violence among patients (15). The clinician must feel safe with the patient in a setting or else it will interfere with the evaluation. In talking to the patient, a wide range of options should be considered, from being alone with the patient with the door closed, to being alone with the door open, to being alone with aides outside of the room, being alone with aides inside the room, to the most extreme option, interviewing the patient while the patient is in physical restraints.

IV. STAFF

In the emergency situation, the staff should be adequate in number and trained to implement seclusion and restraint techniques effectively, appropriately, and safely. The staff should talk to patients in a calm, nonprovocative manner and also listen to patients. As tension increases before violence occurs, even the most psychotic schizophrenic patient may respond to nonprovocative interpersonal contact and expressions of concern and caring. It is important that the staff recognize the warning signs of violence for an individual patient that have preceded violence in the past. A patient may have manifested a specific pattern of behavior or speech before an explosive episode. It may be in the form of pacing in front of the nursing station, repeating the same word or phrase, or some other warning sign known to have preceded violence in the past.

V. USE OF EMERGENCY MEDICATION

Emergency medication is useful for psychotic violent patients and is indicated for nonpsychotic, violent patients when verbal intervention is not appropriate or effective. It may be used instead of seclusion or restraint. It may be used with seclusion or restraint when severe agitation or violence is present to minimize detrimental effects violence may have on patients even though they are secluded or restrained.

A. Antipsychotics

Antipsychotics medication should be used primarily for the management of violent patients who manifest psychotic symptomatology. Occasionally it may be indicted for patients who are not psychotic but who are violent, as in the case of patients with dementia or other organic brain dysfunction, where anxiolytic agents or sedatives may exacerbate the clinical picture (16). In the emergency situation, antipsychotic medication is often given intramuscularly when the psychotic patient is completely out of control. It may be offered by mouth, with the stipulation that if the patient does not take the medication, the medication will be given intramuscularly to manage violence that is a danger to others or to the patient. The use of antipsychotic medication in the nonemergency situation is discussed in Chapter 11.

Soloff (17) reviewed the literature on the use of rapid neuroleptization and the acute management of the violent patient. He indicated that at wide range of drugs can be used in this procedure and that there is general safety and efficacy with rapid neuroleptization. It has been demonstrated effective with schizophrenic and manic patients in terms of improvement of delusions, hallucinations, disorganized thought, and agitation and violence. There are two basic strategies in this approach: the use of high-potency antipsychotic drugs with an anxiolytic or other drug for sedation if necessary versus low-potency antipsychotic drugs for their sedative side effects as well as antipsychotic effects. The use of 20 mg/day of haloperidol has been found to be effective in reducing psychosis, but it may cause side effects such as akathisia (18). Fluphenazine in doses ranging from 0.2 to 0.3 mg/kg/day has produced good responses for the violent psychotic patient (19). Although clozapine is very useful for the management of violent psychotic patients on a long-term basis (20,21) it should not be used for the acute management of violence because it can cause severe hypotension and convulsions.

Although this author favors the use of high-potency antipsychotic drugs with or without concurrent lorazepam, the choice of strategy should also take into consideration the patient's history and physical status. One should attempt to review the patient's previous responses to medication as well as the presence of medical illnesses that may predispose to or be exacerbated by extrapyramidal side effects or orthostatic hypotension. If extrapyramidal side effects are less acceptable, low-potency antipsychotics should be used. If orthostatic hypotension and related side effects are less acceptable, then high-potency antipsychotics are indicated. The physician should be free to change strategy as the patient's medical condition is monitored.

The use of high-potency drugs with rapid neuroleptization often involves haloperidol. There are two approaches with the high-potency neuroleptic strategy. The first is a low-dose approach using haloperidol 5 mg (1 mL) intramuscularly every 4 to 8 hours for a maximum dose of 15 to 30 mg/day. The high-dose approach uses haloperidol 10 mg (2 mL) intramuscularly every 30 minutes with a 24-hour maximum dose of 45 to 100 mg. Most patients treated for violence and acute psychosis will usually need 15 to 60 mg/day. Improvement in terms of decreased violence and hostility is rapid, often within 20 minutes of the initial injection of haloperidol when given as 10 mg intramuscularly.

With rapid neuroleptization, one should be cautious to exclude patients who are delirious or otherwise organically impaired, because the sedative or anticholinergic effects of the neuroleptics may exacerbate such conditions. Likewise, intoxication with alcohol or other sedative drugs is a contraindication to rapid neuroleptization because the patient's level of consciousness may be impaired. Use of these medications in alcohol withdrawal is also contraindicated because they decrease the seizure threshold. Extrapyramidal symptoms such as akathisia may produce a paradoxical reaction, with an increase of agitation and violence. Other serious side effects include neuroleptic malignant syndrome and (very rarely) laryngeal dystonic reaction.

Low-potency antipsychotic medications are used less frequently than the high-potency antipsychotic medications because of problems with orthostatic hypotension and because the sedation obtained by the use of low-potency antipsychotics can also be obtained through the use of lorazepam with high-potency antipsychotic medication. If the low-potency antipsychotic strategy is to be used, chlorpromazine is usually the drug of choice. A test dose of chlorpromazine 10 to 25 mg IM is recommended, and the patient is observed for orthostatic hypotension. If this is not a problem, chlorpromazine should be given 25 mg IM (1 mL) every 4 hours in a low-dose approach or up to 75 mg (3 mL) every 4 hours for the high-dose approach. The maximum daily dose for chlorpromazine given intramuscularly is 400 mg. No more than 3 mL should be injected at any one time because local tissue irritation may result. Vital signs should be monitored. If there is an extreme hypotensive crisis (i.e., the systolic blood pressure is less than 80 mmHg on rising), the patient will require treatment with vasopressors such as metaraminol bitartrate or levarterenol bitartrate. Epinephrine is contraindicated because it may further lower blood pressure in neuroleptic-induced orthostatic hypotension.

Using either approach, once the patient's violence is under control, oral medication may be started using a milligram-for-milligram translation on a 24-hour basis and allowing for further intramuscular doses as needed in case of recurrences of violent behavior. Other clinicians suggest oral doses 1½ times the intramuscular dose administered in the first 24 hours. Oral medication should be given in liquid form and divided into two or more doses, depending on the clinical situation.

B. Benzodiazepines

The benzodiazepines can be used very effectively in emergency situations where violence is in the process of occurring or where it is imminent. Benzodiazepines may be used with the neuroleptic medications for schizophrenics, manics, and patients in other psychotic states (22,23). They may be used alone for the management of nonpsychotic patients. For patients who appear to have some degree of control, they may be offered as oral medication. However, in most emergency situations, benzodiazepines are used intramuscularly. A number of clinicians are cautious about their use because there have been reports of paradoxical violence (24). Aggressive dyscontrol in patients treated with benzodiazepines, with the possible exceptions of clonazepam and alprazolam, appears to be overstated and is not frequent. Approximately 1% of patients have been found to have an increase of hostility or anger when treated with benzodiazepines (25). Patients with borderline personality disorder seem to be at greater risk for having that reaction (26).

For intramuscular use, this author prefers lorazepam because it is reliably and rapidly absorbed from injection sites, unlike diazepam or chlordiazepoxide. Lorazepam is also useful because it produces sedation for a longer period of time than diazepam and remains in the circulation rather than being absorbed into tissues. On the other hand, the half-life of lorazepam is 12 hours, much shorter than that of diazepam, so that accumulation is not as problematic as it is with diazepam. Lorazepam, given by intramuscular injection, rapidly begins to enter the circulation and produces sedation within an hour. The oral administration of lorazepam products more gradual effects, with sedation occurring usually longer than 1 hour and less than 4 hours after administration.

The dose is 2 to 4 mg by mouth or intramuscularly. A subsequent 2- to 4-mg dose can be repeated if there is continued agitation and aggression, at a time depending on the route of administration (i.e., in an hour or so if given intramuscularly or 4 to 6 hours if by mouth). Often this is sufficient to manage violence in the emergency situation. After the emergency has subsided, lower maintenance levels of lorazepam with or without neuroleptics to a maximum of 10 mg/day in three divided doses can be given. Lorazepam up to 4 mg for an average-size person could be given intravenously, but slowly at the rate of 2 mg (1 mL) per minute so as to avoid respiratory depression. This can be repeated in a 10 minutes if needed. This route of administration should be used only in cases of severe violence. Resuscitation equipment and staff able to use this equipment should be nearby, as laryngospasm or respiratory depression are potential side effects.

C. Barbiturates

Lorazepam has largely replaced barbiturates in the control of violence. However, if a barbiturate is used, the barbiturate used to induce sedation or sleep in violent patients in the emergency situation is sodium amobarbital, administered intravenously in 10% aqueous solution. The total dose used is from 200 to 500 mg; the rate of administration should not exceed 1 mL/minute (27). While administering the medication, one should attempt to achieve sedation or sleep without depressing respiration. Because respiratory depression and laryngospasm are possible side effects, resuscitation equipment must be nearby. The beneficial effect of this medication occurs within a few minutes. The dose may be repeated if the patient becomes more agitated and aggressive later. This should be used only in extreme emergencies and usually requires concurrent restraint of the patient while administration of sodium amobarbital is taking place. It is preferable is to use lorazepam with restraint until the medical takes effect instead of giving sodium amobarbital intravenously.

VI. SECLUSION AND RESTRAINT

A. Standards for Seclusion and Restraint

In 1982 the U.S. Supreme Court heard the case of *Youngberg v. Romeo* (28), the latter being a violent, profoundly mentally retarded man who was institutionalized. The court ruled that he could be deprived of his liberty in terms of being restrained if it could be justified to protect others or himself and if the decision was based on the clinical judgment of a professional that was not a substantial departure from professional standards. This case was important because the court deferred to professional judgment rather than a rigid hierarchy of restrictiveness in the management of violence among patients. At the time the court decision was rendered, this author was chairing the Task Force of the American Psychiatric Association (APA) to develop guidelines for the psychiatric uses of seclusion and restraint. These guidelines have been approved by the APA and have set reasonable minimal clinical standards for the management of violence using seclusion and restraint in the context of verbal intervention, involuntary medication, and other factors in the treatment environment (29). The guidelines are expanded on in a book by members of the Task Force (30) and updated in a more recent review article (31). More stringent guidelines at a local level would take precedence, as for a state or individual hospital.

B. Indications for Seclusion or Restraint

Indications for both seclusion and restraint are as follows: (1) to prevent imminent harm to the patient or other persons when other means of control are not effective or appropriate; (2) to prevent serious disruption of the treatment program or significant damage to the physical environment; and (3) to assist in treatment as part of ongoing behavior therapy. Two additional indications pertain solely to seclusion: (4) to decrease the stimulation a patient receives and (5) to comply with a patient's request. The clinical aspects of these indications for seclusion and restraint are discussed below.

One must consider the nature of the danger to the patient and to other persons, what constitutes "imminent" danger, and how one judges that other means of control are not effective or appropriate or that seclusion or restraint is a less restrictive mode of controlling dangerous behavior. The patient can be a danger to himself or herself in two ways: (1) in terms of deliberate suicidal acts or self-mutilation or (2) by a degree of excitement or behavioral dyscontrol that will result in exhaustion or injury if it continues. The patient can be a danger to others by deliberately trying to harm them through assault, using a weapon, or in other ways unintentionally endangering them as a result of marked disorganization of behavior.

Likewise, significant damage to the physical environment or the treatment milieu can be the result of deliberate behavior, as in antisocial or other personality disorders, or the result of grossly disorganized behavior, as in mania. Deliberate attempts to harm others or to damage the environment are often due to psychotic thinking on a functional or organic basis. Most commonly this is manifested as paranoid delusional thoughts, where the assault is seen by the patient as self-defense against others who are perceived as intending to harm him or her.

Disorganized and nondeliberate assault or other dangerous behavior may be the result of a number of clinical entities. This behavior is marked by impulsivity and is often purposeless and uncontrolled activity. For these patients, hallucinations or delusions are often not related to the dangerous behavior. This may be found with nonparanoid schizophrenia, mania, or with organic brain syndromes (e.g., phencyclidine-induced psychosis). Accompanying signs include loss of coherent speech, dysarthria, hyperactivity, fecal smearing and incontinence, screaming, or other manifestations.

If the etiology for the disorganized violent behavior is not known, restraint may be indicated so as to maintain the patient in the drug-free period for purposes of evaluation. Use of seclusion or restraint permits observation over time and differentiation of toxic from functional states. In addition, a violent patient may be preferentially managed in seclusion and restraint because of medical illness or drug allergies that would preclude the use of certain medications to control violent behavior.

Under certain circumstances, seclusion of a patient may be indicated for both the patient's benefit and that of the environment. Certain events, such as destruction of property, uncontrollable screaming or abuse, public masturbation, denudative behavior, uncontrolled intrusiveness on others, or fecal smearing may constitute treatment indications for seclusion or restraint based on environmental needs. Clearly, however, this must be understood in conjunction with the patient's own needs.

Another issue for seclusion and restraint is whether these measures are to be used only once a patient is actually in the process of manifesting dangerous behavior as opposed to whether the staff may use these procedures in anticipation of imminent dangerous behavior by the patient. Once they are familiar with a particular patient, staff may rely on patterns of verbal or nonverbal phenomena that have occurred before violent episodes in the past. This is usually specific for the patient and may include such signs as escalating excited motor behavior, increase in muscle tone, pacing, loud or profane speech, or more subtle manifestations such as the patient asking questions in a repetitive, persistent way.

The use of specific previous patterns of behavior to justify seclusion or restraint must rely on a great deal of familiarity with the individual patient and must be documented.

Seclusion may be used to decrease stimulation, usually for psychotic patients. The quiet atmosphere of the seclusion room is a relief from sensory overload, which may result even when a ward may appear quiet to other patients and staff. Secluding a patient at the patient's own request represents a valid indication. The patient's wish to be in seclusion may be a responsible attempt to prevent sensory overload or to avert an incipient or escalating clinical state that would result in dangerous behavior. However, especially with patients with borderline personality, voluntary self-seclusion may serve regressive pathological rather than therapeutic ends. Other often maladaptive requests for seclusion include those of the adolescent attempting to provoke staff as well as the antisocial patient attempting to test the limits of staff tolerance or to foster a macho self-image. Thus the clinical differentiation of the meaning of a request for seclusion may require that some patients' requests for seclusion be refused and that alternative verbal or other interventions be offered. Other locales in the hospital such as the patient's room, courtyards, or a "music room" may be preferable for voluntary self-isolation.

C. Alternatives to Seclusion or Restraint

In using seclusion or restraint to prevent harm to the patient, other persons, or the environment, the staff must have considered or tried other means of control. Certainly verbal and other interventions such as socialization and recreation should be considered to prevent loss of control prior to resorting to seclusion or restraint. Patients must have continuing opportunities to participate in their environment, to become engaged in activities, and to talk and interact with staff and other patients. Recreational materials and structured activities should be readily available on all inpatient and day-hospital units where patients live or spend their time. Some patients need assistance and prompting to engage in recreational and rehabilitative activities productively. Thus a continuum of active outreach by staff is necessary to ensure that patients are engaged in an appropriate level of activity, given their deficits, assets, and symptomatic handicaps.

In terms of other alternatives, the use of medication as opposed to seclusion or restraint cannot be seen in the context of which option is less restrictive. The decision as to whether one uses medication, seclusion, or restraint to control dangerous behavior must be made in terms of the individual patient. For example, the use of repetitive antipsychotic medication to control dangerous behavior in the developmentally disabled would not be as desirable as using restraint or seclusion first. On the other hand, involuntary medication may be preferred to seclusion and restraint in the case of a paranoid schizophrenic who is acting on paranoid delusions and has not been taking oral antipsychotic medication. With a patient in seclusion (e.g., a manic patient), less medication may be needed as stimulation is decreased.

One should consider the use of constant observation by a staff member to prevent injury to self or others in the inpatient setting. This procedure can be very expensive in terms of staff time and very intrusive for some patients. These decisions should be made on a one-to-one basis since, if the risk of injury is significant enough to warrant close observation, a staff member must be able to react to one patient without abandoning the monitoring of other patients assigned to the staff member. In most institutions, constant observation requires a physician's order. The use of constant observation should be reviewed on a regular basis, at least once a day. The justification for the constant observation must be documented in the patient's record, as should the reason for discontinuing the constant observation. Staff observation of the patient should be recorded on a regular basis—for example, every 15 to 30 minutes. Staff should not interact with the patient excessively or otherwise make the constant observation status pleasurable or gratifying in terms of attention given.

D. Contraindications for Seclusion or Restraint

Seclusion or restraint may be contraindicated because of the patient's clinical or medical condition. The paticnt's unstable medical status—resulting from infection, cardiac illness, disorders of thermoregulation, or metabolic illness—may require close monitoring and close physical proximity of staff such that seclusion is not indicated. For certain such conditions, however, restraint may be valuable (e.g., in neurological problems, such as delirium and dementia, where the patient's vulnerability to reduced sensory input may lead to worsening of the total clinical state, contraindicating seclusion).

Other situations representing relative contraindication to seclusion include those involving patients experiencing reactions to medications; patients who have just taken overdoses and require close monitoring; patients presenting with the symptoms of serious and uncontrollable self-abuse and self-mutilation; and the problem of seclusion rooms that cannot be sufficiently cooled on hot days for patients receiving drugs such as phenothiazines, which impair thermoregulation.

With physical restraint, an adverse effect is circulatory obstruction, which can be minimized by temporarily releasing one of four-point restraints every 5 minutes. Another adverse effect with restraints is aspiration. If a patient is lying on his or her back or is obstructed with restrained, one must guard against aspiration by constant monitoring.

Seclusion of a patient as a purely punitive response is contraindicated. Similarly, a patient should never be secluded for the purpose comfort or convenience of the staff, although it is common for patient and staff distress to coexist. While protection of other patients from harm is a valid indication for seclusion, mere mild obnoxiousness, rudeness, or other unpleasantness to others is not. Finally, although staff anxiety is often a well-validated indicator, through contagion, of actual or incipient dangerousness in a patient, staff anxiety alone should not be a reason for secluding a patient. This distinction is not always easy to make on the clinical scene but may be determined retrospectively by review with the staff.

E. Role of the Physician

Beginning an episode of seclusion or restraint is usually an emergency procedure carried out by the nursing or other staff on an inpatient unit. However, this requires a physician's review and order for continuation. Each institution has specific time parameters regarding review, and the psychiatrist should be familiar with them. The physician should be notified as soon as possible. The Task Force preferred notification within 1 hour after the seclusions or restraint episode begins (31). The physician should see the patient, preferably within 1 hour after the beginning of the seclusion or restraint. When notified by telephone, the physician should indicate approval pending personal examination of the patient. During the visit, the physician should document this in the patient's record. This episode should be reviewed by the patient's physician and treatment team. For each subsequent seclusion or restraint episode for that patient, the physician should be notified within the hour and should see the patient.

A physician should see the secluded or restrained patient as frequently as necessary to monitor any changes in the patient's mental or physical status. Although the frequency of these visits may vary, a visit every 4 hours is recommended. More frequent visits are necessary for certain patients, including those with concurrent medical problems, those receiving medical treatment that may complicate seclusion or restraint, those with organic brain syndrome, and those in situations where hyperthermia may occur and the patient needs to be closely monitored. When the physician sees the patient, the order for continued seclusion or restraint should be justified in terms of its continuation in the patient's record. During the visit, the physician should review the more frequent nursing observations of the patient in seclusion or restraint.

During the visit, a physician should examine the patient and document in the patient's record the reason for continued seclusion or restraint, taking into account the patient's mental and physical status, the degree of agitation, physical and emotional adverse effects of seclusion, and other factors such as staffing and the ability to handle the patient on the open inpatient unit. In some institutions, a large number of violent patients may mean that more than one patient will be in seclusion or restraint at a time. This strains the staff in terms of the need for observation, toileting, and other care of patients who are secluded and restrained. This may detract attention from unsecluded or unrestrained agitated patients. Thus, the condition of the ward, staffing, and types of patients must be considered in relation to whether a patient remains in seclusion or restraint.

It should be noted that guidelines for a specific hospital may be more restrictive than time parameters indicated in this book and that the clinician must adhere to hospital guidelines. The guidelines for seclusion and restraint within a specific hospital should be rehearsed and approved by the hospital staff as well as the legal staff. This includes specific techniques for putting a patient in seclusion, specific time parameters for physician's visits to the patient, and staff monitoring as well as restraint devices such as four-point leather restraints or other devices.

F. Techniques for Seclusion and Restraint

The use of seclusion and restraint techniques places both staff and patients at risk for injury. This may be minimized by rehearsal of these techniques. Once the decision has been made to begin seclusion or restraint of an agitated patient, a seclusion or restraint leader is chosen from among the clinical staff. The leader should indicate the roles to be played by the remaining staff in the seclusion and restraint process. The leader should be chosen for familiarity with the patient or for other factors; for example, a female member of the staff may be more appropriate than a male member of the staff in terms of minimizing provocation and maximizing cooperation of the patient. Female staff members are usually considered less intimidating and less authoritarian than male staff members.

There should be adequate staff to control the patient's behavior if the patient refuses to comply with requests that he or she go into seclusion. This consists of at least five staff members, one for each extremity and one (who can be the seclusion leader) to control the patient's head. The staff should gather around the seclusion leader at the time of first contact with the violent patient. Staff should project an image of confidence and the ability to control the situation should the patient not cooperate. The area should be cleared of all other patients and physical obstructions leading to the seclusion room. Ideally there should be someone to observe the procedure, noting any injuries or difficulties with physical technique. This will make possible a critique of the seclusion or restraint procedure after the episode ends.

The onset of the seclusion or restraint procedure begins with telling the patient the reason for the procedure. The patient is given clear options in a way that is not threatening or provocative. For example, the patient may be told that his or her behavior is out of control and that he or she must go into seclusion so as to regain control. The patient is asked to walk quietly to the seclusion room accompanied by the staff. Having considered other forms of intervention, such as verbal ones or medication alone, further discussion or negotiation at this time is inappropriate. In fact, it may lead to an argument, physical fight, and injuries to the patient as well as staff. The patient is given a few seconds to comply; if the patient does not, the staff begins the seclusion or restraint procedure. At the time of the first contact with the patient and throughout the procedure, the staff must not humiliate or threaten the patient. They must maintain the patient's dignity and self-esteem.

Physical force begins after a prearranged signal from the seclusion leader. Each staff member grabs and controls one of the patient's extremities. Carefully so as not to injure the patient, the staff brings the patient to the ground through a backward motion, and each extremity is restrained at the joint by a member of the team. The patient's head should be controlled to prevent biting or neck injury. The staff should be cautious to avoid injuring the patient or causing pain. Not only is this inappropriate but it may interfere with future therapeutic relationships between the staff and the patient.

After the patient is restrained on the ground, additional staff may be called to assist in moving the patient to the seclusion room or to help apply physical restraints. The staff should lift the patient with the arms pressed into the sides and the legs held tightly at the knees. The head should be controlled and lifted as the back, hips, and legs are lifted.

Once the patient is in the seclusion room, the patient is put on his or her back with the head toward the seclusion door and feet in the opposite direction. Street clothes are removed, and special attention is paid to removing rings, belts, shoes, matches, and other potentially destructive objects. Medication may be injected at this time, while the patient is physically restrained.

The staff exit in a coordinated manner, one at a time, releasing the legs first and the arms last. The last staff member should move quickly in a backward fashion out of the seclusion room door, which is quickly locked. Another way of placing a patient in the seclusion room is to put the patient face down on a mattress with his or her head away from the door. Arms and legs may be brought behind the back, and it is possible for the last member of the team to control arms and legs while the patient is in this position. Again, the last staff member in the seclusion room should quickly release the arms and legs and leave the room. The latter technique may not be advisable for very obese patients, because it may cause respiratory impairment in a face-down position.

After a patient has been placed in seclusion or restraint, the staff should discuss the episode among themselves so as to critique the technique as well as to allow verbalization of any conflicting feelings. The staff should also consider, especially on units where violence is rare, discussing the behavior that led up to the seclusion or restraint episode at community meetings with patients.

G. Monitoring and Caring for the Patient

While the patient is in seclusion or restraint, observations by the nursing staff should be made at least every 15 minutes. This may be done by looking through the window of the seclusion room, especially for severely violent patients. In a written log, the staff should write their observations (e.g., "the patient is quiet," "the patient is walking around the seclusion room," or "the patient is yelling"). These visual checks are important so as to minimize the chance that patients will harm themselves in the seclusion room. Of course, if self-mutilation is a concern, seclusion may not be indicated for the patient or constant observation of the patient in seclusion may be indicated.

A direct visit into the seclusion room is indicated at least every 2 hours. In the case of very violent patients, it is advisable that an adequate number of staff accompany the nursing staff. During these visits, vital signs should be taken; meals, fluids, and toileting needs should be taken care of. All observations and recordings should be documented in the patient's record. In terms of care of the patient, the patient should be allowed to go to the bathroom at least every 4 hours. In certain cases, this may mean taking the patient out of the seclusion room. Again, in the case of very violent patients, adequate staff should be present at that time. In the case of patients in restraints, the restrains will probably have to be removed while the patient is allowed to go to the bathroom. Meals should be brought to the patient at regular intervals when the ward meals are served. Eating utensils, if any, should be blunt; even plastic knives and forks can be used as weapons. The patient should be instructed to sit at one corner of the seclusion room while the meal tray is placed in the seclusion room. If possible, the staff should be present with the patient while the meal is being eaten. This is to allow interpersonal contact with the patient as well as to make observations as to the patient's degree of self-control. Why a patient is being allowed to eat alone should be documented in the patient's record. There should be adequate attention to fluid intake so as to prevent dehydration. Fluid intake should be documented in the patient's record.

The architecture and environment of the seclusion room should be free of hazards. Seclusion rooms are usually empty except for a mattress. The mattress should be constructed of durable foam and not fiber or other materials that patients could use to hang or suffocate themselves. The mattress should not be flammable and patients should be searched for matches prior to being placed in seclusion. The ceiling of the seclusion room should be high, with recessed light fixtures. All walls and ceilings should be made of material that cannot be gouged out.. There should be no sharp edges to windows and no protuberances such as oxygen jets.

The staff should be able to observe every portion of the seclusion room; this may require reflectors. It is important that the staff be able to monitor patients so as to prevent self-mutilation and other injuries. If patients are very hyperactive and there is concern about exhaustion, restraint with or without seclusion should be considered. If it appears that a patient's psychosis has become worse in the seclusion room, one should consider the impact of sensory deprivation in terms of this increase in psychosis. In this case, restraint or constant attention by the staff may be indicated. Table 5 summarizes the process of assessing and monitoring the patient who is put into seclusion or restraint.

H. Release from Seclusion or Restraint

A patient may be released form seclusion or restraint when the patient's behavior is under control and no longer poses a danger to self or others or threatens further disruption of the treatment environment. The ability of a patient to control his or her behavior and to cooperate is evaluated throughout the seclusion episode. For example, during each visit, the patient's ability to respond to a verbal request should be judged. A patient may be asked to sit in a particular part of the seclusion room, or cooperation may be reflected in the patient becoming more amenable to taking oral medication rather than having to have injections. At a higher level, the patient will be able to cooperate with physical examinations, interviews, bathing, toileting, and other procedures.

Release from seclusion is a gradual process. The first step may be opening the seclusion room door for brief periods of time, followed by continued opening of the seclusion room door, to spending time alone in the patient's room, until the patient can be released to the general ward environment. Any evidence of loss of control or lack of cooperation should result in movement back to more restrictive steps in the procedure.

I. Prevention of Inappropriate Seclusion or Restraint

To prevent inappropriate seclusion or restraint or not using these techniques when they should be used, the staff should know their own feelings about violent patients based on countertransference reactions or other emotional reactions to patients (32). As in other areas of psychiatry, negative or inappropriate feelings about patients must be recognized so as not to act on them. The staff should constantly monitor the ward dynamics, particularly in terms of staff conflict, which may translate into inappropriate patient care in the management of violence. The staff should know their own past experiences with violence and how these may affect their treatment of patients. Anger toward a patient for a particular act may be justified, or it may be the result of a countertransference where the patient resembles a significant person from the staff member's past.

A number of defense mechanisms may interfere with the treatment of violent patients and may pose a danger to the therapist and others. Denial of a patient's dangerousness may occur because of the therapist's past experiences with violence or because the patient may be particularly attractive or interesting. On the other hand, a patient may be viewed as more dangerous than he or she actually is because of staff anxiety that is projected onto the patient. Displacement can occur from one patient who is dangerous to another who is not dangerous but who serves as an acceptable scapegoat for a staff member.

Negative reactions to patients on the basis of bias or prejudice are not acceptable. In addition, ward dynamics may result in the inappropriate treatment of violent patients. For example, the staff may feel abandoned by the administration, or the psychiatrist may inappropriately seclude or restrain a particular patient so as to activate procedures where the psychiatrist is required to be on the ward and examine the patient.

To address some of these concerns about the psychodynamics of the staff as well as the patients, it is important to discuss a violent episode once it has occurred. This should be done among the staff as well as with the patient who was violent and among other patients on the ward. This is contrary to what staff usually wish to do. Once the episode is finished, they want to forge about it or deny it. The violent episode should be discussed in terms of what happened, what could have prevented it, why seclusion or restraint was used (if it was), and how the patient or the staff felt in terms of the use of seclusion or restraint.

Most patients will have negative reactions to being secluded and restrained. Among other patients on the ward, it is important to talk about the violent episode and why seclusion or restraint was used for that particular patient, so as to allay other patients' fears that they could be secluded or restrained in the future for no apparent reason.

VII. CONCLUSION

The acute management of violent patients begins with the decision as to whether the patient will respond to verbal deescalation. Patients who are not psychotic and nonorganic may do so, but psychotic or organic patients will probably need medication and/or restraint. A prime consideration is the safety of staff and other patients. Medication can be very useful in the management of the acutely violent patient. High-potency antipsychotics such as haloperidol or fluphenazine can be used for psychotic patients, with lorazepam by mouth or intramuscularly for sedation. Lorazepam alone can be used for nonpsychotic patients. Restraint or seclusion with or without medication can be used to control violent behavior. There are rigorous standards for the use of restraint and seclusion. These address indications and contraindications for the use of restraint and seclusion, the role of the physician in rapidly assessing the patient, and the role of staff in monitoring and caring for patients in restraint and seclusion. Alternatives to restraint or seclusion—such as verbal intervention, medication, and constant observation—should have been used or considered. Putting a patient in restraints or seclusion should be a well-planned and smooth team effort by staff. Staff should be in touch with their feelings toward patients so as to prevent inappropriate restraint or seclusion. Discussion among themselves and discussion with the patient after the emergency has subsided can help in that endeavor.

REFERENCES

1. M.S. Humphreys, E.C. Johnstone, J.F. MacMillan, and P.J. Taylor, Dangerous behavior preceding first admission for schizophrenia, *Br. J. Psychiatry 161*:501 (1992).
2. K. Tardiff and A. Sweillam, Characteristics of assaultive patients in private hospitals, *Am. J. Psychiatry 141*:1232 (1984).
3. A.L. Calcedo-Barba and A. Calcedo-Ordonez, Violence and a paranoid schizophrenia, *Int. J. Law Psychiatry 17*:253 (1994).
4. M. Krakowski, J. Volavka, and D. Brizer, Psychopathology and violence: A review of the literature. *Comp. Psychiatry 27(2)*:131 (1986).
5. J. Junginger, Command hallucinations and the prediction of dangerousness, *Psychiatr. Serv. 46*:911 (1995).
6. M.P. Geller, Sociopathic adaptations in psychotic patients, *Hosp. Commun. Psychiatry 31*:108 (1980).
7. M. Krakowski, A. Convit, J. Jaeger, S. Lin, and J. Volavka, Neurological impairment in violent schizophrenic inpatients, *Am. J. Psychiatry 146*:849 (1989).
8. P. Lindqvist, and P. Allebeck, Schizophrenia and assaultive behaviour: The role of alcohol and drug abuse. *Acta Psychiatr. Scand. 82*:191 (1990).
9. M. Rosenbaum and B. Bennett, Homicide and depression, *Am. J. Psychiatry 143*:367 (1986).
10. R.L. Binder and D.E. McNiel, Effects of diagnosis and context on dangerousness, *Am. J. Psychiatry 145*:728 (1988).
11. W.A. Weiger and D.M. Bear, An approach to the neurology of aggression, *J. Psychiatr. Res. 22*:85 (1988).
12. R.D. Hare and L.M. McPherson, Violent and aggressive behavior by criminal psychopaths, *Int. J. Law Psychiatry 7*:35 (1984).
13. S. Snyder, W.M. Pitts, and A.D. Pokorny, Selected behavioral features of patients with borderline personality traits, *Suicide Life Threat. Behav. 16(1)*:28 (1986).
14. E.S. Barratt, Impulsiveness and aggression, *Violence and Mental Disorder: Development in Risk Assessment* (J. Monahan and H.J. Steadman, eds.), The University of Chicago Press, Chicago, 1994, pp. 61–79.
15. American Psychiatric Association, *Clinician Safety: The Task Force Report #33*, American Psychiatric Association, Washington, DC, 1992.
16. E.F. Coccaro, E. Kramer, Z. Zemishlany, A. Thorne, C.M. Rice, B. Giordani, K. Duvvi, B.M. Patel, J. Torres, R. Nora, R. Neufeld, R.C. Mohs, K.L. Davis, Pharmacologic treatment of noncognitive behavioral disturbances in elderly demented patients, *Am. J. Psychiatry 147*:1640 (1990).

17. P.H. Soloff, Emergency management of the violent patient, *The American Psychiatric Association Annual Review*, vol. 6 (R.E. Hales and A.J. Frances, eds.), American Psychiatric Press, Washington, DC, 1987.
18. T. Van Putten, S.R. Marder, and J. Mintz, A controlled dose comparison of haloperidol in newly admitted schizophrenic patients, *Arch. Gen. Psychiatry 47*:754 (1990).
19. D.F. Levinson, G.M. Simpson, H. Singh, K. Yadalam, A. Jain, M.J. Stephanos, and P. Silver, Fluphenazine dose, clinical response, and extrapyramidal symptoms during acute treatment, *Arch. Gen. Psychiatry 47*:761 (1990).
20. W.H. Wilson, Clinical review of clozapine treatment in a state hospital, *Hosp. Commun. Psychiatry 43*:700 (1992).
21. J. Volavka, J.M. Zito, J. Vitrai, and P. Czobor, Clozapine effects on hostility and aggression in schizophrenia, *J. Clin. Psychopharmacol. 13*:287 (1993).
22. C. Salzman, D. Solomon, E. Miyawaki, R. Glassman, L. Rood, E. Flowers, and S. Thayer, Parenteral lorazepam versus parenteral haloperidol for the control of psychotic disruptive behavior, *J. Clin. Psychiatry 52*:177 (1991).
23. E.S. Garza-Trevino, L.E. Hollister, J.E. Overall, and W.F. Alexander, Efficacy of combinations of intramuscular antipsychotics and sedative-hypnotics for control of psychotic agitation, *Am. J. Psychiatry 146*:1598 (1989).
24. J.D. Little and E.H. Taghavi, Disinhibition after lorazepam augmentation of antipsychotic medication, *Am. J. Psychiatry 148*:1099 (1991).
25. J.T. Dietch and R.K. Jennings, Aggressive dyscontrol in patients treated with benzodiazepines, *J. Clin. Psychiatry* 49:184 (1988).
26. D.L. Gardner and R.W. Crowdry, Alprazolam-induced dyscontrol in borderline personality disorder, *Am. J. Psychiatry 142*:98 (1985).
27. American Medical Association, *AMA Drug Evaluations*, American Medical Association, Chicago, 1986.
28. *Youngberg v Romeo*, 102 Supreme Ct 2452 (1982).
29. American Psychiatric Association, *Seclusion and Restraint: The Psychiatric Uses: Task Force Report No. 22*, American Psychiatric Association, Washington, DC, 1985.
30. K. Tardiff (ed.), *The Psychiatric Uses of Seclusion and Restraint*, American Psychiatric Press, Washington, DC, 1984.
31. K. Tardiff, The current state of psychiatry in the treatment of violent patients, *Arch. Gen. Psychiatry 49*:493 (1992).
32. J.R. Lion and S.A. Pasternak SA. Countertransference reactions to violent patients, *Am. J. Psychiatry 130*:207 (1973).

11
Long-Term Medication for Violent Patients

Burr S. Eichelman
University of Wisconsin–Madison, Madison, Wisconsin

Kenneth Tardiff
Cornell University Medical College, New York, New York

I. INTRODUCTION

The use of long-term psychopharmacological treatment for patients whose mental illness has a violent component has been an area of medical therapeutics that has advanced significantly over the past two decades. In treating violent patients, psychotropic medications can now be utilized in ways that go far beyond the benefit of sedation produced by treatments available in the 1960s with sodium amytal or sedating low-potency antipsychotic medications. Now, specific neurotransmitter systems, even specific receptor systems of those neurotransmitters, can be targeted and manipulated pharmacologically. For example, serotonergic enhancement can be induced by providing increased precursor (giving tryptophan), by blocking the reuptake of serotonin (5-HT) (with drugs like fluoxetine), by reducing catabolism (with monoamine oxidase inhibitors), or by directly stimulating or blocking 5-HT receptors (with drugs like buspirone or mirtazepine). The application of such agents appears to provide utility in reducing the frequency and intensity of destructive behavior in clinically aggressive patients, which, in turn, will allow for the opportunity of enhanced and safer socialization and behavioral interventions. These carry their own positive reinforcement to strengthen still further prosocial, nonviolent, and cooperative behaviors.

This chapter reviews the general strategies for the long-term use of medications in the repetitively violent patient. It does not review the acute "emergency" use of drugs for chemical restraint but rather examines the use of pharmacological agents in the long-term medication of the chronically violent patient. It also reviews, briefly, representative literature and methodology for specific agents currently in the pharmacopeia for violence management.

Medication should be seen as only one component of a treatment plan for violent patients. Other parts of the plan must address factors associated with violence and its prevention. These vary in each case. Strategies to prevent violence must involve work with families and other persons who are potential victims of violence by the patient or who play other important roles in the patient's life. Environmental factors associated with violence—for example, work situations—must be addressed. Psychotherapeutic techniques described in other chapters in this book should be considered.

II. GENERAL PRINCIPLES

For any pharmacological intervention, basic principles should be employed. This is particularly important for the use of medications, which treat symptoms rather than specific disorders, and for treatment, which is often less well researched by well controlled double- blind studies. Critical basic principles for such treatment include the following:

1. Treat the primary illness first.
2. Use objcctive criteria to measure intervention efficacy.
3. In empirically treating patients, have clear beginning and endpoints to assess treatment efficacy.
4. In establishing an empirical psychopharmacological strategy, begin with those drugs with the fewest and least severe side effects.

A. Treat the Illness First

This principle simply mandates the initial choice of pharmacological agent, which begins with agents known to effectively treat the particular disorder. Hence, violent patients who meet diagnostic criteria for schizophrenia should be treated initially with antipsychotic agents before embarking on trials of alternative agents such a beta blockers. Patients who are violent and depressed should be started on antidepressants. Mood stabilizers should be the preferred initial treatment of choice for violent manic patients.

B. Use Objective Criteria to Measure Intervention Efficacy

Violence is episodic and may occur frequently or infrequently. All too often a change in dose or even choice of medication may be implemented on the basis of a single event. If an inpatient assault occurs the evening before a treatment team meeting, there is a high probability that someone will ask the psychiatrist to alter the medication. "Reactive decisions" may not be correct. The episodic nature of aggressive behavior coupled with the delayed efficacy of the medications used requires a more protracted assessment of the patient's behavior. Perhaps the best-known assessment scale for inpatient violence is the Overt Aggression Scale (OAS) (1), which allows for a quantification of aggressive behavior in terms of frequency and intensity. Daily, weekly, or monthly aggression scores can be tracked for a patient, allowing for a better assessment of drug efficacy than can occur "by recollection" at a treatment team meeting. The OAS can be modified for residential or outpatient programs. Or, criteria can be tailor-made for a particular patient and that patient's characteristic violent behavior tracked over time.

C. Have Clear Beginning and Endpoints to Assess Treatment Efficacy

In order to follow this principle, it is necessary to introduce only one pharmacological agent at a time. When a new agent is going to be implemented and evaluated, its trial should have a discrete beginning, followed by dosage titration to therapeutic levels, coupled to an end of the trial and assessment of efficacy. Concretely, this means that the medication should be used at a therapeutic level. If lithium is tried with a blood level of 0.3 mEq/L or valproic acid is used with a blood level of 25 μg/dL, these therapeutic trials will be inadequate for these agents. Once a therapeutic dose is established, assessment should be long enough for a delayed response to be seen. With the exception of rapid responses that occur with benzodiazepines, most "antiaggressive" drug effects approximate more closely than seen with refractory schizophrenics or obsessive-compulsive patients, requiring a response assessment period of 1 to 2 months for a given medication. Determination of drug efficacy for selective serotonine reuptake inhibitors (SSRIs), beta blockers, and mood stabilizers requires this duration of assessment. Keeping patients within such treatment protocols can be challenging when one is faced with pressures for "quick fix" interventions. Finally, if after a period of treatment benefit were observed, that medication would be tapered and discontinued and a new trail of a new agent initiated. Many clinicians seem to build on their patient's treatment, trying an antipsychotic, adding lithium, adding an SSRI, and then adding an anticonvulsant. By the time this polypharmacy is implemented, the cumulative side-effect profile of these agents may have become a significant problem, even perhaps exacerbating the aggressive behavior. Also if, after the addition of the mood stabilizer, the patient improves, the clinician will usually feel that all the medications should be continued when, in fact, only the mood stabilizer is necessary.

Just as in treating depression with medications, clinicians should be aware of potential placebo effects. The hope of successful pharmacological treatment can often alter both staff and patient expectations. This can set into operation new behavioral contingencies which, in turn, can reduce aggressive behavior. In some placebo-controlled studies, placebo response rates have been as high as 60%, underscoring not only how important long-term quantitative assessment is but also how powerful behavioral interventions and social expectations can be in driving behavior.

D. In the Implementation of Innovative Treatment, Begin with the Safest Drugs

Since there are few data to guide clinicians in the initial choice of an antiaggressive medication beyond the caveat of treating the primary illness first, a good rule of thumb is to begin a treatment trial with the safest of agents that have been reported effective in treating aggressive behavior in the particular population to which the patient belongs. For example, for impulsively aggressive patients, one would probably begin with SSRIs before trying mood stabilizers, which, in turn, should be used before turning to antipsychotic drugs (because of the risk of tardive dyskinesia or neuroleptic malignant syndrome). Aggressive schizophrenics might be treated initially with traditional antipsychotic agents and, if unresponsive, with atypical antipsychotic drugs. However, before trying these patients on clozapine—assuming otherwise adequate control of their psychosis—one would insert trials with propranolol or a mood stabilizer. While clinicians might not universally agree, an ordering of agents might look like this:

Low Risk	Moderate Risk	High Risk
SSRIs	Lithium	Clozapine
Benzodiazepines	Beta blockers	
	Valproic acid	
	Antipsychotic agent	

Carbamazepine is a moderate-to high-risk agent, given its uncommon risk of bone marrow suppression.

III. PHARMACOLOGICAL AGENTS

A. Benzodiazepines

The use of benzodiazepines in chemical restraint and in the acute management of the aggressive patient is now part of general practice (2,3). However, these agents may also serve a role in the long-term management of certain patient populations. This may take the form of a direct pharmacological effect but also that of a coping strategy. Nonpsychotic patients who appear to have underlying anxiety disorders (4), or impulsive-aggressive disorders (5) may benefit from chronic benzodiazepine therapy. While not conclusively demonstrated, some benzodiazepines appear to be more effective—for example, oxazepam in preference to diazepam (6) or oxazepam in preference to chlordiazepoxide (7). Doses may be tried at anxiolytic levels and even higher (4) as long as intoxication and disinhibition do not occur. Recently, clinicians have been also trying clonazepam, but its utility thus far is less widely documented (8).

The early use of benzodiapeines was marked with a concern for disinhibition (9). However, if patients are carefully selected so as to exclude alcoholics or violent patients who disinhibit with alcohol, the likelihood of increased aggression on these agents is reduced. The clinical preference for oxazepam and its low level of paradoxical effects might be related to its rate of onset, in contrast to drugs like triazolam, which has a more rapid rate of onset but also a higher incidence of untoward reactions. A new drug, buspirone, has been shown to be effective in managing anxiety. It appears to lack the hypnotic, anticonvulsant, and abuse potential of other antianxiety agents. It does not appear to interact with other sedating drugs, including alcohol. Recommended doses range from 15 to 30 mg/day, beginning with a dose of 5 mg three times a day and increasing by 5 mg every 2 to 3 days. The maximum recommended dose is 60 mg/day.

In addition to "around the clock" treatment, a benzodiazepine can be used as a "coping strategy." Some patients are able to tell when they are about to "explode." Certainly, they can employ behavioral strategies such as walking away. Yet while they are learning other prosocial skills such as assertiveness training or negotiating, they may benefit from the use of short-acting benzodiazepine that functions as a biological coping strategy (i.e., "Go take a pill!"). The use of medication gives the patient an immediate behavioral response as an alternative to aggression. It often works.

Case example: Mr. A, a 57-year-old married businessman, sought help on an outpatient basis for his "temper." He related that on certain days he felt tight and anxious, with an anticipation that it was going to be "one of those days." On such a day he might lose his temper with his wife or secretary, throw objects in a rage, or sweep the top of his desk clean. He was afraid that his outbursts might lead to physical assaults. No organic etiology for these episodes was evident, and no major Axis I diagnosis such as depression, mania, or schizophrenia was noted. The violence was not associated with alcohol. Mr. A was encouraged to use oxazepam, 30 mg, up to four times a day on days when he felt tense and feared losing control. In addition, he was counseled on ways to reduce his work stresses and on techniques of verbal assertiveness. After this intervention, Mr. A reported that he no longer experienced the temper outbursts. However, while intermittent medication proved effective for Mr. A, some patients may need regular daily treatment with benzodiazepines (10).

The side effects of the antianxiety agents and sedatives other than buspirone include sedation, impairment of motor ability, dizziness, and ataxia. Some patients have complained of blurred vision, diplopia, hypotension, amnesia, slurred speech, tremor, urinary incontinence, and constipation. The use of benzodiazepines during the first trimester of pregnancy has been reported to produce developmental abnormalities, including cleft lip with or without cleft palate.

The main side effect associated with anxiolytic agents and sedatives, particularly in patients with a history of violence and personality disorders, is that of abuse and dependence. Physical dependence results in a withdrawal reaction if these medications are discontinued rapidly. This withdrawal reaction may involve aggression and violent behavior as well as other symptoms such as anxiety, irritability, insomnia, tremors, headache, dizziness, anorexia, nausea, vomiting, diarrhea, incoordination, seizures, and depression. The onset of the withdrawal reaction depends on the particular medication and may be anywhere from a day for a short-acting drug such as lorazepam up to a week following cessation of other longer-acting drugs. A gradual reduction of dosage is recommended, namely 5 to 10% a day for 10 to 14 days (11). A long-acting benzodiazepine may be substituted for shorter-acting benzodiazepines. Patients with a history of seizures, alcohol abuse, or abuse of other drugs should be hospitalized for detoxification.

B. Dopamine-Altering Agents

Dopamine antagonists—the traditional antipsychotic agents—have been a mainstay in the treatment of aggressive behavior for psychotic patients, the elderly, and character-disordered patients. While these agents were often effective because of the excessive dosing and sedative side effects, subsequent controlled studies confirm their efficacy in reducing aggressive behavior. In general, high-potency dopamine antagonists are now more commonly used. They have been shown to reduce aggressive behavior in schizophrenic, manic, and mentally retarded patients (12,13) and in conduct-disordered youth (14). Neuroleptic medication should not be used for violent mentally retarded patients unless psychotic symptomatology is part of the clinical picture. The use of long-term neuroleptics for these patients raises the risk of side effects (e.g., tardive dyskinesia) and the concern that learning may be impaired in this group of patients for whom learning is already a major problem.

Haloperidol or fluphenazine are popular because of they can be administered on inpatient units rapidly, in high doses, with minimal side effects, and with safety in terms of not decreasing the seizure threshold in epileptic patients. This is important in cases where subictal activity may coexist with schizophrenia. Of equal importance, to combat noncompliance with haloperidol decanoate and fluphenazine decanoate or enanthate, there is a smooth transition from its use in the emergency situation to oral maintenance levels to long-term depot use (15).

In nonemergency situations for psychotic adult patients, haloperidol should be given 0.5 to 2 mg by mouth for moderate symptoms and 3 to 5 mg by mouth for severe symptoms every 8 to 12 hours until psychotic symptoms are controlled. Doses above 15 mg/day are seldom required. When control has been achieved, the dose is lowered to a minimum effective dose, usually no more than 8 mg/day. Elderly or debilitated patients should be given 0.5 to 2 mg initially, with gradual increments of 0.5 mg. In chronic schizophrenics, higher doses are usually needed for active psychosis, starting with 6 to 15 mg/day in divided doses, with gradual increases until control is achieved. More than 100 mg/day is rarely needed; following control of psychotic symptoms, the dose should be decreased to maintenance levels, usually 15 to 20 mg/day.

Given the frequency of noncompliance and the dire consequences of this (i.e., renewed violent behavior by schizophrenics), serious thought should be given to the use of long-acting depot medication. The initial dose of haloperidol decanoate should be based on the patient's history, physical condition, and response to antipsychotic therapy. Small doses should be given initially and the amount increased as needed. The initial dose of haloperidol decanoate should be 10 to 15 times the previous daily dose in oral haloperidol equivalents, but no more than a maximum initial dose of 100 mg (2 mL) should be given. Usually haloperidol decanoate has been effective when administered at monthly intervals; however, a variation in patient response may cause the clinician to adjust the interval as well as the dose. Lower initial and more gradual adjustments are required for elderly or debilitated patients. Monthly doses greater than 300 mg (6 mL) are rarely if ever indicated.

Fluphenazine should be given to adult psychotic patients, initially 2.5 to 10 mg/day by mouth; when symptoms are controlled, the dose should be reduced to a maintenance level of 1 to 5 mg/day. Elderly or debilitated patients should be given 1 to 2.5 mg/day. The depot fluphenazine preparations should be given to adults initially at 12.5 mg to be followed by 25 mg every 2 to 3 weeks. The maintenance dose depends on the individual patient, but it should not exceed 100 mg every 2 to 3 weeks. Elderly or debilitated patients should be started at 2.5 mg followed by 2.5 to 5 mg every 2 weeks.

If the clinician wishes to choose a neuroleptic with more sedative side effects or if extrapyramidal side effects are problematic, chlorpromazine or other low-potency neuroleptics are recommended. We do not recommend thioridazine for violent psychotic patients because the clinician may want to use propranolol for these patients, and, as discussed below, propranolol increases blood levels of thioridazine and the risk of pigmentary retinopathy. For psychosis, chlorpromazine should be given to adults 25 to 100 mg by mouth every 1 to 4 hours until control of psychotic symptoms has been achieved. Patients with severe psychosis, especially chronic schizophrenia, may require higher initial doses, around 200 mg by mouth every 4 hours. Daily doses exceeding 1 g are rarely needed. Elderly or debilitated patients should be given chlorpromazine at the lower range. If a patient has been on the optimal dose for 2 weeks, the amount should be reduced gradually to a minimum effective dose for maintenance. The average dose for patients under the age of 40 years is 300 to 800 mg/day. Elderly or debilitated patients require one-third to one-half of the usual adult dose.

Aggressive psychotic patients and probably aggressive demented patients should have a trial of treatment with atypical antipsychotic drugs such as risperidone (16). It appears that 5-HT_2 receptor blockade may function like 5-HT_1 receptor stimulation to reduce aggressive behavior. Various reports describe successful treatment of aggressive behavior in schizophrenic patients, autistic patients, and demented patients with risperidone. While it is more problematic because of its risk of agranulocytosis, clozapine has also been shown to reduce aggressive behavior in psychotic patients (17–19). It also appears effective for developmentally disabled as well as brain-injured patients (20,21).

The antipsychotic medications can produce a wide range of adverse side effects, some of which are described briefly below. Extrapyramidal reactions are more common with the high-potency antipsychotic medications. Those that occur early during treatment, usually within weeks, are acute dystonia, akathisia, and parkinsonism. Tardive dyskinesia usually appears after months to years of treatment and occurs with both low- and high-potency neuroleptic medications. Dystonic reactions most frequently occur following parenteral administration of neuroleptics. Acute dystonia appears usually within a few days of treatment and is characterized by abnormal, sustained posturing movements of the neck, jaw, trunk, and eyes, with protrusion of the tongue, spasms of the jaw, and extreme lateral upward gaze of the eyes. It is treated effectively and rapidly by anticholinergic medication.

Akathisia is characterized by a feeling of restlessness, usually in the lower extremities, and an urge to pace up and down. It appears within weeks to a few months after the beginning of neuroleptic medication. The agitation may be interpreted as aggression and violence, thus resulting in increased administration of neuroleptics and a vicious cycle of further agitation (22). The clinician should consider reducing the dose if akathisia occurs or using benzodiazepines or propranolol (23,24). Propranolol 10 to 60 mg/day can also be used to treat the akathisia. Propranolol at these doses has little effect in terms of aggression per se. To treat aggression, it must be used at much higher doses.

Neuroleptic malignant syndrome is a rare reaction characterized by severe muscular hypertonicity and akinesia, dysarthria, and fluctuating levels of consciousness, which can also include stupor and mutism (25). There is a high fever and various autonomic disturbances of heart rate and blood pressure. Accompanying it may be physical exhaustion, dehydration, and pneumonia or pulmonary emboli. The neuroleptic medication should be discontinued immediately and supportive therapy such as control of fever and intravenous fluids should be given. There is some evidence that bromocriptine is effective in doses of 10 to 50 mg/day. Other drugs that have been used include amantadine and a combination of dantrolene and bromocriptine.

Often patients treated with excessive amounts of antipsychotic drug will actually increase the frequency and intensity of their aggressive behavior as they become increasingly organically impaired as a consequence of excessive dosing.

Case example: Ms. D, a 22-year-old woman, attacked her roommate in her college dormitory because she believed the roommate was putting poison into her supply of food in the refrigerator. She was admitted to a psychiatric hospital, where she was found to be delusional and having auditory hallucinations. She attacked staff and other patients whom she believed were poisoning her. The diagnosis was paranoid schizophrenia. Haloperidol 20 mg/day was given. In 2 weeks, she was no longer delusional and her auditory hallucinations ceased. Violence toward others stopped as her mental status improved. After discharge, she was followed by the student health service and began to attend classes. Several months after discharge, her new roommate complained to the dormitory staff that Ms. D was suspicious and complained that the roommate was tampering with her food. The dormitory staff spoke to Ms. D, who admitted to being in treatment. The staff contacted the therapist, who subsequently determined that Ms. D had not been taking her medication for several weeks. Ms. D consented to depot haloperidol and has since been attending classes without any incident for 1 year.

Case example: Mr. F, a 28-year-old man, had been hospitalized in a state hospital constantly for 5 years following a series of hospitalizations for schizophrenia. During hospitalization he was infrequently but extremely violent toward staff and other patients. For example, he broke a nurse's jaw with a direct punch to her face. These violent episodes occurred for no apparent reason. He remained psychotic in terms of vague delusions about God and the destination of the world. His speech and thoughts were disorganized and difficult to comprehend. He had been medicated with a variety of antipsychotic drugs in adequate doses with concurrent carbamazepine and later propranolol. He spent most of his time in four-point restraints. When not in four-point restraints, he was restrained in a chair in the day room. Soon after it was approved for use in the United States, he was given clozapine for several days at 12.5 mg daily, then increases were given at 25-mg increments in the morning and evening over a 25-day period until the daily dose reached 500 mg/day. He was maintained on that dose. In a month it was noted that he was more coherent. He was released from restraints gradually and put on one-to-one observation. He remained in his room except for visits to the recreation room for exercise There were no violent outbursts. After 2 months, he was coherent and not talking about God. He was released into the general ward population.

C. Psychostimulants

Paradoxically, dopamine-enhancing drugs such as methylphenidate may also reduce aggressive behavior. This effect may be indirect and a consequence of treating the underlying condition. Stimulant treatment of aggressive young patients with a diagnosis of attention deficit disorder has been effective in reducing the level of aggressive behavior in some of these individuals (26). As with the effect on attention, these stimulant agents are rapidly effective and individual clinical "trials" can be conducted rapidly—e.g., within 1 week. There have been some reports of the successful use of amphetamines to control aggression in adults with a history of this disorder as well. There were two studies reporting the successful use of amphetamines in delinquent youths: one to control aggression in a group of hospitalized black aggressive delinquents and the other to decrease violence in the classroom for a group of aggressive outpatient boys with antisocial behavior (27,28). Further studies are indicated, and the clinician should proceed with caution in prescribing amphetamines because there is great potential for addiction, abuse, and the production of violent behavior through hyperactivity, emotional lability, or delusional thinking as a result of abuse of psychostimulants.

D. Norepinephrine-Altering Agents

Clonidine, an alpha-adrenergic agonist, reduces the firing of the locus ceruleus neurons, and presumably postsynaptic nonadrenergic activity. It has been used along with stimulants in the treatment of attention deficit children, particularly those with hyperactivity as well as with children with conduct disorder. In both situations case studies have suggested that it concomitantly reduced aggressive behavior (29). Dosing is suggested at levels and rates of increase comparable to those used in treating hyperactive children.

E. Beta-Adrenergic Antagonists

The use of beta blockers in the treatment of aggressive behavior developed from the neurology literature in the mid-1970s. Elliott demonstrated in open with the publication of numerous case reports how substantial doses of propranolol reduced aggressive behavior in patients who had sustained a significant personality change following neurological insult (e.g., the rupture of an aneurysm) (30). These observations were extended to psychiatric patients with "organic syndromes" as well as schizophrenia (31–34). Silver and Yudofsky (35) reviewed a number of control studies, open trials, and case reports on the effectiveness of propranolol in the management of aggressive behavior. Most of the patients studied and responding to propranolol were those with organic brain disease, often with gross impairment secondary to trauma, tumor, alcoholism, encephalitis, Huntington's disease, dementia, Wilson's disease, Korsakoff's psychosis, and mental retardation. In addition, some patients with minimal brain dysfunction or attention deficit have also been reported to respond to propranolol. Nearly all the patients in these studies were refractory to other medications, including neuroleptics, anxiolytic agents, anticonvulsants, and lithium. In a number of cases, concurrent neuroleptic medication was used. Beta blockers are effective for violence associated with traumatic brain injury where psychosis is present, since a number of neurological side effects of antipsychotic drugs may thus be avoided. On the other hand, propranolol can be used in conjunction with antipsychotic drugs for the management of violence in other types of psychotic disorders.

Since these initial reports, nadolol has been shown to be effective in reducing aggressive behavior in schizophrenics and mentally retarded patients (36,37). Metoprolol has been show helpful in treating patients with an intermittent explosive disorder and in cases of aggression associated with mental retardation (38,39). Pindolol, too, has been reported to have similar effects (40). In many cases, the dose of the beta blocker is very high. This suggests that the effect is of a "pharmacological" nature and may include more than the blockade of beta-adrenergic receptors. For example, pindolol has significant serotonergic agonist actions.

Dosing of these drugs requires a gradual increase in daily medication. Dosing of propranolol, for example, generally involves increasing the dose in 20-mg increments daily (in a twice-a-day regimen) and holding the dose at a plateau (e.g., of 240 mg /day) for a period of evaluation. If no response is noted, the dosing is again increased to a higher plateau level (e.g., 480 mg/day). Care must be taken to monitor sympathetic function and hypotension; severe bradycardia requires cessation of treatment. However, most cardiac effects are evident by 300 mg/day. Higher doses rarely seem to effect further changes in cardiac status. Before using propranolol, there should be a thorough medical evaluation of the patient. Patients with the following diseases should be excluded from treatment with propranolol: bronchial asthma, chronic obstructive pulmonary disease, insulin-dependent diabetes, cardiac diseases including angina or congestive heart failure, diabetes mellitus, significant peripheral vascular disease, severe renal disease, and hyperthyroidism.

To withdraw the patient from propranolol, it should be decreased gradually by 60 mg/day until the patient is on a daily dose of 60 mg/day. Then the medication should be decreased at the rate of 20 mg every other day. Propranolol should be decreased even more gradually in patients with hypertension to prevent rebound hypertension. Side effects found with propranolol include hypotension and bradycardia, although these may be managed by decreasing the dose of the drug. Above 300 mg/day there is usually no worsening of bradycardia or hypotension. Depression has been reported rarely by patients receiving propranolol; sedation is sometimes reported as a side effect.

Hypertensive patients should be given propranolol with caution because sudden discontinuation of propranol of may result in rebound hypertension. Propranolol raises the level of phenothiazines. Thus, care must be taken when treating patients concomitantly with thioridazine, since propranolol may raise blood levels of thioridazine threefold. "Safe" doses in terms of risk for retinal injury are not longer valid with concomitant propranolol treatment.

Case example: Mr. P, a 31-year-old married man, had undergone surgery for an aneurysm in the frontal lobe of the brain. Since the surgery, he had suffered from episodic bouts of rage directed at his wife and their property, after which he was remorseful. Those around him described him as a "changed person" during these "attacks." No evidence of ictal activity was found. Mr. P was placed on 240 mg of propranolol daily, given in a divided dose. This regimen markedly attenuated the frequency of his attacks.

Case example: Mr. S, a 23-year-old single man, had been hospitalized for several years on a maximum-security forensic unit for repeated assaultive behavior. He met diagnostic criteria for schizophrenia and had been treated with varying doses of antipsychotic medication. Propranolol was added to his treatment regiment while he was receiving maintenance antipsychotic medication given as fluphenazine decanoate. The dosage of propranolol was increased by 20 mg/day. At a daily dose of 400 mg, Mr S ceased his assaultive behavior. The dosage was gradually increased to 600 mg/day. After several months of aggression-free behavior, Mr S's dosage of propranolol was decreased. At doses below 400 mg/day, he became more agitated and irritable though not assaultive. The dosage was raised again, to above 400 mg/day. Afterward, Mr. S remained essentially free of assaultive behavior and was transferred to a medium-security unit.

F. Serotonin Enhancing Agents

1. Selective Serotonin Reuptake Inhibitors

Research has pointed to an association of low levels of serotonin and 5-hydroxyindoleacetic acid (5-HIAA) and aggressive, impulsive behavior in both externally directed violence and suicide. Both fluoxetine and sertraline have been reported to reduce aggressive behavior in impulsive, personality-disordered individuals (41). Doses are comparable to those utilized in treating depression. Fluoxetine has also been reported effective in the treatment of aggressive behavior, characterized as "anger attacks" in patients with unipolar depression (42). This effect has also been noted in developmentally disabled patients (43). Care must be taken in the initiation of dosing to watch for adverse side effects. Particularly with developmentally disabled patients who may not be verbal, higher doses of SSRIs may produce physical side effects of headache, nausea, or gastrointestinal distress, which may actually lead to an increase in aggressive behavior. Thus, for some patients, 20 mg of fluoxetine may be far more effective than 40 mg.

Some researchers have attempted to increase serotonin levels through the administration of the precursors of serotonin, such as the amino acid tryptophan. Brizer (44) reviewed the literature, including the successful use of tryptophan in a demented 82-year-old woman with agitation and self-destructive behavior. Two additional research studies have pointed to the successful use of tryptophan. One studied 12 aggressive schizophrenic offenders where tryptophan (4 to 8 g/day for 4 weeks) resulted in a decrease of assaultive incidents. The other study found that 4 of 6 patients (5 of whom had neuroleptic-refractory aggression) showed moderate significant improvements in violent behavior while receiving trazodone (50 mg twice a day) plus tryptophan (500 mg twice a day). Tryptophan is a relatively safe medication; its major side effects include nausea and sedation.

2. Mixed Agonists-Antagonists

Trazodone has been reported in open studies to reduce aggressive behavior in demented elderly as well as mentally retarded individuals with Cornelia de Lange syndrome and Down's syndrome with concomitant dementia (45–48). In treating males, attention should be given to the possibility of the development of priapism with trazodone. This side effect has not been reported with the related antidepressant nefazodone. Whether this agent has the same or better efficacy in relation to the attenuation of aggressive behavior remains to be determined.

3. Serotonin Agonists

Buspirone is a 5-HT_{1A} receptor agonist. It has been reported effective in a subpopulation of mentally retarded patients (49). It has also been reported effective in a single, open case report of aggression in association with head injury (50). The same caveat applies for buspirone as for fluoxetine in treating developmentally disabled individuals: namely, to allow adequate evaluation at several dose levels, since higher doses may actually dissipate therapeutic effects observed for some patients at lower doses.

There was considerable optimism over the development of a class of 5-HT_1 agonists labeled "serenics" that demonstrated substantial aggression-inhibiting effects in animal studies. Eltoprazine, one of these agents, was taken into clinical trials. Preliminary results suggested some positive response in schizophrenic patients but a less robust response in developmentally disabled patients (51). However, development of this agent appears to have been halted.

Case example: Mr. JW, a 52-year-old landscaper, described himself as a hot-temperered Irishman. In his second marriage, he became irate and slapped his wife. She charged him with domestic violence and began divorce proceedings. JW was forced to examine his temper and requested medical and psychological help. In addition to joining a group for perpetrators of domestic violence, he began individual therapy to seek tools for managing his anger. He also began taking 50 mg of sertraline daily and reported, after 2 weeks, that he believed this medication "gave him a longer fuse" so that he could implement some of the psychological skills he was beginning to learn in his group and in individual therapy. He eventually sought reconciliation with his wife and entered couples' therapy with her. After approximately 9 months on this medication, he discontinued it because of sexual side effects that could not be fully remedied with intermittent use and concomitant medications. During the period of use, he refrained from assault and "out of control" arguments.

G. Lithium

Long-term use of lithium helps to prevent manic episodes and associated hyperactive aggressive behavior. The use of lithium to manage aggression associated with disorders other than bipolar disorders has been much more controversial. In a double-blind trial testing the effectiveness of lithium in the treatment of aggression in adult mentally retarded patients, Craft et al. found that 73% of patients showed a reduction in aggression during treatment (52). A serum lithium concentration of 0.7 to 1.0 mmol/L was necessary for a clinical effect. The use of lithium was the same as that for the management of bipolar patients. Although there have been other reports of the use of lithium in patients with other disorders, there is a sparsity of double-blind controlled studies (53–57). These patients include those with organic brain syndrome or head injury; aggressive schizophrenics; nonpsychotic, aggressive prisoners; and delinquents and children with conduct or attention-deficit hyperactivity disorders. Some contend that lithium can increase interictal aggression in patients with temporal lobe epilepsy and cause other adverse effects in patients with other seizure disorders and other abnormal electroencephalographic (EEG) changes.

The therapeutic plasma levels for patients on lithium to control aggression range from 0.7 to 1.0 mEq/L. Most patients can be started on 300 mg of lithium carbonate twice a day; this dose can be increased by 300 mg every 3 to 4 days. Plasma levels should be obtained 12 hours after the last lithium dose. Once the therapeutic lithium level has been stabilized, levels should be monitored every month for the first 6 months and every 2 to 3 months afterward. Because congenital abnormalities, particularly heart defects, have been reported, lithium should not be used during pregnancy. It should be used with caution in women of childbearing age. Lithium should not be used in conjunction with iodine or medicines containing iodides (e.g., cough medicines, multivitamin preparations). Indomethacin and phenylbutazone have been shown to elevate serum lithium concentrations.

With serum lithium below toxic levels (which are 1.5 to 2.0 mEq/L), transient mild to moderate side effects may occur. The most common reactions include nausea, diarrhea, malaise, and fine hand tremors. Other common effects reported are thirst, polyuria, polydipsia, and fatigue. Hand tremors may respond to low doses of propranolol.

As one approaches the toxic range of serum lithium levels, drowsiness, vomiting, muscle weakness, ataxia, dryness of mouth, abdominal pain, lethargy, dizziness, slurred speech, and nystagmus are early signs of intoxication. At levels above 2 mEq/L, symptoms include anorexia, severe nausea and vomiting, blurred vision, fasciculations, clonic movements of the whole body and limbs, hyperactive tendon reflexes, choreoathetoid movements, toxic psychosis, syncope, EEG changes, acute circulatory failure, stupor, and coma. The last stages of lithium toxicity are manifest by generalized convulsions, oliguria, and death.

Long-term administration of lithium has resulted in impaired renal function and, rarely, persistent neurological deficits. Thus long-term lithium treatment for violence should be embarked on after serious consideration. Since lithium is excreted by the kidneys, it should be used cautiously in patients receiving diuretics or those on low-salt diets. Precautions should be taken when lithium is used in the elderly because renal function usually declines with age. Leukocytosis has been reported, it is usually not serious and can be reversed with discontinuation of lithium treatment. If lithium is used concurrently with neuroleptic medications, blood levels of the neuroleptic medication should be monitored.

H. Carbamazepine and Other Anticonvulsants

Carbamazepine is approved as an anticonvulsant medication for complex partial seizures as well as generalized clonic-tonic seizures and other types of partial seizures. Although it is not recommended as the anticonvulsant of first choice, it is very popular because of its to fewer side effects, such as sedation, as compared with phenytoin and barbiturates (58).

A number of case studies and open drug trials have indicated that carbamazepine is probably effective for the management of aggression in several different types of psychiatric patients. In a double-blind crossover study of 13 chronic psychiatric patients, 10 of whom were schizophrenic, Neppe reported beneficial effects in terms of decreasing aggressive episodes (59). Although the patients were not epileptic, they did have temporal lobe EEG abnormalities. The patients were treated with neuroleptics, anticholinergics, antidepressants, and benzodiazepines. The dose of carbamazepine was 200 mg three times a day. Luchins reported on an open carbamazepine trial in seven chronic psychiatric inpatients, six of whom were schizophrenics (60). None of the patients had EEG abnormalities. He reported that six of the seven patients had fewer aggressive episodes on carbamazepine than either before or after the drug. All the patients were concurrently treated with neuroleptic drugs. Mattes et al. found that carbamazepine is very effective in decreasing aggression in patients with psychiatric diagnoses other than schizophrenia. These include personality disorders, conduct disorders, and some organic disorders. Later noncontrolled studies have confirmed that carbamazepine is effective in treating violent patients without epilepsy (61–64). Caution should be given to the use of carbamazepine in patients with gross brain damage or mental retardation because there have been reports of paradoxical worsening of aggression in this group.

In conclusion, there is some evidence that carbamazepine may be effective in terms of managing aggression and irritability in patients with overt seizures, both complex partial seizures and generalized seizures; in schizophrenic patients with and without EEG abnormalities; and in other types of patients with episodic violence without gross brain damage or mental retardation.

Early reports about carbamazepine causing thrombocytopenia, agranulocytosis, and aplastic anemia have not been supported, and these side effects appear to be rare. Nevertheless, monitoring of hematological parameters and liver function is essential in addition to a complete medical evaluation. Complete blood cell and platelet counts are recommended before treatment and every 2 weeks for the first 2 months of treatment and every 3 months thereafter. Liver function tests should include serum glutamic-oxaloacetic transaminase (SGOT), serum glutamic-pyruvic transaminase (SGPT), lactate dehydrogenase (LDH), and alkaline phosphatase. These tests should be repeated every month early in treatment and every 3 months thereafter. Patients with leukopenia, thrombocytopenia, or liver disease should not be treated with carbamazepine (65).

Some patients treated with carbamazepine report side effects such as nausea, drowsiness, vertigo, ataxia, blurred vision, and diplopia, which are usually mild and decrease when the dosages decrease. There are other less frequent toxic consequences of treatment, such as jaundice, renal effects, nystagmus, skin reactions, thyroid effects, and memory impairment (66). In approximately 5% of patients, carbamazepine is discontinued due to toxic reactions. Dyskinetic movements such as dystonia, dyskinesias, and other extrapyramidal reactions are rare and self-limited if the medication is withdrawn or the dosage decreased.

For an anticonvulsant response with carbamazepine, the therapeutic serum levels must be from 8 to 12 ng/mL. The usual method for treatment of seizures is to prescribe 100 to 200 mg twice a day for 1 week and then to increase the dose by 100- to 200-mg increments and measure serum levels when daily doses of 400 to 600 mg are achieved. It is not uncommon for patients with seizure disorders to take up to 1200 mg/day. The onset of therapeutic effects is within the first days or weeks after treatment is initiated.

Patients without seizure disorders have benefited from carbamazepine at doses of approximately 600 mg/day. Once the therapeutic level is reached and a response is obtained, blood levels of carbamazepine should be monitored every month for the first 3 months and then every 3 months thereafter. Other anticonvulsants have been tried in the control of aggression with inconsistent results. Positive findings have included the use of diphenylhydantoin in the treatment of aggressive mentally retarded children, violent nonepileptic male adults (half of whom had EEG abnormalities), and adults with episodic dyscontrol syndrome (67,68).

Valproate has been found to be effective for a violent patient who could not be treated with carbamazepine (69).

IV. CONCLUSION

A number of medications can be used in the long-term treatment of violent patients. These drugs are used in conjunction with other forms of treatment, such as psychotherapy and education. Antipsychotic drugs are used to treat psychosis associated with violence. Other drugs—such as lithium, propranolol, carbamazepine, and serotonin reuptake inhibitors—can be used for episodic violence due to a number of disorders. A baseline of violence and evaluation of the effect of medication is necessary. Dosages should be adequate and the course of treatment should be of sufficient duration before a trial of medication is said to be ineffective. No doubt, new antipsychotic drugs and other drugs for violence will be developed in the future.

REFERENCES

1. S.C. Yudofsky, J.M. Silver, W. Jackson, et al., The Overt Aggression Scale for the objective rating of verbal and physical aggression, *Am. J. Psychiatry 143*:35 (1986).

2. P.A. Bick and A.I. Hannah, Intramuscular lorazepam to restrain violent patients, *Lancet 1*:206 (1986).
3. C. Salzman, A.I. Green, F. Rodriguez-Villa, et al., Benzodiazepines combined with neuroleptics for management of severe disruptive behavior. *Psychosomatics 27(suppl)*:17 (1986).
4. J. Lion, Benzodiazepines in the treatment of aggressive patients. *J. Clin. Psychiatry 40*:70 (1979).
5. R. Monroe, *Episodic Behavioral Disorders*. Harvard University Press, Cambridge, MA, 1970.
6. C.R. Brown, The use and misuse of anxiolytics in the violent, aggressive individual, *New Frontiers in Psychotropic Drug Research* (S. Fielding and R.C. Effland, eds.), New York, Futura, 1979, pp. 241–258.
7. G. Gardos et al., Differential actions of chlordiazepoxide and oxazepam on hostility, *Arch. Gen. Psychiatry 18*:757 (1968).
8. K. Tardiff, *Assessment and Management of Violent Patients*, 2d ed., American Psychiatric Press, Washington, DC, 1996.
9. J.M. Tobin, I.F. Bird, and D.F. Boyle, Preliminary evaluation of Librium in the treatment of anxiety reactions, *Dis. Nerv. Syst. 21(Mar suppl)*:11 (1960).
10. B. Eichelman, Toward a rational pharmacotherapy for aggressive and violent behavior. *Hosp. Commun. Psychiatry 39*:31 (1988).
11. R.I. Shader and D.J. Greenblatt, Drug therapy: use of benzodiazepines in anxiety disorders. *N. Engl. J. Med. 328*:1398 (1993).
12. B.L. Leventhal and H.K.H. Brodie, The pharmacology of violence, *Biobehavioral Aspects of Aggression* (D.A. Hamburg and MB Trudeau, eds.), Alan R. Liss, New York, 1981, pp. 85–106.
13. T.M. Itil and A. Wadud, Treatment of human aggression with major tranquilizers, antidepressants, and newer psychotropic drugs, *J. Nerv. Ment. Dis. 160*:83 (1975).
14. T.M. Itil and A. Wadud, Treatment of human aggression with major tranquilizers, antidepressants, and newer psychotropic drugs, *J. Nerv. Ment. Dis. 160*:83 (1975).
15. J.M. Kane, Compliance issues in outpatient treatment. *J. Clin. Psychopharmacol. 5 (suppl)*:22S (1985).
16. S. R. Marder and R.C. Meibach, Risperidone in the treatment of schizophrenia, *Am. J. Psychiatry, 151*:825 (1994).
17. W.H. Wilson and A.M. Claussen, 18-month outcome of clozapine treatment for 100 patients in a state psychiatric hospital, *Psychiatr. Serv. 46*:386 (1995).
18. J. Volavka, J.M. Zito, J. Vitrai, and P. Czobor, Clozapine effects on hostility and aggression in schizophrenia, *J. Clin. Psychopharmacol. 13*:287 (1993).
19. J.A. Chiles, P. Davidson, and D. McBride, Effects of clozapine on use of seclusion and restraint at a state hospital, *Hosp. Commun. Psychiatry 45*:269 (1994).
20. J.J. Ratey, C. Leveroni, D. Kilmer, C. Gutheil and B. Swartz, The effects of clozapine on severely aggressive psychiatric inpatients in a state hospital, *J. Clin. Psychiatry 54*:219 (1993).
21. M.L. Michals, M.L. Crismon, S. Roberts, et al., Clozapine response and adverse effects in nine brain-injured patients, *J. Clin. Psychopharmacol. 13*:198 (1993).
22. M.L. Crowner, R. Douyon, A. Convit, P. Gaztanaga, J. Volavka, and R. Bakall, Akathisia and violence, *Psychopharmacol. Bull. 26*:115 (1990).

23. W.W. Fleischhacker, S.D. Roth, and J.M. Kane, The pharmacologic treatment of neuroleptic-induced akathisia, *J. Clin. Psychopharmacol. 10*:12 (1990).
24. J.F. Lipinski, G.S. Zubenko, B.M. Cohen, and B.J. Barreira, Propanolol in the treatment of neuroleptic-induced akathisia, *Am. J. Psychiatry 141*:412 (1984).
25. S.N. Caroff, S.C. Mann, A. Lazarus, K. Sullivan, and W. MacFadden, Neuroleptic malignant syndrome: Diagnostic issues, *Psychiatr. Ann. 21*:130 (1991).
26. R.P. Allen, D. Safer, and Covil, Effects of psychostimulants on aggression, *J. Nerv. Ment. Dis. 160*:138 (1975).
27. L. Eisenberg, R. Lachman, P.A. Walling, et al., A psychopharmacologic experiment in a training school for delinquent boys, *Am. J. Orthopsychiatry 33*:431 (1963).
28. B.M. Maletzsky, The episodic dyscontrol syndrome, *Dis. Nerv. Syst. 35*:543 (1974).
29. J.M. Zavodnick, Combined drug therapy debate, *J. Am. Acad. Child Adolesc. Psychiatry 36*:1 (1997).
30. F.A. Elliott, Propranolol for the control of belligerent behavior following acute brain damage. *Ann. Neurol. 1*:489 (1977).
31. R.M. Greendyke, D.B. Schuster, and J.A. Wooton Propanolol in the treatment of assaultive patients with organic brain disease. *J. Clin. Psychopharmacol.* 4:282 (1984).
32. S. Yudofsky, D. Williams, and J. Gorman, Propranolol in the treatment of rage and violent behavior in patients with chronic brain syndromes, *Am. J. Psychiatry 138*:218 (1981).
33. D.T. Williams, R. Mehl, S. Yodofsky, et al., The effect of propanolol on uncontrolled rage outbursts in children and adolescents with organic brain dysfunction. *J. Am. Acad. Child Psychiatry 21*:129 (1982).
34. P.J. Sorgi, J.J. Ratey, and S. Polakoff, Beta-adrenergic blockers for the control of aggressive behaviors in patients with chronic schzophrenia, *Am. J. Psychiatry 143*:775 (1986).
35. J.M. Silver and S. Yudofsky, Propanolol for aggression: Literature review and clinical guidelines. *Int. Drug Newsl. 20*:9 (1985).
36. M. Alpert, E.R. Allan, L. Citrome, G. Laury, C. Sison, and A. Sudilovsky, A double-blind, placebo-controlled study of adjunctive nadolol in the management of violent psychiatric patients, *Psychopharmacol. Bull. 26*:367 (1990).
37. S.A. Polakoff, P.J. Sorgi, and J.J. Ratey, The treatment of impulsive and aggressive behavior with nadolol, *J. Clin. Psychopharmacol. 6*:125 (1986).
38. J.A. Mattes, Metoprolol for intermittent explosive disorder. *Am. J. Psychiatry 142*:1108 (1985).
39. T. Kastner, K. Burlingham, and D.L. Friedman, Metoprolol for aggressive behavior in persons with mental retardation, *Am. Fam. Physician 42*:1585 (1990).
40. R.M. Greendyke and D.R. Kanter, Therapeutic effects of pindolol on behavioral disturbances associated with organic brain disease: a double-blind study, *J. Clin. Psychiatry 47*:423 (1986).
41. E.F. Coccaro, J.L. Astill, J.I. Herbert, et al., Fluoxetine treatment of impulsive aggression in DSM-III-R personality disordered patients, *J. Clin. Psychopharmacol. 10*:373 (1990).
42. M. Fava, J.F. Rosenbaum, J.A. Pava, et al., Anger attacks in unipolar depression:

Part 1. Clinical correlates and response to fluoxetine treatment. *Am. J. Psychiatry 150*:1158 (1993).
43. P.I. Markowitz, Effect of fluoxetine on self-injurious behavior in the developmentally disabled: A preliminary study, *J. Clin. Psychopharmacol. 12*:27 (1992).
44. D.A. Brizer, Psychopharmacology and the management of violent patients, *Psychiatr. Clin. North Am. 11*:551 (1988).
45. D.M. Simpson and D. Foster, Improvement in organically disturbed behavior with trazodone treatment. *J. Clin. Psychiatry 47*:191 (1986).
46. E. Pinner and C.L. Rich, Effects of trazodone on aggressive behavior in seven patients with organic mental disorders, *Am. J. Psychiatry 145*:1295 (1988).
47. M. O'Neil, N. Page, W.N. Adkins, et al., Tryptophan-trazodone treatment of aggressive behavior, *Lancet 2*:859 (1986).
48. A. Gedye, Serotonergic treatment for aggression in a Down's syndrome adult showing signs of Alzheimer's disease. *J. Ment. Defic. Res. 35*:247 (1991).
49. J. Ratey, R. Sovner, A. Parks, et al., Buspirone treatment of aggression and anxiety in mentally retarded patients: A multiple-baseline, placebo lead-in study. *J. Clin. Psychiatry 52*:159 (1991).
50. A.M. Levine, buspirone and agitation in head injury, *Brain Inj. 2*:165 (1988).
51. J. Tiihonen, P. Hakola, J. Paanila, and M. Turtiainen, Eltoprazine for aggression in schizophrenia and mental retardation, *Lancet 341*:307 (1993).
52. M. Craft, I.A. Ismail, D. Krishnamurti, et al., Lithium in the treatment of aggression in mentally handicapped patients, *Br. J. Psychiatry 150*:685 (1987).
53. J.P. Tupin, D.B. Smith, T.L. Clanon, L.I. Kim, A. Nugent, and A. Groupe, The long-term use of lithium in aggressive prisoners, *Comp. Psychiatry 14*:311 (1973).
54. M.H. Sheard, Lithium in the treatment of aggression, *J. Nerv. Ment. Dis. 160*:108 (1975).
55. M.H. Sheard, J.L. Marini, C.I. Bridges, and E. Wagner, The effect of lithium in impulsive aggressive behavior in man, *Am. J. Psychiatry 133*:1409 (1976).
56. Luchins DJ, Dojka D. Lithium and propanolol in aggression and self-injurious behavior in the mentally retarded, Psychopharmacology Bulletin 1989, 25:372–375.
57. M.B. Glenn, B. Wroblewski, J. Parziale, L. Levine, J. Whyte, and M. Rosenthal, Lithium carbonate for aggressive behavior or affective instability in ten brain-injured patients, *Am. J. Phys. Med. Rehabil.* 221 (1989).
58. R.W. Evans and C.T. Gualtieri, Carbamazepine: a neuropsychological and psychatric profile, *Clin. Neuropharmacol. 8*:221 (1985).
59. V.M. Neppe, Cabamazepine as adjunctive treatment in nonepileptic chronic inpatients with EEG temporal lobe abnormalities, *J. Clin. Psychiatry 44*:326 (1983).
60. D.J. Luchins, Carbamazepine for the violent psychiatric patient, *Lancet 1*:766 (1983).
61. J.A. Mattes, Carbamazepine for uncontrolled rage outbursts, *Lancet 2*:1164 (1984).
62. J.A. Mattes, Comparative effectiveness of carbamazepine and propranolol for rage outbursts, *J. Neuropsychiatry Clin. Neurosci. 2*:159 (1990).
63. J.A. Mattes, J. Rosenberg, and D. Mays, Carbamazepine versus propanolol in patients with uncontrolled rage outbursts: A random assignment study, *Psychopharmacol. Bull. 20*:98 (1984).

64. V.M. Neppe, B.R. Bowman, and K.S. Sawchuk, Carbamazepine for atypical psychosis with episodic hostility, *J. Nerv. Ment. Dis. 179*:439 (1991).
65. J.M. Silver and S.C. Yudofsky, Psychopharmacology and electroconvulsive therapy, *The American Psychiatric Press Textbook of Psychiatry* (J.A. Talbott, R.E. Hales, and S.C. Yodofsky, eds.), American Psychiatric Press, Washington, DC, 1988.
66. K.J. Meador, D.W. Loring, O.L. Abney, M.E. Allen, G.E. Moore, E.Y. Zamrini, and D.W. King, Effects of carbamazepine and phenytoin on EEG and memory in health adults, *Epilepsia 34*:153 (1993).
67. Barratt ES. The use of anticonvulsants in aggression and violence, *Psychopharmacol. Bull. 29*:75 (1993).
68. E.S. Barratt, T.A. Kent, S.G. Bryant, and A.R. Felthous, A controlled trial of phenytoin in impulsive aggression (letter), *J. Clin. Psychopharmacol. 11*:388 (1991).
69. L.P. Kasper, J.P. Seibyl, and J.H. Krystal, Valproate management of psychosis in a patient with carbamazepine-induced hyponatremia, *J. Clin. Psychopharmacol. 12*:137 (1992).

12
Psychological Issues in Treatment: Transference and Countertransference

Gary J. Maier
Mendota Mental Health Institute, Madison, Wisconsin

I. INTRODUCTION

We live in an aggressive era. Aggressive behavior of outpatients shows alarming increases. In nearly all states, the standards that govern civil commitment have been narrowed to mental illness and dangerousness. As a result, psychiatric hospitals now house a subset of patients: those that are irritable, angry, and aggressive (1,2). Managing aggressive behavior, however, is still in the "shadow" of psychiatry for a number of reasons, including underdeveloped clinical theory, uncoordinated training, and poor management of staff countertransference reactions (3). Because aggressive events are threatening and cause injury, the normal reactions of fear and anger have also hindered rational progress in making the work environment safe. The very techniques required to manage aggression—seclusion, physical restraint, ambulatory restraint, and chemical restraint—activate unpleasant feelings because they strike at our basic values of freedom and dignity. When seclusion becomes the principal way to manage the acutely aggressive patient, it is easy to conclude that out of sight (seclusion) is out of mind (denial). Denying that a significant number of our patients are aggressive is a critical factor that impedes progress in the management and treatment of these patients (4).

But society as a whole does not deny that battered citizens have a right to justice; the criminal justice model provides penalties for criminal behavior and more and more tries to compensate victims for losses (see Fig. 1). The extreme case of criminal behavior illustrates that society recognizes that disputes arouse feeling and that anger can lead to aggressive behavior. Society has, therefore,

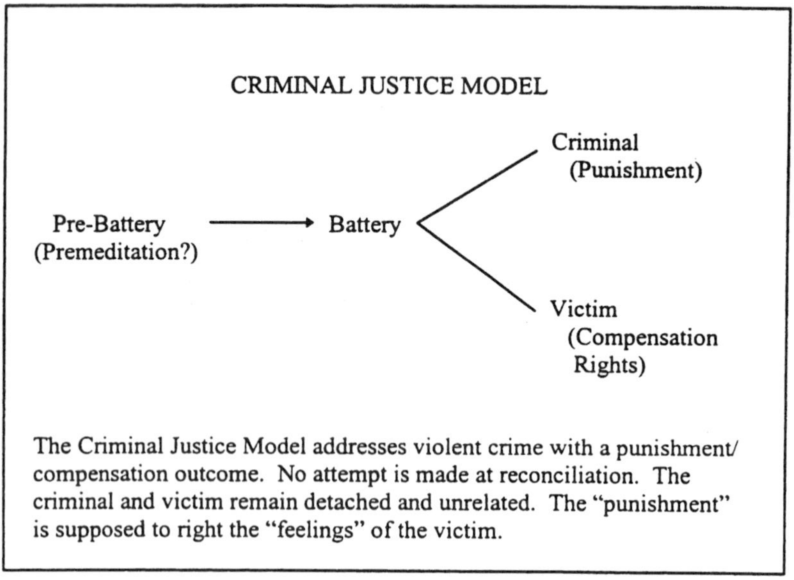

Fig. 1 Criminal justice model.

implemented the rules of debate so that disputes can be resolved in an orderly way. Robert's Rules of Order have been adopted by most democracies to allow opposing opinions to clash without disorder. The issue of interpersonal argument leading to aggression is just now becoming a major focus of study. What happens in a fight and the dynamics of abusive relationships are slowly becoming more understandable.

While many continue to deny the impact of aggressive behavior on victims, including ourselves, that denial is eroding for others. Surveys like that by E. Poster and J. Ryan have demonstrated that there is a nationwide concern among nursing staff about safety (5). The American Psychiatric Association (APA) published the report of their task force on clinician safety in 1993 and concluded that while we know little about patient aggression, we do know that hospitals and clinics can be unsafe areas in which to work (6). Programs like the Assaulted Staff Action Program (ASAP) in Massachusetts are growing (7). Further scientific studies now support the commonsense observation that "postdisaster debriefing" interventions decrease the psychological distress that can follow a disaster, including a physical assault (8). Training staff to work in a potentially unsafe work environment and caring for staff immediately after a traumatic event will be shown to be the best way to prevent long-term reactions.

This chapter describes the origins of the development of transference and countertransference feelings and then describes approaches to managing countertransference, including the use of immediate debriefing and group process meetings, here called Me-Time. Formal programs exist that address these issues are briefly described.

II. UNDERSTANDING THE ORIGIN OF THE PSYCHOLOGICAL ISSUES RAISED BY AGGRESSION

Clinical observation of patient-patient aggression has led to the realization that the elements of each aggressive event follow a similar course. Further observation has led to the conclusion that while the course of single aggressive events is similar, the course of events that occur when there are repeated episodes of aggression have similar but unique phases. From these observations a comprehensive clinical model for understanding and managing aggression was developed (9–11). It consists of two dynamic processes: the process that occurs during a single aggressive event, called *the linear aggression sequence*, and the more complex process that results when aggression becomes repetitive, called *the aggression cycle*.

A. Aggression Sequence of a "Fair Fight"

When a patient attacks, the assault is obviously "unfair." That is, the aggressor takes advantage of the potential victim and, if no other factors are involved, such an unfair attack will create a victim and thus negate the hope of a mutually acceptable resolution to what turn out to be the disputed issues. The criminal justice model then becomes the arena for dispute resolution. A fair fight, by contrast, is a process of dispute resolution that maintains mutual self-esteem while offering the parties the hope of a mutually acceptable outcome. While a fair fight may include threats and abusive statements aside from obvious physical aggression, the phases of the aggression process can be the same as those that occur in an outright battery. These processes are identified to separate them from a special type of aggressive relationship called an "abusive relationship." The dynamics of an abusive fight are discussed below to bring more clarity to their boundaries, to alert the clinician to the needs of both abusers and the abused, and to underpin the fact that some staff abuse patients and that some patient aggression is a response to staff abuse (12).

Aggression occurring in a medical setting can be regarded as a linear process that may be broken into six phases: preaggression, aggression, control, diagnosis and assessment, treatment and management, and the postaggression phase called the aggression postmortem (see Fig. 2). Because the first three phases of the aggression sequence can flow into each other in a rapid fashion and can cause physiological arousal in the staff, they have been difficult to separate. Further,

THE LINEAR AGGRESSION SEQUENCE

("FAIR-FIGHT")

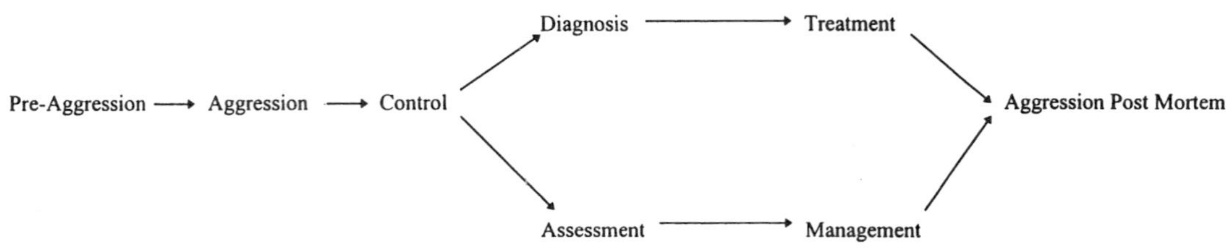

The Linear Aggression Sequence consists of the six phases above. The difference between the two tracts of the latter phases is often a source of confusion. In prisons and on the street, Security Guards, Prison Guards, Police, SWAT members, and Military teams are charged with the responsibility of controlling and managing aggressive persons. In medical settings, staff share this responsibility. They use similar interventions. They are also able to diagnose and treat these patients, and to the degree that aggressive behavior is part of the illness, treatment reduces aggression. The aggression post-mortem phase recognizes the need to document each aggressive event, unfettered by incipient countertransference feelings which often contaminate fact finding that can lead to better management and treatment techniques.

Fig. 2 The linear aggression sequence.

these phases are at times not clearly differentiated, so staff reactions to them can also become confused and interventions can become misplaced. Phases four and five are bimodal. Two separate but related functions occur during each phase. Finally, the aggression postmortem phase recognizes the need to document and review each aggressive event in order to develop better management and treatment techniques. The following description of the characteristics and boundaries of each phase will outline the general structure of these processes. Because the processes can be complex, this outline can only present an approximation of the phases themselves.

1. Preaggression Phase

The origins of this phase can vary with one's theoretical orientation (13). According to analytic theory, the expression of infantile aggression awaits the first tooth (14). A behaviorist may limit the origins of the phase to the various contingencies in operation moments before the aggression erupted. Harris and Varney (16) have reported that patient-patient aggression is usually the product of direct interaction between patients, whether real or perceived. Patients report a number of reasons they aggress against each other. These range from a simple "payback" for a previous transgression to the acting out of a command hallucination. Tanke et al.(15) have demonstrated that the Brief Psychiatric Rating Scale (BPRS) can be used to identify patients who will aggress but who do not give verbal cues prior to their aggression; research of this type has not yet resulted in the development of reliable etiological typologies. Whatever the origins, the preaggression phase typically ends with either a verbal (gestural) threat or a physically aggressive act.

2. Aggression Phase

The aggression phase begins with a verbal threat or an act of physical aggression (17). While neither medical nor psychiatric dictionaries define the word *fight*, common sense tells us that this phase involves punches, kicks, bites, and scratches. Often one patient is the manifest aggressor and another patient (or staff) is the manifest victim. The phase continues until the aggressor regains self-control or the staff intervene and subdue him or her. When staff members witness the onset of this phase, they must intervene, either by talking down or taking down the aggressor patient. This phase involves engaging the patient until the staff have established control. This phase can be as short as the time it takes a patient to make a verbal threat or as long as it takes a SWAT team to gain control over an aggressive patient who has taken a hostage (18).

3. Control Phase

During the control phase, the aggressive behavior is stopped, either because the patient develops self-control or because of the intervention of the staff. In situations where staff arrive after the patient has stopped his or her aggressive act, the control phase is synonymous with the development of self-control by the patient, and the resulting ability to act responsibly. In other situations, staff must actively intervene to stop the aggression, which often means they must physically control the patient (19). In these situations, control is initiated and maintained through physical and/or chemical restraint and, as appropriate, seclusion. When the patient has finally regained self-control, the staff may impose a probationary period during which the patient must demonstrate that he or she can and will accept staff directions. This period often occurs while the patient is secluded. The control phase ends when the staff give the patient the responsibility for self-control in the open milieu.

Aggression constitutes a psychiatric emergency (20). The act of aggression breaks the trust that is the bond of the therapeutic alliance. One cannot provide therapy to a person who is trying to kill him or her (21,22). Consequently staff become empowered to utilize police powers during the control phase. At the same time, the patient loses certain rights. It is for this obvious reason that it is important to distinguish between the concepts of control and management, which *are not* based on trust, and treatment or therapy, which *are* based on trust. This fundamental, basic difference is not sufficiently understood by administrators, training directors, or patient advocates.

4. Diagnosis and Assessment

There is a difference between diagnosis and assessment. Using the medical model, diagnosis is reserved for the process of determining the presence of medical or psychiatric illness. Unfortunately medical and psychiatric diagnosis is usually of little value in determining the probability of future aggression because aggressive behavior is not pathognomonic of any specific disorder, and, worse, aggression can be associated with any medical or psychiatric disorder. Diagnosis follows the traditional medical and psychiatric process and is based on history, physical examination, laboratory tests, the patient's mental status, neurological examination, psychological tests, and other special medical procedures, such as computed tomography (CT), roentgenography, electroencephalography (EEG), and so on. The process can take from a few days to several weeks and may include clinical trials on medication. Diagnoses are stated in the DSM-IV format (23).

The term *assessment* is reserved for the process of determining the probability that a patient will become aggressive in the immediate future (hours, days, or weeks). Assessment for aggression potential is done by a review of the patient's history of aggressive behavior at home, at school, and at work; in hospitals, correctional facilities, or the armed services. The relationship between the aggressive behavior and environmental and situational factors is important. The description of aggressive behaviors outlined in the Overt Aggression Scale by Yudofsky et al. (24)—aggression against others, aggression against property, threats towards others, and aggression against self—are useful in establishing meaningful clinical categories. These categories can be utilized to look for clusters or patterns that then help to determine the long-term management plan. While past behavior is still the most reliable predictor of future behavior, patients who manifest behavior from more than one category are often more dangerous than those who have only one pattern of aggression (25).

5. Treatment and Management Phase

The term *treatment* is used in the classic medical sense. It refers to all the traditional approaches used to help the mentally ill and includes psychotherapy, psychopharmacology, and some behavioral approaches based on learning theory. When aggressive behaviors are closely associated with the psychiatric illness (e.g., paranoid schizophrenia), treating the illness will often significantly reduce the aggression. In this paradigm the aggressive behavior is considered to be a sign of illness, because the treatment does, or appears to, correct the primary pathology. Frequently, however, the aggressive behavior is characterological, learned, or only coincidentally associated with the psychiatric condition. In these cases the terms *manage* and *management* are used to refer to the interventions. These terms refer to approaches used to exert external control over aggressive behavior. Talk-down and take-down procedures, seclusion, and ambulatory restraints are good examples. Clinicians may need to continue specific treatment and/or management techniques to help a patient maintain behavioral control for short periods of time or for the indefinite future.

6. Aggression Postmortems

Following each aggression of any significance, an independent fact finder should review all aspects of the aggressive event and then meet with the principals involved in order to fully understand from their perspectives what happened, what might have prevented it, and—once started—what would have brought it under control more quickly and with less trauma. Following this procedure will allow each aggressive event to become a learning event, not just a traumatic event. A report should result that will describe the incident and its the outcomes and make recommendations to senior clinicians and administrators about issues that can range from staffing patterns to the need for audio or video surveillance in a particular area or the need for referral to an employee victim program (26,27). Careful review of these data over time, can not only suggest new ways to intervene but also identify patterns of aggression unique to the specific unit or facility that will suggest alternate ways of responding. Following up with staff who have been injured as they return to duty is another function of these postmortems (28).

III. AGGRESSION SEQUENCE OF AN ABUSIVE FIGHT

A. Irritability

The description of a fair fight in Section II.A above is necessary in order to understand how a fair fight can devolve into an abusive fight (see Fig. 3). The dynamics of a fair fight change to abuse when the "irritable" aggressor uses the issues to beat up the self-esteem of the abused. The disputed issues are no longer the focus. The self-esteem of the abused becomes the focus, as in the following: "You are on Prolixin, not Haldol." "You don't know what you're talking about. You're stupid!" The example shows how the aggression stage transforms into the power and control stages ("You're stupid; I can say anything I want to you") so the abuser can then exercise control over the abused. The dynamics of power and control supplant the dynamics of respectful dispute. Remember, a fair fight is a process that maintains mutual self-esteem and offers the hope of resolution with an outcome acceptable to both parties. It is about the issues and not about self-esteem. An abusive fight ends with a staff "winner" and a patient "loser." This subtle shift in the focus of an argument makes it difficult to point out exactly how some staff members abuse patients, setting up retaliatory aggression by the patient.

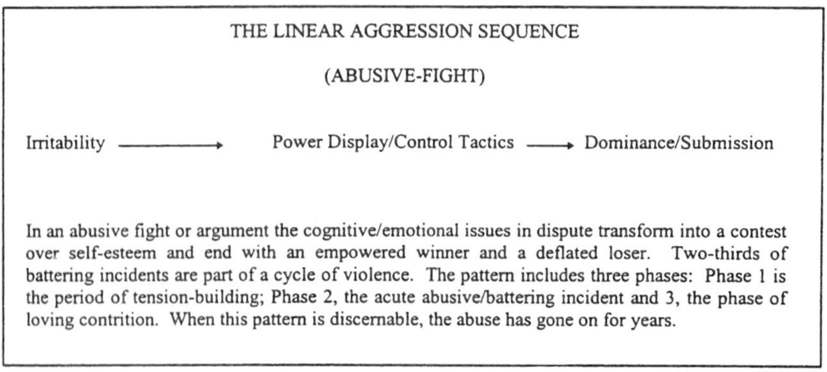

Fig. 3 The linear aggression sequence.

B. Power Display Control Tactics

Table 1 lists common control tactics used by abusers and the psychological impact of the tactics on the abused. (These are best illustrated in abusive marriages.*) These include, in order of increasing intensity, private criticism and withholding of praise, leading to doubt and hurt; public criticism, leading to shame or humiliation; withholding accountability, leading to loss of trust; verbal threats, which can begin a process of fear, verbal and physical tirades, or tantrums (i.e., power displays), leaving the abused feeling helpless; and finally physical aggression, which can lead to fears of death. In the process of a relationship where a staff member uses these "tactics" on a patient (man or a woman?), any or all can be used in any order at any time. The staff will establish dominance and the patient will become timid and submissive. Over time, the patient will adopt the victim role and, when the staff is around, will feel that he or she is "walking on eggshells." The process will continue as long as the staff denies the abuse or the impact of these tactics on the patient and the patient also denies being victimized (29). Since patients have less real power than therapists, it can take a significant effort to bring the abuse to the attention of a supervisor.

To confuse the picture, the abuser often keeps up a good appearance on the ward. The abuser may appear respectful. If a male, he may have a stable work record and be a good provider. He may be a family man and quite social. Unfortunately the abuser is not only limited in his approaches to managing patients but his work pattern may mirrors the pattern he exhibits at home.

C. Dominance/Submission

Without effective interventions, each abusive event ends with the abuser in a dominant position and the abused left submissive. Efforts at "processing" or clarifying the issues are usually unproductive because the staff denies the abuse and the patient is not powerful enough to press the case. The abused may try to rectify the process by suggesting a talk with a third party. This, too, is usually met with effective resistance. Thus an abusing staff member may go on abusing pa-

---

*In fact, in an abusive relationship, when the woman can no longer deny the physical abuse, she will cling to the positive aspects of the relationship—i.e., "He says he loves me. He's sorry. He doesn't want to break up. He'll change." But with greater examination, even these are seen as hollow. This can result in a crisis of "trust," so that she will have trouble trusting any relationship. When she complains of abuse but stays in the relationship, friends and family say "Then you deserve what you get." They blame the victim, which further isolates her from her natural support group. If she decides to leave, he says "Look at all I have done for you!" "How can you do this to me?" and "Explain that to the kids!" these lines create more guilt feelings and make it more difficult to persevere in leaving (30).

Table 1 Power, Control, and Abuse: Tactics and Results

Abuser: Control Tactics		Abused: Emotional Impact	
1.	Private criticism	1.	Doubt, uncertainty
2.	Withholding praise	2.	Doubt, uncertainty
3.	Public criticism	3.	Shame, humiliation
4.	Withholding accountability	4.	Loss of trust
5.	Verbal abuse	5.	Insult, fear, humiliation
6.	Verbal threats	6.	Insult, fear, humiliation
7.	Tantrums/tirades	7.	Fear, helplessness
8.	Physical assault	8.	Fear, hopelessness, injury, death

tients for years before he or she is caught. Therefore administrators and senior clinicians must look for the softer signs of abuse. These may take the form of frequent patient complaints or grievances, indicating that there is fire in all the smoke. As noted above, sometimes apparently unprovoked aggression by a patient is a sign that the patient is being abused, just as an adolescent suicide attempt can signal abuse. Whereas a cycle of violence with three discernible phases can be identified in abusive marital relationships (i.e., phase 1, tension building; phase 2, the acute abusive/battering incident; and phase 3, the phase of loving contrition), phase 3 cannot be overtly shared in a controlled environment like a hospital because of the possibility of being fired. When a cycle of abuse occurs in an inpatient setting, the regular reappearance of complaints, disruptive behavior, and unexplained changes in the mental status of a patient may be the only clues.

IV. AGGRESSION CYCLES

The second part of the model consists of identifying the processes that occur when aggression becomes repetitive (see Fig. 4). While several authors (31–33) have described cyclic patterns of aggression, these patterns have not been incorporated into a general model, nor have the authors focused on the critical role that staff countertransference plays in maintaining the cyclic process. The following describes these processes from the perspective of the staff, with specific reference to the need to identify and resolve staff feelings. The description of the physical aggression cycle from the patients' perspective is described in this comprehensive model (11,34,35).

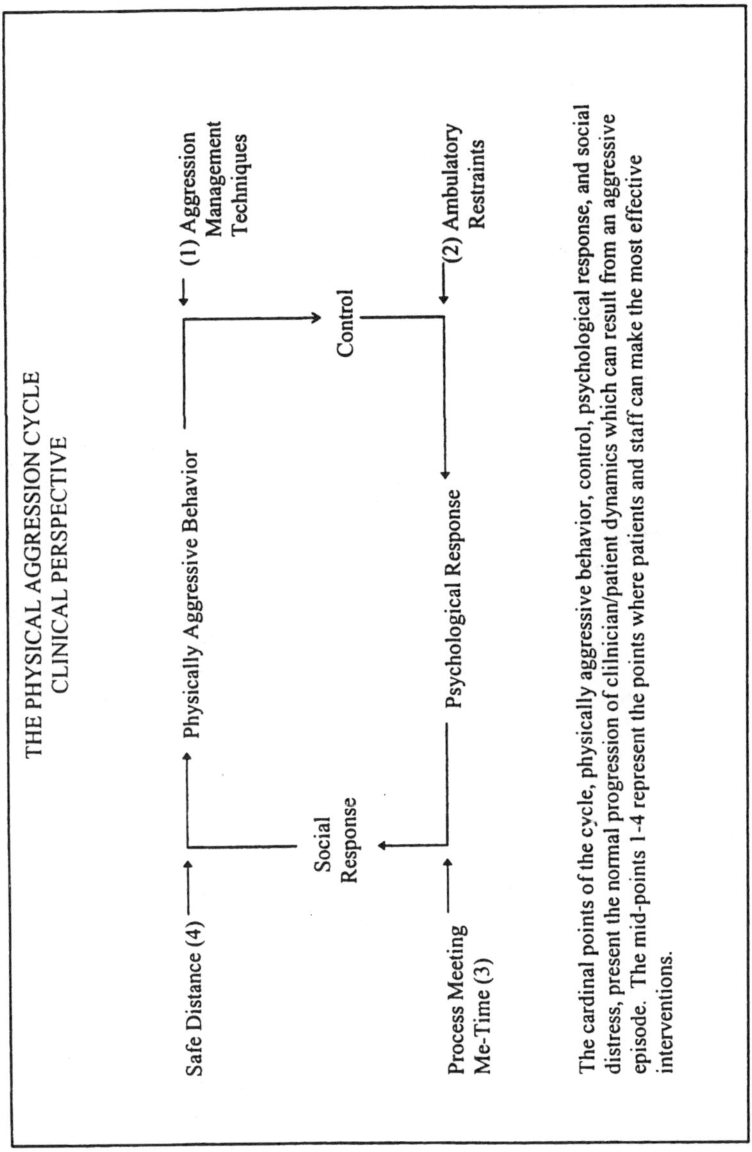

Fig. 4 The physical aggression cycle clinical perspective.

A. Description of the Cycle

Physical aggression often results in the chain of events illustrated in Fig 4). The first three phases of the process are the same as in the linear process. Staff respond rapidly to the patient-aggressor. They secure him by talk down or take down and, if necessary, control him by placing him in seclusion.

After the aggression is controlled, staff will spontaneously inquire about possible physical injuries. They will not ask whether coworkers were frightened by the aggression or were angry that the patient put them in such jeopardy. If they recognize that they have these feelings themselves, they wait until after work to share them. Because the usual process of dealing with aggression in the work setting does not include discussion about staff feelings of fear, anger, rage, or a sense of helplessness, these feelings may go undetected and unresolved, but they do not go away (36,37).

The secluded patient is usually released from seclusion before the staff have time to process what conscious feelings they can identify. Staff and other patients will prepare for the secluded patient's return with unresolved feelings. It is the accumulation of denied feeling that contributes to the creation of a cyclic process. These unresolved staff countertransference feelings* take over the process. As a result, when the patient is released from seclusion, some staff (and some patients) will remain physically and emotionally distant, thereby minimizing therapeutic contact. The distrust and anger the staff and other patients feel may be evident to the patient and cause him to feel alienated. Given this response, it is likely that a small incident will evoke another act of aggression and begin the cycle again (38).

B. Interventions

As the description of the cycle suggests, all the interventions exercised in controlling and managing a single aggressive episode are also appropriate in managing the early phases of cyclic aggression. The key difference is the role that countertransference feelings play (8,9,39,40). They become the limiting factor in the ability of the staff to continue to provide humane care. Consequently, it is the responsibility of the administrator of the facility and of the individual staff to recognize the presence of these feelings and to provide a mechanism whereby they can be resolved (41,42). So while the staff must be well trained in aggression management skills, have well-designed seclusion rooms available, have chemical restraint available, and, as appropriate, be prepared to use physical re-

---

*The term *countertransference reaction* in this paper refers to any staff feelings, conscious or unconscious, derived from the patient/staff relationship. The paper deals only with the fear, anger, hate, and rage spectrum of feelings because they are specifically aroused by aggression.

straint, they also need to know that the administration and their immediate supervisors understand their feelings and are willing to give them the opportunity to express and resolve them. The process of resolving countertransference feelings is described below.

When staff are able to process their feelings as they develop instead of remaining fearful or angry at the patients and therefore distancing themselves from them, they develop the healthy martial arts concept of "safe distance" (43). This means that they have given themselves the right to work safely with the patients. Consciousness has been raised. When this occurs, the staff and patient can develop trust because the staff no longer deny that at times they experience powerful negative feelings; therefore these feelings no longer unconsciously govern the relationship. Trust becomes possible, and then other forms of treatment can develop (44,45).

C. Case Example and Discussion

A recently admitted female patient with a suspected diagnosis of schizophrenia began pacing up and down the corridor of a locked civil unit. By the time the staff noticed this behavior and decided to assess the patient, she had begun yelling at patients in an indiscriminate manner and, at the same time, appeared to be talking to persons unknown. One of the female staff walked out to contact the patient. As she walked up to the patient, the patient suddenly stepped toward her and yelled "Get away from me, you slut!" Surprised, the staff member stepped back as the patient brushed by her. She followed the patient down the hall and at the same time motioned to the staff in the nursing station to come out to assist. The patient, who sensed she was being followed, turned around and yelled again. The staff member stopped, but this was not enough. The patient began yelling obscenities and began walking toward the staff member, who looked to see if help was coming from the nursing station. She could not see anyone on their way, but then wanted to pay attention to the patient who continued to advance toward her. She quickly made a decision to see if the patient would respond to her voice. She did not know the patient's first name so she said, in a voice loud enough to catch the patient's attention but not so loud that it would frighten her, "Stop yelling. I'm not going to harm you. Stop." This seemed to catch the patient's attention and at the same time seemed to alert the other staff because one of them appeared in the corridor. They made eye contact, which said, "Get help."

Meanwhile the patient continued to escalate. She kept up her verbal attack on the female staff member and increased the intensity of her threats. The staff member tried again to talk to her. "I hear you. I am not going to harm you." She could see three of her teammates moving slowly down the corridor toward them. The patient sensed their movement and turned sideways so she could see everyone. Another patient tried to enter the corridor from her bedroom but was quietly told to return to her room.

It appeared as though the patient were calming down, but out of the blue she yelled and lunged at the female staff member before her. The staff member stepped back and cushioned the force of the attack with her leg, but both women fell to the floor. The other staff members joined them in seconds and after about a minute of scuffling, the patient was bound.

Now in control, the staff gently told the patient, who was still yelling obscenities, to calm down. When it was clear that she would not, they called for help, bound her in leather restraints, and carried her to the seclusion room. The psychiatrist arrived just as the staff were going to leave the seclusion room. He did a quick assessment, agreed with the need for seclusion, and went to the nursing station to write the order. The staff then evacuated the seclusion room. The female staff member who was attacked discovered that she had a sore elbow and a small cut on her face. The nursing supervisor agreed to send her to the medical clinic, where her injuries were assessed and treated. She returned to work the next day.

The following day the psychiatrist, nurse, and safety officer who made up the Aggression Postmortem Committee, reviewed the incident and made the following report:

> *Description of the Incident*: The talk-down and seclusion of a female patient on the admission unit on Jan. 7, 1996, was managed in a humane, ethical manner. The staff saw the preaggressive behavior (pacing, yelling) as potentially threatening. They sent one of the staff to assess the patient, who suddenly escalated from verbal abuse and threats to a physical assault. While the staff tried to talk the patient down, the patient appeared to be attending to internal stimuli and did not respond. Before the staff could assemble to manage the patient in a more controlled manner, she attacked. The staff were forced to take the patient to the floor. One staff member was injured, sent to the clinic, and returned to work the next day. The patient was not injured. The incident was uneventful after the patient was placed in seclusion. Recommendations: (a) The patient had a history of sudden attack, especially on females. The history should have been available to the staff. (b) Because there did not appear to be any immediate risk to staff or other patients, the staff could have planned their intervention more carefully. The need for more help could have been considered sooner. (c) The staff could have sent two members to assess the patient, since there were three staff people available at the time. (d) The injury was caused by the hard floor. The floors on the patient units in the admission building should be carpeted. (e) One staff member should be assigned to monitor all patient behavior in the day room and in the principal corridor. (f) Video surveillance might be a more cost-effective way to achieve the same goal. (g) Staff would benefit from a refresher course on talking down escalating patients.

The example and postmortem report are typical of countless aggressive incidents. While the example cannot be comprehensive, we think these comments are relevant. The example illustrates the usual sequence of events. The staff member did try to talk to the patient. She also tried to alert the other staff, who seemed to have forgotten about her mission. There were three staff people present; this is one more than the staffing pattern at many facilities. There was a "plan." That is, the staff noticed the aberrant behavior and planned to assess it. The sudden attack is also typical. It is nearly impossible to tell when an agitated patient is going to attack. The best guide to prevention is to recognize that verbal abuse and verbal threats are clear signs that the process may escalate if not managed very carefully. This is not to fault the staff, since these incidents can change from controlled to out of control in a matter of seconds. The "take-down" was in reality a "pile-on." These are never pretty interventions. Staff members know this and do not expect that they will be second-guessed about their performance after the event. Finally, reports like this one make administrators happy, but they can fail the staff. It may be the impersonal nature of such reports that has given them a bad name with line staff. Nevertheless, there is useful information in such reviews.

V. TRANSFERENCE AND COUNTERTRANSFERENCE

The psychiatric literature clearly demonstrates that fear and anger are the most common countertransference reactions aroused in staff who work with aggressive patients (46,47). In fact, for staff who work with repetitively aggressive patients in closed systems such as inpatient units, fear and anger are the principal long-term occupational hazards of their work (48). It is not surprising that staff feel frightened and angry at patients who threaten (49,50), injure (51), and try to kill (52,53) them. What is surprising is how frequently these feelings are left unchecked or unattended by the staff, so that they become the driving force behind nearly every decision made regarding the patients. Perhaps it is because staff have significant difficulty tolerating strong feelings of fear, anger, helplessness, and frustration that their most common response is to deny them (54). Because unresolved countertransference reactions significantly affect individual patient care, they are, in our opinion, the primary reason that the management of aggressive patients remains part of the "dark side of psychiatry." Before we can properly understand how staff react to aggressive patients, it is necessary to understand the stages involved in the escalating behavior of an agitated patient. The process of escalation described below is a more detailed description of the preaggression, aggression, and control phases of the linear aggression sequence. This description focuses specifically on the patient's behavioral changes and associated feelings and the staff's feeling response. It is intended to clarify how patients escalating to aggression transfer their feelings onto the targets of their aggression.

A. The Process of Transference

Table 2 describes a five-stage process that an aggressive patient may go through when escalating toward physical aggression. The left-hand column demonstrates five behavioral stages, which, consecutively, include minor motor changes, verbal abuse/threats, major motor changes, physical aggression, and relaxation. These five behavioral stages are commonly associated with a range of patient feelings. These stage-specific feelings are anxiety/frustration, hostility, anger, rage, and, finally, exhaustion. Not every patient experiences these feelings and the feelings do not proceed in this order for every case. Nonetheless, the process of the behavioral stages and their associated feelings, as presented in Table 2, is common enough to be identified as the typical order of escalation that can result in physical aggression and control.

Physical aggression causes significant physiological arousal in patients or staff who may be the target of attack. The analytic concept *transference* (55) has traditionally referred to unconscious feelings originating from relationships that were significant in the patient's earlier life and then are transferred onto the therapist. This concept can be applied to the aggressive patient as well (56). Patients who are aggressive transfer their feelings (usually anger or rage) in a physical manner onto their victims. The escalating process of psychological arousal results in the physical projection, or transference, of the feelings onto the actual body of the victim.

With the above as a foundation, consider the typical reaction of staff to the five stages of escalation experienced by the patient. When the staff observe minor motor changes that may indicate feelings of anxiety and frustration, they approach the patient in an empathic manner. When the patient surprises staff by responding with verbal abuse or threats of physical harm, they respond by becoming anxious and concerned. Next, as the patient escalates to major motor

Table 2 Stages of Escalation

Behavioral States	Associated Feelings	Clinician Responses
Minor Motor	Anxiety	Empathy
Verbal Abuse Verbal Threats	Hostility	Anxiety
Major Motor	Anger	Fear/Anger
Aggression	Rage	Counter/Aggression
Exhaustion	Relaxation	Frustration

behavior, the staff most typically feel fearful and, in retrospect identify this stage as the one at which they began to feel anger. The very fact that the patient at this stage is pacing rapidly, invading other people's space, and making verbally abusive and threatening comments is alarming and frightening. If the patient escalates to actual physical aggression, the staff is empowered to contact that patient and subdue him or her if necessary. Feelings of self-preservation can be typical during this stage.

The counteraggression required to subdue a patient in the process of injuring or attempting to injure can jolt the staff member into the shocking awareness that he or she could become a killer in self-defense. The average clinician finds it very difficult to maintain this awareness. Nevertheless, aggression, if severe enough, can arouse murderous impulses in staff. The extreme discomfort accompanying the realization that one could be transformed into a killer—given the right circumstances—may account for the fact that staff often build up such strong denial around the whole issue of managing patient aggression.

Once the aggressor is sufficiently controlled, exhausted, and perhaps beginning to relax, the staff are also able to physically relax. However, following aggression, they will not be able to release the intense feelings aroused in them as a result of the physical experience. Typically they feel frustrated. The staff, therefore, go through a series of feeling changes as the stages of escalation progress, except that end where the patient began, in frustration.

A review of the third column in Table 2 shows that staff go through the feeling processes of empathy and then move to anxiety, fear, anger, counteraggression, and finally frustration. In a real sense the staff reactions in their sequence trail behind the patients' feelings, making it plausible to postulate that the patients' feelings are transferred to staff when the staff become the target of their aggression. Staff who experience this feeling chain repeatedly, without a means of support, will, in turn, develop chronic countertransference reactions. All too often the psychological reactions of staff to each single aggression are minimized. By minimizing the impact of aggression on staff, a subtle denial takes place, which ultimately will handicap staff in their development of effective approaches to the prevention, management, and treatment of aggressive behavior. If staff are consumed by unresolved feelings of fear and anger toward patients, they will not be able to see clearly how to develop more humane and effective interventions (57).

B. A Countertransference Policy and Procedure

In order to identify and work through countertransference feelings resulting from aggression, it is incumbent on psychiatric facilities to have a policy governing the process for all levels of staff. This policy should derive from a study of incidents of aggression events (58–61) and result in a description of the characteristics of repetitive aggressors (62). Emphasis should be given to the current intervention strategies that favor the least restrictive alternative but are, at bottom, safe (63,64). The facility should state its intent to protect staff and patients by stubbornly developing a humane environment (65) that minimizes risk (66). Finally, the policy must be supported by the top administrative staff because they realize the significant impact that aggression can have on the ability of staff to provide humane care (67). The policy should be explained to all new employees and should include the following basic information:

1. Working with aggressive patients will, at time, arouse intense personal feelings of fear and anger, among other feelings (39,68–70).
2. Staff are *expected* to identify and share these feelings with their peers and supervisor (71–74).
3. The clinical administration will provide four forums where these feelings can be discussed. They are (a) during the development of patient treatment plans, (b) at team meetings, (c) during "Me Time," and (d) during individual supervision.
4. Should these feelings cause a change in the ability to provide humane treatment to a patient, staff will be expected to address the issues that prevent them from delivering humane care. The personnel process may be utilized to facilitate required change, including referral to the Employee Assistance Program.
5. If, over time, a staff person is unable to manage feelings such as fear and anger and this is noticeable in work performance, he or she may be expected change work areas.

Having identified four forums where these feelings can be processed, staff are encouraged and trained to develop greater facility in dealing with their feelings. Further, in the structure called Me Time, discussed below, they are given permission to describe how they feel about the patients in any manner they find satisfying for their emotional needs.

C. Stages of the Countertransference Process

The stages of escalation describe the feeling process of an individual aggression episode. When individual aggression multiplies to repeated aggressions, a different intrapsychic countertransference process evolves. Table 3 illustrates a six-stage sequence in the evolution of countertransference feelings as they move from acceptable conscious awareness to unconscious denial and acting out. These stages are discernibly different and indicate a growing intensity of feeling that progressively challenges the psychological defenses of the staff.

Table 3 shows the means by which the visible signs of each stage are assessed by the individual staff member and others. Glancing down Table 3 to

Table 3 Stages in the Development of Countertransference Feelings[a]

Conscious					Unconscious	
Sequence	Neutral to→ Hopeful Attitude (i.e., Empathy) ↓	Percolating → Negative Feelings (e.g., Fear & Anger)	Contained → Feelings (e.g., Dislike to Hate) ↓	Defenses (e.g., → Denial to Projection) ↓	Expressed Acting → Out Against Others (e.g., Patients & Peers) ↓	Rationalization (e.g., Secret Guilt, Shame) ↓
Personal Intervention	Self ↓	Self ↓	Self & Peers ↓	Self, Peers, & Staff ↓	Self & Supervisor ↓	Self & Therapist ↓
Intervention Outcomes	Accept Feelings	Acknowledge Feelings	Reality Checks Feelings	Acknowledge & Express Feelings to Others	Express Towards Patient Appropriately	Resolve, Understand, Self-Acceptance

[a]Staff countertransference reactions, if left unchecked, will proceed through the six-stage sequence above. For each staff member, there is a personal intervention which, if successful, will lead to predictable, healthy outcomes.

"Personal Intervention," it can be seen that, in the initial stages, simple personal assessment or awareness of the development of negative feelings is sufficient to manage them. But as the feelings intensify and strain the individual psychological defense system, it may be that peers and other staff as well as the supervisor are required to assist in managing feelings too weighty to be handled by any person alone (75). Finally, if the above interventions fail and the feelings grow in intensity and complexity, personal therapy may be in order as a means to offer resolution and holistic self-acceptance (76).

1. Countertransference Sequence: Neutral to Hopeful Attitude

Most staff bring a neutral, hopeful, or empathic attitude to their first encounter with a patient. Having chosen their profession, staff quickly learn that they are required to relate to strangers called *patients* (clients, inmates, etc.). The initial interview can be revealing. Often significant information about the patient and staff surfaces. Typically, in the first encounter, staff are less judgmental, more tolerant, and—when emotionally challenged—less vulnerable. The original innocence of the first encounter usually reveals an acceptance of a broad range of feelings about the patient. Sometimes, of course, one feels an immediate acceptance or rejection of the patient because of personal factors (e.g., the patient reminds the staff person of a significant other). In such situations the staff person may be aware of the second stage—of the emergence of percolating feelings. When intense (and usually negative) feelings such as fear or anger spring into consciousness, immediate self-management is required.

2. Countertransference Sequence: "Negative" Feelings

In the more typical situation, especially during the "honeymoon" phase of relationships with difficult patients, feelings generated in the initial encounter are more likely to slowly appear in consciousness. The staff get to know the true nature of the patient. These feelings can be viewed as "percolating," meaning that they more or less bubble up a bit at a time.

When this process begins, the staff person, in becoming aware that the feelings are there, may not be able to manage them in a satisfactory manner. Full acceptance is a rare occurrence. This is not surprising, because the very fact that the feelings are percolating may not be a reflection of a direct relationship between the staff person and the patient's stimulus. Rather, percolating feelings bubble up into awareness because they tend to be unmanageable within the staff's own defense system, and the patient acts as a stimulus to activate unconscious feelings in the staff, which first developed in previous relationships.

In the best-case scenario, the percolating feelings are fully accepted. More often than not, the nature of the feelings and the interplay of personal factors signals that full acceptance will take time. But their full acknowledgment can be brought forth and recognized. A healthy resolution at this stage is for the staff members to acknowledge that a patient is generating intense feelings that are difficult for them to fully accept and integrate.

3. Countertransference Sequence: Feeling Containment

As countertransference feelings grow in intensity, staff members may have difficulty acknowledging them as the principal means of managing them. Often there is a struggle in the psyche to contain the strong feelings in a conscious and then not so conscious manner. In the third stage of feeling containment, staff members can no longer count on their own self-assessment of feelings because, to a significant degree, they cannot tolerate or even cognitively acknowledge the feelings. Conscious containment becomes the best mode of coping. While the staff person consciously tries to cope by not expressing or acting on negative feelings, such a personal management approach may not be completely successful. Reality checks with peers about the feelings may validate their existence because of the more objective perceptions of another person. Reality checks from peers can be the feedback that the current self-management strategy is effective or that another coping response should be pursued.

Unconscious defenses are in play all the time. Obviously, when containment is the chief method of coping, the feelings are beyond the healthiest psychological checks and balances. The psychological defenses may be placed into overdrive. It is not difficult to see that more exposure to the patient in an unmodified context will result in a further evolution of the countertransference process. The strength of the countertransference feeling aroused will begin to press more fully into unconscious psychological defenses.

Feeling containment can be explained by imagining that a staff is like a "vase" with a finite capacity for holding feelings. As the staff move from one day to the next, they will ultimately "fill up" on their feelings. Once feelings rise to the level of the vase's lip, there is nowhere else for them to go but "out." Therefore, staff contain feelings as long as they can, and then their unconscious has to find a way to release them. The release may occur through direct or indirect ways. It may occur at work against peers or patients or somewhere in their personal lives. Regardless, release of negative feelings will take place once the staff can no longer contain them by maintaining a healthy intrapsychic balance.

4. Countertransference Sequence: Unconscious Defenses

For reasons that are unclear, denial and projection are the unconscious defenses that tend to become activated when powerful countertransference reactions build up. If the first mechanism, denial, could be translated into words, the following might be stated, "Yes, I am frightened by this patient and I've tried to put it out of my mind because I don't like that feeling. While I know on some level that this patient frightens me, I've contained that feeling so well that I no longer feel it. Therefore, I don't feel frightened, since there is no longer anything to frighten me." Since, by definition, psychological defenses are unconscious, it is quite likely that denial is in operation in such cases. The danger in this progression is the false sense of security resulting from a feeling that is no longer felt but nonetheless is "known" at some level. When our feelings become blocked through this powerful denial mechanism, our normal alert system to dangerous aspects of our environment is significantly impaired.

In the defense of projection, a staff member may attribute his or her own fear to the patient in a way that could be translated into words such as, "Yes, I used to be frightened of this patient, but now I can see that he is actually more afraid of me than anything else. Therefore he is pretty weak and I don't have to be concerned about him." Because of this projection, the fear in the staff person can no longer act as an alerting mechanism when the patient might really be threatening aggression. When staff fear is projected onto the patient as though the patient actually were the one who was frightened, the staff person, at the least, will be set up to mismanage the patient and, at the most, will exacerbate aggression.

It is at this stage that the concept of *Me Time* becomes operational. During this specially designated time of the workday, the staff are expected to pour out some of their feelings so as to drain off emotions that might affect their work performance negatively. If staff openly express themselves during these meetings and receive feedback from peers, their conscious awareness of feelings may reappear. In this way defenses such as denial and projection can be identified and staff have the opportunity not only to experience the release of contained emotions but also to reintroduce more effective coping mechanisms.

5. Countertransference Sequence: Acting Out

The entrance of unconscious mechanisms is often first recognized when the acting-out behavior that inevitably accompanies these mechanisms results in the mismanagement or abuse of patients. Acting out (77) can be observed in several different ways. Complaints by the patients about particular staff may increase. Other staff may note the unhealthy nature of the relationship and try to intervene. In the worst-case scenario, actual patient abuse is witnessed and other staff are obligated to report the behavior.

When this occurs, the supervisor and possibly other authorities must become involved (78). Informal or formal discussions/interactions with peers and other staff are no longer sufficient. The supervisor must review the relevant data, but with a focus on the staff person's countertransference process. When this is done in a professional way, the staff member should be able to identify his or her feelings, share them with the supervisor, and finally express them in an appropriate manner.

The supervisor, of course, may discover that the acting-out behavior has arisen not just from interactions with the patient but also from other staff dynamics or personal issues like family problems, alcohol abuse, etc. When other factors appear to be in play, a referral to an employee assistance program or to a counselor may be necessary. The key to this type of referral will likely arise from the assessment that the staff member not only has other personal problems connected to poor work performance but that these problems are minimized as well. Overuse of rationalizations as an explanation for acting-out behaviors is a common indication whereby this process can be recognized.

6. Countertransference Sequence: Rationalization

Facing limits within themselves is difficult for all people, including those with professional training (79). When rationalizations or other, similar explanations are overused to minimize the impact of a staff member's inappropriate behavior toward patients (or others), the threshold for personal therapy has been met. The most common time for staff to begin a rationalizing process is when they have made a particularly punitive response to an unsavory patient. Staff may secretly feel guilt about having acted out on a patient but will not easily let go of a harsh decision without intervention. The principal intervention question is "What is this patient's behavior doing to your decision-making ability?" If there are no frank discussions among staff about how their feelings affect their decisions, a chronic pattern of decision making based on powerful countertransference reactions take place. This may result in anything from a perpetually bad attitude to patient abuse. It is possible, with supervision, for staff to adopt the viewpoint that the most difficult patients are the ones who will "teach" them the most about their personal deficits. With such a perspective, staff can gain a better understanding about themselves as well as provide better patient care.

Consideration must also be given to the fact that some staff do not have the interpersonal skills to work with patients who elicit strong negative feelings. For some staff, no amount of intervention would appropriately diffuse negative countertransference reactions. It may be well known to everyone working with a particular staff person that he or she simply does not seem able to cope emotionally with a specific patient. The best guidance here is to counsel the staff to identify these deficits so they can, at a minimum, respond to them in a neutral manner. The fact is that some staff are better at working with some patients than with others. When staff cannot resolve negative countertransference issues and the maladaptive behavior that results from them, it may be time to discuss transfer to a less intense environment or, if the problem is severe enough, consider termination.

VI. RESOLVING COUNTERTRANSFERENCE FEELINGS/ PREVENTING POSTTRAUMATIC STRESS DISORDER

Every effort must be made to encourage staff to learn how to understand and attenuate the process of escalating aggressive behavior and to work through the stages of countertransference that result from it (80). The process of resolving these feelings begins with a conscious awareness that countertransference exists. This is tantamount to saying that the denial generally associated with this process has been consciously acknowledged and that a full-faced attempt to prevent and resolve countertransference feelings through ongoing discussions is expected and valued. The discussions are sanctioned to occur on an informal and formal basis (81).

The informal discussion occurs throughout the day among all levels of staff. These are dialogues that occur in the corridor, nursing station, staff break room (but away from the patients), at lunch, and after work. In these discussions the staff simply acknowledge how they feel toward individual patients or toward the whole patient group. These discussions are invaluable and establish a general climate that will legitimize all types of feelings, good and bad, from hate to love. However, as informal discussions, they can hardly be effective in bringing intrangient countertransference reactions into awareness so that they can be resolved.

The literature has shown that structured programs directed at attenuating the development of long-term countertransference feelings do have impact. Staff at Mendota Mental Health Institute, in Madison, Wisconsin, have developed a program called Staff Assistance for Employees (SAFE) (82). When the staff face any major crisis, whether it is suicide, a serious assault, or some other potentially threatening incident, a volunteer staff member usually of the same discipline, is identified to talk with each staff member involved in the incident as soon as possible. The purpose of this buddy approach is to make a contact directly with the person who has experienced the trauma in order to form a trusting relationship with them so that they can be prompted to discuss their initial reaction to the stress privately and to establish a relationship whereby the peer will continue to monitor how the staff member is doing in regard to resolving the incremental reaction that will occur in the following days as they have memories of the traumatic event and as they form attitudes about the safety of the workplace in regard to the stress. The SAFE program has been in effect for several years and has received high ratings from staff. It is similar in its goals to those described in the paper by Chemtob et al. (8).

Chemtob et al. describe a field study on the impact of debriefing on the psychological stress suffered by persons who have been subjected to a stressful event. They looked at two groups of subjects who were exposed to Hurricane

Iniki in Hawaii and who were assessed before and after participating in multihour debriefing groups. Their conclusions were that the effectiveness of the postdisaster psychological interventions were clear and led to the identification of further areas of training and research that would better prepare people for the management of stress.

Similarly, Flannery et al. describe a report on a program to help staff cope with psychological sequelae after assault by patients (7). This program, called the Assaulted Staff Action Program (ASAP), also featured immediate debriefing on ongoing staff processing group for staff that had been assaulted. This program helped staff members to develop a greater sense of control over their feelings. They built up a support network to help them work through and prevent the appearance of symptoms of posttraumatic stress disorder (PTSD). They were able to return to the workplace in a more timely manner and, in general, the issues that sometimes confound such programs and, that is confidentiality and whether ASAP team members were working with them rather than for the administration became clarified. Aside from the SAFE Program at Mendota Mental Health Institute, we have also identified as a need on our Management Unit, where we have placed the most repetitively aggressive patients, for regular processing meetings called Me Time.

Me Time is a regularly scheduled semisupervisory session that occurs among all levels of staff under the direction of the unit supervisor(s). Me Time is recommended to take place for a minimum of 1 hour per week, but up to 1 hour per day on units with high rates of aggression. In general the goal of Me Time is to consciously tune into the feeling processes of staff. It may be a difficult process in itself and will likely be met with typical resistances such as silence, anger, projection, and rationalization. When staff are allowed to meet in a confidential manner on a regular basis, however, a process will evolve in which staff will come to trust each other enough to share their real feelings. There are only a few simple rules. First, all nursing and clinical staff must attend. Past the attendance rule and the fact that racist and sexist comments are not acceptable, staff are encouraged to express themselves in language that is meaningful and satisfying to them. They may talk about individual patients, the current patient group, their peers, their own idiosyncratic issues, or anything else that may be on their minds. The process of encouraging free expression and working through staff differences when life and death are at stake is beyond the scope of this chapter. Consider the following example.

A typical example of the process of a Me Time is that of resolving staff splitting (83) about the management and treatment approach for a patient. In this scenario staff feelings are polarized, with one group wanting to approach the patient as heartless "hard hats" who act like Nazis, while the other group, the "bleeding hearts," want to approach the patient like forgiving nuns. These polar opposite approaches toward the patient can be very difficult to resolve unless the supervisor(s) understand that time is needed to allow the staff to reconcile their differences. Staff cannot be protected from the process of their own struggle. Instead, supervisors should allow the struggle to take place. With proper regulation, supervisors should encourage the staff to express the range of their opposed feelings. This sometimes painful process will move toward the resolving phase, where reasonable management decisions results. The processing step for the staff becomes understanding the affect that has polarized the staff and seeing that it is imperative to discharge it before any risk-taking decisions are made.

A. "Me Time": How It Works

The first step of resolution, therefore, is to allow both sides to express themselves as completely as possible. After this catharsis, the silent majority usually begin to moderate their polar positions toward some central position. Through the work of the unit supervisors and those staff that are not as emotionally aroused, a compromise position can be determined. Since risks need to be taken with patients who have been aggressive, the compromise position is the most reasonable one that the feelings of staff will allow, given the strength of their polarized positions. Such decision making is called "taking a reasonable risk." The concept of reasonable risk taking means that decisions are not made from feelings but from reason. Most important though, is the philosophy that before any decisions about aggressive patients are made, all staff are given the opportunity to free themselves from emotions that would only cloud good decision making.

On occasion, informal and semiformal processes of working through countertransference cannot affect the intensity of the countertransference that an individual staff person may feel. In situations such as this, the countertransference must be addressed in the most formal forum, that of individual supervision. In this forum the individual supervisor will have an opportunity to discuss the work performance of the staff member as it relates to the staff member's feelings for selected patients. The supervisor can also make an assessment of issues that may be unresolved in the staff member's persona life, which may be appearing at work. It is not uncommon for staff who are experiencing stress in their personal lives to act it out at work. Once the work performance has been properly assessed, supervisors can suggest appropriate ways for the employee to make corrections in the work area. They may also need to refer the individual to the Employee Assistance Program for further counseling. At times it may be appropriate for a supervisor to suggest that the employee seek private counseling and even therapy.

The broad-range approach described above of informal, semi-formal, and formal ways of addressing countertransference issues complies with the goals of an established countertransference policy and can greatly contribute to providing an environment free of patient abuse. It may also be the key ingredient to helping staff remain emotionally healthy while working with potentially aggressive patients (84,85).

B. Case Example and Discussion

The staff of an inpatient unit serving acutely ill patients expressed concern to the unit supervisor about a recently admitted patient who had been manifesting some symptoms of agitation and hostility toward patients and staff. In the Friday afternoon team meeting, they worried that the patient would continue to escalate and become more problematic over the weekend. The supervisor listened to them politely but ultimately stated that they were "overconcerned" about this patient and that no special precautions needed to be taken. By Friday evening the patient had challenged several patients to fight him and had been verbally abusive to staff. While everyone was on alert to potential problems, no plan had been established to deescalate the situation. During the lunch hour on Saturday, when the unit was minimally staffed, the patient became very hostile and started to threaten everyone. The staff attempted to talk him down but he refused to comply with their redirection. The patient continued to escalate. In response, a disorganized and understaffed take down was attempted. In the fracas, the charge nurse received a broken nose and one of the aide staff suffered a sprained back.

On Monday the busy unit supervisor arrived for the regularly scheduled Me Time, knowing that the staff would be angry about the aggression on the weekend. The supervisor opened the meeting by ignoring their pressing feelings and started to tell the staff about some concerns raised by the dietary department. The staff, well acquainted with the process of Me Time, stopped the supervisor because they wanted to talk about the recent aggression and staff injuries. The supervisor, in an attempt to deflect the discussion away from the feeling level, tried to switch the discussion to the patient's diagnosis, so they could formulate a modified treatment plan. The staff, however, persisted in discussing their feelings about how, in the Friday meeting, they had expressed serious concerns about the patient's preaggression symptoms and how the supervisor had dismissed the need for preventive action. They expressed anger to the supervisor for dismissing their input during Friday's meeting and for appearing unconcerned about the injury to the staff.

After several attempts to deny and deflect the staff's feelings, the supervisor realized his mistake and admitted that the staff's reactions to the way the situation had been managed were legitimate. The discussion then progressed to the staff's feeling that felt the supervisor did not give them enough input into the management of potentially serious circumstances involving patient and staff safety. The staff reported that they felt disrespected because the supervisor did not trust their judgment about patients. The supervisor responded that he felt very accountable for the care of patients and therefore could not relinquish his responsibility easily. In further discussion, the supervisor and the staff carefully walked through the decision-making process of the last aggression and considered how the incident could have been managed better. The staff stated that they were willing to work together with the supervisor about these important issues but that the supervisor had to do a better job taking their concerns seriously. The staff pointed out that the supervisor actually would be more responsible if he trusted them more and acted on some of their suggested interventions.

This typical but ideal example illustrates several important points. First, managing inpatient aggression requires multidisciplinary skills, those of line staff and those of the trained clinician. Respectful communication is essential between all levels of staff and is the best way to prevent aggression. While it is always easy to second guess decisions, in the above case the principal decision maker, the unit supervisor (who could be a psychiatrist, psychologist, or one of several disciplines) made an effort to listen to the staff concerns but failed to solicit specific reasons or specific precautions before labeling their fears as an "overconcern." Learning how to identify the behaviors of a potentially aggressive patient that may reliably contribute to a plan of prevention, from the feeling staff have that they are at risk, is critical in the preaggression phase. The aggression postmortem should pick up this dissonance and suggest guidelines that could lead to better communication between the levels of staff. The example cannot describe in a detailed way the replay of the whole process. This Me Time, however, did give the line staff an opportunity to vent their anger toward one of their "superiors." These staff are always at the bottom of the authority/power hierarchy. But they often have good ideas and exercise good judgment when faced with unpredictable circumstances. It is important that they feel supported. While it may even be true that one or more of the staff have a tendency to overreact in such situations, which is not suggested in the example, this is the kind of issue that other staff might bring up. The staff usually will not support each other if they themselves believe that a patient was provoked into self-defense by the staff's need to overcontrol the patient. At the same time, the supervisors are not always on the hot seat. In fact, most often they are in a position to relieve staff-staff impasses. They are often the power brokers who can help shape staff opinion, practice, or values. Me Time then becomes an inservice for all staff and an opportunity for healing rifts among staff. Team building is an important part of the process. While every Me Time is not an encounter, the very fact that the opportunity is there, on a regularly scheduled basis, lets all levels of staff know that they do not need to wait for a crisis to express their concerns to their supervisors or to each other. And that is the principal strength Me Time.

VII. SUMMARY

Managing the intense reactions that are a natural response to aggressive behavior is difficult, at best, for all levels of staff working in inpatient settings. Before we can rationally plan to identify and work through these intense emotions, we must come to know and understand the processes producing them. The model presented at the beginning of this chapter is a first step in describing the phases of aggression. Understanding these phases makes it possible to focus more intensely on the specific process of escalation. This process is the one that carries the energy transfer from the patient to the staff. Staff are emotionally traumatized by each aggressive event. The accumulation of unresolved "negative" emotion cannot but factor into the way staff relate to patients. Recognition of this fact led to the formulation of the dynamics of aggression cycles. Unresolved staff countertransference feelings govern the rhythm of aggression on many inpatient units. This notwithstanding the fact that admission units get out-of-control, actively psychotic people as their new patients.

Understanding that the accumulation of unresolved countertransference feelings plays a significant role in defining the humane quality of the environment of the unit makes it incumbent on those who work with aggressive patients to develop methods to prevent and work through such feelings. This will necessarily mean that some form of policy and/or training will need to be developed. The countertransference policy and procedure, and the structure called *Me Time*, are the two clinical/administrative responses recommended to address these concerns. There are many other aspects of aggression management that are relevant to this issue, but the interventions described above are necessary elements in any comprehensive approach to the management of staff feelings toward aggressive patients.

REFERENCES

1. H. Carmel and M. Hunter, Staff injuries from inpatient violence. *Hosp. Commun. Psychiatry 40*:41 (1989).
2. J.R. Lion and W.H. Reid (eds.), *Assaults WIthin Psychiatric Facilities*, Grune & Stratton, New York, 1983.
3. J.R. Lion, Training for battle: Thoughts on managing aggressive patients, *Hosp. Commun. Psychiatry 38*:882 (1987).
4. G.J. Maier and G.J. Van Rybroek, Offensive images: Managing aggression isn't pretty (editorial), *Hosp. Commun. Psychiatry 41*:357 (1990).
5. E.C. Poster and J. Ryan, A multiregional study of nurses' beliefs and attitudes about work safety and patient assault, *Hosp. Commun. Psychiatry 45*:1104 (1994).

6. *Clinician Safety* (W.R. Dubin and J.R. Lion, eds.), American Psychiatric Association Task Force Report #33. American Psychiatric Press, Washington, DC, 1993.
7. R.B. Flannery, Jr., P. Fulton, J. Tausch, and A.Y. DeLoffi, A program to help staff cope with psychological sequelae of assaults by patients. *Hosp. Commun. Psychiatry 42*:935 (1991).
8. C.M. Chemtob, S. Tomas, W. Law, and D. Cremniter, Postdisaster psychosocial intervention: A field study of the impact of debriefing on psychological distress, *Am. J. Psychiatry 154*:415 (1997).
9. G.J. Maier, L.J. Stava, B.R. Morrow, G.J. Van Ryboek, and K. Bauman, A model for understanding and managing cycles of aggression among psychiatric patients, *Hosp. Commun. Psychiatry 38*:520 (1987).
10. G.J. Maier, G.J. Van Rybroek, D.M. Doren, E.A. Musholt, and R.D. Miller, A comprehensive model for understanding and managing aggressive inpatients, *Am. J. Cont. Educ. Nurs., Sec. C*, 1988, pp. 1–16.
11. G.J. Maier, *Management Approaches for the Repetitively Aggressive Patient* (D. Sledge and A. Tasman, eds.), Clinical Challenges in Psychiatry, American Psychiatric Press, Washington, DC, 1993.
12. G.J. Maier, Understanding the Dynamics of Abusive Relationships. *Psychiatric Times 9*:26 (1996).
13. J. Monahan, *The Clinical Prediction of Violent Behavior* (DHHS Publ No (ADM)81-921, National Institute of Mental Health, Rockville, MD, 1981.
14. F.S. Perls, *Ego, Hunger and Aggression*, Vintage Books, New York, 1947.
15. E.D. Tanke and J.A. Yesavage, Characteristics of assaultive Patients Who do and do not provide visible cues of potential violence. *Am. J. Psychiatry 142*:1409 (1985).
16. G.T. Harris and G.W. Varney, *Assaults and Assaulters in Psychiatric Facilities*, Grune & Stratton, New York, 1983.
17. G.J. Maier, Managing threatening behavior: The role of talk down and talk up. *J. Psychosoc. Nurs. 34*:25 (1996).
18. J.T. Turner, Hostage-takers in health care settings: The violent patient. *Psychiatr. Clin. North Am. 4*:649 (1988).
19. *Intervention Options Continuum (IOC)*, Mendota Mental Health Institute Training Department, 301 Troy Drive, Madison, Wisconsin 53704.
20. K. Tardiff, *Concise Guide to Assessment and Management of Violent Patients*, American Psychiatric Press, Washington, DC, 1989.
21. E. Revitch, Patients who Kill their physician. *J. Med. Soc. N.J. 76*:429 (1979).
22. LV. Annis and C.A. Baker, A psychiatrist's murder in a mental hospital, *Hosp. Commun. Psychiatry 37*:505 (1986).
23. American Psychiatric Association, *Diagnostic and Statistical Manual of Mental Disorders*, 4th ed., American Psychiatric Association, Washington, DC, 1994.
24. S.C. Yudofsky, J.M. Silver, and W. Jackson, The overt aggression scale for the objective rating of verbal and physical aggression, *Am. J. Psychiatry 143*:35 (1986).
25. F.C. Depp, Violent behavior patterns on psychiatric wards, *Aggress. Behav. 2*:395 (1976).
26. J. Dawson, M. Johnson, and N. Kehiayan, Response to patient assault: A peer support program for nurses. *J. Psyhosoc. Nurs. Ment. Health Serv. 26*:8 (1988).

27. G.J. Maier, Understanding the dynamics of abusive relationships, *Psychiatr. Times* 9:26 (1996).
28. *Management's Response to Violence in the Workplace*, Wisconsin's Statewide Employee Assistance Program (EAP).
29. A. Jones and S. Schechter, *When Love Goes Wrong*, Harper Perennial, New York, 1992.
30. G. McCarthy, *Getting Free: A Handbook for Women in Abusive Relationships*, The Seal Press, Seattle, 1982.
31. S.G. Kaplan and E.G. Wheeler, Survival skills for working with potentially violent clients, *Soc. Casework J. Contemp. Soc. Work* 339 (1983).
32. J.J. McGee, Gentle teaching, *N.Z. J. Ment. Retard. 40*:13 (1985).
33. R.T. Rada, The violent patient: Rapid assessment and management, *Psychosomatics 22*:101 (1981).
34. R.L. Binder, The use of seclusion on an inpatient intervention unit, *Hosp. Commun. Psychiatry 30*:266 (1979).
35. R.L. Binder and S.M. McCoy, A study of patients' attitudes toward placement in seclusion, *Hosp. Commun. Psychiatry 34*:1052 (1983).
36. G. Adler, Helplessness in the helpers, *Br. J. Med. Psychol. 45*:315 (1972).
37. J.R. Lion and S.A. Pasternak, Countertransference reactions to violent patients. *Am. J. Psychiatry 130*:207 (1973).
38. R.D. Alaron, A.A. Bancroft, and T.D. Daniels, Dynamics of the inpatient psychiatric setting. *Psychiatr. Ann. 18*:102 (1988).
39. P.L. Giovacchini, *Countertransference Triumphs and Catastrophes*, Jason Aronson, New York, 1989.
40. J. Sandler, A. Holder, and C. Dare, Basic psychoanalytic concepts, IV: Countertransference. *Br. J. Psychiatry 117*:83 (1970).
41. M. Lakovics, A classification of countertransference phenomena and its application to inpatient psychiatry, *Psychiatr. J. U. Ottawa 10*:132 (1984).
42. Mendota Mental Health Institute: *General Policy #22, Countertransference Issues*, Forensic Center, Policy Manual. Mendota Mental Health Institute, Madison, WI, 1989.
43. A. Westbrook and O. Ratti, *Akido and the Dynamic Sphere*, Charles E. Tuttle, Rutland, VT, 1980.
44. K.H. Johansen, The impact of patients with chronic character pathology on a hospital inpatient unit, *Hosp. Commun. Psychiatry 43*:842 (1983).
45. P.J. Schroeder, Recognizing transference and countertransference, *J. Psychosoc. Nurs. Ment. Health Serv.* 23:21 (1986).
46. D.B. Colson, J.G. Allen, and L. Coyne, An anatomy of countertransference: Staff reactions to difficult psychiatric hospital patients, *Hosp. Commun. Psychiatry 47*:923 (1986).
47. M.L. Lanza, The reactions of nursing staff to physical assault by a patient, *Hosp. Commun. Psychiatry 43*:44 (1983).
48. M.L. Lanza, How nurses react to patient assault, *J. Psychosoc. Nurs. Ment. Health Serv. 23*:6 (1985).

49. D.L. Fink, Threats and Assaults Against Residents, paper presented at the 143rd Annual Meeting of the American Psychiatric Association, New York, May 14, 1990.
50. R.D. Miller, The harassment of forensic psychiatrists outside of court, *Bull. Am. Acad. Psychiatry Law 13*:337 (1985).
51. H. Carmel and M. Hunter, Staff injuries from inpatient violence, *Hosp. Commun. Psychiatry 40*:41 (1989).
52. L.V. Annis and C.A. Baker, A psychiatrist's murder in a mental hospital, *Hosp. Commun. Psychiatry 47*:505 (1986).
53. D.M. Turns and E.M. Gruenberg, An attendant is murdered: The state hospital responds, *Psychiatr. Q. 47*:487 (1973).
54. J. Sandler, C. Dare, and A. Holder, Basic psychoanalytic concepts: III. Transference. *Br. J. Psychiatry 116*:667 (1970).
55. G.J. Van Rybroek and G.J. Maier, Aggressive inmates: Hitting critical components of management, *Correct Care 1*:7, (1987).
56. J. Sandler, C. Dare, and A. Holder, Basic psychoanalytic concepts: VIII. Special forms of transference, *Br. J. Psychiatry 117*:561 (1970).
57. R.B. Cornfield and S.D. Fielding, Impact of the threatening patient on ward communications, *Am. J. Psychiatry 137*:616 (1980).
58. F.C. Depp, Violent behavior patterns on psychiatric wards, *Aggress. Behav. 2*:295 (1976).
59. J.R. Lion and W.H. Reid (eds), *Assaults Within Psychiatric Facilities*, Grune & Stratton, New York, 1983.
60. J.M. Silver and S.C. Yudofsky, Documentation of aggression in the assessment of the violent patient, *Psychiatr. Ann. 17*:375 (1987).
61. L.F. Sparr, Incident Reporting is Key to Managing Violence in Hospitals, *Psychiatric Times*, April 1989.
62. J.W. Barber, P. Hundley, and E. Kellog, Clinical and demographic characteristics of 15 patients with repetitively assaultive behavior, *Psychiatr. Q. 59*:213 (1988).
63. S.M. Glynn, L.L. Bowen, and B.D. Marshall, Jr., Compliance with less restrictive aggression-control procedures, *Hosp. Commun. Psychiatry 40*:82 (1989).
64. J.A. Infantino and S. Musingo, Assaults and injuries among staff with and without training in aggression control techniques, *Hosp. Commun. Psychiatry 36*:1312 (1985).
65. J.G. Gunderson, Defining the therapeutic proesses in psychiatric milieus, *Psychiatry 41*:327 (1978).
66. D.J. Drummond, L.F. Sparr, and G.H. Gordon, Hospital violence reduction among high-risk patients, *J.A.M.A. 26*:2531 (1989).
67. L.S. Lehmann, M. Padilla, and S. Clark, Training personnel in the prevention and management of violent behavior, *Hosp. Commun. Psychiatry 34*:40 (1983).
68. L.F. Brown, Staff countertransference reactions in the hospital treatment of borderline patients, *Psychiatry 43*:333 (1980).
69. J.E. Groves, Taking care of the hateful patient, *N. Engl. J. Med. 298*:883 (1978).
70. L.H. Strasburger, Countertransference with psychopathic patients. *Psychiatric News*, November 1987.
71. L.B. Boyer, Countertransference with severely regressed patients, *Countertransference* (L. Epstein and A. Feiner, eds.) Jason Aronson, New York, 1979, pp. 347–373.

72. L. Epstein, The therapeutic function of hate in the countertransference, *Countertransference*. L. Epstein and A. Feiner, eds.), Jason Aronson, New York, 1979, pp. 213–234.
73. P.L. Giovacchini, Countertransference with primitive mental states, *Countertransference*, L. Epstein and A. Feiner, eds.), Jason Aronson, New York, 1979, pp. 235–265.
74. R.J. Marshall, Countertransference with children and adolescents, *Countertransference* (L. Epstein and A. Feiner, eds.), Jason Aronson, New York, 1979, pp. 407–441.
75. D.W. Winnicott, Hate in the Counter-Transference, *Int. J. Psychoanal. 30*:699 (1949).
76. W. Wilber, *No Boundary: Eastern and Western Approaches to Personal Growth*, New Science Library, Boston, 1981.
77. J. Sandler, A. Holder, and C. Dare, Basic Psychoanalytic Concepts: IV. Countertransference, *Br. J. Psychiatry 117*:83 (1970).
78. W.T. Merkel and C.A. Pillard, Applying modern management principles to clinical administration of a behaviorally oriented inpatient unit, *Hosp. Commun. Psychiatry 38*:153 (1987).
79. G.J. Maier, M.J. Bernstein, and E.A. Musholt, Personal coping mechanisms for prison clinicians, *J. Prison Jail Health 8*:29 (1989).
80. J. Heider, *The Tao of Leadership*. Bantam Books, New York, 1985.
81. C.M. Monroe, G.J. Van Rybroek, and G.J. Maier, Decompressing aggressive inpatients: Breaking the aggression cycle to enhance positive outcome, *Behav. Sci. Law 6*:543 (1988).
82. *Staff Assistance for Employees Program*. Mendota Mental Health Institute, Madison, WI, 1997.
83. G.O. Gabbard, Splitting in hospital treatment. *Am. J. Psychiatry 144*:444 (1989).
84. K. Minkoff and R. Stern, Paradoxes faced by residents being trained in the psychosocial treatment of people with chronic schizophrenia. *Hosp. Commun. Psychiatry 36*:859 (1985).
85. K. Tardiff, *Assessment and Management of Violent Patients*, American Psychiatric Press, Washington, DC, 1989.

13
Psychotherapeutic Treatment of Violence

Marilyn Lewis Lanza
Edith Nourse Rogers Memorial Veterans Hospital, Bedford; Boston University School of Medicine, Boston; and Boston University School of Public Health, Boston, Massachusetts

I. INTRODUCTION

The psychotherapeutic treatment of violence is a particularly difficult activity. It lacks the glamour of assessment and is definitely not the "quick fix" approach. Psychotherapy with violent individuals does not allow a clinician to make one rapid assessment with the hoped for outcome that disaster has been avoided. Rather, this assessment must be made continually. One does not feel clever, omnipotent etc.—all the countertransference feelings that need to be processed but are pleasurable just the same. Psychotherapy with violent people puts one in touch with one's own vulnerability: for example, the fear of making a mistake in judging how safe the patient is at a particular point in time either during a specific therapeutic maneuver or when considering issues such as discharge. A sense of vulnerability is also felt in considering one's own safety. Psychotherapy with the violent patient means getting to know the patient well, putting oneself in his or her shoes and giving up the attitude of "us versus them." Disquieting experiences for therapists include getting in touch with their own rage and finding that they begin to like the aggressor.

In order to perform therapy with the violent patient, clinicians must understand a violent person's motives for violence. Clinicians must step into the shoes of the aggressor and reconstruct his or her unique perspective, no matter how odd or strange it may be. Clinicians must recreate the world of the violent person, with all its fears and apprehensions, with its hopes and ambitions, with its strains and stresses. Clinicians must allow themselves to consider that violence is often a two-person game. Even where the victim does no more than appear at the wrong time and place, his or her contribution is essential for the consummation of his or her destruction. And usually more than mere physical presence is involved. Common sense and law are attracted to the image of passive victims mauled by spontaneously malevolent aggressors. In the world of violence, however, the situation is rarely that simple (1). The clinician's role is to explore the complex world of aggression with the patient. To be highly effective, clinicians also need to explore the complicated feelings and attitudes of their own aggression.

This chapter includes the following:

1. A literature review of individual, group, and couples/family treatment of violence (hospital assault as well as domestic violence). Outcome studies are cited when available. Most attention has been given to group therapy as a treatment modality. This reflects group as the treatment of choice in the literature and may also be indicative of clinicians' discomfort with aggression and practice of referring these persons to others.
2. The pros and cons of "mandatory reporting".
3. Recommendations for conducting psychotherapy with violent people.

II. OVERALL COMMENTS ON THERAPY WITH THE VIOLENT PATIENT

The goal of therapy with the violent person is to alter self-image and develop alternative response patterns (2). Violent patients tend to have an image of themselves as persons to be feared and to have limited patterns of imagination and fantasy that might inhibit alternative responses. They must learn to identify patterns of escalation in violence and learn to disengage at the early phase of escalation (3). Psychotherapy should provide insight as to why these patients must use violence as a means of expression. Often, they have difficulty expressing their feelings and conflicts. Issues common in the treatment of violent patients are low self-esteem in terms of money, sex, and authority. Tardiff (3) concluded that some violent patients respond to long-term psychotherapy. These patients are generally nonpsychotic and have primarily personality disorders or intermittent explosive disorders.

III. INDIVIDUAL THERAPY

There is a range of opinion concerning the efficacy of psychotherapy with violent patients. Studies of efficacy are few or have produced results that are difficult to evaluate (4). In a study of 110 nonpsychotic opiate addicts randomly assigned to drug counseling alone or drug counseling with psychotherapy, outcomes of psychotherapy were examined in four groups: those with opiate dependence (OP) alone (*N*=16); OP plus depression (*N*=16); OP plus depression plus antisocial personality disorder (*N*=17); and OP plus antisocial personality disorder (*N*=13). All groups showed improvement in several areas (e.g., drug use, employment, legal status, psychiatric function) except the group with OP plus antisocial personality disorder, which showed improvement only on ratings of drug use. The authors concluded that the poor response to psychotherapy seen in this group was attributable to difficulties these patients have in forming meaningful relationships (5).

Limited success in the treatment of antisocial personality, disorder can be attributed to the patient's lack of motivation, tendency to externalize, and habitual distrust of authority (6). Although Gunderson (6) recommended therapies that depend on peer pressure and socially corrective experiences rather than individual therapy, he conceded that psychotherapy may be helpful when residential placement (including prison), which limits antisocial behaviors, invokes in the patient feelings of emptiness, depression, and anxiety. Gabbard (7) also argued against outpatient individual psychotherapy of the severely antisocial patient, stating that it is doomed to fail because the lack of containment in institutional settings allows affect to be discharged via action and because the patient's dishonesty prevents the therapist from knowing what is really going on in his or her life. He acknowledged a continuum of antisocial character pathology, with some points along the continuum being more amenable to treatment, and suggested the use of psychological testing to evaluate the patient's object relations and superego development before attempting psychotherapy with inpatients. Kernberg (8), in a discussion of the limits of treatment, maintained that deterioration or absence of superego functions found in antisocial personalities precluded treatment with analytically oriented psychotherapy.

Although recommendations are proposed about the type of patient who will (and will not) do well in psychotherapy, studies have not always supported the expected relationship between personality traits and success in treatment (9). With caveats, therefore, some experts propose that psychoanalytically oriented therapy or other psychodynamic treatments can be useful. Reid (10) suggested that psychotherapy can facilitate symptom relief and defensive restructuring in patients with antisocial personalities. Individual psychotherapy with patients with severe borderline personality disorder who act out in assaultive and self-destructive ways can also be valuable in defining the therapeutic issues, studying countertransference, and improving psychotherapeutic techniques (11). Even mild psychopathically disturbed patients may benefit from weekly individual therapy (12). Meloy defined the treatable patient as one who can form attachments and whose level of superego pathology, using the six levels described by Kernberg (13), is not too severe. Meloy (12) identified five clinical features that contraindicate psychotherapy (Table 1) and offered other guides for the assessment of severity of psychopathic disturbance.

While psychoanalytic psychotherapy was recommended for violent patients in some cases, others suggested adding some elements of a behavioral-cognitive approach, such as limit setting and cognitive dialogue concerning the consequences of violent behavior. The latter is especially useful in helping the impulsive patient learn to examine the cost-benefit ratio of alternative coping strategies (14). A predominantly supportive, rather than expressive, focus was recommended with patients who lack psychological mindedness or who have severe personality disorders with a tendency to act out, impaired object relations, tenuous ability to form a therapeutic alliance, and/or poor impulse control (7).

One of the first goals of psychotherapy with the violent patient is assessing motivation and the reason for seeking treatment (15). Although it is preferable to accept a patient who is motivated by the negative impact of violent behavior on his or her life or by feelings of guilt and remorse, it is more likely that the patient is being coerced in some way to enter treatment, which does not necessarily consign the treatment to failure (4,15). Another important initial goal is helping the patient develop self-control of emotions and behavior. This includes giving the patient the phone number of the local emergency department, a hot line, or the therapist's pager. As the patient learns to verbalize rather than act on feelings, any violent behavior can be analyzed (15). In the treatment of aggressive patients, there is often an initial phase when aggression appears to cease. The therapist is endowed with attributes that represent the opposite of the patient's inner state. Accordingly, strength is obtained by contact with the therapist, and the patient finds the ability to function without becoming aggressive (15).

In a discussion of the management of assaultive adolescents, Marohn (16) advises helping patients experience affect as part of themselves, with the goal of learning to manage affect and use it as a basis for communication and self-

Table 1 Interpersonal or Intrapsychic Features That Contraindicate Psychotherapy

1. A history of sadistic, aggressive behavior that resulted in serious injury, maiming, or death to the victim.
2. A complete absence of any remorse, justification, or rationalization for such behavior.
3. Intelligence either in the very superior or mildly mentally retarded range.
4. A historical absence of any capacity or inclination to form an emotional attachment to another person.
5. An intense countertransference fear of predation on the part of the experienced clinician without any overt behavior on the patient's part.

Source: From Ref. 12.

understanding, thereby converting motor behavior to verbal behavior. Tardiff (15,17) emphasizes the importance of the development of affective awareness, enabling the violent patient to avoid being either flooded with affect or remaining oblivious to it. The patient must learn to identify early physiological warning signs such as rapid heartbeat, flushed face, or sweating, so that he or she can respond appropriately (e.g., by taking a walk, calling the therapist, or finding someone to talk to) (14,15,17).

Violent patients must learn to extend their fantasies beyond the violent acts they envision to the consequences of those acts. The therapist can facilitate this by asking the patient to relate in a step-by-step manner the events before, during, and after the violent act. This process should include eliciting information about the setting, the people involved, what will happen to the patient afterward, how others will feel, and possible disastrous outcomes (4). The patient should even be encouraged to fantasize in some detail about what it will be like to be in jail, attend a funeral, or lose his or her job or significant others (15).

A long-term goal is the development of insight regarding the dynamics of violence, which empowers the patient to deal psychologically with a potentially violent situation (15,17). The patient's attention must be repeatedly drawn to issues of self-esteem and vulnerabilities elicited by precipitants to a violent episode. The patient should be encouraged to discuss concerns or weaknesses without fear of the retaliation or humiliation that he or she may have encountered in the past (15). The therapist should remain mindful of the patient's environment outside the office and intervene as an advocate for the patient when appropriate (17).

There is general agreement in the literature about the importance of establishing, at the outset, a firm frame for the therapeutic relationship that will control the threat of acting out. Initial contracts and limit setting regarding the patient's behavior help to establish such a structure (4,8,11,14,17). The therapist should take care not to set up contract conditions to which the patient cannot possibly adhere (4). Limit setting may stimulate fantasies of omnipotence about the therapist that will have to be resolved, but without this the patient will be condemned to repeating earlier patterns of aggressive behavior (11).

Limit setting may at times include involving the criminal justice system (11,12). Threats must be addressed in a safe environment, with honesty both about the fear or anxiety they engender in the therapist as well as acknowledgment of their illegality and the steps the therapist is prepared to take. Furthermore, the therapist must endeavor to ensure his or her own safety and that of office personnel. A means of communication with the receptionist, through a code word or buzzer system, should be established, with a set plan for responding to a violent situation. The therapist should learn some basic techniques of self-defense and should assess the office environment for potential sources of injury and protection (15,17).

Change in the nature of the transference is the most critical and potentially dangerous aspect of work with aggressive patients. The therapist must monitor this set of feelings because it can change as a function of the patient's primitiveness. The therapist must constantly assess whether the patient poses a danger to him or her.

Countertransference also requires evaluation. The countertransference is the most important indicator of the relationship between patient and therapist, although one easily subject to distortion in the case of violence. Countertransference reactions to violent patients vary from denial of danger or fear to projection of anxiety onto the patient, so that he or she seems more dangerous than he/she really is; devaluing the antisocial patient as untreatable; a false belief that a therapeutic alliance exists when it does not; helplessness—which may become transformed into rage toward the patient and be expressed as withdrawal or through reaction formation as excessive attention, rescue fantasies, or heroic attempts to "fix" the patient; and hatred and the wish to destroy (12,17). It is helpful in dealing with such feelings to discuss them with other experienced colleagues or in case consultation (4,10). It is especially helpful, in attempting to assess the risk the patient poses to others, to have the patient seen in consultation (17).

Awareness of both the patient's initial overidealized view of the therapist and the patient's use of projective identification is essential (10). The patient projects hatred and rage onto the therapist and unconsciously attempts to provoke the therapist into the role of torturer and then to control the therapist to limit his or her dangerousness. Under extreme circumstances, the patient may find reality intolerable, and psychopathic transferences—deception, pseudocommunication, and affect storms expressed in dissociated forms—ensue (8). Kernberg (8) describes the antisocial personality as "a characterological structure so dominated by hatred that primitive, split-off idealizations are no longer possible, the world is populated exclusively by hated, hateful, sadistic persecutors, and to triumph in such a terrifying world can only occur by becoming oneself a hateful persecutor as the only alternative to destruction and suicide" (p.708). Adler (11) calls this the "devour-or-be-devoured" (p.211) position, explaining that wishes for intimacy lead to the terror of annihilation or to frustration followed by rage.

Although the rage must be uncovered, the therapist should take care not to directly confront the patient's grandiosity, upon which his internal cohesiveness depends. Interpretations of transference should be grounded in the here and now rather than in events of early childhood (10). Drawing on the experience of several therapists who have treated violent patients, Gabbard (7) has developed six basic principles of technique (Table 2).

Progress is very gradual and often depends on the ego strength the patient has or develops, allowing him or her to learn to delay and to verbalize rather than act out (4). Resistances (e.g., manipulative cycling, deception, malignant pseudo-

Table 2 Basic Principles of Technique for Therapy with Antisocial Patients

1.	The therapist must be stable, persistent, and thoroughly incorruptible.
2.	The therapist must repeatedly confront the patient's denial and minimization of antisocial behavior.
3.	The therapist must help the patient to connect actions with internal states.
4.	Confrontations of here-and-now behavior are more effective than interpretations of unconscious material from the past.
5.	Countertransference must be rigorously monitored to avoid acting out by the therapist.
6.	The therapist must avoid having excessive expectations for improvement.

Source: From Ref. 7.

identification, and sadistic control) are to be expected as the patient experiences therapy as a threat to his or her grandiose self-concept (12). Success must be redefined to include modest improvement (14).

IV. GROUP THERAPY

A. The Outcome of Aggressive Behavior in Response to Group Therapy

Schramski and coworkers (18) reported a successful experience using group therapy as a treatment modality to help adults in a correctional facility cope with their anger. Anger therapy was compared with three other groups—psychodrama, values clarification, and decision making—as well as with a control group. The anger therapy group was significantly different from the other treatment groups in encouraging the expression of intragroup and individual conflicts and was distinctly less oriented than the other groups toward structured activities and leader directiveness (18). By using the Group Environment Scale (19), those in anger therapy were found to improve significantly (10 to 15%) over those in the control group on the subscales of Autonomy and Personal Problem Orientation as well as on the dimension of Obsessive-Compulsive and Depression. The anger therapy group had the highest mean rating score for cohesion, suggesting that this group fostered a high degree of group togetherness (18).

An interesting follow-up report by Homant (20) on initial improvement in the institutional behavior demonstrated by prisoners in group therapy as compared with control subjects showed that this improvement did not continue 10 years later. Homant (20) suggested that (a) institutional behavior may be a poor predictor of follow-up adjustment and (b) groups need to be specific in their goals, methods, and target populations. More follow-up study is needed to determine the efficacy of group therapy. It may be that its utility is for more immediate goals, as for improving inpatient behavior on such outcomes as assault.

State hospital wards designated as "violent" (at least one assault or battery each day) or "peaceful" (several days or weeks passing without a violent incident) were compared (21). A characteristic of peaceful wards was that staff were engaged in therapy groups with patients. Violent wards had little staff/patient interaction or few therapy groups.

Positive results were found for a psychoeducational group offered to veterans suffering from posttraumatic stress disorder (22). Participants showed a significant drop in both state and trait anger.

Group therapy was found to be effective for nonviolent sex offenders. Some 65% (*N* = 36) had not been convicted of further sex offenses at the end of the 10-year study period. Many of the offenders demonstrated a high degree of commitment to the group, and group attendance ran consistently at over 70% (23). The objectives of the group were to discuss mutual problems, reduce feelings of isolation and abnormality, confront members with the effects of their behavior, provide strategies for the management of sexual feelings, and promote wider social contacts as part of the process of disengaging from the group.

A quasi-experimental design examined postconviction recidivism rates for men convicted of wife assault (24). Fifty men who completed a 16-week treatment program has a 4% recidivism rate for a posttreatment period of up to 3 years. A comparable group who were not treated had a 40% recidivism rate in the same period. Thus the "success" rate was 36%.

Lower recidivism rates for participants as opposed to controls were reported for a psychoeducational group for abusive husbands (25). The program was said to be much less structured than most psychoeducational groups and allowed for "insight, growth, spontaneous interaction, helping to build relationships and group solidarity." The promotion of members sharing ideas and providing mutual support was very important in view of the social isolation of many abusive men. An important finding is that nonrecidivists had higher scores on depression (they were less depressed) than recidivists.

Lanza (26) recently completed a 6-month randomized clinical trial conducted in a Department of Veterans Affairs Medical Center to determine if psychodynamic group psychotherapy decreases the occurrence of physical assault by male group members. Group members showed decreased expression of anger at follow-up, increased effort to control anger at follow-up, and decline in aggressive behavior (striking, kicking, pushing, pulling hair, physically attacking others). Control subjects demonstrated no change in level of angry feelings, increased expression of anger at follow-up, decreased effort to control anger at follow-up, and no change in aggressive behavior. Stein and Brown (27) reported that group therapy is not effective for mentally ill offenders. The researchers found that forensic patients have personality characteristics that preclude the development of therapeutic group dynamics. Denial of responsibility undermined the individual's recognition of the group as potentially beneficial. As they did not see themselves as part of the problem, these patients had no desire to increase their self-understanding. Their inability to form attachments inhibited cohesiveness and altruism among group members. The lack of transference indicated that neither the group members nor the leaders were highly valued in the eyes of the other members. The inability to trust others prevented them from feeling safe enough to take risks within the group; thus catharsis rarely occurred. True empathy, like true relatedness, was precluded by their egocentricity.

B. Stages of Group Development for Men and the Expression of Aggression

Based upon a review of the literature of stages of group development, men's issues in groups, and hostility related to group stages, the author developed the following framework, entitled "Stages of Group Development for Men and the Expression of Aggression" (28).

There are five stages, entering, early, reactive, mature, and termination.

1. Entering the Therapy Group

To begin in a group, men sense having betrayed masculine identifications and having returned to an earlier attachment and identification with mother. On entering a psychotherapy group with women present, the male patient is confronted consciously by his competitive and aggressive wishes and fears and unconsciously by his dependent yearnings and counterdependent defenses (29,30). A man among the other men in the presence of women is caught between his wish to be noticed and chosen by the women and his need to connect with the other men. He may also be in touch with anger toward women for the power they have exercised in his life (31).

2. Early Stage

The early phase of group psychotherapy is characterized by confusion, mistrust, and a lack of safety. Feelings of anxiety, dependency, and helplessness are experienced. Sources of hostility include overwhelming anxiety, vulnerability to attack, prejudice and fear of exclusion, loss of control, and narcissistic injury (32).

a. Overwhelming Anxiety. Stranger anxiety, fear of exposure, and resultant shame contribute to the tension characteristic of a new group. Feelings of powerlessness stimulate impulses to act. Common violent responses might be self-image compensating to promote low self-esteem (1).

b. Vulnerability to Act. Group fosters the emergence of the irrational, uncivilized parts of each member. Attempts to dehumanize others may be seen (1).

c. Prejudice and Fear of Exclusion. Since it is terrifying for a group of strangers to get together in the same room, prejudice provides the illusion of knowing the other and reduces anxiety. Since prejudging is a violation of another's uniqueness, it often elicits angry responses.

d. Loss of Control. In the beginning of the group experience, members sense how little control they have over many things, such as when members speak, who gets listened to, etc. This loss of control can lead to a generalized irritability and subsequent hostility.

e. Narcissistic Injury. While a blow to self-esteem can occur in any group phase, this is one of the most frequent causes of hostility in early group development. Inevitably some event or empathic failure reveals the leader's inability to prevent narcissistic injury, soothe hurt, or contain projected anger (33). The leader may see any of the aggressive behaviors in "self-preserving strategies" and "approaches to dehumanize others" (1).

In response to dependent wishes—which are heightened by the presence of women, by the experience of the group itself as "mother" (34), and by transference to the parental leader—counterdependent responses become prominent. Flight, withholding, withdrawal, and distancing are common responses and will begin to be recognized as parallel to behavior in other relationships (35). Men may form a subgroup to protect themselves from the demands of women and the group leader (36). This ritual boundary forms a collective barrier against the affective contagion of the larger group, allowing men to achieve intimacy among themselves and then to function better as part of a larger group.

3. Reactive Stage

Anger is common during the reactive phase. Issues of control and power characterize interpersonal transactions. There is ambivalence and uneven commitment about belonging to the group. There is much projection (30). Individual differences and interpersonal dislikes that were submerged in the beginning phase, in an attempt to achieve cohesion, now find uncomfortable expression. Members comment about traits or behaviors that they do not like. At this stage, the emphasis is placed on justified fault finding rather than confronting and examining in oneself what it is that makes one angry at another person. This unconscious process of projection intensifies such confrontations (33). According to Fried (37), individuation has begun and is always accompanied by hostility and aggression. The latter two serve as reinforcement for the emerging self that is now taking on a separation struggle from the leader and the others. Sources of hostility include self-confrontation through another, sibling rivalry, transference, and premature termination (33). Aggression in the form of self-preserving strategies and attempts to dehumanize others continue (1).

a. Self-Confrontation Through Another. Members attack those traits in others that they find unacceptable in themselves through the process of projective identification. Unlike projection, where unacceptable thoughts, feelings and so on are placed upon others and then avoided, in projective identification one person makes another the container for those unwanted aspects. The projector then identifies with these disowned parts by focusing on traits now believed to reside in the other.

b. Sibling Rivalry. This is a source of hostility when a new member is added and between earlier members. In the first case, "another sick child will receive too much attention." In the second case, members believe that the leader has a favorite or that he or she is "so professional," he or she regards everyone equally.

c. Transference. Angry portions of members' past relationships are repeated in the group, particularly in this phase, when control and power issues dominate.

d. Premature Termination. Premature termination evokes the greatest hostility during this phase. It poses a greater risk if powerful transference reactions occur before secure membership has been established.

4. Mature Stage

At this point members have made a place for themselves, and they are able to be open about issues of power and authority and the risk of becoming dependent. They are able to tolerate rejection and protect themselves from aggression. Gradually the male members become able to recognize their transferential projections onto the group process and their distortions of it, its members, and the leader (31). Collusive deals and alliances are revealed. It is in the sorting out of projections—with each member owning his or her respective disowned portions—that the most important work in group therapy is accomplished (33). Strong attractions and repulsions toward members and the leader become accessible during this phase of increased differentiation. Fears and wishes around engulfment, sadistic impulses, and wishes for phallic prominence are openly acknowledged. For many men the group can become a unique experience where they may be able to bring forth their true selves despite their shame and fear. This acceptance may give rise to surges of sadness, anger, and grief as they begin to feel the previously unfelt losses of their lives (31).

According to Gans (33), there is much less anger during the mature phase than during earlier phases. Anger can arise from two common phenomena: subgrouping and self-disclosure (33). Subgrouping arises from the belief of two or more members that they can derive more gratification from a relationship with each other (either within or outside the group) than from one with the entire group. Other members, who experience exclusion, betrayal, or oedipal defeat, become angry. Self-disclosure can be intentional or unconscious and can result in misunderstanding, judgmentalism, or aversion (33). The shamed member may then attack the group. Table 3 describes process, content, and leader implications by group phase.

C. Recommendations for Conducting Group Psychotherapy with Assaultive Patients

A particularly detailed and useful description of the leader's role in addressing aggression in group therapy was presented by Ormont (38). He began the discussion by addressing the universal ambivalence all people experience about aggression. Although patients may repress or misdirect their aggression, they need it to function. The leader's job is to help them unblock aggression so they can infuse it into their everyday expression.

Ormont (38) summarized steps in group psychotherapy to help patients learn to deal with their aggression.

1. Identify the group members' defenses against feeling and verbalizing irritation and frustration, especially toward the group leader.
2. Decide what the appropriate interventions are to make the group comfortable with all its feelings, including aggression.
3. Consider the feelings of the therapist and what he or she can possibly think and do when barraged by the aggression of eight or ten people.

Ormont (38) concluded that if the therapist is successful, group members' anger can be converted into a powerful force that can serve them throughout their entire lives in a multitude of ways.

1. Role of the Leader

The leader helps patients manage their aggression by "detoxifying" (39) and "containing" (40) it. The leader accepts their aggressive feelings as manageable and demonstrates that he or she will not retaliate. When anger is addressed and dealt with successfully in group therapy, inward freedom and flexibility result (33).

The leader who keeps the group relatively free of humiliation is seen as trustworthy. This is particularly important, since men experience shame as they reveal their secret fears and inadequacies (31).

Men will respond in the group to the degree that the leader recognizes well-learned adaptive skills in their defensive distancing, intellectualizing, and avoidance. According to Krugman and Osherson (31), by affirming the strengths that men have shown, despite their limitations, self-esteem is preserved enough to permit men to explore alternate means of coping and interacting.

Table 3 Model—Phases of Group Therapy for Assaultive Men

PHASE	PROCESS	CONTENT	LEADER IMPLICATIONS
ENTERING	• Competitive, dependent & counterdependent feelings • Confrontation • Betrayal of masculine identifications, returning to earlier attachment & identification with mother	• Is it safe to be here? • Resistance to joining	• Maintain group boundaries • Set contract • Group as a whole focus
EARLY	• Confusion • Mistrust • Anxiety • Dependency • Helplessness • Shame • Male subgrouping, against women • Denial	• Self-image compensating • Dehumanize others • Loss of control • Narcissistic injury • Flight • Withholding • Withdrawal • Distancing	• Maintain group boundaries • Set contract • Group as a whole focus • Leader inquiries to individual members
REACTIVE	• Anger • Ambivalence • Projection • Blaming others • Loss of mother too great, male subgrouping serves as a male mother	• Self-confrontation through another • Sibling rivalry • Transference • Premature termination • Identify & acknowledge feelings • Coping strategies • Increased cohesion	• Maintain group boundaries • Set contract • Group as a whole focus • Leader inquiries to individual members
MATURE	• Open about issues of power and authority • Risk becoming dependent • Explore transferential projections and distortions • Collusive deals and alliances are revealed • Fears & wishes around engulfment & sadistic impulses are acknowledged • Lessening of denial • Sorting out projections, each member owning his respective disowned portions • Reentry into the larger group	• Explore conscious & unconscious feelings intrapsychically, interpersonally & toward the entire group • Acceptance of vulnerable & shameful parts of themselves • Understand own responsibility in aggression/violence • Acknowledge the personal cost of violence • Lessening of displacement • Appropriately express feelings • Coping strategies	• Maintain group boundaries • Set contract • Group as a whole focus • Leader inquiries to individual members
TERMINATION	• Sadness • Loss • Anger • Ambivalence about ending • Hope for future	• Acknowledge sadness & loss • Explore importance of members, group, & leader • A time of ending and beginning	• Maintain group boundaries • Set contract • Group as a whole focus

Key issues for accomplishing this are modeling authority, countertransference and projective identification, preparation for the group, group contract including group as a whole approach, and patient selection.

2. Modeling Authority

Modeling authority based upon confidence in their own experience helps anxious men develop a sense of safety in the group. One of the crucial balancing acts the leader must perform is to support the men's characteristic approach to examining behavioral problems and looking for solutions while prompting them to examine this activity as a way to avoid feelings (31).

A female leader of a men's group presents particular issues for exploration. For many men, female authority is either maternal or unfamiliar. Men often experience conflict over their regressive desire for nurturing and then deny their shameful wishes and take a controlling and pseudomature attitude (31) .

Men may fear to identify with a woman leader because their sense of masculinity is threatened. Violent offenders often make denigrating comments about women (26,41). The female leader must be aware enough to work through her own inferiority feelings as well as her ambivalence about the role and status conflict in order to face the challenges that will necessarily be presented by the group (42).

Gans (32,33) suggests that it is crucial for the leader to avoid power struggles with the member who begins to challenge authority. Instead, the leader might appreciate that this member is often speaking for the group as a whole.

3. Countertransference and Projective Identification

Countertransference involves unresolved feelings of the therapist stirred up by a patient's transference. Countertransference feelings include competitive and retaliatory impulses as well as shame and humiliation. Gans (33) points out that the group attack on the leader's self-esteem is due to the thwarting of the leader's narcissistic wish to know all, love all, and heal all. In group work with men who have brutalized women and children, the female leader may feel contempt and revulsion; she may have difficulty feeling safe and allowing a full airing of what must be shared (31). To complicate the countertransference reactions, the men often appear terribly deprived and needy. The leader's internal dilemma is how to offer empathic contact on one hand while wishing for distance on the other.

The leader's willingness to deal with anger in group therapy will vary with his or her own early family experience, which is each leader's first group experience (33). Aversion on the therapist's part is a dangerous affect, as it results in psychological abandonment of the patient

Examples of countertransference problems include the following: (a) Group leaders may be unaware of the extent of their need for admiration and thus may miss the hate underlying the group's idealization of them. (b) Leaders may be so frightened by the extent of their dislike for one member (perhaps as a result of containing the entire group's hatred of that member) that they resort to reaction formation, experiencing the hated patient as beloved. Ideally, in response to group hostility, the leader should determine if the hostility being expressed is a resistance to group work or an integral part of it, protect the object of attack by drawing hostility onto herself where indicated, or shift the onus of responsibility for the hostility onto the group (33).

Leader mistakes in the face of hostility include the following (33):

Demonstrating preference for a "good" group rather than a hostile one by encouraging politeness rather than authenticity

Responding to an attack with retaliation

Through reaction formation, turning retaliatory impulses into apparent warmth, thus relinquishing the opportunity to understand her anger

Colluding with the group in scapegoating a hated member

Encouraging premature closure of hostile expression

Masochistically submitting to group hostility because she is unconscious of her guilt and need for punishment

Because of the leader's need to be liked, not seeing hostility in the form of disguised idealization

Responding to the hated patient with psychological termination, despite the patient's apparent interest, or with actual abandonment

Failing to set limits and permitting abusive interactions to continue because of an inability to distinguish destructive from healthy expressions of hostility

D. Preparation for the Group

To encourage referrals, the leader should meet with the heads of the clinical services and psychiatric unit nurse managers to describe the group and referral criteria. The group will receive less institutional resistance if there is strong endorsement by hospital management. This type of group will thrive best in hospitals where aggressive patient behavior is acknowledged as a serious concern.

Despite endorsement of and support for an "anger" group, there is often much anxiety, including the leader's. The leader may be initially excited about the group and at the same time overwhelmed at the complexity and enormity of the task, therefore experiencing a variety of self-doubts. Staff anxiety may be expressed in questions about the leader's knowledge in conducting this type of group and the presence of security during the group.

The issue of safety should be acknowledged in the group purpose, contract, and informed consent letter. Patients should be interviewed in a standardized, environmentally safe and secure area. In addition, attention should be given, during individual patient evaluation and screening sessions with the leader, to the patient's ambivalence about any group experience including this one, the anticipated "pros and cons" of this group, likely areas of resistance, and the importance of working in the group particularly at those times that seem to the patient to be the most problematic. Education about how a group works and what members experience is vital to help the patient form sufficient alliance with the leader to overcome the more negative aspects of group experience, such as anxiety, feeling different, and/or feeling shame.

Boundaries are considered essential to maintain safety. Attention to any violations in the group contract is required. The role of leaders, group participants, and any observers must be very clear.

1. Group Contract

Pay scrupulous attention to the contract so that members begin to incorporate it. Bion's concept of the container is central. The group structure defines "what is in and what is out." The container must be wide and deep enough for the work to be done (40). Two dangers in a group stem from affect that is out of control and affect that is not tapped (43). The group as "container" must allow an optimal level of containment of affect, allowing participants to work with the anger. The successful management of anger in a group therapy setting can lead to substantial progress on many levels: enhancing closeness, facilitating forgiveness, freeing up energy, and encouraging healthy assertiveness. Anger that remains unprocessed can lead to deep stubbornness and a resentment that can be extremely refractory to therapeutic intervention, manifesting itself as vengeance, contempt, verbal abusiveness, passive-aggressive behavior, and even violence (33). The leader's task is to build a group that is well defined contractually; this promotes a well-functioning group while supporting obsessional defenses in the face of a new and highly ambiguous situation (31). For example, start and end on time. Pay attention to and comment on the acting out rather than the verbalizing of aggression—e.g., getting out of one's chair, punching hand with fist. A limit-setting contract (e.g., no physical violence, no touching in the group) coupled with an attitude of containment helps men who are concerned about aggression, that of others as well as their own (31).

Violations of the group contract are destructive if they go unprocessed. Early in the life of the group, the group permits and forgives contractual violations in its members and becomes angry with and tries to discourage the leader who comments on the group's indulgence of such behaviors (33). By shifting the focus of attention from the offending member to the entire group, the leader confronts group resistance, interrupts developing hostility, and invites the group to assume greater ownership of its own process (33). Conversely, groups characterized by an absence of anger often have leaders who fail to monitor breaches of the contract. Such groups, however, often have high dropout rates, and their members tend not to feel safe enough to share their shameful feelings.

Focusing on the underlying process taking place in the group rather than on one particular member (group-as-a-whole approach) (30) often protects a member from further exposure while helping all members explore their part in the behavior exhibited by that particular member. For example, to focus on the issue of anger, it is important, when a shamed member attacks the group, for the leader to support the vulnerable member and help the group focus on and explore the feelings that interfered with its capacity for empathy. Once the group is running, patients begin to express evidence of the internalized contract by addressing contract violations themselves.

2. Patient Selection

MacKenzie and Prendergast (44) highlight the importance of excluding patients who are psychotic or sociopathic or who are abusing substances. McKay (45) rules out people for anger control groups who are severely depressed and describe suicidal thoughts and impulses, people with a history of physical violence, or people who have paranoid beliefs that influence their anger responses. Those who would have been excluded by McKay make up most of a group of inpatients used in a pilot study by Lanza (26). Other exclusionary criteria depend on whether the group is conducted on an inpatient or outpatient basis. With inpatient groups, there is more control over patient behaviors, and this may permit the inclusion of patients who have questionable motivation, use the group to "prove" their nonviolence for legal reasons, or have a history of high lethality. Abbott (46) similarly asserted the need to determine the propensity for the group member to act out in ways dangerous to victims before engaging such a member in outpatient treatment. Through appropriate selection of patients, the chances of encountering destructive expression of hostility are minimized. The best predictor of a positive outcome for groups dealing with violence/aggression is the willingness of a client to honestly examine and admit the consequences of poor anger control (45).

Destructive expressions of hostility (calcified anger) usually involve a sustained violation of the contract coupled with no demonstrated intention over time of taking responsibility for and working on such behavior. Examples include the following: (a) repeated, gratuitous, and hateful attacks on another member, the leader, or the entire group; (b) breaches of confidentiality; (c) sexual acting out; (d) destroying personal property or physically harming another member or the leader; and (e) prolonged silence (months or years) as an expression of hostility.

V. COUPLES/FAMILY THERAPY

The inclusion of an aggressive person in couples or family therapy requires careful and thorough assessment. Everyone must be safe in the process. It is not unusual for the therapist to be unaware of the violence occurring at the same time the family unit is involved in therapy. There can be a tragic collusion of silence. For example, the aggressor and other family members may not raise the issue of violence. The victims may feel afraid, believe that this is "normal," or that they are part of the problem. The therapist may collude by not exploring the possibility adequately.

If there is adequate monitoring and a guarantee that the aggressor will not physically attack or threaten others, family therapy can be very useful. It must be kept in mind that people are not unidimensional; therefore the aggressor may also be a vital and loved family member. Effective couples/family therapy can explore the cause, patterns, and effects of violence. Alternative family coping styles can be explored.

Many violent families remain intact. Helping them to love and relate to each other in a nonviolent way may be the best therapeutic result. However, it must be remembered that it is the aggressor who is responsible for his or her aggression. Family members are not to be scapegoated with blame.

VI. COMBINED TREATMENTS

Several authors advocate the use of a multisystem approach as opposed to just one treatment modality. Borduin et al. (47), in focusing on the treatment of serious juvenile offenders, found that multisystem therapy produced better results than individual therapy in improving key family correlates of antisocial behavior and in ameliorating adjustment problems in individual family members. Davis and Boster (2) advocate using a combination of social learning theory, cognitive psychotherapy, and creative therapy. An interesting example of a multisystem approach is the Attachment-Based Program for Conduct Disorder reported by Moretti and colleagues (48). Youths exposed to prolonged adverse socialization experiences develop attachment representations that lead them to anticipate rejecting and abusive social experiences. The nature of their attachment experiences leaves little for them to internalize to ensure emotional and behavioral self-regulation. Consequently, they rely heavily on others for these functions. In working with these youths, the authors attempt to focus the attention of the immediate and wider community on attachment issues that underlie the youth's behavior rather than on the behavior problems alone. The program involves a 30-day residential stay for the youth and involvement with the family and community groups.

VII. PROS AND CONS OF MANDATORY REPORTING

A final note of caution regarding the treatment of violent persons is the controversy surrounding mandatory reporting. Most clinicians have been made aware of the mandatory reporting laws for various types of abuse in their states. The intent of the laws is to protect victims. Long-term psychotherapy with violent patients brings the dilemma about the requirement for mandatory reporting into clear focus. Only clinicians who have never dealt with the complexities of treating a violent prone person indicate that following the mandatory reporting requirement is simple and clear. Ambivalence about mandatory reporting is related in the findings of a national survey in which approximately one-fourth of the professionals who participated failed to report child abuse because the family had already accepted treatment (49).

To begin, mandatory reporting involves the therapist in a personal conflict of interest. There is conflict about encouraging the patient to disclose information that then makes him or her vulnerable to penalty. This is a problem despite the fact that the clinician has told the patient in the very first session about the limits of confidentiality and privileged information. Second is pressure on the clinician to report all instances of suspected child abuse, often to avoid personal liability. This may skew professional judgment, forcing the therapist to weigh his or her own legal interests against the therapeutic needs of the patient (50).

Recent reports also indicate that mandatory reporting can have a detrimental effect upon reducing abuse. For example, the findings of a study at Johns Hopkins University found that a broad mandatory child-abuse reporting statute reduced the number of child abusers who voluntarily sought treatment (51). This presumably has the effect of increasing the rate of child abuse and is counterproductive if the goal of the statute is to rehabilitate child abusers (52).

VIII. CONCLUSION

Psychotherapeutic treatment of violent persons may occur both on an inpatient and an outpatient basis. Outpatient treatment can take place in an institution or a private practice. Initial treatment for the violent person may be to attend a psychoeducational program focused on aggression awareness and management. Assertiveness training can also be helpful.

Clinicians dealing with violent persons must pay particular attention to making sure that the diagnosis for depression has not been missed. Untreated depression often underlies violent behavior, particularly in the case of abusers.

Clinicians may also encounter knowledge of a patient's violence after the patient has been in treatment with the clinician for some time. This presents its own set of problems. Many times clinicians learn, after several years of therapy and after the patient has grown to trust them, about past or current violent acts. All clinicians need to be familiar with their state's mandatory reporting laws, review with each patient the limits of confidentiality during the first therapy session, and have access to both good clinical supervision and legal consultation.

In conclusion, psychotherapeutic treatment of the violent person is an arduous but extremely important task. As clinicians, we all bear responsibility for supporting the viability of the endeavor. While many clinicians may not have the skill or motivation to learn to treat violent persons, society needs clinicians, collectively, to support those who can provide such treatment. This may mean simply knowing about and referring violent patients to appropriate long-term psychotherapies. If none exist, actively encourage their development. Clinicians working with violent people are often working in relative isolation and with minimal support. Working with perpetrators does not receive the same public and professional support as does working with victims.

Clinicians must give up the tendency to dichotomize treatment and resist the pull of polarized thinking—either good or evil, victim or perpetrator. Polarizations break ideas down into neat categories and seemingly clear choices. It is also insidiously destructive, creating a wedge between people by making their differences seem insurmountable (53).

ACKNOWLEDGMENT

I wish to acknowledge the contribution (by Sally Guy, R.N.) to the material on individual therapy with the violent patient. Ms. Guy is a psychiatric nurse on the New England Medical Center/Bay Cove Community Treatment Team and a graduate student at Northeastern University School of Nursing.

REFERENCES

1. H. Toch, *Violent Men: An Inquiry into the Psychology of Violence.* American Psychological Association, Washington, DC, 1992.
2. D.L. Davis and L. Boster. Multifaceted therapeutic interventions with the violent psychiatric inpatient, *Hosp. Commun. Psychiatry 39*:867 (1988).
3. K. Tardiff, The current state of psychiatry in the treatment of violent patients, *Arch. Gen. Psychiatry 49*:493 (1992).
4. D.J. Madden, Psychotherapeutic approaches in the treatment of violent persons, *Clinical Treatment of the Violent Person*, (L.H. Roth, ed.) Guilford Press, New York, 1987, pp. 54–78.
5. G.E. Woody, A.T. McLellan, L. Luborsky, and C. O'Brien, Sociopathy and psychotherapy outcome, *Arch. Gen. Psychiatry, 42*:1081 (1985).

6. J.G. Gunderson, Personality disorders, *The New Harvard Guide to Psychiatry* (A.M. Nicholi, Jr., ed.), Harvard University Press, Cambridge, MA, 1988, pp. 337–350.
7. G.O. Gabbard, *Psychodynamic Psychiatry in Clinical Practice: The DSM-IV Edition*, American Psychiatric Press, Washington, DC, 1994.
8. O. Kernberg, Aggression, trauma, and hatred in the treatment of borderline patients, *Psychiatr. Clin. North Am. 17*:701 (1994).
9. H.R. Conte, R. Plutchik, S. Picard, and T. Karasu, Can personality traits predict psychotherapy outcome? *Compr. Psychiatry 32*:66 (1991).
10. W.H. Reid, The antisocial personality: A review, *Hosp. Commun. Psychiatry 36*:831 (1985).
11. G. Adler, *Borderline psychopathology and its treatment*, Jason Aronson, New York, 1985.
12. J.R. Meloy, *The Psychopathic Mind: Origins, Dynamics, and Treatment*, Jason Aronson, Northvale NJ, 1988.
13. O.F. Kernberg, *Severe Personality Disorders: Psychotherapeutic Strategies*, Yale University Press, New Haven, CT, 1984.
14. M.H. Stone, Psychotherapy in patients with impulsive aggression, *Impulsivity and Aggression* E. Hollander and D.J. Stein, eds., John Wiley & Sons, Chichester, England, 1995, pp. 313–331.
15. K. Tardiff, Violence, *The American Psychiatric Press Textbook of Psychiatry*, 2d ed. (R.E. Hales, S.C. Yudofsky, and J. A. Talbott, eds.), American Psychiatric Press, Washington, DC, 1994, pp. 1273–1295.
16. R.C. Marohn, Management of the assaultive adolescent, *Hosp. Commun. Psychiatry 43*:622 (1992).
17. K. Tardiff, *Concise Guide to Assessment and Management of Violent Patients*, American Psychiatric Press, Washington, DC, 1996.
18. T.G. Schramski, C.A. Feldman, D.R. Harvey, and M. Holman. The Comparative evaluation of group treatments in an adult correctional facility, *J. Group Psychother. Psychodrama Sociometry 36*(4):134 (1984).
19. R.H. Moos, *Group Environment Scale Manual*, 2d ed., Consulting Psychologists Press, Palo Alto, CA, 1981.
20. R.J. Homant, Ten years after: A follow-up of therapy effectiveness. *J. Offender Counsel. Serv. Rehabil. 10*(3):51 (1986).
21. P. Katz and F.R. Kirkland, Violence and social structure on mental hospital wards, Psychiatry 53:262 (1990).
22. A.A. Gerlock, Veterans' responses to anger management interventions, *Issues Men. Health Nurs. 15*:393 (1994).
23. A.G. Cook, A.F. Fox, C.M. Weaver, and F.G. Rooth, The Berkeley Group: Ten years' experience of a group for non-violent sex offenders, *Br. J. Psychiatry 158*:238 (1991).
24. D.G. Dutton, The outcome of court-mandated treatment for wife assault: A quasi-experiental evaluation, *Violence Victims, 1* (3):163 (1986).
25. S.E. Palmer, R.A. Brown, and M.E. Barrera. Group treatment for abusive husbands: Long term evaluation. *Am. J. Orthopsychiatry 62* (2):276 (1992).

26. M.L. Lanza, H. Satz, J. Stone, and H. Kayne, Assessing the impact of group treatment for aggressive inpatients, *Group 19*:195 (1996).
27. E. Stein and J.D. Brown, Group therapy in a forensic setting, *Canad. J. Psychiatry 36*:718 (1991)
28. M.L. Lanza, H. Satz, J. Stone, and H. Kayne. Developing psychodynamic group treatment methods for aggressive, *Issues Ment. Health Nurs. 17*:5 (1996).
29. Y.M. Agazarian, Phases of group development, *The Visible and Invisible Group* (Y.M. Agazarian, R. Peters, and P. Kegan, eds.), Routledge, London, 1981, pp. 124–147.
30. J.S. Rutan and W.N. Stone, *Psychodynamic Group Psychotherapy*, 2d ed. Guilford Press, New York, 1993.
31. S. Krugman and S. Osherson, Men in group therapy, *Group Therapy in Clinical Practice* (A. Alonson and H.I. Swiller, eds.), American Psychiatric Press, Washington, DC, 1993, pp. 393–420.
32. J Gans, On the use of hostility in groups, *Int. J. Group Psychother. 39*:499 (1990).
33. J.S. Gans, Dealing with anger in psychodynamic group therapy, *Direct. Psychiatry 14(12)*:1 (1994).
34. S. Scheidlinger, On the concept of the mother-group, *Int. J. Group Psychother. 244*:17 (1974).
35. R. Fine, Understanding men's emotional problems, *Troubled Men.* (R. Fine, ed.), Jossey-Bass, San Francisco, 1988, pp. 1–24.
36. T. MacNab, What do men want? Male rituals of initiation in group psychotherapy, *Int. J. Group Psychother. 40*:139 (1990).
37. E. Fried, Individuation through group psychotherapy, *Int. J. Group Psychother. 4*:450 (1970).
38. L.R. Ormont, The leader's role in dealing with aggression in groups, *Int. J. Group Psychother. 34*:553 (1984).
39. H.D. Kibel, Inpatient group psychotherapy, *Group Therapy in Clinical Practice* (A. Alonso and H.I. Swiller, eds.), American Psychiatric Press, Washington, DC, 1993, pp. 93–109.
40. W.R. Bion, *Learning from Experience*. Basic Books, New York, 1962.
41. R. Eisenman, Denigration of a victim in group psychotherapy by violent vs seductive sex offenders, *Psychol. Rep. 72*:413 (1993).
42. A. Alonso and J.S. Rutan, Women in group therapy, *Int. J. Group Psychother.* 29:481 (1979).
43. H. Bernard, Anger and Aggression in group treatment: Contrasting views, Presentation at N.S.G.P. Thirteenth Annual Regional Conference, Wellesley College, Wellesley, MA, June 18, 1994.
44. A. MacKenzie and J. Prendergast, Domestic violence offender groups, *Focal Group Psychotherapy* (M. McKay and K. Paleg, eds.), New Harbinger Publications, Oakland, CA, 1992, pp. 419–459.
45. M. McKay, Anger control groups, *Focal Group Psychotherapy*, (M. McKay and K. Paleg, eds.), New Harbinger Publications, Oakland, CA, 1992, pp. 163–194.
46. B.R. Abbott, Group therapy for adult incest offenders and adolescent child molesters, *Focal Group Psychotherapy* (M. McKay and K. Paleg, eds.), New Harbinger Publications, 1992, pp. 359–417.

47. C.M. Borduin, L.T. Cone, B.J. Mann, S.W. Henggeler, B.R. Fucci, D.M. Blaske, and R.A. Williams, *J. Consult. Clin. Psychology 63*:569 (1995).
48. M.M. Moretti, R. Holland, and Peterson, Attachment-based program for conduct disorder. *Can. J. Psychiatry 39*:360 (1994).
49. D. Finklehor and G. Zellman, Flexible reporting options for skilled child abuse professionals, *Child Abuse Neglect 15*:335 (1991).
50. R.D. Miller, and R. Weinstock, Conflict of interest between therapist-patient confidentiality and the duty to report sexual abuse of children, *Behav. Sci. Law 5*:161 (1987).
51. F.S. Berlin, H.M. Malin, and S. Dean, Effects of statutes requiring psychiatrists to report suspected abuse of children. *Am. J. Psychiatry 148*:449 (1991).
52. M Smith-Bell and W.M. Winslade, Privacy, confidentiality, and privilege in psychotherapeutic relationships, *Am. J. Orthopsychiatry 64*(2): (1994).
53. K. Hardy, Embracing both/and, *Networker* 42 (1995).

14

Posttraumatic Stress Disorders in Victims of Violence

Matthew J. Friedman
National Center for Posttraumatic Stress Disorder, White River Junction, Vermont, and Dartmouth Medical School, Hanover, New Hampshire

Martha S. was a 32-year-old single white, graduate of a prestigious northeastern business school, now embarked upon a highly successful career at a major midwestern corporation. She lived alone in an upscale garden apartment that had security guards on duty around the clock. One night, after returning home from a dinner party, she entered her living room to discover two bearded men in shabby clothes robbing her apartment. Before she could flee or cry out, the taller of the two grabbed her by the hair, covered her face with a pillow, and threw her down on the couch. While he held her down, his partner tore off her clothes and raped her. When he was done, his partner did the same. When the partner had finished, he pulled out a knife and stabbed her through the ribs so deeply that the knife penetrated her heart. She remembers how terrified she was throughout the episode, the excruciating pain in her chest from the knife wound, and the overwhelming fear that she was about to die. She has no further memories of the two assailants who escaped with her television, jewelry, and other prized possessions. What she does remember is the blood oozing out of her chest. She remembers how it smelled and how warm and slippery it was as she crawled on her belly across the living room rug, somehow getting through the front door, and reaching her neighbor's apartment across the hall. She does not really remember ringing his doorbell or telling him what had happened. She must have succeeded, however, since an ambulance was called and she was rapidly transported to the hospital. She survived the open-heart surgery and convalesced without complications.

After discharge from the hospital she went immediately to her hometown in New England to stay with her mother for several months until she felt strong enough to return to work. She was very optimistic on the eve of her return back to the Midwest. She enjoyed the plane trip and felt good on the taxi ride in from the airport. When she entered her apartment, however, she was overwhelmed by growing anxiety, especially in the living room. When darkness fell, the anxiety escalated to terror. She began to have vivid recollections of her two assailants and from time to time thought that she actually saw them hiding behind the living room curtains, although she knew that her mind was playing tricks on her. She also knew that she could not stand to be alone in her apartment and left to spend the night with a girlfriend who lived nearby.

She never returned to her apartment except to get her things and move elsewhere. Even in her new lodgings, however, she felt unsafe, especially after dark, and had frequent nightmares about the rape. It was difficult for her to perform at work as before. Her attempts to focus on work were constantly interrupted by trauma-related images and she could not experience the old excitement and enjoyment of the vocational challenges that she had relished months before. She found herself obsessed with fears about her personal safety. Whereas previously she had been open, adventurous, and gregarious, she was now fearful, withdrawn, suspicious, and jumpy. She abruptly discontinued what had been a satisfying sexual relationship with a man for whom she cared, and she became panic-stricken when bearded men, especially bearded men wearing shabby clothes, came anywhere near her.

Martha S. is suffering from posttraumatic stress disorder (PTSD). Based on recent epidemiological data (1), 10.4% of all American women and 5% of all American men will also develop PTSD at some point in their lives. Using this clinical vignette as the frame of reference, this chapter begins by describing the clinical phenomenology and diagnostic criteria for this disorder. Next, it reviews the epidemiology of PTSD, especially when it has been precipitated by interpersonal violence. Understanding the pathophysiology of PTSD is of great importance from both a scientific and clinical perspective. Scientifically, the abnormalities associated with PTSD can best be understood as manifestations of fundamental psychological processes that mediate learning and appraisal and as manifestations of fundamental neurobiological mechanisms that mediate coping, and adaptation to stress. Clinically, a rational approach to PTSD treatment can be conceptualized only by designing interventions that specifically address the complex pathophysiology of this disorder. Following a review of current PTSD treatment, the chapter describes some major controversies in the field of psychotraumatology. Finally, an agenda for future research is presented.

I. CLINICAL PHENOMENOLOGY AND DIAGNOSTIC CRITERIA

Individuals can only develop PTSD if they have been exposed to a traumatic event. As operationalized in the fourth edition of the *Diagnostic and Statistical Manual of Mental Disorders* DSM-IV (2) and shown in Table 1 (as the "Al" criterion), traumatic events "involve actual or threatened death or serious injury, or a threat to the physical integrity of oneself or others." Certainly the near lethal and sexual assault experienced by Martha S. meets this definition, as does exposure to war, torture, genocide, nuclear attack, natural disasters, or industrial accidents. When PTSD was first introduced as a diagnostic entity in the DSM-III (3), it was thought that such events were "beyond the range of normal human experience." Alas, we have learned since that time that exposure to trauma is not a rare event. As shown in Table 2 (abstracted from Ref. 1), more than half of all American men (60.7%) and women (51.2%) have been exposed to at least one traumatic event in the course of their lives. With respect to interpersonal violence (rape, molestation, physical attack, and physical abuse), twice as many women (33.2%) as men (17.8%) have been traumatized. This difference may be responsible for the higher PTSD rates observed among women than men, as discussed further on.

All adverse events are not traumatic. Indeed, very painful stressors such as divorce, failure, rejection, serious illness, financial reverses, and the like do not meet the DSM-IV A1 criterion. Serious psychological reactions to such vicissitudes of life are characterized as adjustment disorders rather than PTSD. This dichotomization between traumatic and other stressors is based on the assumption that although most individuals have the ability to cope with ordinary stress, their adaptive capacities may be overwhelmed by a traumatic stressor.

Clinical experience with the PTSD diagnosis has shown that most people who are exposed to a catastrophic event do not develop PTSD. Indeed, there are vast individual differences regarding the capacity to cope with a traumatic event, and different people may have different psychological responses to the same catastrophe. Such observations have prompted a recognition that trauma, like pain, is not an external phenomenon that can be completely objectified. Like pain, the traumatic experience is filtered through a cognitive and emotional process called *appraisal.* Therefore, the same event may be appraised by some as a severe threat, while others will consider it a challenge with which they can cope. Because appraisal plays such an important role in the psychological processing of a catastrophic event, DSM-IV added the "A2" criterion (Table 1) to the definition of trauma; "the individual's response must involve an intense emotional reaction such as fear, helplessness, or horror." In other words, exposure to a catastrophic event can be considered traumatic only if such exposure precipitates an intense

Table 1 Proposed DSM-IV Criteria for PTSD

A. The person has been exposed to a traumatic event in which both of the following have been present:
   (1) the person has experienced, witnessed, or been confronted with an event or events that involve actual or threatened death or serious injury, or a threat to the physical integrity of oneself or others
   (2) the person's response involved intense fear, helplessness, or horror. Note: in children, it may be expressed instead by disorganized or agitated behavior

B. The traumatic event is persistently reexperienced in at least one of the following ways:
   (1) recurrent and intrusive distressing recollections of the event, including images, thoughts, or perceptions. Note: in young children, repetitive play may occur in which themes or aspects of the trauma are expressed
   (2) recurrent distressing dreams of the event. Note: in children, there may be frightening dreams without recognizable content
   (3) acting or feeling as if the traumatic event were recurring (includes a sense of reliving the experience, illusions, hallucinations, and dissociative flashback episodes, including those that occur upon awakening or when intoxicated). Note: in young children, trauma-specific reenactment may occur.
   (4) intense psychological distress at exposure to internal or external cues that symbolize or resemble an aspect of the traumatic event
   (5) physiologic reactivity upon exposure to internal or external cues that symbolize or resemble an aspect of the traumatic event

C. Persistent avoidance of stimuli associated with the trauma and numbing of general responsiveness (not present before the trauma), as indicated by at least three of the following:
   (1) efforts to avoid thoughts, feelings, or conversations associated with the trauma
   (2) efforts to avoid activities, places, or people that arouse recollections of the trauma
   (3) inability to recall an important aspect of the trauma
   (4) markedly diminished interest or participation in significant activities
   (5) feeling of detachment or estrangement from others
   (6) restricted range of affect (e.g., unable to have loving feelings)
   (7) sense of a foreshortened future (e.g., does not expect to have a career, marriage, children, or a normal life span)

D. Persistent symptoms of increased arousal (not present before the trauma), as indicated by at least two of the following:
   (1) difficulty falling or staying asleep
   (2) irritability or outbursts of anger
   (3) difficulty concentrating
   (4) hypervigilance
   (5) exaggerated startle response

E. Duration of the disturbance (symptoms in B, C, and D) is more than one month.

(*continued*)

Table 1 Continued

F. The disturbance causes clinically significant distress or impairment in social, occupational, or other important areas of functioning.

Specify if:

Acute: if duration of symptoms is less than three months

Chronic: if duration of symptoms is three months or more

Specify if:

With Delayed Onset: onset of symptoms at least six months after the stressor

emotional reaction. This is certainly true for Martha S., who was terrified, painfully injured, and fearful that she would die during her terrible ordeal. Although appraisal is an important issue in many catastrophic events, such as accidents and natural disasters, the experience of most people exposed to interpersonal violence usually meets the DSM-IV definition of trauma.

The "B" or reexperiencing criterion includes symptoms that are perhaps the most distinctive and readily identifiable manifestations of this disorder. For individuals with PTSD, the traumatic event remains, sometimes for decades or a lifetime, a dominating psychological experience that retains its power to evoke panic, terror, dread, grief, or despair in the face of intrusive daytime recollections, traumatic nightmares, and psychotic re-enactments known as PTSD flashbacks. For Martha S., such reexperiencing flashbacks were so severe that she had

Table 2 Lifetime Prevalence of Trauma Experience

Trauma	Men (%) ($N = 2812$)	Women (%) ($N = 3065$)
Any trauma	60.7	51.2
Number of traumas		
1	25.6	26.3
2	14.5	13.5
3	9.5	5.0
4	10.2	6.4
Rape[a]	0.7	9.2
Molestation[a]	2.8	12.3
Physical attack[a]	11.1	6.9
Physical abuse[a]	3.2	4.8
Combat	6.4	0.0
Threat with weapon	19.0	6.8
Accident	25.0	13.8
Natural disaster with fire	18.9	15.2

[a]Interpersonal violence.

Source: Adapted from Ref. 1.

to move from her apartment, could not keep her mind on her work, and altered her behavior and lifestyle significantly. PTSD symptoms are often triggered by stimuli or situations that are reminiscent of the initial traumatic event. For that reason, researchers can reproduce PTSD symptoms in the laboratory by exposing affected individuals to stimuli associated with the original traumatic event (4,5). That is why fear conditioning has been proposed as one conceptual model for PTSD (6). Martha S. exhibited this phenomenon in a number of ways. First, she became initially symptomatic when reexposed to the stimuli of her apartment, where she had been raped and almost murdered. Her symptoms intensified at night (the time of the trauma), when it became dark. She became so terrified that she had PTSD flashbacks in which she "saw" her assailants hiding behind the curtains. She terminated a sexual relationship, which she had previously enjoyed, partly because stimuli associated with sexual activity triggered intolerable recollections of the rape. Finally, her new fear of bearded men, based on this distinguishing facial characteristic of both assailants, shows how trauma-related stimuli can change the behavior of a woman who had never exhibited such fears before she was raped and almost killed. This also illustrates how PTSD patients appraise the world as a dangerous place and become easily alarmed by any stimulus that has become associated with the traumatic experience.

The "C" or avoidant/numbing criterion consists of symptoms reflecting behavioral, cognitive, or emotional strategies by which PTSD patients attempt to reduce the likelihood that they will expose themselves to trauma-related stimuli or, if exposed, will minimize the intensity of their psychological response. Behavioral strategies include avoiding any situation in which PTSD patients perceive a risk of confronting such stimuli. In its most extreme manifestation, avoidant behavior may superficially resemble agoraphobia, because the person with PTSD is afraid to leave the house for fear of confronting reminders of the traumatic event(s). For Martha S., avoidant behaviors included moving out of her apartment, avoiding social situations, terminating a sexual relationship, and avoiding bearded men.

Numbing symptoms are psychological rather than behavioral strategies by which individuals reduce or obliterate the conscious experience of trauma-based memories and feelings. Such symptoms include amnesia for traumatic events, dissociation, feelings of detachment, and a restricted range of affect. Individuals with PTSD cannot tolerate strong emotions, especially those associated with the traumatic experience. They separate the cognitive from the emotional aspects of psychological experiences and perceive only the former. Such "psychic numbing" is an emotional anesthesia that makes it extremely difficult for people with PTSD to participate in meaningful interpersonal relationships. That is another reason why Martha S. terminated her relationship with the man with whom she had previously enjoyed a very satisfactory emotional and sexual relationship.

Criterion "D" includes arousal symptoms such as insomnia, irritability, and inability to concentrate (all exhibited by Martha S.); these are often found in other anxiety disorders such as panic and generalized anxiety disorder. Hypervigilance and an exaggerated startle response (both also exhibited by Martha S.) are more characteristic of PTSD. Hypervigilance is a manifestation of the traumatized person's perpetual surveillance of his or her environment to detect any signs of danger that might provoke another traumatic episode. The hypervigilance in PTSD may sometimes become so intense as to appear like frank paranoia. The agitation and jumpiness seen in PTSD patients is a manifestation of the exaggerated startle response, a hard-wired neurological reflex that is abnormally resistant to extinction in patients with this disorder (6,7).

Martha S. also met the "E" criterion, because her symptoms persisted for more than a month, and the "F" criterion, because her PTSD caused clinically significant distress and impairment in several functional domains.

II. EPIDEMIOLOGY

In the National Comorbidity Survey, Kessler and associates (1) reported that the lifetime prevalence of PTSD among American men and women was 5.0 and 10.4% respectively. As shown in Table 3, lifetime prevalence among men and women who have actually been traumatized is 8.1 and 20.4%, respectively. It is important to emphasize, in this regard, that the majority of people exposed to a traumatic event do not develop PTSD. For women, especially, exposure to interpersonal violence (rape, molestation, physical attack, and physical abuse) is particularly predictive of the later development of PTSD. Rape is a relatively rare

Table 3 Association of Specific Traumas with PTSD

Trauma	Men (%) (*N* = 2812)	Women (%) (*N* = 3065)
Any trauma	8.1	20.4
Rape[a]	65.0	45.9
Molestation[a]	12.2	26.5
Physical attack[a]	1.8	21.3
Physical abuse[a]	22.3	48.5
Combat	38.8	–
Threat with weapon	1.9	32.6
Accident	6.3	8.8
Natural disaster with fire	3.7	7.5

[a]Interpersonal violence.
Source: Adapted from Ref. 1.

event for men (0.7%) as compared with women (9.2%), as shown in Table 2; however, when it does occur, it is much more likely to cause PTSD among men (65.0%) than among women (45.9%), as shown in Table 3. These data also demonstrate that exposure to interpersonal violence is more likely to cause PTSD than a traumatic event that lacks a human perpetrator, such as a natural disaster with fire.

In general, epidemiological research on PTSD has focused on a limited number of selected populations at risk, such as military veterans, sexual assault survivors, and natural disaster survivors (see comprehensive review, Ref. 8, for further references), although a few investigators have studied the prevalence of PTSD among victims of crime (9,10). Even the literature on the Nazi holocaust has been inconsistent in relating its results to PTSD (see Refs. 11 and 12). In general, much less attention has been paid to cohorts exposed to domestic violence, urban violence, physical abuse, child abuse, or other traumas. Indeed, from a PTSD perspective, it is frustrating to contemplate the large literature in the abuse and violence field because it usually does not go far enough. It is not enough to know whether an individual has been exposed to sexual/physical abuse or domestic/urban violence, since the majority of traumatized people do not develop PTSD.

From this perspective, it is equally important to know whether a given traumatic experience resulted in PTSD or not. Therefore, it is encouraging that a number of recent reviews have conceptualized interpersonal violence from a PTSD perspective with respect to partner violence (13–16); child abuse (16–18); torture (19,20); and shooting and hostage situations among children (21). In epidemological research on infectious diseases, both vector (infectious agent) and host (susceptibility to infection) factors are considered important. We must do the same in PTSD research and address both vector (traumatic exposure) and host (vulnerability to PTSD) factors.

In order to understand why some traumatized people develop PTSD while most do not, it is useful to consider three different domains in which individual differences may affect vulnerability: appraisal tendencies, constitutional/genetic variables, and specific risk factors. First, as noted earlier, the appraisal or subjective response to a traumatic event may differ from one individual to another. Some people may be more likely to perceive situations as frightening or threatening than others. That is why the DSM-IV definition of trauma has been expanded to stipulate that exposed individuals must experience "intense fear, helplessness, or horror" (the "A2" criterion) for that exposure to be considered "traumatic." Second, Yehuda and McFarlane (22) have hypothesized that there is a constitutional vulnerability that distinguishes traumatized people who develop PTSD from the majority of traumatized people who never exhibit the disorder. It is interesting, in this regard, to consider the early work of Cohen and associates (23) on World War II veterans with "neurocirculatory asthenia" (NCA).

Many if not most of these veterans appear to have had what would now be called PTSD. After characterizing the medical and psychiatric symptoms of these individuals, Cohen et al. went on to conduct family studies, since they had concluded that there was a genetically mediated vulnerability for NCA (24). In that regard, it might be said that almost 50 years ago, Cohen et al. anticipated Yehuda and McFarlane's hypothesis regarding a constitutional vulnerability to PTSD. Evidence for a genetic risk for developing PTSD has also been obtained from a study of male monozygotic twins who served in Vietnam and were compared with their identical siblings who also served in the military but not in Vietnam (25).

III. RISK FACTORS FOR PTSD

The third domain in which individuals differ with respect to vulnerability to develop PTSD concerns specific risk factors. In considering risk factors for PTSD, it is useful to divide them into pretraumatic, traumatic, and posttraumatic categories. Pretraumatic risk factors that have been identified in a number of studies (see review by Fairbank et al., Ref. 8) include (a) familial psychiatric illness; (b) parental poverty; (c) childhood trauma (e.g., sexual assault, parents separated or divorced before child reached age 10); (d) childhood behavior disorder; (e) neuroticism; (f) introversion; (g) prior psychiatric disorder; (h) adverse life events before and after the trauma; (i) being female and between the ages of 36 and 50; (j) being concerned about finances; and (k) having had prior physical health problems. In the National Comorbidity Survey (1), PTSD was most prevalent among women, the previously married, and persons of lower socioeconomic status.

Such pretraumatic risk factors play a small but significant role in predicting PTSD prevalence. Much more important predictors are aspects of the traumatic event itself: severity of exposure; whether a person was injured during the episode; for Vietnam veterans, whether the individual witnessed or participated in atrocities (26); and for rape victims, whether the victim had prior acquaintance with the perpetrator or whether her life was threatened at the time of the rape (27). Indeed, a robust finding in almost all PTSD research has been a linear dose-response curve between severity of the trauma and the later development of PTSD (28–30) (see Ref. 8 for other references).

Characteristics of the posttraumatic environment have also been shown to be related to the later development of PTSD. Among Vietnam veterans, low levels of postmilitary social support and dysfunctional patterns of social interaction have been shown to increase the risk for PTSD (26–31). Similar findings regarding the deleterious impact of low posttraumatic social support have been shown for rape victims (32,33). Finally, there has been considerable speculation regarding the importance of rapid posttraumatic clinical interventions such as critical incident stress debriefing (CISD). Mitchell (34) has maintained that when CISD is provided as soon after the trauma as possible, it will prevent the later development of PTSD. This is currently a matter of controversy, however, as discussed below.

IV. COMORBIDITY

If an individual meets diagnostic criteria for PTSD, it is likely that he or she will exhibit at least one other DSM-IV disorder (28,35). In the National Comorbidity Survey, a lifetime history of at least one other psychiatric disorder was found in approximately 80% of all men and women with lifetime PTSD. Among men and women with PTSD, lifetime prevalence of comorbid disorders was approximately 48% for major depressive disorders, 22% for dysthymia, 16% for generalized anxiety disorder, 30% for simple phobia, and 28% for social phobia. Women exhibited greater lifetime prevalence of panic disorder (12.6 to 7.3%) and agoraphobia (22.4 to 16.1%), while men exhibited greater lifetime prevalence of alcohol abuse/dependence (51.9 to 27.9%), drug abuse/dependence (34.5 to 26.9%), and conduct disorder (43.3 to 15.4%) (1).

We have argued elsewhere (36) that high rates of comorbid disorders associated with PTSD may actually reflect shortcomings of a nosology (e.g., DSM-IV) that is predicated entirely on phenomenological observations. For example, there is strong neurobiological evidence suggesting that the major depressive disorder (MDD) usually associated with PTSD is different with respect to adrenocortical function from true melancholia. MDD patients without PTSD are often dexamethasone nonsuppressors, while those with PTSD are often dexamethasone supersuppressors (37). In other words, PTSD plus MDD may not reflect two comorbid disorders (as dictated by current DSM-IV diagnostic decision rules) but rather a depressive subtype of PTSD that is neurobiologically distinct from classic melancholia, or MDD. These considerations may also apply to certain anxiety disorders when they are comorbid with PTSD. Clearly, this is an important and exciting focus for future research.

V. LONGITUDINAL COURSE AND CHRONICITY

Studies of World War II military veterans and Dutch anti-Nazi resistance fighters have shown that PTSD can persist for decades (see review, Ref. 38). Furthermore, symptoms may actually worsen rather than improve over time. Data from the National Comorbidity Survey suggest that approximately 40% of patients with lifetime PTSD are unlikely to recover whether or not they have ever received treatment. For others, the longitudinal course, as with other chronic medical and psychiatric disorders, is a series of remissions and relapses. When a patient with lifetime PTSD who had been clinically asymptomatic suddenly begins to exhibit the full PTSD pattern of clinical symptoms, the immediate precipitant is usually a situation that resembles the original trauma in a significant way. For example, we might expect that a fully recovered Martha S. who had been asymptomatic for many years might experience a relapse were she again exposed to sexual harassment or assault or even if she learned that her daughter had been sexually traumatized.

As with other medical and psychiatric disorders, PTSD may differ in severity from one person to the next. Some people with this disorder are able to lead productive and fulfilling lives. Others, however, may develop a persistent incapacitating mental illness marked by severe and intolerable symptoms; marital, social, and vocational disability; and extensive use of psychiatric and community services. Such people can often be found on the fringes of society, in homeless shelters, or enrolled in public-sector programs designed for patients with persistent mental illnesses such as schizophrenia, from whom they are superficially indistinguishable (39).

VI. CROSS-NATIONAL AND CROSS-CULTURAL CONSIDERATIONS

The epidemiological and comorbidity data presented previously are derived from studies of American men and women. Surveys of PTSD in other nations have yet to be done. Extrapolating from current research findings, however, it seems likely that PTSD prevalence will be much higher in nations where the probability of exposure to interpersonal violence and war is great. Indeed, nations such as Rwanda, Bosnia, and Cambodia, in which unspeakable violence has been perpetrated within a genocidal context, can be expected to exhibit PTSD prevalence that greatly exceeds that found in the United States.

There have been a number of criticisms of the PTSD diagnosis from a cross-cultural perspective. These include (a) conceptualizing PTSD as a culture-bound syndrome; (b) rejecting PTSD for failing to incorporate unique psychohistorical dimensions that define the meaning of trauma; and (c) rejecting PTSD as a construct because it pathologizes a normal and healthy rehabilitative process that is more suitably characterized as cultural bereavement. We disagree with these criticisms and have argued elsewhere that the PTSD construct has both culture-bound and universal dimensions (40). That is not to say, however, that there may not be other culture-specific idioms of distress, such as *calor* or *atiques de nervios*, that may fall outside strict DSM-IV diagnostic criteria but are significant indicators of clinically significant posttraumatic distress in their own right (41). In this regard, PTSD may be only one of a spectrum of posttraumatic syndromes that need further explication in future research and clinical practice.

VII. PATHOPHYSIOLOGY

A thorough discussion of the current state of knowledge on the pathophysiology of PTSD is beyond the scope of this chapter. A more comprehensive overview can be found in our recent book (42). Kardiner (43) first proposed that "traumatic neurosis" among World War I veterans was a physioneurosis marked by autonomic hyperarousal, exaggerated startle reflexes, and disturbed sleep. Kolb (6), invoking Kardiner's seminal observations, suggested that altered limbic system functioning produced by trauma-induced fear conditioning represented a fundamental abnormality in PTSD. Since then, a number of biobehavioral models have been proposed for PTSD including inescapable stress, fear conditioning, failure of extinction, behavioral sensitization, and kindling (44–47). We have proposed that humans exposed to catastrophic stressors utilize the same neurobiological mechanisms that are activated following exposure to a less severe, "normal" stressor. We have further proposed that failure to cope with traumatic stress successfully has significant neurobiological consequences (42). It is necessary to understand these abnormalities, and once understood, to develop interventions that will apply this fundamental knowledge to clinical situations. The search for effective treatments demands that fundamental laboratory paradigms—heretofore utilized only in basic research on learning, appraisal, stress, and coping—be modified so that clinical abnormalities associated, with PTSD may be subjected to the most rigorous laboratory investigations.

VIII. TREATMENT

Many therapeutic approaches have been advocated for PTSD, including psychodynamic therapy (48); cognitive-behavioral therapy (49); pharmacotherapy (50); group, family, couples, and inpatient treatment (51,52); and treatment for patients dually diagnosed with PTSD and alcoholism/substance abuse (53). Herman (27) has shown that therapists working with patients who have survived different kinds of traumatic events (war, natural disasters, etc.) generally agree that therapy can be divided into three phases: (a) establishing trust, safety, and "earning the right to gain access" to carefully guarded traumatic material (54; p. 806); (b) trauma-focused therapy—exploring traumatic material in depth and titrating intrusive recollections with avoidant/numbing symptoms (55); and (c) helping the patient disconnect from the trauma and reconnect with family, friends, and society. It should be noted that patients who reach the third phase have achieved some resolution of trauma-specific concerns and are ready to concentrate, almost exclusively, on here-and-now issues concerning marriage, family, work, and other current issues (27,54,56).

Marmar and associates (48) have suggested that there are five identifiable posttraumatic syndromes, each requiring a different treatment approach: normal stress response, acute catastrophic stress reaction, uncomplicated PTSD, PTSD comorbid with other disorders, and posttraumatic personality. The *normal stress response* occurs when healthy adults who have been exposed to a single discrete traumatic event in adulthood experience intense intrusive recollections, numbing, denial, feelings of unreality, and arousal. It has become generally (but not universally—see below) accepted that most individuals will achieve complete recovery following rapid posttraumatic individual or group interventions such as critical incident stress debriefing (CISD) (34,57,58). Often a single 2-hour group debriefing experience is all that is needed. Such sessions begin by describing the traumatic event. They then progress to an exploration of survivors' emotional responses to the event. Next, there is an open discussion of symptoms precipitated by the trauma. Finally, there is a resolution, in which survivors' responses are normalized and adaptive coping strategies are identified. Recent studies, however, have challenged the effectiveness of CISD. Kenardy and associates (59) reported that Australian emergency workers did not benefit from debriefing following an earthquake, while Bisson (60) reported that British burn trauma victims randomly assigned to CISD had worse outcomes than those who did not receive debriefing. In view of the general worldwide belief in the efficacy of CISD and the lack of randomized clinical trials to support this belief, this is a very important area for current and future research.

Acute catastrophic stress reactions are characterized by panic reactions, cognitive disorganization, disorientation, dissociation, severe insomnia, tics and other movement disorders, paranoid reactions, and incapacity to manage even basic self-care, work, and interpersonal functions (61). Treatment includes immediate support, removal from the scene of the trauma, use of anxiolytic medication for immediate relief of anxiety and insomnia, and brief supportive, aggressive, dynamic psychotherapy provided in the context of crisis intervention (48).

Uncomplicated PTSD may respond to group, psychodynamic, cognitive, behavioral, pharmacological, or combination approaches. During the past 10 years we have come to appreciate the powerful therapeutic potential of positive peer group treatment as practiced in Vet Centers for military veterans and in rape crisis centers for sexual assault and domestic violence victims. Peer groups provide an excellent therapeutic setting for trauma survivors because the participants' posttraumatic emotions, memories, and behaviors are validated, normalized, understood, and destigmatized. They are able to risk sharing traumatic material in presence of the safety, cohesion, and empathy provided by fellow trauma survivors. It is often much easier to accept confrontation from a fellow sufferer who has impeccable credentials as a trauma survivor than from a professional therapist who never went through those experiences personally. When group members achieve greater understanding and resolution of traumatic themes, they must next integrate such themes with their current lives and focus on the present rather than the past (27,56).

In brief psychodynamic psychotherapy, trauma survivors focus on the traumatic event itself. Through the retelling of the traumatic event to a calm, empathetic, compassionate and nonjudgmental therapist, the patient achieves a greater sense of self-cohesion, develops more adaptive defenses and coping strategies, and more successfully modulates the intense emotions that emerge during therapy (48). The therapist must constantly address the linkage between posttraumatic and current life stress by helping the patient to identify current life situations that set off traumatic memories and exacerbate PTSD symptoms.

There are two cognitive-behavioral approaches: exposure therapy and cognitive-behavioral therapy (CBT). Exposure therapy includes systematic desensitization on the one hand and imaginal and in vivo techniques such as flooding on the other. In general, flooding has been much more effective than systematic desensitization. The second approach, cognitive-behavioral therapy, includes a variety of anxiety-management training strategies for reducing anxiety, such as relaxation training, stress inoculation training, cognitive restructuring, breathing retraining, biofeedback, social skills training, and distraction techniques (62,63). Foa and associates (64,65) have shown that flooding and anxiety management training are both effective for rape victims with PTSD. They have also speculated that a CBT approach including a combination of exposure and cognitive restructuring might be the most effective one for PTSD (66).

Group treatment has long been a mainstay of PTSD treatment, although there are few systematic evaluations of it. An important exception is the work of Resick and associates (52), who have conducted a series of clinical trials of group psychotherapy with rape victims with PTSD. Their approach is called cognitive processing therapy (CPT), which includes education, exposure, and cognitive components. This group approach shares many of the components used by Foa and associates in individual CBT therapy.

Given our expanding understanding of the many neurobiological abnormalities associated with PTSD (42), pharmacotherapy appears to have a place in PTSD treatment. From a practical perspective, there is no question that drugs can provide some symptomatic relief of anxiety, depression, and insomnia, whether or not they ameliorate core PTSD intrusive and avoidant/numbing symptoms. At this time no particular drug has emerged as a definitive treatment for

PTSD, although medication is clearly useful for symptom relief, thereby making it possible for patients to participate in group, psychodynamic, cognitive-behavioral, or other forms of psychotherapy. In most but not all randomized clinical trials, improvement has been achieved with antidepressants such as imipramine, amitriptyline, phenelzine, and fluoxetine. Results have been mixed, probably because of cohort differences in PTSD severity and chronicity. Promising results in uncontrolled trials indicate that further testing is warranted for antiadrenergic agents such as clonidine and propranolol and for anticonvulsant/antikindling agents such as carbamazepine and valproate (50). I have suggested (67) that the most effective pharmacotherapeutic approaches in the future may involve drugs that address the unique pathophysiology of PTSD. In this regard, corticotropin releasing factor (CRF) antagonists, currently being developed for human trials, appear to be an extremely promising family of drugs to test with PTSD patients.

PTSD comorbid with other DSM-IV Axis I disorders is actually much more common than uncomplicated PTSD. As noted earlier, PTSD is usually associated with at least one other major psychiatric disorder, such as depression, alcohol/substance abuse, panic disorder, and other anxiety disorders (1). Sometimes the comorbid disorder is the presenting complaint that requires immediate attention. At other times, the PTSD appears to be the major problem. In general, the best results are achieved when both PTSD and the comorbid disorder(s) are treated concurrently rather than one after the other. This is especially true for PTSD and alcohol/substance abuse (53,68). Treatment previously described for uncomplicated PTSD should also be used for these patients.

Posttraumatic personality disorder is found among individuals who have been exposed to prolonged traumatic circumstances, especially during childhood, such as childhood sex abuse. These individuals often meet DSM-IV criteria for diagnoses such as borderline personality disorder, somatoform disorder, and dissociative identity disorder (multiple personality disorder). Such patients exhibit behavioral difficulties (such as impulsivity, aggression, sexual acting out, eating disorders, alcohol/drug abuse, and self-destructive actions), emotional difficulties (such as affect lability, rage, depression, panic), and cognitive difficulties (such as fragmented thoughts, dissociation, and amnesia). Treatment generally focuses on behavioral and affect management in a here-and-now context, with emphasis on family function, vocational rehabilitation, social skills training, and alcohol/drug rehabilitation. Long-term individual and group treatments have been described for such patients by Herman (27), Koller et al. (69), and Scurfield (56). Dialectical behavior therapy, a cognitive behavioral group approach developed by Linehan and her associates for chronically suicidal borderline patients (70), may also have a role in the treatment of posttraumatic personality disorder. Trauma-focused treatment should be initiated only after long therapeutic preparation. Inpatient treatment may be needed to provide adequate safety and safeguards before a therapeutic exploration of traumatic themes is undertaken. The three phases of treatment described earlier apply to these patients as well as those with uncomplicated PTSD, but treatment may take much longer, may progress at a much slower rate, and may be fraught with much more complexity than with other traumatized patients.

IX. CONTROVERSIES

PTSD is inherently a controversial field. Since many traumas are public events that are perpetrated by people, it is reasonable to consider how such human-induced human suffering might be prevented. Although we must continue the search for the ideal anti-PTSD drug, clinical outcomes in PTSD may ultimately be more responsive to changes in public policy. Issues such as gun control, protection of children, safety for battered women, reduction of crime, and United Nations peacekeeping operations all have a direct bearing on the potential risk and prevalence of PTSD. In my opinion, prevention of trauma is a legitimate pursuit for the medical professional and one that should be taken seriously. Many colleagues disagree. They believe that professional activities should be restricted to the clinic. Public policy advocacy, they argue, is a private initiative that should be kept separate from professional actions. This controversy can be addressed and resolved only by each clinician individually.

Three other controversies have attracted considerable attention. The first concerns the efficacy of CISD following acute exposure to rape, war, or natural disasters. As noted previously, CISD has been generally accepted as an intervention that should be made available as soon as possible after acute traumatization. It is surprising, perhaps, that CISD has become so universally accepted despite the lack of data from randomized clinical trials demonstrating its efficacy. Indeed, as noted earlier, two recent studies suggest that CISD is either ineffective (59) or actually worsens PTSD symptoms (60) instead of preventing the later development of PTSD, as is generally believed. Obviously, much more research is needed. However, as we ask ourselves how CISD could have attracted so many strong adherents in the absence of convincing data, the answer may lie in the low prevalence of PTSD among individuals exposed to natural disasters (Table 3). If most people exposed to natural disasters will never develop PTSD, then most people exposed to natural disasters who receive CISD will never develop PTSD. The pertinent question, therefore, is whether individuals most likely to develop PTSD will have more favorable outcomes if they receive CISD. Clearly we must move beyond clinical impressions and descriptive studies to rigorous randomized trials if we hope to understand whether CISD can actually prevent the later development of PTSD among acutely traumatized individuals.

A trauma-related controversy that has been fueled by forensic rather than clinical activity concerns the question of "recovered memories." Adults who had been sexually assaulted as children sometimes have no memories of these childhood assaults (71). Sometimes, such missing traumatic memories later become accessible, so that patients regain access to discrete recollections of such childhood events as father-daughter incest (72). In some cases, there is irrefutable evidence that such childhood trauma actually occurred. In many other cases, there is no proof regarding the actuality of the alleged sexual contact. It is reported that approximately one-third of such "recovered memories" have emerged during the course of psychotherapy, whereas most such memories are triggered by life events that include aspects of the initial trauma (73). (Such a scenario is entirely consistent with current models of PTSD as stimulus-driven memories, feelings, or behavior.) Some patients who claim to have regained traumatic memories of this nature have confronted parents whom they now regard as perpetrators of childhood sexual trauma. In some cases they have taken parents to court for these alleged abuses. Sometimes the accused parents vehemently deny that such events ever occurred and maintain that these "traumatic memories" are really emblematic of a "false-memory syndrome" manufactured in the course of therapy. Loftus (74) has written extensively about the problem of authenticating such rediscovered, previously repressed memories. Williams (71), on the other hand, has shown that women who were sexually assaulted during childhood (documented by recorded visits to hospital emergency rooms) are sometimes unable to recall such traumatic events. Although a comprehensive review of this issue is beyond the scope of this chapter, there is general agreement that (a) memory, especially childhood memory, is fallible but not necessarily incorrect; (b) documented traumatic events are sometimes forgotten; and (c) forgotten memories of documented traumatic events are sometimes "recovered" (75–79). When we move from generalities to specifics, especially in a courtroom, it is often difficult to meet legal standards of proof regarding the veracity of a specific traumatic memory. This is especially so when the alleged perpetrator denies participating in such an event, and when there is neither additional evidence nor another witness to support the plaintiff's case. This hotly debated issue has theoretical, clinical, and forensic implications that will have to be sorted out in the future.

Finally, clinicians who work with victims of prolonged trauma, such as incest and torture, argue that such patients suffer from a clinical syndrome that is not adequately characterized by the PTSD construct. Although most patients in this category meet PTSD diagnostic criteria, it is argued that their primary problem is not PTSD. Instead, Herman (80) has proposed a new syndrome, which she has named "complex PTSD," characterized by problems with impulsivity, affect regulation, dissociative symptoms, self-destructive behavior, abnormalities in sexual expression, and somatic symptoms. Identification and treatment of these patients has been described previously (posttraumatic personality). The question is whether complex PTSD is distinct from PTSD and whether it should have its own diagnostic identity. After much discussion, it was decided not to include complex PTSD in the DSM-IV. The controversy has stimulated a number of research initiatives. It is expected that this issue will be revisited during development of the next revision of the DSM-IV.

X. LOOKING AHEAD

As noted earlier, most PTSD research and most clinical applications of that research have focused on military veterans, rape victims, and survivors of natural disasters. That research has, on the one hand, deepened our understanding of fundamental biobehavioral mechanisms and, on the other, promoted the development of promising therapeutic interventions. It is time to expand this focus to other domains, with special attention to interpersonal violence and abuse.

Since the majority of traumatized people do not develop PTSD, we must try to identify risk and protective factors concerning the psychological impact of trauma. We must try to understand whether there is something unique about the trauma of interpersonal violence, something that generates a distinctive pathophysiology, and something that will require a different kind of clinical intervention than has been found effective for PTSD patients exposed to other kinds of trauma. The PTSD field has grown rapidly. There are many animal models, laboratory paradigms, assessment instruments, and conceptual approaches. A rich body of experimental and clinical data has already been developed. It is a good time to make a major effort to apply this knowledge so as to increase our understanding of the psychological impact of interpersonal violence.

REFERENCES

1. R.C. Kessler, A. Sonnega, E. Bromet, M. Hughes, and C.B. Nelson, Posttraumatic stress disorder in the National Comorbidity Survey, *Arch. Gen. Psychiatry 52*:1048–1060 (1995).
2. American Psychiatric Committee on Nomenclature and Statistics, *Diagnostic and Statistical Manual of Mental Disorders*, 4th ed., American Psychiatric Association, Washington, DC, 1994.
3. American Psychiatric Commitee on Nomenclature and Statistics, *Diagnostic and Statistical Manual of Mental Disorders*, 3d ed., American Psychiatric Association, Washington, DC, 1980.
4. P.F. Malloy, J.A. Fairbank, and T.M. Keane, Validation of a multimethod assessment of post-traumatic stress disorders in Vietnam veterans, *J. Consult. Clin. Psychol. 51*:488 (1983).
5. R.K. Pitman, S.P. Orr, D.F. Forgue, J.B. deJong, and J.M. Clairborn, Psychophysi-

ologic assessment of post-traumatic stress disorder imagery in Vietnam combat veterans, *Arch. Gen. Psychiatry 44*:970 (1987).
6. L.C. Kolb, A neuropsychological hypothesis explaining post-traumatic stress disorders, *Am. J. Psychiatry 144*:989 (1987).
7. A.Y. Shalev, S.P. Orr, T. Peri, S. Schreiber, and R.K. Pitman, Physiologic responses to loud tones in Israeli patients with posttraumatic stress disorder, *Arch. Gen. Psychiatry 49*:870 (1992).
8. J.A. Fairbank, W.E. Schlenger, P.A. Saigh, and J.R.T. Davidson, An epidemiologic profile of post-traumatic stress disorder: Prevalence, comorbidity, and risk factors, *Neurobiological and Clinical Consequences of Stress: From Normal Adaptation to Post-traumatic Stress Disorder* (M. J. Friedman, D. S. Charney, and A. Y. Deutch, eds.), Lipincott-Raven, Philadelphia, 1995, pp. 415–427.
9. D.G. Kilpatrick, B.E. Saunders, L.J. Veronen, C.L. Best, and J.M. Von, Criminal victimization: Lifetime prevalence, reporting to the police, and psychological impact, *Crime Delinq. 33*: 479 (1987).
10. F.H. Norris, Epidemiology of trauma: Frequency and impact of different potentially traumatic events on different demographic groups, *J. Consult. Clin. Psychol. 60*: 409 (1992).
11. H. Krystal and Y. Danieli, Holocaust survivor studies in the context of PTSD, *PTSD Res. Q. 5*:1 (1994).
12. R. Yehuda, Comments on the lack of integration between the holocaust and PTSD literatures, *PTSD Res. Q 5*:5 (1994).
13. M.P. Koss, L.A. Goodman, A. Browne, L.F. Fitzgerald, G.P. Keita, and N.F. Russo (eds.), Physical and psychological outcomes of partner violence, *No Safe Haven: Male Violence Against Women at Home, at Work, and in the Community*, American Psychological Association, Washington, DC, 1994, pp. 69–93.
14. B.M. Houskamp, Assessing and treating battered women: A clinical review of issues and approaches, *New Dir. Ment. Health Serv. 64*:79 (1994).
15. S.J. Woods and J.C. Campbell, Posttraumatic stress in battered women: Does the diagnosis fit? *Issues Ment. Health Nurs. 14*:173 (1993).
16. D.A. Wolfe and P. Jaffe, Child abuse and family violence as determinants of child psychopathology, *Can. J. Behav. Sci. 23*:282 (1991).
17. V.V. Wolfe and J. Birt, The psychological sequelae of child sexual abuse, *Adv. Clin. Child Psychiatry 17*:233 (1995).
18. J. Kaufman, Child abuse, *Curr. Opin. Psychiatry 9*:251 (1996).
19. R.J. McIvor and S.W. Turner, Assessment and treatment approaches for survivors of torture, *Br. J. Psychiatry 166*:705 (1995).
20. A.P. Reeler, Is torture a post-traumatic stress disorder? *Torture 4*:59 (1994).
21. R.H. Rozensky, I.H. Sloan, E.D. Schwarz, and J.M. Kowalski, Psychological response of children to shootings and hostage situations, *Children and Disasters* (C. F. Saylor, ed.), Plenum Press, New York, 1993, pp. 123–136.
22. R. Yehuda and A.C. McFarlane, Conflict between current knowledge about posttraumatic stress disorder and its original conceptual basis, *Am. J Psychiatry 152*:1705 (1995).
23. M.E. Cohen, P.D. White, and R.E. Johnson, Neurocirculatory asthenia, anxiety neurosis, or the effort syndrome, *Arch. Intern. Med. 81*:260 (1948).

24. M.E. Cohen, D.W. Badal, A. Kilpatrick, E.W. Reed, and P.D. White, The high familial prevalence of neurocirculatory asthenia, *Am. J. Hum. Genet. 3*:126 (1951).
25. J. Goldberg, W.R. True, S.A. Eisen, and W.C. Henderson, A twin study of the effects of the Vietnam War on posttraumatic stress disorder, *J.A.M.A. 263*:1227 (1990).
26. A. Fontana and R. Rosenheck, A causal model of the etiology of war-related PTSD, *J. Traum. Stress 6*:37 (1993).
27. J.L. Herman, *Trauma and recovery*, Basic Books, New York, 1992.
28. R.A. Kulka, W.E. Schlenger, J.A. Fairbank, et al. (eds.), *Trauma and the Vietnam War Generation*, Brunner/Mazel, New York, 1990.
29. I. Winfield, L.K. George, M.S. Swartz, and D.G. Blazer, Sexual assault and psychiatric disorders among women in a community population, *Am. J. Psychiatry 147*: 335 (1990).
30. J.H. Shore, E.L. Tatum, and W.M. Vollmer, Psychiatric reactions to disaster: The Mount St. Helen's experience, *Am. J. Psychiatry 143*: 590 (1986).
31. B.K. Jordan, W. Schlenger, R. Hough, et al., Lifetime and current prevalence of specific psychiatric disorders among Vietnam veterans and controls, *Arch. Gen. Psychiatry 48*: 207 (1991).
32. B.M. Atkenson, K.S. Calhoun, P.A. Resick, and E.M. Ellis, Victims of rape: Repeated assessment of depressive symptoms, *J. Consult. Clin. Psychol. 50*:96 (1982).
33. A.W. Burgess and L.L. Holmstrom, Adaptive strategies and recovery from rape, *Am. J. Psychiatry 136*:1278 (1979).
34. J. Mitchell, When disaster strikes. . . . The critical incident stress debriefing process, *J Emerg. Med. Serv. 8*:36 (1983).
35. J.R.T. Davidson and E. Foa (eds.), *Post-traumatic Stress Disorder: DSM-IV and Beyond*, American Psychiatric Press, Washington, DC, 1993.
36. M.J. Friedman and R. Yehuda, Post-traumatic stress disorder and comorbidity: Psychobiological approaches to differential diagnosis, *Neurobiological and Clinical Consequences of Stress: From Normal Adaptation to PTSD* (M. J. Friedman, D. S. Charney, and A. Y. Deutch, eds.), Raven Press, New York, 1995, pp. 429–446.
37. R. Yehuda, D. Boisoneau, M.T. Lowy, and E.L. Giller, Dose-response changes in plasma cortisol and lymphocyte glucocorticoid receptors following dexamethasone administration, *Arch. Gen. Psychiatry 52*:583 (1995).
38. P.P. Schnurr, PTSD and combat-related psychiatric symptoms in older veterans, *PTSD Res. Q. 2*:1 (1991).
39. M.J. Friedman, and R.A. Rosenheck, PTSD as a persistent mental illness, *The Seriously and Persistently Mentally Ill: The State-of-the-Art Treatment Handbook* (S. Soreff, ed.), Hogrefe & Huber, Seattle, WA, 1996, pp. 369–389.
40. M.J. Friedman, and J.M. Jaranson, The applicability of the PTSD concept to refugees, *Amidst Peril and Pain: The Mental Health and Well-Being of the World's Refugees* (A. J. Marsella, T. H. Borneman, S. Ekblad, and J. Orley, eds.), American Psychological Press, Washington, DC, 1994, pp. 207–228.
41. A.J. Marsella, M.J. Friedman, E.T. Gerrity, and R.M. Scurfield (eds.), *Ethnocultural Aspects of Posttraumatic Stress Disorder: Issues, Research, and Clinical Applications*, American Psychological Association Press, Washington, DC, 1996.
42. M.J. Friedman, D.S. Charney, and A.Y. Deutch (eds.) *Neurobiological and Clini-*

cal Consequences of Stress: From Normal Adaptation to PTSD, Raven Press, New York, 1995.
43. A. Kardiner, The traumatic neuroses of war, *Psychosom. Med. Monograph I-II*: National Research Council, Washington, DC, 1941.
44. D.S. Charney, A.Y. Deutch, J.H. Krystal, S.M. Southwick, and M. Davis, Psychobiologic mechanisms of post-traumatic stress disorder. *Arch. Gen. Psychiatry 50*:294 (1993).
45. Davis, Animal models of anxiety based on classical conditioning: The conditioned emotional response and fear potentiated startle effect, *Pharmacol. Ther. 47*:147 (1990).
46. R.M. Post, S.R.B. Weiss, and M.A. Smith, Sensitization and kindling: Implications for the evolving neural substrates of post-traumatic stress disorder, *Neurobiological and Clinical Consequences of Stress: From Normal Adaptation to PTSD* (M. J. Friedman, D. S. Charney, and A. Y. Deutch, eds.), Raven Press, New York, 1995, pp. 203–224.
47. B.A. van der Kolk, M. Greenberg, H. Boyd, and J. Krystal, Inescapable shock, neurotransmitters, and addiction to trauma: Toward a psychobiology of post-traumatic stress, *Biol. Psychiatry 20*:314, (1985).
48. C.R. Marmar, D. Foy, B. Kagan, et al., An integrated approach for treating post-traumatic stress, *American Psychiatric Press Review of Psychiatry, Vol. 12* (J. M. Oldham, M. B. Riba, and A. Tasman, eds.), American Psychiatric Press, Washington, DC, 1993, pp. 239–252.
49. E.B. Foa, B.O. Rothbaum, and C. Molnar, Cognitive-behavioral therapy of PTSD, *Neurobiological and Clinical Consequences of Stress: From Normal Adaptation to PTSD* (M. J. Friedman, D. S. Charney, and A. Y. Deutch, eds.), Raven Press, New York, 1995, pp. 483–494.
50. M.J. Friedman and S.M. Southwick, Towards pharmacotherapy for PTSD, *Neurobiological and Clinical Consequences of Stress: From Normal Adaptation to PTSD* (M. J. Friedman, D. S. Charney, and A. Y. Deutch, eds.), Raven Press, New York, 1995, pp. 465–482.
51. M.B. Williams and J.F. Sommer (eds.), *Handbook of Post-Traumatic Therapy*, Greenwood Press, Westport, CT, 1994.
52. P.A. Resick and M.K. Schnicke, Cognitive processing therapy for sexual assault victims, *J. Consult. Clin. Psychol. 60*:748 (1992).
53. L. Kofoed, M.J. Friedman, and R. Peck, Alcoholism and drug abuse in patients with PTSD, *Psychiatric Quarterly 64*:151 (1993).
54. J.D. Lindy, Focal psychoanalytic psychotherapy, *International Handbook of Traumatic Stress Syndromes* (J. P. Wilson and B. Raphael, eds.), Plenum Press, New York, 1993, pp. 803–809.
55. M.J. Horowitz (ed.), *Stress response syndromes*, 2d ed., Jason Aronson, New York, 1986.
56. R.M. Scurfield, Treatment of PTSD in Vietnam veterans, *International Handbook of Traumatic Stress Syndromes* (J. P. Wilson and B. Raphael, eds.), Plenum Press, New York, 1993, pp. 879–888.

57. K. Armstrong, W. O'Callahan, and C.R. Marmar, Debriefing Red Cross disaster personnel: The multiple stressor debriefing model. *J. Traum. Stress 4*:481 (1991).
58. B. Raphael (ed.), *When Disaster Strikes*, Basic Books, New York, 1985.
59. J.A. Kenardy, R.A. Webster, T.J. Lewin, V.J. Carr, P.L. Hazell, and G.L. Carter, Stress debriefing and patterns of recovery following a natural disaster, *J. Traum. Stress 9*:37 (1996).
60. J.I. Bisson, Critical incident stress debriefing: Does it work? Presented at the Twelfth Annual Meeting, International Society for Traumatic Stress Studies, San Francisco, CA, November 9–13, 1996.
61. C.R. Marmar, Brief dynamic psychotherapy of post-traumatic stress disorder, *Psychiatr. Ann. 21*:405 (1991).
62. L. Hyer (ed.), *Trauma victim: Theoretical Issues and Practical Suggestions*, Accelerated Development, Muncie, IN, 1994.
63. E.B. Foa and D.B. Riggs, Post-traumatic stress disorder in rape victims, *American Psychiatric Press Review of Psychiatry, Vol. 12* (J. Oldham, M. B. Riba, and A. Tasman, eds.), American Psychiatric Press, Washington, DC, 1993, pp. 273–303.
64. E.B. Foa, B.O. Rothbaum, T. Murdock, et al., The treatment of PTSD in rape victims, *J. Consult. Clin. Psychol. 59*:715 (1991).
65. B.O. Rothbaum, E.B. Fog, D.S. Riggs, et al., A prospective examination of post-traumatic stress disorder in rape victims, *J. Traum. Stress 5*:455 (1992).
66. E.B. Foa, Personal communication, September 19, 1995.
67. M.J. Friedman, Drug treatment for PTSD: Answers and questions, *Ann. NY Acad. Sci.* (in press).
68. F. Abueg and J. Fairbank, Behavioral treatment of the PTSD substance abuser, *Post-traumatic Stress Disorder: A Behavioral Approach to Assessment and Treatment* (P. A. Saigh, ed.), Pergamon Press, New York, 1991.
69. P. Koller, C.R. Marmar, and N. Kanas, Psychodynamic group treatment of post-traumatic stress disorder in Vietnam veterans, *Int. J. Group Psychother. 42*:225 (1992).
70. M.M. Linehan, D.A. Tutek, H.L. Heard, and H.E. Armstrong, Interpersonal outcome of cognitive behavioral treatment for chronically suicidal borderline patients, *Am. J. Psychiatry 151*:1771 (1994).
71. L.M. Williams, Recall of childhood trauma: A prospective study of women's memories of child sexual abuse, *J. Consult. Clin. Psychol. 62*:1167 (1994).
72. J.L. Herman and E. Schatzow Recovery and verification of memories of childhood sexual trauma, *Psychoanal. Psychol. 4*:1 (1987).
73. J.L. Herman and M. Harvey, Adult memories of childhood trauma: A chart review, Presented at Trauma and Memory: An International Research Conference, University of New Hampshire, Durham, NH, July 26–28, 1996.
74. E.F. Loftus, The reality of repressed memories, *Am. Psychol. 48*:518 (1993).
75. D.M. Elliott and J. Briere, Posttraumatic stress associated with delayed recall of sexual abuse: A general population study, *J. Traum. Stress 8*:629 (1995).
76. D.S. Lindsay and J.D. Read, Psychotherapy and memories of childhood sexual abuse: A cognitive perspective, *Appl. Cogn. Psychol. 8*:281 (1994).
77. E.F. Loftus, S. Polonsky, and M.T. Fullilove, Memories of childhood sexual abuse: Remembering and repressing, *Psychol Women Q. 18*:67 (1994).

78. J. Metcalfe and W.J. Jacobs, A "hot-system/cool-system" view of memory under stress, *PTSD Res. Q. 7*:1 (1996).
79. K.S. Pope, Memory, abuse, and science: Questioning claims about the false memory syndrome epidemic, *Am. Psychol. 51*:957 (1996).
80. J.L. Herman, Complex PTSD: A syndrome in survivors of prolonged and repeated trauma, *J. Traum. Stress 5*:377 (1992).

15
Domestic Violence

Leah J. Dickstein
University of Louisville School of Medicine, Louisville, Kentucky

In the current intensely time-limited medical model in which most physicians practice, writing a prescription for symptomatic relief of posttraumatic stress disorder and other anxiety and depressive symptoms takes less time than asking questions and listening to emotion-laden responses about domestic violence. However, the result of saving time in the short term is that patients will probably live in frustration with chronic, unremitting symptoms while returning endlessly for refills or medication changes or perhaps self-medicating, causing distress to their physicians as well.

Domestic violence is the great mimicker of the late twentieth century, as was tuberculosis in the early 1900s. Formal medical recognition of the importance of this problem led to the Association of American Medical Colleges' January 1997 publication of a supplement to its journal, *Academic Medicine*, entitled, *Educating the Nations' Physicians About Family Violence and Abuse* (1). Furthermore, at the December 1996 AMA House of Delegates Meeting, Resolution 303 was amended to read "Education of Medical Students *and Residents* About Domestic Violence Screening" (2).

Domestic violence, i.e., abuse in our homes, was an ongoing problem without a name until 1981, when the first National Day of Unity against domestic violence was observed annually until 1984. Then, seven days in October were designated Domestic Violence and Educational Awareness Week. In 1987, this annual public recognition event was expanded to the observance of the entire month by its sponsors, the National Coalition Against Domestic Violence (NCADV). NCADV is an organization of battered women's shelters and support groups, simultaneously offering ongoing education to the public, including a 24-hour Domestic Violence Hotline, 1-800-333-SAFE, for information and shelter referral (3).

Clearly, the recognition of domestic violence as a widespread issue resulted from the Second Women's Movement for Equality in the 1960s. Unfortunately but expectedly, there has been recent backlash toward the rights and needs of women, not only in the ongoing prevalence of domestic violence but also in misinformation presented in the media, i.e., "women are just as violent as men, if not more so" (4). The facts, as reported by Gelles, are that "the majority of female assault cases involve women who are responding to physical and/or psychological provocation." Furthermore, "men who beat their wives, who use emotional abuse and blackmail to control their wives, and are then hit or even harmed, cannot be considered to be battered men" (5).

A handgun in the home is 43 times more likely to kill a family member than to be used in self-defense. Of all murdered women, 30% are murdered by their known male partners. If a woman leaves an abusive situation, she runs a 75% increased risk that her former partner will murder her.

I. HISTORICAL PERSPECTIVE

In a 1985 Medical College of Virginia report, a paleopathology team identified a much higher incidence of fractures (30 to 50%) among females than among males (9 to 20%) in mummies that were 2000 to nearly 3000 years old. These fractures, primarily of the skull, were caused by lethal blows as a result of peacetime personal violence (6). The Code of Hamurabi (1800 B.C.) officially decreed that a wife was subservient to her husband. In ancient Rome, around 750 B.C., husbands were allowed to physically discipline their wives for various offenses, often unspecified. These women were considered to be their husbands' legal property, since the wife did not exist as a legal individual (7). Fortunately for others, Theodora, Justinian's empress and coleader of Byzantium from A.D. 508 to 548, was active in women's causes; among other things, she ensured the prevention of physical abuse of women by their husbands (8). Spouse and child abuse, the first and second most common forms of domestic violence, arrived in the colonies with the Puritans. Early Americans laws,

> based on the old English common law doctrines, permitted wife-beating for the purpose of correcting behavior deemed inappropriate by husbands. In effect until the end of the nineteenth century, the Rule of Thumb Law permitted a husband to beat his wife with a stick no larger than the circumference of his thumb! In 1910, the first International Women's Day was instituted to focus on the issue of domestic violence. In the 1970s, a Pennsylvania town ordinance prohibited a husband from beating his wife after 10:00 p.m., or on Sundays (9).

II. CURRENT PERSPECTIVE

At a press conference on September 30, 1993, Senator Barbara Boxer (D-Calif.) and Representative Ron Wyden (D-Ore.) announced the introduction of the Domestic Violence Identification and Referral Act. This bill adds to Title VII of the Public Health Service Act to provide training for competency of health professions students to identify, examine, treat, and refer patients who are domestic violence victims (10). In 1996, it was further extended to ensure that priority in funding to all health sciences center schools and training programs require students to be trained in all issues related to domestic violence (11). The Federal Bureau of Investigation (FBI) estimates that in the United States:

1. A woman is beaten every 15 seconds.
2. Among all women who use emergency rooms, 21% are battered.
3. Almost half of all injuries suffered by women seen in emergency rooms are due to battering, yet only 4% are recognized and offered appropriate treatment.
4. Among all murdered women, 30% are killed by their husbands, boyfriends, or ex-partners.
5. Battering is a cause of half of the suicide attempts by African-American women and one out of four suicide attempts by all women (12).

In addition, the 1986 National Institute of Justice study revealed that:

6. More than 1.7 million people annually face a spouse with a gun or a knife.
7. Approximately 2 million people annually are beaten by their spouses.
8. Of the 18,692 United States homicides in 1984, some 8.4% (i.e., 1570 victims) involved one spouse killing another. (13)

These statistics highlight the fact that some form of domestic violence occurs in the United States in half our homes at least annually.

III. DEFINITION

Domestic violence most often represents spouse abuse. In 95% of cases, women are the victims in physical, emotional, psychological, sexual, and economic forms of abuse. All forms of abuse are used to perpetuate fear, intimidation, inappropriate control, and power by the perpetrator, who, almost all the time, is a man.

To begin to learn the process of evaluating patients for evidence, by history, of domestic violence, we must understand that there is no typical woman victim, and 2 to 4 million women are victims annually. Abuse can begin in utero because pregnant women are the most common victims. No age group is immune, including the most recently identified and most neglected group, the elderly (14).

Race, ethnicity, and religion or faith are also categories within which there are no unaffected groups. Religious leaders may be highly respected in their professional roles while abusing spouses and children and "acting out" behind closed doors. A recent book (*The Shame Borne in Silence: Spouse Abuse in the Jewish Community*, Mirkov Publications, Pittsburgh, 1996) by Dr. Abraham Twerski, rabbi-psychiatrist, concerns domestic violence in the Jewish community. Sexual orientation—whether heterosexual, gay, lesbian or bisexual—does not affect the occurrence of violence; it is prevalent in all sexually intimate relationships, whether formal marital bonds exist or partners simply live together or apart but have a significant relationship.

Domestic violence occurs across all socioeconomic, political, and apolitical groups, as it does across all levels of educational attainment from among those who are illiterate to those with Ph.D., J.D., and M.D. degrees who are university senior administrators and local, national, or international organization leaders. For those women who do not work outside the home, vulnerability can be greater and ability to leave can be less, although, with courage, they often take the children or only themselves if they are childless and escape to family or friends and to the more than 1500 women's shelters nationwide. However, there are more than 3000 animal shelters!

Among women professionals, they may have been victims of violence before, during, and/or after their professional training. Many left abusive relationships and, then, often as single parents, entered college and completed their professional education. Dr. Martin Symonds, psychiatrist–psychoanalyst and deputy surgeon to the New York City Police Department, has identified the issue of recognition of "duel career" versus "dual career" marriages by careful history taking rather than by assumption without questioning the patient.

Women attorneys and Ph.D.s working in academic or in other sites, as well as women politicians, even in Congress, have more recently revealed personal histories of domestic violence and report having waited for varying amounts of time until they left the abuser and courageously moved on with their lives and careers. It is not unusual for professionals to function well in their work and to be abusers or victims at home. Poet Laureate Robert Penn Warren, Kentucky-born, has written of a childhood with a frightening mother and an uninvolved father and then the cruel and mentally ill first wife whom he divorced. Margaret Mitchell, author of the classic love story, *Gone With The Wind*, revealed a history of physical and sexual abuse inflicted by her first husband. A woman medical student and victim retorted to a question about reaching out for help with "The police would have taken action after I was dead!" Another left a professional husband because he refused treatment for dual diagnosis of substance abuse and mental illness and threatened to kill her. He would allow one of their young children to sit on his lap and drive in order to frighten and control her. Restraining orders were issued for years to protect the children at school and all of them in another city. Finally divorce stopped the abuse. Later, after psychiatric treatment, she and the children achieved notable professional careers.

IV. ETIOLOGY

Domestic abuse is a behavior learned across the life cycle—in childhood, adolescence, and adulthood—as victim, observer, and perpetrator. Some 95% of abuse against girls and 80% against boys is perpetrated by men. New York City psychoanalysts Drs. Alexandra and Martin Symonds developed two models of violence in marriage. In the more common, the man, unprovoked to violence by the woman, is immature, compulsive, explosive, and inarticulate; violence is his guiltless solution to any conflict because he feels powerless. Domestic violence arises in the second model in a "Who's Afraid of Virginia Woolf relationship," in which two people seem unable to resolve their psychological relationship conflicts any other way (15). Victimizers and at times victims lack effective verbal and nonverbal communication skills. Equally pertinent, these partners have been stereotypically socialized as to sex role—i.e., mis-socialized, about "appropriate" roles for women and men—and these myths too often lead to potential and actual abuse. This error in socialization includes the myths that women are raised to be helpless for their own care while simultaneously being inordinately pleasing and helpful to others, at all cost to themselves. These women victims are taught early and often to suppress anger and assertiveness and instead cry, eat, and use alcohol and illicit and prescribed tranquilizers. The men are missocialized to be powerful and to control, at any cost, these missocialized, apparently helpless and powerless women, as they themselves deny their normal and vulnerable dependency feelings, which they swallow with alcohol or relieve with violence to maintain a "stiff upper lip."

The book, *Myths of Masculinity*, by psychologist, Dr. Joseph Pleck, delineates these and other errors in socialization that often lead to domestic violence (1). The book, *Toward A New Psychology of Women*, by the leading pioneer in defining women's unique mentally healthy interpersonal relationship styles, psychiatrist-psychoanalyst, Dr. Jean Baker Miller, refutes the myth that women are overly emotionally dependent, because interrelatedness is a key and constructive life concern (17).

Finkelhor also identifies three aspects of male sex-role socialization that increase the likelihood of potential abuse of women:

1. Difficulty acquiring a nonsexual, intimate, interpersonal relationship, whereas women learn this behavior early, as they are more likely to care for small children.

2. Men's socialization to choose younger, smaller, less powerful individuals as sex partners, whereas women seek older, powerful partners.
3. Men are socialized to feel that weakness and subordination are erotic stimuli. (18)

Developed in 1991 and revised in 1996 to include racial and ethnic equity, this author's formula for both professionals, patients, and the public to clearly understand the issues related to gender equity is succinctly formulated as $REGE=A^5VE^2M^2B$. It stands for *racial*, *ethnic*, and *gender equity* are based on one's *awareness, attitudes, assertiveness, advocacy, and action*, times one's values, listening with *ears* tuned to equity, *eyes* seeing equity clearly, times *minds* thinking equitably, then with equitable words spoken from *mouths* and finally, all result in *behavior* which is equitable and just!

V. TREATMENT

A major issue for treating professionals to consider includes the "transference factor"—i.e., that more than 80% of Americans think physicians can play a role in helping to control and reduce domestic violence. An equally important issue is our "countertransference." Treating professionals must have the courage to consider the possibility and then to ask, listen, and respond appropriately in all areas related to domestic violence, but we can do this only if we first recognize any past or current abuse in our own personal lives. Only then can professionals listen to rather than deny this behavior in their patients' lives as well as in their own.

Professionals in many fields, beyond all fields of medicine, should be trained and mandated to accept responsibility to evaluate all patients, clients, detainees, students, parishioners, and all others for domestic violence histories. Evaluation sites in which this diagnosis can and should be made include:

1. All emergency rooms
2. Inpatient sites
3. Primary care outpatient sites
4. Obstetrics-gynecology offices, clinics, hospital beds
5. Surgical sites: general and subspecialty
6. Dental offices
7. Optometry offices
8. Social service sites
9. Schools
10. Work sites
11. Religious institutions

12. Community sites
13. The police/legal system

VI. KEYS TO DIAGNOSIS OF A HISTORY OF DOMESTIC VIOLENCE

Observation of generalized anxiety and posttraumatic stress disorder symptoms—including noting dissociation during the sessions and facial and body expressions—is necessary. Excluding eating, nicotine and substance abuse, of the more than 23 million Americans with anxiety disorders, trauma experiences like domestic violence are the most unrecognized cause. Patients must also be observed in the waiting room, in the presence of their significant others, and listened to on the telephone. They must be carefully reevaluated when lack of expected improvement or poor treatment response to medication and psychotherapy, if indicated, are noted. Furthermore, researchers have found that abuse histories are not "put in patients' belief systems" by well-trained professionals. Current national concerns about "planting abuse histories" have, in fact, been attributed to poorly trained and unlicensed therapists.

Early diagnosis can be made if patients are questioned carefully and empathically during the first and following evaluation and treatment sessions. If the patients' presenting symptoms persist, health professionals must supportively ask again about domestic violence experiences. Legal issues and referrals for safety are clearly early and important treatment issues. All patients, alone in the treatment setting with the professional, must be asked simple, direct, open-ended questions, allowing silent time for their hesitation, shame, and fear to respond truthfully. Moreover, some patients were raised in homes where parents ignored them and their needs and did not listen to or protect them. Consequently, they continue to fear not being believed and, if believed, then fear having to take action. Silence is not golden in relation to domestic violence. We must not assume its historical absence for the patient. Indeed, the issue must be left open-ended. Patients' good eye contact, or lack thereof, when asked the following questions—as well as voice tone revealing shame, fear, distrust or relief when telling—must all be noted.

It is well to start with a general statement, such as "Many people are hurt by someone they love and may live with. When you fight, how does it happen? Are you ever afraid? How safe and/or comfortable psychologically and physically do you feel at home?

The following patient vignette clarifies this point: During "medicine check" clinic appointments, patients should be asked about their current lives, with whom they live and interact closely, and how they spend their time. A 60-year-old woman, having responded several years ago to such questions, had said that she wrote stories and was then connected by the attending psychiatrist to a local writer, who helped her publish a story. Recently, the patient called the psychiatrist's medical school office to reveal that her husband was beating her, as he had for decades. She had adult professional children locally who know yet who took no action. This call was reported immediately to the proper authorities, i.e., Adult Protective Services. Unfortunately, the patient refused to leave her husband and home and reported later that the physical abuse had lessened. Clearly the situation was not resolved, but the patient called because she believed she could be heard by someone who had made time for her before.

Domestic violence may precipitate first-time psychiatric symptoms, including somatization disorder, or increased symptoms in those with preexisting or underlying psychiatric disorders. Three phases of victim reaction include:

1. Shock, disbelief, denial
2. Terror state, where the patient's behavior appears infantile as she clings to the perpetrator and remains friendly to him
3. Depression, withdrawal, silence, and becoming house-bound

Emergency room health professional staff must be trained to carefully evaluate every patient they treat. At the University of Louisville School of Medicine, William Spafford Smock, M.D., formulated a new specialty, forensic medicine, with a 1-year fellowship that began in 1993 and which now exists nationally to ensure that all forms of violence are recognized as health issues, especially in emergency rooms (20).

Common remote and/or recent symptoms include:

1. Suicide attempts (50% by African-American women and 25% by all women).
2. After years of abuse, women victims may then attempt to and in fact do sometimes murder their abusers. Carmen found an abuse history, up to 50%, in psychiatric inpatients, especially in adult women and teenage boys (18).
3. Alcohol and substance abuse, including nicotine and caffeine,are commonly used and abused by perpetrators and victims. Women victims are more likely to begin alcohol and drug abuse secondarily to their abuser's insistence.
4. Feelings of isolation and inability to cope are common.
5. All forms of depressive and anxiety disorders are common, including panic disorder with and without agoraphobia, generalized anxiety disorder, obsessive compulsive disorder, phobic disorders, and posttraumatic stress disorder (PTSD) as well as eating disorders, including anorexia, bulimia, their combination, obesity, sleep disorders includ-

ing initial insomnia, repeated awakenings, and requests for sleeping pills, and sexual disorders.

The two categories of PTSD should be reviewed with every patient, that is,

1. Hyperarousal with: intrusive recall, hypervigilance, flashbacks, nightmares and night terrors; the sleep disorders; irritability, agitation, anger and its dyscontrol: and decreased concentration
2. Blunted affect: avoidance, depersonalization, derealization, dissociative behavior and state, numbing, flat affect, anhedonia, and paresthesias

Child victims often turn to lying, and female adolescent victims may act out sexually. A recently reported rare form of child abuse, "Munchausen by proxy," was reported by Yale faculty and at other academic centers. In this instance, an abused child's mother convinced physicians that there were medical problems, which led to distressing medical workups and potentially dangerous medication trials. In fact, the child had no medical problems and the mother had lied in order to inflict painful medical evaluation on the child (21).

Abused children's mothers are often seriously ill with general medical or psychiatric disorders. Thus they feel helpless to intervene when their partners or others perpetrate the violence. Child perpetrators may abuse power, be violent, and have sexual feelings toward the child victim. However, not all men perpetrators were abused, especially young abusers.

Fortunately, outcome studies have shown that more than half of child victims function normally in adulthood and only 20% suffer very acute mental illness. A January 1997 television interview with 20-year-old David Rothenberg, who uses only the name "David" now, enabled him to recount that in his parents' child custody dispute; his angry father doused 6-year-old David with kerosene and set him ablaze in a motel. Still visibly scarred and after years of treatment, he has become a filmmaker, has "moved on with his life," and even visits others in hospitals to serve as a role model.

With a safe atmosphere established with the patient and with clear and honest introspection completed and in control by the health professionals for themselves, one should ask the following: "How many of these things has your partner done to you?"

1. Ignored your feelings?
2. Ridiculed or insulted your gender as a group?
3. Ridiculed or insulted your most valued beliefs, your religion, race, heritage, or class?
4. Withheld approval, appreciation, or affection as punishment?
5. Continually criticized you, called you names, shouted at you?

6. Humiliated you in private or public?
7. Refused to socialize with you?
8. Kept you from working, controlled your money, made all decisions?
9. Refused to work or share money?
10. Took car keys or money away from you?
11. Regularly threatened to leave or told you to leave?
12. Threatened to hurt you or your family?
13. Punished or deprived the children when angry at you?
14. Threatened to kidnap the children if you left?
15. Abused, tortured, or killed pets to hurt you?
16. Harassed you about imagined affairs?
17. Manipulated you with lies and contradictions?
18. Destroyed furniture, punched holes in walls, broke appliances?
19. Wielded a weapon in a threatening way?
20. Abused you physically by pushing, hitting, punching, pounding, being bitten, tied up or down, throwing, dragging, cutting, shooting, choking, shoving, slapping, kicking, assaulting with a weapon?
21. Is there a gun in your home? Does your partner or adolescent/child have one?
22. Refused to help when victim is sick, injured?
23. Used intimidation, coercion and extortion in your relationship?
24. Do you have any body scars from someone trying to hurt you on purpose, or from you trying to hurt yourself because others have hurt you before? (Too often patients who self-mutilate are diagnosed with borderline personality disorder. In fact, as Dr. Judith Herman has emphasized in her book *Trauma and Recovery* and in this author's clinical experience, low self-esteem and identifying with the aggressor, as well as countertransference issues, should identify this for what it really is—posttraumatic stress disorder behavior (22).
25. Locked you up or out? (23)

The following additional questions are from child abuse expert Dr. Jean Goodwin's work. She supports research demonstrating that in 85% of cases, the child knows the perpetrator.

26. When you were a child, did anyone do anything to you that you thought was sexual and that made you feel uncomfortable?
27. As a child, did you ever worry about the mental state of a caretaker, run away from home, think about suicide? (Asking about victims' early experiences helps them make connections to learning about and accepting that violence occurred, thereby decreasing their guilt and

increasing their desire to change and, especially for child victims, not to repeat this abuse by imitation as adult perpetrators or victims.)

28. Do you have nightmares or bad dreams about something bad that happened to you?
29. Have you ever used drugs or alcohol to get numb? (This behavior is especially common among teens, adult women, and some abused men.)
30. Have you ever "tranced out," "lost time," "left your body," or "flown away?"' (24)

VII. SPECIAL ISSUES

To avoid the potentially dangerous trap for patients of assuming stereotypes, professionals must know that domestic violence occurs in all geographic and community locations—i.e. rural, urban, and suburban environments, in crowding and isolation. The latter factor, isolation from nuclear and extended family because of the continuing high mobility rate in the United States, adds to the lack of connections to others beyond the victim's current home. Additionally, the woman may have no close friends or come to know her neighbors and thus lacks the information and support that might enable her to leave and report the violence; she has no one to turn to and no place to go. Her apparent lack of connections may be based on her own fear or stem from the fact that the male abuser does not want the woman to relate to others, fearing that she might reveal the truth. Her fear worsens her already low self-esteem, as fear does in children who are isolated.

Victimizers as well as victims fits into every category: stepparents; live-in partners to single parents; recent immigrants with their own distinct cultural mores and additional stressors of lack of language, jobs, job skills, or money; children abusing other relatives or stepchildren, siblings, step-siblings; and adolescents on drugs who abuse their parents. Approximately 4% of the elderly in the 1980s, the most recently identified victim group, suffer most from neglect. Most elderly victims are women oven the age of 75. The Elder Assessment Instrument is a valid test to appraise the elders' needs. Their abusers are usually adult children, often overworked or greedy for their parent's assets; they are also often angry, frustrated, and immature. Therefore they withhold food, medicine, and medical care and hit or threaten their elders. Occasionally, elderly partners or paid caretakers also abuse the elderly. The handicapped of all ages and both sexes are also subject to abuse.

Poverty can be a factor, yet all economic strata are noted among victims and abusers. Alcohol and substance abuse are commonly noted; therefore, dual diagnosis of substance abuse in the abuser and victimization of the partner must be ruled out. At times, the abuser forces the victim to become a substance abuser as well. Thus, dual diagnosis must be ruled out in all involved. Furthermore, it is well known that women can tolerate only one-third the amount of alcohol as can men. Consequently, they become alcohol-dependent more quickly and lose more positive self-esteem and control sooner.

Domestic violence is often a missed or incorrect diagnosis among patients treated in general medical practice. For example, a gynecological checkup in an adult woman may reveal a scarred cervix from child sexual abuse but may be ignored by the health professional; the patient consequently is not questioned specifically about a possible history of abuse. Some women patients may dissociate during a vaginal examination and again the physician may ignore this behavior. Women may present with chronic urinary tract infections consequent to abuse and be treated with medications but without the taking of a thorough psychiatric and social history.

The impact of domestic violence—i.e., chronic stress—affects the immune system. Disorders such as lupus, rheumatoid arthritis, and other immune system disorders as well as chronic pain symptoms and syndromes have been noted to be exacerbated by chronic stress. Patients who present with these immune system diseases must be carefully evaluated for early and/or current abuse. Unquestionably, child abusers can be anyone from any part of the child's life: biological, adoptive, stepgrandfathers, fathers, live-in boyfriends, visiting boyfriends, uncles, babysitters, children or partners of these individuals, grandmothers, mothers, aunts, lesbian partners, religious and scout leaders, teachers, neighbors, or coaches. Three children die daily and more babies are born with defects due to battering in utero than due to lack of immunization.

VIII. TREATMENT ISSUES

As treating professionals, we must not be judgmental. We must not say, too early in treatment, "Why do you stay?" Rather, patients should be encouraged to relate the violence experience and praised when they do. The majority who stay say that they do it for the children, have neither money nor job, and got married "for better or worse," and to "love, honor, and obey."

The therapist must be supportive and patient, clearly and early telling patients the laws, give emergency telephone and shelter numbers, and advise victims to put multiple copies of these contacts in safe places with money, clothing, important papers, and identification.

Important statements to make to patients who are victims of domestic violence include "Let's make a safety plan" and "you can change your situation; there is a better way to live without fear."

Medication alone, medication given prematurely, or overmedication in place of a correct diagnosis of domestic violence is wrong, though apparently, in the short term, it is expedient in place of and/or in addition to psychotherapy.

Instead, in psychotherapy, the value of power, its uses and misuses must be defined and taught. Patients can learn to deal constructively with anger via words, the arts, and sports—i.e., constructive thinking and acting.

Both victims and victimizers, must learn about the correct flexible roles for women and men in the home, together with respect for self, for power related to women and men, and respect for women's and men's chosen appropriate similar, different, and unique roles based on gender equity, as already outlined. Indirect effective treatment can be accomplished with office, waiting room, and rest-room pamphlets labeled "to be taken" as well as wall posters and books in the waiting room that define and describe domestic violence and give the same emergency telephone numbers and addresses. Patients may take this information before they have the courage to reveal their traumas, despite having been asked. However, the presence of the material in the office communicates clearly that the professional is aware and willing to help.

Dr. Victor Strasburger, Chief of Adolescent Medicine at the University of New Mexico, calls "electronic child abuse" what the American Academy of Pediatrics also found, that repeated exposure to graphic sexuality and violence desensitizes children to violence and distorts their understanding of sexuality. Clearly, these effects are similar for people of all ages.

All forms of the media, including television, the Internet and beyond—i.e., films, music, magazines, tabloid journalism, catalogues with tee-shirt logos, and shop displays—too frequently encourage, sensationalize, and exploit sexuality, violence, and abuse of power solely for profit.

Even respected news media use a sports and war vocabulary that can incite aggression and which can then spread to other life areas—e.g., "Beat, battle, defend, kill, maim," "a man of few words and fierce punches." A current film, whose ad displays a woman holding a gun behind a man, is entitled, "Thin Line Between Love and Hate."

Linguist Dr. Deborah Tannen's books *You Just Don't Understand: Women and Men in Conversation* and *9 to 5* are useful to explain differences in meanings of the same words to women and men and how they may miscommunicate both at work and in their personal lives. Women and men must also learn effective nonverbal communication skills (25,26).

Treatment must include acute emergency room care when necessary. A classic study by Carmen et al. of 60 consecutive women patients treated in an emergency room found that, when asked at the initial visit, only one patient said her injuries were due to domestic violence. With follow-up care, all 60 finally revealed the same truth (26). Some 21% of all women who use emergency rooms are battered. Half of all emergency room injuries seen are due to battering, but only 4% are recognized and the women offered treatment for domestic violence as well as for bruises and broken bones.

For the victim, brief and/or psychodynamic psychotherapy is key. Tissues, paper and pens, pencils and crayons to draw with are quite helpful to patients who cannot begin verbally. These nonverbal techniques can help women victims recall events and acknowledge painful emotions. Patients should be encouraged to recall dreams and nightmares—even fragments can be useful to begin psychodynamic psychotherapy work. Patients should be encouraged to keep journals and bedside notebooks and pens so that they can record the nightmare or dream easily on awakening, before it is suppressed or repressed, and bring it to therapy sessions. The psychotherapist's interpretations given early and consistently can be very encouraging and helpful for the patient: for example, "I wonder if . . ." and "it seems to me that . . . ." Cognitive behavioral therapy to reduce anxiety symptoms and modify behavior is another useful treatment option.

Women victims should be seen in individual or same-sex group therapy. For the perpetrator, individual or same-sex group therapy is strongly recommended. It is most important that in almost all instances family, couple, and dyadic therapy be delayed until the patient's belief systems and behaviors have changed permanently from belief in inequality for women and abuse of power by men to the more appropriate gender equity and respect already described.

If a patient is noncompliant with treatment, the professional must contact the patient and, in a special session, help her recall what has not been shared that may be blocking appropriate and effective treatment.

IX. TREATMENT FOR MEN: THE EMERGE MODEL

Since the 1970s in Boston, Adams and his group have developed a profeminist effective treatment paradigm for male abusers based on first confronting men's excuses for violence while simultaneously helping to increase their personal costs and the consequences for continued violence. The Emerge program includes legal involvement—i.e., mandated court referral to ensure that the men enter and complete treatment, which consists first of individual sessions for several months of psychological work. Then group therapy follows for 9 to 12 months, during which the men learn to accept responsibility for their behaviors and, additionally, learn about and accept antisexist and therefore correct gender-equitable beliefs.

The ultimate treatment goal is that the men's personal actions should reflect their changed personal values. Insight-oriented therapy is an important opportunity for the male batterers to work through early unresolved personal conflicts and impaired egos, along with poor impulse control, and inability to deal with anxiety, but it does not specifically address men's violence against women.

Adams outlines the often overlooked similarities between violence and alcohol or drug abuse—i.e., these behaviors cannot be interpreted away and are self-perpetuating unless directly confronted and challenged. For therapists working with abusers and victims, it is useful to note research that has shown men to be better listeners when interacting with female coworkers or their female spouses.

Adams and Penn indicate that "education for practice of self-assertion, and other alternative skills simply will not necessarily induce batterers to stop utilizing their inappropriate control skills" (the battering). Such educational programs must also be accompanied by strengthened social and legal sanctions against continued violence, along with specific attention to the abusers' inherent sexist expectations and behavior.

The profeminist model, developed by Adams, defines violence in its broadest terms as "any act that causes the victim to do something she does not want to, prevents her from doing something she wants to do, or causes her to be afraid." Violence—plus intimidating acts such as punching walls, verbal threats, and psychological abuse—can achieve the same results, while psychological abuse itself includes behavior that directly undermines the self-determination or self-esteem of the other person. When combined with physical abuse, covert acts serve to subliminally remind the victim of the potential for repeated violence. The Emerge program, initiated in several similar groups across the country, includes the expectation that the men make safety plans which minimize the possibility for continued violence.

Adams (27) has identified five stages through which abusers progress as they relinquish their abusive control over their partners:

1. *Denial* that he is responsible for his violence
2. *Anger* at her for labeling it a problem
3. *Bargaining* to retain some control
4. *Depression* and *confusion* over how to feel or act differently
5. *Acceptance* that he cannot control others

After this, individual and possibly couples therapy can take place to continue working on change. Finally, all health professionals must keep detailed records and report all cases according to their state's laws.

X. CLINICAL VIGNETTES

The following clinical vignettes are examples of the broad diversity of domestic violence in our society and in the professions; they are offered to dispel stereotypes so that better diagnosis of this public health problem will occur on a regular basis.

1. A male graduate student came to treatment with moderate anxiety and revealed that his male music teacher had sexually abused him in his latency years. His educated, caring parents disbelieved him, and the episodes continued until another male child told his parents, who reported the offender and who was then remanded to jail.
2. A male graduate student came to treatment because of marital problems, which eventually ended in a divorce he did not want but was sought by his mentally ill wife. He courageously revealed that he had been sexually abused by his educated mother, who had a substance abuse problem, as did his father. Until entering treatment, he dealt with his posttraumatic stress disorder symptoms intermittently by driving on highways at over 100 miles per hour and participating in occasional inappropriate exhibitionist sexual behavior.
3. A man, prominent in the community, was referred for consultation because of a substance abuse problem and depressive symptoms. Under hypnosis, the patient revealed that he had experienced childhood sexual abuse by his father in their basement while his mother prepared dinner upstairs in the kitchen.
4. A professional woman, diagnosed with dissociative identity disorder, revealed a history of childhood sexual, psychological and physical abuse by a professional father while her mother was emotionally uncaring and suffered from an untreated substance abuse disorder. Only the unconditional, consistent love of a grandmother kept her from becoming "The fist of anger or revenge." Toning and chanting with a musicologist to decrease anxiety symptoms—along with antianxiety medication, art therapy, including a scream box, weekly counseling with a social worker, and psychiatric treatment every 3 weeks, which included psychodynamic psychotherapy and medication treatments—enabled the patient to slowly and consistently work through the traumas and begin to build positive self-esteem and a constructive and contented life.
5. A nontraditional West Virginia woman osteopathic student, separated from her abusive long-term boyfriend, who was the father of her children, had notified school officials and the police of his past violent behavior and constant threats, but he kidnaped and murdered her and then killed himself.
6. A widow over 60 years of age, grandmother, and retired physical therapist, who was wheelchair-bound with severe rheumatoid arthritis and on medication, was part of a special 4-hour, 20-week group therapy program led by Josephine Rhodes, peer counselor, with the

present author as cotherapist. Techniques used included imagery, art therapy, education about the disease, snacks, and psychotherapy. With the imagery work, the patient recalled preschool sexual abuse by her father. Six years after treatment, she was independently mobile and on no medication.

7. A woman physician suffered from depressive symptoms in professional school and entered treatment; she was later divorced twice, bore one child and was murdered by her husband during an argument. Her professionally successful, educated parents (deceased) had had their own untreated substance abuse disorders.
8. A woman graduate student lost the sight of one eye as a child when a brother hit her with a golf club, though he had beaten her for years before that, until she entered high school. Her parents did nothing to protect her because "he had problems," and "it was no one's business."
9. A woman graduate student complained of being unable to have sexual relations with her respectful fiancé without using one or two alcoholic drinks first. Therapy uncovered child abuse by her "respected and caring" father while with her "caring" mother was in the home.
10. A woman graduate student, in treatment for major depressive disorder, did not reveal her sexual abuse by her older male sibling for a number of years until an ill parent died in order not to upset the caring parents, especially the one who was ill.
11. An older undergraduate student, diagnosed with dissociative identity disorder and academically very successful, revealed to her 16th therapist that her father, mother, and oldest brother during her childhood as well as a previous psychiatrist and a primary care physician in adulthood had sexually abused her when she sought medical treatment.
12. Seen in an outpatient clinic, a very intelligent 40-year-old single mother suffering from severe posttraumatic stress disorder, anxiety, and depressive symptoms revealed on questioning early psychological abuse by her mother and older brothers. Ongoing psychodynamic psychotherapy plus toning, medication, journaling, and artwork reduced all symptoms, enabling the patient to take control of her life and establish positive relationships.
13. According to the media, a little girl had been abused by an uncle; as seen on television, he was led off to 30 years in jail, saying simply, "I'm sorry."
14. On the advice of a dean, a woman student reported to the health sciences center psychiatrist that her husband had threatened to murder

her on the previous night. The university police were called to accompany her to the courthouse.

15. A woman student revealed that her father had impregnated her while she was an early adolescent. He aborted her and had her help him to dispose of the fetus in their garbage.
16. Finally, a woman patient with panic and depressive symptoms finally kept her "medication only" clinic checkup after missing 40 appointments in 2 years. Now she was extremely anxious and had run out of medicine. Recently she had taken out an emergency protective order against her husband because of his physical abuse and had gone to a shelter with her young children. She returned to their home because he said "We'll work it out." The attending psychiatrist took the time to ask about early life, and the obviously intelligent woman said that her caring and beloved father was divorced from her mother because he could not help her with her substance-abuse problems. As an only child, she ran away early and married to stop the cycle whereby her drug-abusing mother abused her psychologically. She appeared relieved after recounting these early and current experiences. She was referred for therapy and promised to keep the appointment.

Another useful treatment resource can be books written for victims, perpetrators, and interested others. The Courage to Change Press (28) publishes a number of self-help books which, when given to patients to read outside of the treatment session, can reinforce their understanding and working through of issues dealt with in therapy. Furthermore, patients' reading may encourage them to bring new issues to therapy. If patients see these and other books in the waiting room, they may gain confidence to read about the issues independently because they realize the therapist thinks these books can be useful. Examples include the following:

1. *The Courage to Heal*
2. *A First Book for Survivors of Child Sexual Abuse*
3. *Silently Seduced: When Parents Make Their Children Partners*
4. *Beyond Survival: A Writing Journey for Healing Childhood Abuse*
5. *Unchained Memories*
6. *Women Who Hurt Themselves*
7. *Abused Boys*
8. *Reclaiming Your Life*
9. *Incest and Sexuality*
10. *Outgrowing the Pain Together*
11. *The Verbally Abusive Relationship*
12. *No Visible Wounds*

13. *Before It's Too Late*
14. *The Batterer*
15. *Breaking Free from Domestic Violence*
16. *Betrayal Trauma*
17. *You Can't Say That To Me!*
18. *Children of Trauma*
19. *When the Bough Breaks*
20. *The Me Nobody Knows*
21. *How Long Does it Hurt?*

Beyond the early treatment sessions, as patients work through their legitimate emotions consequent to the experienced abuse, it is important that therapists, through interpretations and discussion, help patients learn, for their present and future lives, what factors and behaviors can enable them to have healthy relationships. Psychologist Dr. Judith Wallerstein's excellent book *The Good Marriage* (29) outlines nine tasks that domestic violence victims, and victimizers may be completely unaware of and should learn about:

1. Detach from one's family of origin, commit to the relationship, and build new and different connections to the family of origin.
2. Build togetherness through intimacy and expand the sense of self and include the other.
3. Expand the circle to include children (only by choice).
4. Confront the inevitable developmental challenges, manage stressors and tragedies.
5. Build a safe relationship so both can express differences, anger, and conflict, which are inevitable, and ways to resolve them (i.e., constructively). Conflict alone does not destroy a marriage. (This author would add: Look for and work towards the "hardiness" of a significant relationship.)
6. Establish an imaginative and pleasurable sex life.
7. Share laughter and humor, keep interests in the relationship alive.
8. Provide mutual emotional nurturance and encouragement.
9. Sustain the innermost core of the relationship with recall (aloud) of courtship and early marriage as well as the current reality. Thus, maintain the simultaneous double image of past and present. (This author would add: Look for the "goodness of fit" of partners' temperaments, like Dr. Stella Chess's parent and child paradigm of "goodness of fit" (30).

Patients must understand that frequent, honest, and ongoing verbal communication includes listening, speaking, understanding, respecting, and tolerating differences and saving good memories, not anger. They must expect changes at different life stages and at different times in each other and to expect the unexpected and still care. We must help patients develop and demand from and for themselves and others what psychiatrist Dr. Robert Coles has detailed in his book *Moral Intelligence* (31).

The message that domestic violence is all-pervasive and must be eliminated has begun to reach into communities, governments, and many organizations. In 1995, the American Medical Association (AMA) Alliance began the SAVE program: Stop America's Violence Everywhere. As professionals, we must ensure that there are specific treatment options for the medical community, professionals, their significant others, and their children as well. As there are Alcoholics Anonymous groups for health professionals, perhaps there needs to be the same option for domestic violence victims and their significant others.

Psychiatrist-psychoanalyst Dr. Cornelia Burwell Wilbur, pioneer of the identification and treatment of child abuse resulting in dissociation in childhood and across the life cycle, not only successfully treated the well-known patient "Sybil" but taught countless numbers of therapists to do the same. From Dr. Wilbur's library after her death in 1992, this author received a book called *Branching Out: Thoughts About Purpose*, by Judy Tower. Tower's inscription to Dr. Wilbur read, "My gratitude for you and your work which enabled others to believe in people like me" (32). The book's last line reads, "I am special, significant, and have a purpose."

We all want to enable our patients to feel special and significant and to have a purpose as they heal from whatever forms of domestic violence they have lived through. With our current professional knowledge and patients' and the public's better understanding of what is involved, together they can heal and "Before they make a fist, they can make a better choice" to not use violence or be violent or tolerate violence in their homes (33).

Finally, educating the public of all ages and everywhere must become a high public health priority. The AMA Physician's Campaign Against Family Violence has distributed physician guidebooks, the *Physician Guide to Media Violence*, and a pin to wear that states, "It's OK! Talk to me about family violence." When drivers' licenses are renewed, at gas stations, on public transportation, when tax forms are filed, wherever health care is administered, in all shops, at all levels of education, from day care to graduate schools, people must be educated directly and indirectly and made aware of all forms of domestic violence and what to do about it.

Since 1984, this author has supervised second-year medical students who teach middle school students about S.T.E.P. (Students Teaching Early Prevention), i.e., steps to early prevention of illness. Students receive training and elective credit as they talk about diet, exercise, and drug dangers; then, with parental consent, they allow the gloved children to touch diseased hearts and lungs.

The children "get it." Another elective, STOP and START, is in development, about stopping violence and starting constructive communication. We must incorporate similar age- appropriate programs everywhere. All forms of the media must take part. From a phrase on the front page of every daily newspaper to sports and other television programs and in all community sites, all must become more aware of stopping violence and starting other more constructive ways of communicating! Only then, with informed public and health professionals in our communities, can the epidemic and scourge of domestic violence be decreased and avoided.

REFERENCE

1. E.J. Alpert and S. Cohen, eds., *Educating the nation's physicians about family violence and abuse, Acad. Med. (suppl.) 72*(1):1 (1997).
2. APA delegate summary of AMA House of Delegates meeting, APA, Washington, DC, February 25, 1997.
3. National Coalition Against Domestic Violence (NCADV), 2401 Virginia Avenue N.W., Washington, DC, 20037.
4. J. Leo, Things that go bump in the home, *U.S. News World Rep.* May 13, 1996.
5. M. Strauss, R. Gelles, and S. Steinmetz, *Behind Closed Doors: Violence in the American Family*, Anchor Press/Doubleday, Garden City, NY, 1980.
6. Violence Among the ancients, *Am. Med. News Rep.* December 9, 1986, p. 11.
7. Code of Hammurabi, *The New Encyclopedia Britannica*, Vol. 5, 1990, p. 669.
8. J. Chicago, *The Dinner Party: Needlework, Embroidery, Our Heritage*, Anchor Books/Anchor Press/Doubleday, Garden City, NY, 1980.
9. D. Williams-White, Self-Help and advocacy: An alternative approach to helping battered women, *Family Violence Emerging Issues of a National Crisis* L.J. Dickstein and C.C. Nadelson, eds.), American Psychiatric Press, Washington, DC, 1989, p. 48.
10. B. Boxer and R. Wyden, Domestic violence legislation introduced 1993, American Association Medical Colleges, *Washington Highlights, 4(37)*:5 (1993).
11. B. Boxer, R. Wyden, and C. Morella, The Domestic Violence Identification and Referral Act 5.101, H.R. 884, in J. Haynes Douglas NOW Legal Defense and Education Fund Meeting Announcement and Issue Update, March 12, 1997, p.3.
12. L. Gaines and P. Kraska, *Drugs, Crime, and Justice: Contemporary Perspectives*, Waveland Press, Propect Heights, IL, 1997.
13. L.J. Dickstein, Spouse abuse and other domestic violence, *Psychiatr. Clin. North Am. 11(4)*:611 (1988).
14. J.L. Uva, *Am. Med. News*, December 9, 1996, p. 23.
15. M. Symonds, personal communication, February 1997.
16. J. Pleck, *The Myth of Masculinity*, MIT Press, Cambridge, MA, 1981.
17. J.B. Miller, *Toward a New Psychology of Women*, 2d ed., Beacon Press, Boston, 1986.

18. D. Finkelhor, Many myths said to surround child sex abuse, *Psychiatr. News*, January 15, 1988, p. 28.
19. E. Hilberman, C.B. Fullen, and S. Call, Overview: The wife-beater's wife reconsidered, *Am. J. Psychiatry 137*:1336 (1980).
20. W.S. Smock, Personal communication, March 1997.
21. J. Rosenberg, *Am. Med. News* December 16, 1996, p. 16.
22. J. Herman, *Trauma and Recovery: The Aftermath of Violence*, Basic Books, New York, 1992.
23. National Coalition Against Domestic Violence, Washington, D.C.
24. J. Goodwin, Family violence: Principles of intervention and prevention, *Commun. Psychiatry 36*:1074 (1985).
25. D. Tannen, *You Just Don't Understand: Women and Men in Conversation*, William Morrow, Ballantine, NY, 1990.
26. E.H. Carmen, P.P. Ricker, and T. Mills, Victims of violence and psychiatric illness, *Am. J. Psychiatry 141*:378 (1984).
27. D. Adams and A. McCormick, Men unlearning violence: Group work with men who batter, *The Abusive Partner* (M. Roy, ed.), Van Nostrand Reinhold, New York, 1982.
28. *Courage to Change: Catalog for Life's Changes*, P.O. Box 2140, Cranberry Twp., PA 11066.
29. J. Wallerstein and S. Blakeslee, *The Good Marriage*, Houghton Mifflin, Boston, 1995.
30. S. Chess, Early childhood development and its implications for analytic theory and practice, 33rd annual Karen Horney lecture, *Am. J. Psychoanaly. 46(2)*:123 (1986).
31. R. Coles, *Moral Intelligence of Children*, Random House, New York, 1997.
32. J. Tower, *Branching Out: Thoughts About Purpose*, Tower Publication, Oshkosh, WI, 1989.
33. YMCA billboard, "Before You Make A Fist, Make A Choice," St. Louis, MO, October 14, 1995.

BIBLIOGRAPHY

A.M.A. Diagnostic and Treatment Guidelines on Elder Abuse and Neglect, A.M.A., Chicago, 1997.

M.Z. Goldstein, Elder neglect, abuse and exploitation, in L.J. Dickstein, C.C. Nadelson, eds. *Family Violence: Emerging Issues of a National Crisis*, American Psychiatric Press, Washington, D.C., 1989, pp. 101–124.

K. Tardiff, ed., The Violent Patient, *Psychiatric Clin North Am 11(4)*:1 (1988).

E. Stark and A. Flitcraft, *Women at Risk: Domestic Violence and Women's Health*, Sage Publications, Thousand Oaks, CA

C. Warshaw, Domestic violence: Changing theory, changing practice, *J. Am. Med. Women's Assoc. 51(3)*:87 (1996).

16
Rape and Sexual Assault of Adult Women

Dawn M. Hughes and Marylene Cloitre
Cornell University Medical College, New York, New York

I. INTRODUCTION

Sexual victimization attacks women's deepest vulnerabilities and often results in lasting psychological effects. This chapter defines various forms of sexual victimization and explores the breadth of the problem of rape and sexual assault experienced by adult women. We also identify sequelae of rape-related trauma, including disturbances in psychological, cognitive, and interpersonal functioning. Finally, we provide information regarding issues of assessment and treatment of women who have been sexually victimized and conclude with professional considerations in treating the sexual assault victim.

II. DEFINITION OF RAPE

The legal definition of forcible rape utilized in the Federal Bureau of Investigation's (FBI's) *Uniform Crime Reports* is "carnal knowledge of a female forcibly and against her will. Assaults or attempts to commit rape by force or intent are also included; however, statutory rape (without force) and other sex offenses are excluded" (1). Penetration of the victim, typically vaginal, anal, and sometimes oral, is typically required to legally to establish the crime of rape. Although the major tenets of the legal definition of rape remain consistent, reform statutes do vary from state to state. To obtain rape prevalence data, the National Women's Study also utilized a conservative definition of rape, described as "an event that occurred without the woman's consent, involved the use of force, and involved sexual penetration of the victim's vagina, mouth, or rectum" (2). Generally, when someone known or unknown to a woman forces or coerces her to engage in sexual intercourse against her will and without her consent, it is rape. Sexual assault includes attempted rape, where penetration of the vagina, anus, or mouth is not completed, and molestation, such as kissing, fondling, and cunnilingus.

Sexual victimization research unequivocally dispels the myth that women are attacked and sexually assaulted by an unknown assailant in a dark alley. In fact, *stranger rape* is by far the *least* common of rape crimes. In one study, only 22% of rapes were committed by a perpetrator unknown to the victim (2). Far more common is *acquaintance rape*, which involves a victim and assailant who are known to one another, such as a neighbor, coworker, or friend. The term *date rape* is reserved for situations in which force and coercion are used to obtain sexual relations within the interpersonal context of an intimate relationship. Date rape is as serious as other forms of rape and is particularly prevalent among college women. When victim and perpetrator are spouses, it is known as *marital rape*.

Other forms of noncontact sexual victimization include voyeurism, exhibitionism, and sexual harassment. It is worth noting that these are high-frequency and usually low-intensity forms of victimization. Typically, women do not present for treatment because of these behaviors exclusively, but such acts may trigger strong emotional reactions in women with prior histories of sexual assault. Although these are important areas of concern and a cause of significant distress among women, they are not addressed in this chapter.

III. THE SCOPE OF THE PROBLEM

A. Incidence

Incidence data on rape—the number of reported rapes per year—are compiled and documented annually in the FBI's *Uniform Crime Reports* (UCR). In 1995, the FBI documented that 97,464 rapes and attempted rapes were reported to law enforcement agencies (1). This number indicates that 72 out of 100,000 American females were reported rape victims and that *one forcible rape occurs every 5 minutes*. However, it is generally agreed that UCR statistics represent a gross underestimation of actual rape crimes, since the majority of rapes and attempted rapes are *never* reported to authorities (2,3). In fact, researchers have documented rates nearly five times larger than those reported by the FBI or the U.S. Department of Justice, which includes reported and unreported rapes (2). Large-scale community studies that utilize well-trained interviewers and sensitive questioning tend to enhance disclosure and therefore yield more accurate estimates of sexual victimization.

B. Prevalence

A multitude of well-designed research studies investigating sexual violence against women have been conducted during the last two decades. The consensus among investigators is that rape and sexual assault against women is highly prevalent. The results of the National Women's Study, a 3-year longitudinal examination of approximately 4000 women, estimates that 12 million women have experienced forcible rape at some time in their lives (2). *This represents one out of eight women.* It is worth noting that although childhood sexual abuse, including rape, is not addressed in this chapter, the aforementioned study revealed that the majority of rapes (62%) occurred in victims under the age of 17.

Several methodologically sound studies have documented comparable rates of adult sexual victimization. Russell's large-scale community survey uncovered that 44 % of adult women had been victims of rape or attempted rape and that 14% experienced marital rape (4). In an examination of primary care patients, Koss and coworkers found that 20% of these women had experienced at least one completed rape (5). In an examination of the prevalence of marital rape, two community sample studies found between 9 (2) and 14% (4) of women indicated that they were forced to engage in sexual relations with their husband against their will.

Researchers utilizing telephone interviews revealed a sexual assault rate of only 9% (3). However, when these investigators recruited a subsample of these women for personal interviews, much higher prevalence rates emerged, with 54% of women indicating that they had been sexually assaulted, 23% raped, and 13% reporting an attempted rape. The above results suggest that when methodology is explicit and researchers are sensitively trained, women are more likely to disclose assault experiences, thereby allowing studies to yield accurate rates of victimization.

Prevalence rates are notably higher among college women. An alarming 54% of college women reported some type of unwanted, forced sexual contact, with 15% reporting rape and 12% reporting attempted rape (6). Approximately 78% of a sample of college women reported an experience of sexual assault within a dating context (7). Most recently, a prospective study of college women found that 18% of women surveyed experienced some form of sexual assault during one semester (a 9-week interval), with 7% reporting rape or attempted rape (8).

Surveys of clinical populations have also revealed higher rates of sexual assault. Recently, researchers documented that 22% of a large sample of female psychiatric inpatients reported at least one adult sexual assault (9). Two prior studies documented higher rates among female inpatients, perhaps due to a broader definition of sexual assault, with 38 (10) and 58% (11) of women reporting a sexual assault in adulthood.

In sum, depending on the research study, methodology, and definitions used, findings suggest that anywhere from *one out of eight* to *one out of two* women will be sexually victimized sometime in their life,.Undeniably, the crime of rape and sexual assault is an all too common experience in women's lives.

C. Risk Factors

Research has failed to identify personality characteristics that reliably differentiate victims from nonvictims (12). Vulnerability to rape was predicted by external variables beyond the woman's control or in the woman's past or by factors that were inherently unpredictable. For example, research has identified certain risk factors that may increase a woman's vulnerability to assault; these include youth, the use of alcohol, enrollment in college, and a history of childhood victimization.

A history of childhood sexual assault may place a woman at risk for subsequent adult victimization (4,12). Research has demonstrated that women who had been sexually abused as children were 2.4 times more likely to be sexually assaulted as adults (13). A more recent study revealed that the risk of assault among women with a sexual abuse history was 3.1 times higher for psychiatrically hospitalized women and that childhood physical abuse was also related to further victimization (9). In attempting to understand this phenomenon, it has been posited that early childhood victimization may increase a person's tolerance for future abusive situations. Women who were abused as children are therefore not masochistic, nor do they actively seek out abuse. Rather, childhood abuse is known to result in feelings of powerlessness, impaired self-efficacy, depression, and reduced coping skills, all of which may increase susceptibility to subsequent victimization (13,14).

Another factor that may place women at risk for sexual victimization is age. Younger women are more likely to be assaulted. Only 13% of rape victims in one study were 25 years of age or older at the time of the attack (2). In fact, the group with the highest ratio of sexual assaults comprised women between the ages of 11 and 17, accounting for 32% of women in the National Survey, with 18- to 24-year-olds representing 22% of the sample.

College women are at increased risk for rape and sexual assault, especially during their first year. This group is particularly susceptible for three primary reasons. First and most obvious is the fact that college women are in the age range that has been documented to account for a majority of sexual assaults. Second, the presence of alcohol on college campuses has been associated with a greater threat of rape and attempted rape. It has been documented that one-third to two-thirds of perpetrators and almost half of victims had consumed alcohol prior to the assault (15,16). The use of alcohol may serve as a disinhibitor for the male perpetrator and be used as a strategy to reduce resistance on the part of the woman (17). In addition, alcohol may decrease a woman's ability to comprehend the dangerousness of a situation, lower her physical ability to ward off her aggressor, and/or diminish her cognitive ability to say no to unwanted intercourse (4). Third, it has been suggested that the organization of fraternities and membership in them creates a social structure that encourages male domination over women, thus heavily contributing to coercive and often violent sex or rape (18,19).

IV. TRAUMATIC SEQUELAE OF SEXUAL VICTIMIZATION

The aftermath of sexual victimization affects a woman's psychological, cognitive, and interpersonal functioning. Symptomatic responses immediately following rape are common and may resolve without intervention (20). However, for approximately half of all rape victims, this initial distress develops into a chronic symptom pattern characterized by posttraumatic stress disorder and related symptoms such as anxiety, fears, depression, somatic complaints, a sense of powerlessness, low self-esteem, and problems with sexual intimacy. The following section identifies the most common psychiatric diagnoses associated with rape as well as typical affective, cognitive, and interpersonal problems.

A. Diagnoses

1. Posttraumatic Stress Disorder

Posttraumatic stress disorder (PTSD) is a constellation of symptoms that arise in response to a traumatic event. This diagnosis was originally applied to war veterans who exhibited a myriad of psychological symptoms after serving in combat. However, a growing body of literature over the last 15 years has identified PTSD in populations other than combat veterans, such as crime victims (21), battered women (22,23), and victims of rape and sexual assault (20,24).

In order to receive the diagnosis of PTSD, individuals must satisfy the criterion of having been exposed to a traumatic event that involved actual or threatened death or serious injury or a threat to their physical integrity. Further, the person's response to the trauma must involve intense fear, helplessness, or horror. Rape and sexual assault are among the criteria listed in the *Diagnostic and Statistical Manual of Mental Disorders*, 4th ed. (DSM-IV), as stressful life events capable of causing PTSD (25).

Posttraumatic stress disorder is classified among the anxiety disorders. The hallmarks of PTSD are organized into three symptom clusters: intrusion, avoidancc, and physiological arousal. Intrusive symptoms occur when the individual has recurrent and distressing recollections of the trauma. This can occur in a waking state in the form of flashbacks or in a sleeping state in the form of assault-related dreams or nightmares. Such reexperiencing of the trauma occurs spontaneously and often in response to a trigger or external reminder of the trauma. For example, in passing the location of the rape or one similar to it, an assault victim may become flooded with persistent images of her attack and experience psychological distress, as evidenced by an increased heart rate and perspiration. Since this intrusive process occurs involuntarily and an immediate connection to the assault is not made, the victim often feels a pervasive sense of loss of control.

The second cluster of PTSD symptoms involves avoidance behaviors. Assault victims generally expend much effort on avoiding specific thoughts and feelings associated with the trauma, often resulting in a restricted range of affect, emotional numbing, and detachment from others. Victims often develop strategies to elude reminders of their assault, such as avoiding elevators if that was the locality of the rape. Such avoidance interferes with the process of accommodation and integration of the experience.

The third symptom cluster of PTSD is increased arousal. Women with rape-related PTSD are frequently in a state of physiological hyperarousal characterized by difficulties with attention and concentration, insomnia, motor restlessness, and overall irritability. Hypervigilance is a common arousal feature, since rape victims frequently feel unsafe and may engage in constant yet unwarranted surveillance of their surroundings.

It has been estimated that 3.8 million adult American women have PTSD as a result of rape (2). Other studies have documented PTSD lifetime prevalence rates of 57 % of women who were raped and 11% of women who were molested (3). One week following an assault, 94% of victims satisfied the symptom criteria for PTSD, whereas less than half (47%) met the criteria after 3 months (20). Such results suggest that for some women, a reduction in PTSD symptoms occurs naturally over time without treatment. However, the condition of a substantial number of women who do not seek treatment does not improve and may deteriorate. Research has suggested that if victims continue to meet the criteria for rape-related PTSD 2 months after the attack, they are unlikely to recover spontaneously (20). Chronic posttraumatic stress disorder can be a debilitating disorder, interfering with a woman's normal, everyday functioning.

2. Acute Stress Disorder

The symptom picture of acute stress disorder is analogous to that of PTSD as detailed above except for two notable distinctions. Acute stress disorder, unlike PTSD, includes the presence of dissociative reactions where the victim experiences numbing, detachment, derealization, and/or a sense of depersonalization. The second difference is the length of time the constellation of symptoms is present. A diagnosis of acute stress disorder can be assigned immediately following the traumatic event if symptoms are present for a minimum of 2 days. The diagnosis expires 4 weeks following the traumatic event. Therefore, if a woman is seen immediately after rape with posttraumatic symptomatology and satisfies the criteria for acute stress disorder, she would receive the diagnosis until a period of 1 month had expired. If at that time posttraumatic symptoms persisted, a change in classification to PTSD would be warranted.

Questions remain as to whether a dissociative response is a normal, immediate reaction to trauma or whether it may be a key predictor of long-term disruption in functioning (26). It would be useful to be able to identify those at risk for chronic PTSD through this new diagnostic category, and if this were done, to ascertain whether early intervention and treatment reduced the likelihood of long-term difficulties. The inclusion of acute stress disorder in the DSM-IV remains in its infancy; future research is required to establish data as to the prevalence and utility of this diagnosis.

B. Affective Complaints

1. Anxiety and Fears

Comorbid conditions among rape victims, such as anxiety and fears, are frequently encountered in addition to PTSD. Panic attacks and simple phobias can constitute symptomatic responses to sexual victimization and are best explained through behavioral conditioning. A rape victim who was assaulted in her car may try to avoid cars altogether, developing a simple phobia. Since cars are inherently difficult to avoid without a significant disruption in daily functioning, generalized anxiety may result. Such anxiety may heighten in response to exposure to other rape-related stimuli, sometimes resulting in a panic attack. If these panic attacks occurred on a more regular basis and at unpredictable times, a rape victim might feel afraid to leave her home altogether, resulting in a more severe case of panic disorder with agoraphobia. Given the high rate of comorbidity, all anxiety disorders should receive thorough attention and be evaluated within the framework of a victimization history.

Fears and related anxiety are prominent features seen immediately after assault. Victims describe feeling scared, worried, confused, and helpless, all of which contribute to intense anxiety. Rape-related fears often persist after that time and may be difficult to extinguish. Common rape-related fears are (1) fears of future attack, such as being alone or having someone behind you; (2) fears of stimuli or items directly related to the rape, such as a weapon or tough-looking male; and (3) fears of the consequences of rape, such as talking to the police or medical professionals (27). It is important that these fear-based symptoms be interpreted as responses to rape and not pathologized as paranoid thinking.

2. Depression and Suicidal Ideation

Depressive symptomatology is commonly encountered among women who have experienced rape or sexual assault. Research has revealed that 30% of rape victims have experienced at least one major depressive disorder in their lives (2). Victims often experience a loss of their belief in the safety of the world, justified sadness regarding the assault, and overall feelings of apathy or alexithymia. These feelings may develop into a major depressive disorder, especially if the victim has postponed seeking treatment for a significant length of time or has limited sources of social support.

Depressive symptomatology must be regarded seriously and be accurately assessed, since suicidal ideation is frequently encountered among victims of sexual assault. Recent research has documented that rape victims were approximately four times as likely to contemplate suicide and 13 times as likely to have attempted suicide than women who have not been the victims of a crime (2).

C. Cognitive Functioning

Sexual victimization can greatly affect a woman's cognitive processes, including her thinking patterns and perceptions of life. In an attempt to make sense of her victimization, three previously held beliefs about the world, herself, and others are questioned: (1) the belief in personal invulnerability; (2) the perception that the world is a meaningful place; and (3) the perception of oneself as positive (28). The extent to which the individual succeeds or fails in integrating her assault represents an integral part of healing.

Many people adhere to a common belief that "nothing like that [rape] can happen to me." Although most people are keenly aware of crime in society, they often hold strongly to a belief of personal invulnerability. This permits them to navigate the world free of the stress and anxiety that would arise if danger were constantly perceived. After sexual assault, rape victims no longer feel invulnerable; they struggle with a lost sense of safety and feeling of helplessness. The fear of recurrence is a particular cause of emotional distress among rape victims (29). Hence, a goal of treatment is to regain a sense of safety, moderated by the knowledge and experience that negative and very threatening events can happen.

In order to exist in an unpredictable and chaotic world, most people tend to adopt the view that "things happen for a reason." This perception can typically offer solace in the wake of the incomprehensible. However, justification for why bad things happen may not always be found. Once having been victimized, one may no longer see life as being meaningful or based on principles of fairness or justice. Such a loss of meaning can be a major contributor to depressive symptomatology.

When the cognitive assumptions of invulnerability and meaning fail and the victim is unable to accommodate to the rape psychologically, she begins to question her own self-worth. Self-esteem is replaced by feelings of helplessness and powerlessness. Victims of assault frequently blame themselves for their victimization, for example, by saying "I shouldn't have walked home alone." Two types of blame have been identified, characterological and behavioral; both appear to be related to recovery from victimization (30). Behavioral self-blame refers to a victim's critical analysis of her behavior, as evidenced by the above statement. On the other hand, characterological self-blame involves a victim's negative attributions regarding her fundamental character—e.g., "I must be such a bad judge of people to let this happen to me." The latter has been associated with greater depressive symptomatology and a more difficult recovery from victimization.

Self-blame is a common reaction to sexual assault and is complicated by the sociocultural context of rape which often assigns the victim some responsibility for her own victimization. Cultural myths, stereotypes, and beliefs about rape create a climate that affects a victim negatively (31). Common rape myths include the following: "Only bad girls get raped," "Any woman can resist a rape if she really wants to," and "Only sex-starved strangers commit rape in dark alleys." Although empirical evidence regarding the prevalence and characteristics of rape discredits these myths, family members, friends, and professionals alike may adhere to a belief system that can result in dismissal of a victim's rape-related distress. Legal and medical involvement following the assault may be experienced as insensitive, blaming, and unsupportive, which may exacerbate the victim's own struggle with feelings of low self-worth and self-blame.

Long after the psychological symptomatology subsides, sexual assault can profoundly alter the way a woman approaches and thinks about her life. Therefore treatment, either through psychotherapy or support groups, can be critical in helping victims make necessary cognitive adaptations regarding assumptions of invulnerability, meaning, and self-esteem.

D. Behavioral Problems

1. Interpersonal Adjustment

Within months following an assault, rape victims have been found to have difficulty in their family, intimate, professional, and cultural activities. Rape can produce long-term effects of discord within the family unit and marital dyad (3). Perhaps the longest-lasting problem of social adjustment faced by victims of rape is sexual dysfunction (32–34). Approximately 60% of rape victims reported a disruption in their normal sexual functioning immediately following their assault (34), and for many women, sexual dysfunction continues years after the assault. Studies indicate that as many as one-third of women who were 4 to 6 years postvictimization felt that their sexual functioning had not returned to the preassault level (33). Flashbacks or intrusive images of the assault may be triggered through sexual contact with one's partner, creating distress and subsequent avoidance of sexual contact altogether. This pattern of avoidance can result in further impairment of other aspects of the victim's intimate relationship.

2. Substance Abuse

Sexual assault victims have a higher likelihood of abusing drugs and alcohol than women without assault histories (2). Substances are typically used as a form of self-medication to ward off distressing emotions related to the assault, such as intense anxiety, intrusive imagery, and loss of control. Abuse of all substances—including alcohol, cocaine, cannabis, and legally or illegally obtained prescription medications; such as opiates and benzodiazepines—must be thoroughly evaluated.

V. ISSUES IN ASSESSMENT

Given the widespread prevalence of victimization of women, it is extremely likely that clinicians will encounter an assault victim during an initial evaluation or intake. It is also highly likely that many women with assault histories are receiving treatment from mental health professionals who are unaware of their clients' prior victimization. For this reason, awareness of assessment issues regarding interpersonal violence, including rape and sexual assault, is essential and must be integrated as part of an overall clinical assessment. This information is critical to determine an accurate clinical formulation, understand presenting complaints and symptom profile within the context of victimization, and implement the most effective course of treatment.

A. Clinical Sensitivity to Sexual Victimization

Since research has demonstrated that sexual victimization can be a leading etiological agent in the formation of PTSD, anxiety, depression, substance abuse, and interpersonal dysfunction, clinicians need to be sensitive to the effects of victimization in their assessment. Questions regarding the nature and type of assaults experienced should be behaviorally based (35). Sensitive wording to gather sexual assault information has been helpful in eliciting disclosure. Conservative questions such as "Have you ever been raped?" often produce an underestimation of victimization experiences, since many women do not label their experience as "rape" (36). A general rule is do *not* use the word *rape* (37). A more agreeable method of assessment, proposed by Kilpatrick (35), includes a normalization of the experience, such as "It is now generally recognized that some things happen to women that are unpleasant, such as being forced to do something sexual that they did not want to. Has anything similar to this ever happened to you?" Or, more simply, "Have you ever been threatened or forced to do something sexual or have intercourse when you did not want to?"

It is important to be aware that many women have never previously discussed their victimization, and a clinician's comprehensive assessment may represent a first-time disclosure. Myths, stereotypes, and the stigma associated with rape all contribute to the reluctance of women to seek mental health services. In a recent study of college women, more than half of those raped *told no one* of their sexual victimization (5). Two-thirds of women in a national survey were extremely concerned that their families might find out about the rape and about people thinking it was their fault (2). Thus, a woman may not want to disclose her experience because she is apprehensive about the reaction she may receive. She may be fearful of the implication of blame.

There are other reasons why women may not want to talk about experiences of sexual victimization. In general, assault victims go to great lengths *not* to think or talk about their assault, so as to avoid feelings of distress and anxiety that often follows. Also, a rape victim may not connect her current state of distress with her victimization and see little utility in offering such intimate information. Thus, clinicians need to be open, nonjudgmental, and accepting in their responses, displaying genuine empathy and support. If a safe, comfortable, and trusting atmosphere is created, disclosure will be more likely.

B. Suicide and Homicide

Of primary importance in the assessment of the victim of sexual assault is her ability to keep herself safe. As stated previously, suicidal ideation is common among rape victims, especially immediately after the assault (2). Standard suicidal assessment is appropriate, such as determining actual intent, available means, lethality, and history of prior attempts. Assessment of available means, such as the possession of a weapon, is warranted, since a gun or knife may have been purchased after the assault as a means of protection from revictimization. Clearly, if a client is unable to contract for safety, appropriate steps need to be taken to protect her, which may include a brief hospitalization.

Homicidal ideation should also be assessed. The rape victim may have intense anger and thoughts of retribution toward her assailant. Again, assessment of available means, lethality, and prior history is required. Potential for violence toward others, although rare, needs to be evaluated.

C. Psychiatric History

A thorough assessment of the rape victim includes obtaining a standard psychiatric history, such as prior treatment, hospitalizations, and medications. Such information can prove invaluable in determining any preexisting (prior to the assault) disorders or conditions. It may also further the clinician's understanding of the chronicity of posttraumatic symptomatology. In addition, a high rate of comorbidity of anxiety, depressive, and substance abuse disorders exist with rape-related PTSD and should be thoroughly evaluated. Family psychiatric illness also needs to be part of a comprehensive assessment.

A psychosocial history of the rape victim should be obtained as well. The client's strengths, coping techniques, and social support are variables that may mediate or buffer the development and maintenance of posttraumatic reactions. Other stressors in the client's life not directly related to the trauma—including financial difficulties, job-related stress, relationship discord, family illness, or an unstable living situation—may also affect her psychological functioning and ability to cope.

D. Current Assault History

A thorough evaluation of the most recent sexual assault should be conducted. This includes determining the type of sexual assault experienced, such as completed or attempted rape or completed or attempted molestation. Assault characteristics include assessing the victim's age at the time of the assault, the relationship to the perpetrator (acquaintance, boyfriend, relative, stranger), threatened or actual use of force, the presence of a weapon, the degree of sustained injury, chronicity (single versus multiple incidents), and the degree to which the victim feared death. Additionally, inquiry regarding the initial psychological effects following the rape is critical since initial distress may be related to future functioning (24). The way in which a client's perceptions and belief system have been altered by her victimization may yield helpful information regarding treatment options.

E. Lifetime Trauma History

The assessment of multiple traumas across the life span represents a significant component of a comprehensive assessment, especially since empirical findings have revealed that a majority of women with adult assault experiences were either physically or sexually abused as children. Prior victimization experiences include childhood physical or sexual abuse, prior rapes in adulthood (including date or marital rape), and domestic violence (current, past, and witnessed within the family of origin). Women who have complicated trauma histories, especially trauma occurring in the early developmental years, may be at risk for more intractable difficulties in the cognitive, behavioral, and symptomatic domains.

Although a detailed trauma history is often beneficial in understanding a particular client's symptom profile, the clinician must be sensitive enough to balance the need for information with the client's willingness and emotional readiness to discuss potentially distressing and anxiety-provoking details of her life.

While history gathering is important, disclosure must be voluntary. A client should never be forced to discuss details of her sexual victimization experiences if she chooses not to.

F. Psychometric Instruments

1. Structured Clinical Interview

In our clinic, we utilize two trauma-specific modules, the Adult Interpersonal Violence Module (38) and the Childhood Interpersonal Violence Module (39), both of which provide the clinician with a framework to fully assess current and past assault histories and characteristics. Both instruments have demonstrated reliability. Other structured clinical interviews, on which the development of our modules was based, include the Sexual Assault History Initial Interview (40) and the Child Maltreatment Interview Schedule (41).

The Structured Clinical Interview for DSM-IV Axis I Disorders (SCID) is a comprehensive method to assess and confirm DSM-IV diagnoses (42). The SCID is clinician-administered and contains questions specific to DSM-IV criteria to ensure that major Axis I diagnoses are thoroughly evaluated.

2. General Measures

Two self-report measures that are routinely administered to assess depression and anxiety, respectively, are the Beck Depression Inventory (BDI) (43) and the State-Trait Anxiety Inventory (STAI) (44). The Symptom Checklist—Revised (SCL-90-R) is a brief self-report measure of overall psychological distress (45) and has also been widely used in trauma populations. The SCL-90-R contains a Crime-Related Posttraumatic Stress Disorder subscale, which consists of 28 items constructed to measure posttraumatic symptomatology among women who have been assaulted (46).

3. Trauma-Specific Measures

The following measures are commonly utilized research and clinical instruments, with demonstrated reliability and validity, to assess PTSD and trauma-related distress. The Impact of Events Scale (IES) was one of the earliest instruments developed to assess current intrusion and avoidance dimensions of PTSD (47). The IES is a brief self-report instrument of 15 items; it has been found useful in the detection and prediction of PTSD with a variety of trauma populations. A more recent measure, the PTSD Symptom Scale (PSS), was designed to assess all the specific symptoms of PTSD necessary to diagnose the disorder according to DSM-III-R criteria (48). This measure is a semistructured interview of 17 questions that target the severity of the three primary clusters of PTSD: intrusion, avoidance, and arousal. The PTSD Symptom Scale has been validated with assault victims and has demonstrated reliability. Both the IES and the PTSD Symptom Scale are designed to measure PTSD following a traumatic event; they are not specific to rape. The Rape Aftermath Symptom Test (RAST) is a 70-item self-report instrument specifically designed assesses rape-related fears and associated psychological symptomatology (49). The RAST has been successful in discriminating between victims and nonvictims for up to 3 years following the assault (50).

VI. TREATMENT IMPLICATIONS

The clinical treatment of the sexual assault victim may differ depending upon the length of time postassault. Rape victims who seek immediate intervention typically present at rape crisis centers at the request of emergency room nurses or physicians, law enforcement officials, the district attorney's office, or a family member or friend. However, the majority of women who have been victimized do not seek treatment from mental health professionals, and only 4% of college students utilized rape crisis centers (51). Nonetheless, approximately 48% of rape victims have eventually sought treatment due to persistent symptoms that failed to diminish over time (52).

In light of these findings, it is most likely that a rape victim will be evaluated in the chronic phase, often many years after the assault. Clinicians will be confronted with evaluating and treating nonrecent and perhaps more complex assault cases. This chapter discusses acute treatment strategies for rape and sexual assault only briefly. For detailed information regarding crisis intervention and single-session rape debriefing, readers are directed elsewhere (37).

A. Acute Intervention

The most important aspect in treating the victim of a recent rape is to address emergent needs. Rape represents a medical emergency and must be treated as such. The rape victim should be referred to the nearest hospital or physician of her choice so that her medical condition can be thoroughly assessed. She may have sustained injuries, whether or not such injuries are obvious. Preventive treatment for sexually transmitted diseases, AIDS, and pregnancy is imperative. Additionally, forensic evidence can be collected, which is essential for future criminal prosecution.

A second component in treating an assault victim in crisis is the provision of support. The first contact a woman has after rape can be instrumental in determining whether she will seek therapeutic services in the future. If her emotional distress is minimized or she feels blamed for her attack, she will be less likely to seek additional treatment. Therefore, it is important for the clinician to display acceptance, genuine support, and empathy. The victim should be reassured of her safety, with statements such as "You are safe now" and "I'm sorry this happened to you." The clinician should dismiss potential feelings of self-blame, such as "No matter what happened, you did not deserve to be a victim of a crime." The victim should be clearly informed that her sexual assault was a crime and against the law. Furnishing her with the number of a local rape crisis center can be indispensable in providing her legal assistance and overall support. The mobilization of the client's social support network is important. She may need assistance notifying family, spouse, or friends of her current situation and may choose to have them accompany her to the hospital.

Victims of rape and sexual assault also require basic education regarding the immediate psychological effects of victimization. They should be informed that nearly every woman who has been raped or sexually assaulted will experience some psychological distress or problems. Common responses include nightmares, fear, the need to talk about the assault continually, sadness, and numbness. Prospective information provides the assault victim with knowledge regarding the origins of her symptoms and may deter feelings of loss of control or of "going crazy." She should be encouraged to seek assistance from friends or family members who will demonstrate appropriate support. With the client's consent, a family member or close friend may benefit from an explanation of the common effects of victimization as well as suggestions to on how to extend support.

B. Psychotherapeutic Treatment of Sexual Assault

The ultimate goal of therapy for the victim of sexual assault is to facilitate healing from the traumatic effects of victimization (53). This is accomplished through the establishment of a supportive therapeutic relationship, reduction of posttraumatic and related symptomatology associated with the rape, accession and integration painful memories of the event, and processing of altered perceptions and beliefs.

The empirical literature regarding treatment of rape and sexual assault has predominantly assessed cognitive-behavioral models of interventions. These treatments typically consist of short-term interventions of approximately 12 weeks. Studies indicate that Stress Inoculation Training (SIT), Prolonged Exposure (PE), and Cognitive Processing Therapy (CPT) have established efficacy in relieving posttraumatic stress disorder stemming from rape and sexual assault (54–57). These five treatment approaches are discussed in the following.

1. Stress Inoculation Training (SIT)

Stress inoculation training was one of the first structured treatments for the victim of sexual assault (57). The focus of SIT is to enhance coping skills for reducing anxiety-related symptomatology and behaviors. The treatment typically begins with an education phase in which clients are provided with a learning-based rationale for fears and anxiety. They are taught that because sexual assault involves intense fear and is potentially life-threatening, their bodies react in an automatic manner, which involuntarily affects physiology, cognition and behavior. These automatic responses then become paired with relatively innocuous stimuli, such as the locality of the rape, and higher-order fear is created. For example, a rape victim may report experiencing intense anxiety and physiological hyperactivity when confronted with using an elevator, the site of her attack. A conditioned fear to elevators may develop as a result of the assault. Educating individuals about the generalization of fear helps to empower them by broadening their understanding of the development and maintenance of fears and anxiety.

In SIT, assault victims are taught controlled breathing and muscle relaxation (58) to reduce physiological fear reactions such as increased heart rate, rapid breathing, dizziness, trembling, and muscle tension. SIT also provides the client with the basics of cognitive therapy, which identifies extreme and maladaptive beliefs stemming from the assault. Fear based reasoning such as "I will never be safe again" and "All men are bad" are analyzed as understandable but overgeneralized and unlikely to facilitate recovery from sexual assault. In order to counter rumination or negative thinking, thought stopping (59) and guided self-talk (60) are utilized. Role playing is useful in helping women to learn or consolidate behavioral skills in assertiveness and other areas that may have been undermined by an assault experience. The length of treatment is approximately 12 to 14 weeks. Through repeated and sometimes daily practice of the aforementioned skills and techniques, clients regain mastery over their feelings and cognitions related to the assault.

2. Prolonged Exposure (PE)

Exposure therapy is based upon the premise that in order to alleviate fear and anxiety, memory for the assault must be activated and thoroughly relived (54). Initial exposure to the feared memory is intended to produce extremely high levels of arousal and anxiety. However, such intense feelings cannot be physiologically sustained and, as a result, repeated recollection of the rape occurs without hyperarousal or physiological distress. Repeated exposure to the memory of the rape in a safe environment and without hyperarousal is believed to significantly alter an assault victim's perceptions of danger and fear regarding rape-related events, thus alleviating PTSD symptomatology.

Exposure involves a retelling of the rape or assault within the safe confines of a therapy office. Clients are encouraged to bring their victimization experience to awareness as vividly as possible and to describe it aloud in the present tense, as if it were occurring at that moment. Therapists assist by ensuring safety and providing support. Narratives are audio-taped and clients are instructed to listen to their stories outside the sessions on a daily basis. The course of treatment typically consists of 9 biweekly sessions of 90 minutes each. Aside from the first two therapy sessions, which focus on information gathering and providing an explanation of the treatment, all remaining sessions are devoted to reliving the assault scenarios.

3. Cognitive Processing Therapy (CPT)

Cognitive processing therapy was developed to address rape-related PTSD; it includes three primary components: education regarding post-rape reactions (e.g., PTSD), exposure to the trauma memory, and cognitive restructuring (55). CPT begins by providing the client with psychoeducation regarding common rape reactions and symptoms. She is then asked to write a narrative (journal) telling what it means to her to have been sexually victimized. In this way, the exposure component is achieved outside of session; later, reading it aloud during therapy sessions often activates intense affect. Clients are then encouraged to explore perceptions about themselves and others that may have changed as a result of the rape and how this may affect current symptomatology and functioning. With the therapist's guidance, clients are encouraged to identify and process "stuck points"—negative beliefs that often have a significant impact on a woman's functioning, such as "I can never take a train because I might be raped."

CPT can be distinguished from prolonged exposure in that it elicits memories of the trauma (exposure) and then directly identifies maladaptive beliefs associated with it. This process allows for the provision of corrective information and attributions that would not be achieved by an exposure therapy alone. Resolution of rape-related fears and negative beliefs associated with these fears are the targeted goals of this treatment.

4. Critique of Cognitive-Behavioral Approaches

The empirical investigation of treatment for sexual assault has disproportionately included behaviorally based, short-term approaches (66). These brief intervention programs have received criticism for being most efficacious in cases of single assault (37). Women who have previous histories of childhood abuse or multiple sexual assaults in adulthood may have more intractable and profound alterations in their perceptions about themselves and others and require longer-term interventions. For example, women with incest histories are often excluded from CPT because of researchers' awareness that these women may benefit most from establishing a trusting relationship with a therapist, which would not be optimally achieved in brief treatment (67).

Further, cognitive and behavioral treatments of adult sexual assault have primarily focused on the alleviation of PTSD, anxiety, and fears. Other difficulties have been noted in this population, such as sexual dysfunction, interpersonal difficulties, and depression but have not received ample attention in treatment outcome literature. We are currently investigating therapeutic interventions for women with multiple sexual assault experiences, including those in childhood, that address difficulties in affect regulation and interpersonal dysfunction. Preliminary analyses reveal that a slightly longer (18 weeks) multidimensional treatment, which provides skills training in interpersonal effectiveness and emotional management in addition to more traditional PTSD interventions, is effective in reducing problems in a variety of symptom domains.

SIT, prolonged exposure, and cognitive processing therapy all have been empirically proven to be effective in the reduction of PTSD symptomatology. However, none of these approaches has been demonstrated to be superior to any other. Psychoeducation, coping skills, cognitive restructuring, a retelling of the assault, and rebuilding of assumptions are all important treatment components and would prove beneficial in any therapy with victimized women. It is important to note, however, that CPT and prolonged exposure are distinct treatment protocols that require specialized training. A clinician, therefore, should not attempt an exposure technique alone without other safeguards in place. Researchers utilizing PE are cognizant that exposure therapy may not be appropriate for all assault victims and have detailed exclusion criteria for participation in this treatment. Inappropriate use of exposure can result in increased symptomatology and, more seriously, increased suicidal ideation. Instruction and training manuals in PE and CPT can be obtained by contacting the researchers directly.

5. Other Treatment Considerations

For some assault victims, treatment must not focus solely on symptom reduction. A good proportion of sexual assault victims fails to meet criteria for PTSD. These individuals would be excluded from participating in the majority of current research protocols that are bound to the PTSD diagnosis. The mere absence of PTSD does not imply that rape victims do not suffer from legitimate distress related to their assault but rather that they may not be best suited for short-term, PTSD-focused interventions. Psychodynamic approaches and other long-term insight-oriented therapies have been underrepresented in treatment outcome studies. This is perhaps due to methodological problems, such as difficulty operationalizing treatment technique and the expense involved in researching longer treatments. Long-term approaches can be extremely helpful in rebuilding connections with others (beginning with the therapist), since interpersonal connectedness is often severed when the source of the trauma is the result of human action. Long-term therapy may facilitate healing by allowing the client to access her memory of the assault at her own pace and to have a period of mourning, for many victimized individuals feel a part of them has died, a legitimate and often underaddressed aspect of victimization (53).

Supportive counseling groups typically offered at rape crisis centers and women's clinics are perhaps the most frequently used methods of intervention yet the least empirically investigated. Rape crisis centers represent a "grass-roots" and feminist product of the 1970s and have been influential in criminal justice reform, legal advocacy, and overall social reform regarding rape. Rape crisis centers are perhaps solely responsible for initiating rape crisis hotlines, immediate emergency assistance, hospital and court accompaniment, and peer support groups. Being part of a larger organization sensitive to issues of sexual assault helps to reduce isolation, provide clear support, provide validation of feelings and experiences, counteract self-blame, and allow for shared experiences and interpersonal connection (37). Rape victims have noted that being an advocate for social change regarding the overall empowerment of women in American society, such as participating in "Take Back the Night" marches, has proved instrumental in their recovery from victimization.

The goal of future research is twofold: (1) to develop more effective treatments for a greater number of women and (2) to continue to increase our understanding of which specific treatment components are the most helpful for a particular type of client. Of course, no one approach is appropriate for all assault victims. Therapists must ultimately rely on clinical judgment in determining which modality or combination of modalities would best serve a particular client's needs. In all, the clinical and empirical treatment literature is optimistic and victims of rape and sexual assault have received assistance in healing from the traumatic effects of victimization.

C. Psychopharmacological Treatment

Pharmacotherapy can be an effective adjunct to psychotherapy in the alleviation of symptoms associated with rape and sexual assault. The goal of medication is the reduction of PTSD symptomatology, including anxiety, intrusive imagery, sleep difficulty, arousal, depression, and numbing. Medication can stabilize affective states and reduce autonomic arousal, which may enhance everyday functioning and improve participation in psychotherapy.

The empirical investigation of pharmacotherapy for PTSD has produced mixed results. The double-blind controlled studies that do exist regarding medication management of PTSD have been conducted with male combat veterans, and the results obtained may not generalize to other trauma populations (61). There are no controlled studies with female rape victims exclusively. Preliminary results from an open clinical trial of sertraline in the treatment of rape-related PTSD, however, demonstrated reduction of PTSD and related symptoms (62). For symptomatic relief of intrusive imagery, drugs that reduce autonomic arousal may be helpful, such as a benzodiazapine or clonidine. Tricyclic antidepressants, such as amitriptyline and imipramine, and the selective serotonin reuptake inhibitors (SSRIs), such as fluvoxetine and sertraline, have also been found helpful in the treatment of chronic PTSD. For a more detailed description of the pharmacological treatment of PTSD, the reader is directed elsewhere (63,64). In all, clinicians must rely on the available body of literature in conjunction with clinical experience.

VII. PROFESSIONAL CONSIDERATIONS

Rape and sexual assault are topics likely to produce strong reactions in clinicians. Feelings of personal vulnerability, helplessness, and guilt are common responses to working with this population. Clinicians must be cognizant of their own biases, stereotypes, and adherence to rape myths if they are to effectively evaluate or provide therapeutic services to women who have been victimized. If unaddressed, such feelings are likely to affect the therapeutic process negatively, leaving the clinician feeling unskilled and the victim unheard or unsupported.

Clinicians who routinely encounter women with assault histories must be aware of personal reactions to hearing about the trauma, such as vicarious traumatization (65). Bearing witness to clients' horror, suffering, and pain can result in "burnout" if left unaddressed. Furthermore, traumatized individuals, especially those who have been repeatedly victimized, often experience difficulties in effectively communicating their feelings and relating to others, including the therapist. If these difficulties are misinterpreted as therapeutic resistance or taken "personally," clinicians may find themselves harboring anger toward their clients and feeling frustrated with the course of treatment. Compared to other treatment populations, trauma victims often require more time (such as between-session interventions); such treatment takes more emotional energy as it requires the processing of devastating and horrifying events in the victim's life. In order to buffer the effects of vicarious traumatization, the therapist should diversify his or her caseload, engage in self-care—such as proper nutrition, sleep, and exercise—and obtain peer support and supervision.

Second, working with traumatized individuals, specifically women who have experienced sexual victimization, is an area of increasing specialty and training. If the clinician's knowledge and experience are lacking, additional training and supervision, may be indicated. Alternatively, a referral to a specialty clinic, rape crisis center, or practitioner who has demonstrated experience in working with this population may be warranted. Following these guidelines will increase the likelihood that the treatment of the trauma client will be successful and rewarding.

REFERENCES

1. Federal Bureau of Investigation, *Uniform Crime Reports*, U.S. Department of Justice, Washington, DC, 1995.
2. National Victim Center, *Rape in America: A Report to the Nation*, Arlington, VA, 1992.
3. D.G. Kilpatrick, B.E. Saunders, L.J. Veronen, C.L. Best, and J.M. Von, Criminal victimization: Lifetime prevalence, reporting to police, and psychological impact, *Crime Delinq. 33*:479 (1987).
4. D.E.H. Russell, *Sexual Exploitation*, Sage, Newbury Park, CA, 1984.
5. M.P. Koss, W.J. Woodruff, and P.G. Koss, Criminal victimization among primary care patients: Prevalence, incidence and physician usage, *Behav. Sci. Law 9*:85 (1991).
6. M.P. Koss, C.A. Gidycz, and N. Wisniewski, The scope of rape: Incidence and prevalence of sexual aggression and victimization in a national sample of higher education students, *J. Consult. Clin. Psychol. 55*:162 (1987).
7. C. Muehlenhard and M. Linton, Date rape and sexual aggression in dating situations: Incidence and risk factors, *J. Couns. Psychol. 34*:186 (1987).
8. C.A. Gidycz, C.N. Coble, L. Latham, and M.J. Layman, Sexual assault experience in adulthood and prior victimization experiences: A prospective analysis, *Psychol. Women Q. 17*:151 (1993).
9. M. Cloitre, K. Tardiff, P.M. Mazuk, A.C. Leon, and L. Portera, Childhood abuse and subsequent sexual assault among female inpatients. *J. Traum. Stress 9*:473 (1996).
10. A. Jacobson and B. Richardson, Assault experiences of 100 psychiatric inpatients: Evidence of the need for routine inquiry, *Am. J. Psychiatry 144*:908 (1987).
11. J.B. Bryer, B.A. Nelson, J.B. Miller, and P.A. Krol, *Am. J. Psychiatry 144*:1426 (1987).
12. M.P. Koss and T.E. Dinero, Discriminant analysis of risk factors for sexual victimization among a national sample of college women, *J. Consult. Clin. Psychol. 57*:242 (1989).
13. G. Wyatt, D. Guthrie, and C. Notgrass, Differential effects of women's child sexual abuse and subsequent revictimization, *J. Consul. Clin. Psychol. 60*:167 (1992).
14. D. Finkelhor and A. Browne, The traumatic impact of child sexual abuse: A conceptualization, *Am. J. Orthopsychiaty 55*:530 (1985).
15. B. Lott, M.E. Reilly, and D.R. Howard, Sexual assault harrassment: A campus community case study, *Signs J. Women Culture Soc. 8*:296 (1982).
16. W. Wilson and R. Durrenberger, Comparison of rape and attempted rape victims, *Psychol. Rep. 50*:198 (1982).

17. D. Richardson and G. Hammock, The role of alcohol in acquaintance rape, *Acquaintance Rape: The Hidden Crime* (A. Parot and L. Bechhofer, eds.), Wiley, New York, 1990.
18. S. Copenhaver and B. Grauerholz, Sexual victimization among sorority women: Exploring the link between sexual violence and institutional practices, *Sex Roles 24*:31 (1991).
19. P.Y. Martin and R.A. Hummer, Fraternities and rape on campus. *Gender Soc. 3*:457 (1989).
20. B.O. Rothbaum, E.B. Foa, D.S. Riggs, T. Murdock, and W. Walsh, A prospective examination of posttraumatic stress disorder in rape victims, *J. Traum. Stress 5*:455 (1992).
21. D.G. Kilpatrick, B.E. Saunders, A. Amick-McMullan, C.L. Best, L.J. Veronen, and P.A. Resick, Victim and crime factors associated with the development of posttraumatic stress disorder, *Behav. Ther. 20*:199 (1989).
22. M.C. Astin, K.J. Lawrence, and D.W. Foy, Posttraumatic stress disorder among battered women: Risk and resiliency factors, *Violence Victims 8*:17 (1993).
23. M.A. Dutton, *Empowering and Healing the Battered Woman: Assessment and Treatment*, Springer, New York, 1992.
24. D.G. Kilpatrick, L.J. Veronen, and C.L. Best, Factors predicting psychological distress among rape victims, *Trauma and Its Wake: The Study and Treatment of Posttraumatic Stress Disorder* (C.R. Figley, ed.), Brunner/Mazel, New York, 1985 pp. 113–141.
25. American Psychiatric Association, *Diagnostic and Statistical Manual of Mental Disorders*, 4th ed., Washington, DC, 1994.
26. C.V. Dancu, D.S. Riggs, D. Hearst-Ikeda, B.G. Shoyer, and E.B. Foa, Dissociative experiences and posttraumatic stress disorder among female victims of criminal assault and rape, *J. Traum. Stress 9*:253 (1996).
27. D.G. Kilpatrick, P.A. Resick, and L.J. Veronen, Effects of a rape experience: A longitudinal study, *J. Social Issues 37*:105 (1981).
28. R. Janoff-Bulmann, The aftermath of victimization: Rebuilding shattered assumptions, *Trauma and Its Wake: The Study and Treatment of Post-traumatic Stress-Disorder* (C.R. Figley, ed.), Brunner/Mazel, New York, 1985, pp. 15–35.
29. A.W. Burgess and L.L. Holmstrom, Crisis and counseling requests of rape victims, *J. Nurs. Res. 23*:196 (1974).
30. R. Janoff-Bulmann, Characterological versus behavioral self-blame: Inquiries into depression and rape, *J. Personal. Soc. Psychol. 37*:1798 (1979).
31. M.R. Burt, Cultural myths and support for rape, *J. Personal. Soc. Psychol. 38*:217 (1980).
32. J.V. Becker, G.G. Abel, and L.J. Skinner, The impact of sexual assault on the victim's sexual life, *Victimol. Int. J. 4*:229 (1979).
33. A.W. Burgess and L.L. Holmstrom, Rape: Sexual disruption and recovery, *Am. J. Orthopsychiatry 49*:648 (1979).
34. E.M. Ellis, K.S. Calhoun, and B.M. Atkeson, Sexual dysfunctions in victims of rape, *Women Health 5*:39 (1980).
35. D.G. Kilpatrick, Rape victims: Detection, assessment and treatment, *Clin Psychol. 36(4)*:92 (1983).

36. M.P. Koss, The hidden rape victim: Personality, attitudinal, and situational characteristics, *Psychol. Women Q. 9*:193 (1985).
37. M.P. Koss and M.R. Harvey, *The Rape Victim: Clinical and Community Interventions*, Sage, Newbury Park, CA, 1991.
38. M. Cloitre and R. Hand, Adult interpersonal violence module, unpublished protocol, 1996.
39. M. Cloitre and R. Hand, Childhood interpersonal violence before age 18 module, unpublished protocol, 1996.
40. P.A. Resick, Reactions of female and male victims of rape and robbery, Final Report, NIJ Grant No. MH37296, National Institute of Justice, Washington, DC, 1987.
41. J. Briere, *Child Abuse Trauma: Theory and Treatment of Lasting Effects*, Sage, Newbury Park, CA, 1992.
42. M.B. First, R.L. Spitzer, M. Gibbon, and J.B. Williams, *Structured Clinical Interview for DSM-IV Axis I Disorders*, New York State Psychiatric Institute, New York, 1996.
43. A.T. Beck, C.H. Ward, M. Mendelsohn, J. Mock, and J. Erbaugh. An inventory for measuring depression, *Arch. Gen. Psychiatry 4*:561 (1961).
44. C.D. Spielberger, R.L. Gorsuch, and R.E. Lushene, *Manual for the State-Trait Anxiety Inventory (Self-Evaluation Questionnaire)*, Consulting Psychologist Press, Palo Alto, CA, 1970.
45. L.R. Derogatis, *Symptom Checklist 90—Revised: Administration, Scoring, and Procedures Manual*, 2d ed., Clinical Psychometric Research, Towson, MD, 1988.
46. B.E. Saunders, C.M. Arata, and D.G. Kilpatrick, Development of a crime-realted posttraumatic stress disorder scale for women within the Symptom Checklist-90-Revised, *J. Traum. Stress 3*:439 (1990).
47. M. Horowitz, N. Wilner, and W. Alvarez, Impact of events scale: A measure of subjective distress, *Psychosom. Med. 41*:209 (1979).
48. E.B. Foa, D.S. Riggs, C.V. Dancu, and B.O. Rothbaum, Reliability and validity of a brief instrument for assessing posttraumatic stress disorder, *J. Traum. Stress 6*:459 (1993).
49. D.G. Kilpatrick, Rape Aftermath Symptom Test, *Dictionary of Behavioral Assessment Techniques* (M. Hersen and A.S. Bellack, eds.), Pergamon Press, Oxford, UK, 1988, pp. 366–367.
50. D.G. Kilpatrick, C.L. Best, L.J. Veronen, M.H. Ruff, G.A. Ruff, and J.C. Allison, The aftermath of rape: A three-year longitudinal study, paper presented at the annual convention of the American Psychological Association, Los Angeles, 1995.
51. M.P. Koss, Hidden rape: Sexual aggression and victimization in a national sample of students in higher education, *Rape and Sexual Assault* (A.W. Burgess, ed.), Garland, New York, 1988, pp. 3–35.
52. E.M. Ellis, B.M. Atkeson, and K.S. Calhoun, An assessment of long-term reactions to rape, *J. Abnormal Psychology 90*:263 (1981).
53. J.L. Herman, *Trauma and Recovery*, Basic Books, New York, 1992.
54. E.B. Foa, B.O. Rothbaum, D.S. Riggs, and T.B. Murdock, Treatment of posttraumatic stress disorder in rape victims: A comparison between cognitive-behavioral procedures in counseling, *J. Consult. Clin. Psychol. 59*:715 (1991).

55. P.A. Resick and M.K. Schnicke, Cognitive processing therapy for sexual assault victims, *J. Consult. Clin. Psychol. 60*:748 (1992).
56. P.A. Resick, C.G. Jordan, S.A. Girelli, C.K. Hutter, and S.M. Dvorak, A comparative outcome study of behavioral group therapy for sexual assault victims, *Behavior Therapy 19*:385 (1988).
57. L.J. Veronen and D.G. Kilpatrick, Stress management for rape victims, *Stress Reduction and Prevention* (D. Meichenbaum and M.E. Jaremko, eds.), Plenum, New York, 1983, pp. 341–374.
58. E. Jacobson, *Progressive Relaxation*, University of Chicago Press, Chicago, 1938.
59. J. Wolpe, *Psychotherapy by Reciprocal Inhibition*, Stanford University Press, Stanford, CA, 1958.
60. D. Meichenbaum, *Cognitive Behavioral Modification*, General Learning Press, Morristown, NJ, 1974
61. B.A. van der Kolk, D. Dreyfuss, M. Michaels, D. Shera, B. Berkowitz, R. Fishler, and G. Saxe, Fluoxetine in posttraumatic stress disorder, *J. Clin. Psychiatry 55*:517 (1994).
62. B.O. Rothbaum, P.T. Ninan, and L. Thomas, Sertraline in the treatment of rape victims with posttraumatic stress disorder, *J. Traum. Stress 9*:865 (1996).
63. M.J. Friedman and S.M. Southwich, Towards pharmacotherapy for PTSD, *Neurobiological and Clinical Consequences of Stress: From Normal Adaptation to PTSD* (M.J. Friedman, D.S. Charney, and A.Y. Deutch, eds.), Raven Press, New York, 1995, pp. 465–482.
64. J.R.T. Davidson and B.A. van der Kolk, The psychopharmacological treatment of posttraumatic stress disorder, *Traumatic Stress: The Effects of Overwhelming Experience on Mind, Body, and Society* (B.A. van der Kolk, A.C. McFarlane, and L. Weisaeth, eds.), Guilford Press, New York, 1996, pp. 510–524.
65. K.W. Saakvitne and L.A. Pearlman, *Transforming the Pain: A Workbook on Vicarious Traumatization*, Norton, New York, 1996
66. P.A. Resick, and M.K. Schnicke, Treating symptoms in adult victims of sexual assault, *J. Interpers. Violence 5*:488 (1990).
67. P.A. Resick and M.K. Schnicke, *Cognitive Processing Therapy for Sexual Assault Survivors: A Therapist's Manual*, Sage, Newbury Park, CA, 1993.

17

Patterns of Violence Transmission in Physically and Sexually Abused Children

Arthur H. Green†
Columbia University College of Physicians and Surgeons, New York, New York

I. INTRODUCTION

Child maltreatment has been a major public health problem in the United States ever since mandatory reporting laws were enacted in 1965, and it has dramatically increased during the past decade. The total number of reports has increased by 49% since 1986. The rate of reporting of abuse and neglect involving children has also increased by 15% between 1990 and 1995, from 40 per 1000 children to 46 per 1000. In 1995, there were 996,000 confirmed cases of maltreatment; 249,000 children were physically abused, 109,560 were sexually abused, and 537,840 were neglected (I). The aim of this chapter is to explore the relationship between the physical and sexual abuse of children and other forms of violencc in our society, including criminal and assaultive behavior, homicide, suicide, sexual offending, spouse abuse, and the maltreatment of children in the next generation. Brief case vignettes are utilized to describe some of the typical sequelae of child abuse and how the maltreated child evolves into a violence-prone adolescent and adult. The intergenerational transmission of violence is explored from the perspectives of psychodynamic, social learning, and attachment theory within the context of new psychobiological findings associated with posttraumatic stress.

†Dr. Green passed away November 25, 1998.

II. PHYSICAL ABUSE LEADING TO AGGRESSIVE AND ASSAULTIVE BEHAVIOR

Aggressive and assaultive behavior have frequently been observed in physically abused children of all ages. George and Main (2) observed physically abused toddlers from ages 1 to 3 in a day care setting and reported that they physically assaulted their peers twice as often as the nonabused controls, and they also harassed and assaulted their adult caregivers. The abused toddlers were also less likely to approach caregivers in response to friendly gestures. Bousha and Twentyman (3) demonstrated that abused and neglected preschool children observed while interacting with their parents at home displayed more verbal and physical aggression and fewer positive behaviors than non-maltreated controls.

Hyperaggressive behavior in abused children of school age was reported by Green (4). He cited their identification with their violent parents, which facilitated the use of "identification with the aggressor" as a major defense against feelings of anxiety and helplessness. Livingston (5) reported a significantly higher incidence of conduct and oppositional disorders in physically abused children than in nonabused control subjects admitted to an inpatient psychiatric facility. Famularo et al. (6) also found a higher incidence of oppositional behavior and conduct disorder in abused children ranging from 5 to 10 years old than controls. The abused children also exhibited a high incidence of posttraumatic stress disorder (PTSD) and attention deficit hyperactivity disorder (ADHD). Scerbo and Kolko (7) reported that the aggressive behavior in physically abused children referred for disruptive behavior disorders were associated with the presence of internalizing problems measured by the Child Behavior Checklist.

Case Illustration: Juan, a 13-year-old youngster, gave a glass of lye to Benny, his 5-year-old half-brother. This child drank the liquid and was hospitalized in critical condition with severe burns and a perforated esophagus. Juan had returned to his mother's house in New York from Puerto Rico 2 years before this incident. He had been living with his father and stepmother, who had physically abused and neglected him. His pent up anger at having been maltreated by his father and abandoned by his mother was displaced onto Benny who was the mother's favorite. Juan admitted his jealousy of Benny, and his wish to "burn his guts." He then showed his therapist scars on his back from burns inflicted by his father.

III. PHYSICAL ABUSE LEADING TO DELINQUENT AND CRIMINAL BEHAVIOR

Criminal and assaultive behavior has also been demonstrated in physically abused adolescents. Truscott (8) found that violent behavior in a group of inpatient juvenile offenders was related to verbal and physical abuse by their fathers. In studies of incarcerated adolescent juvenile offenders, Lewis et al. (9) and Geller and Ford-Somma (10) found that the offenders who committed crimes of violence had higher incidence of physical abuse in childhood than the nonviolent offenders. In a similar type of study, Tarter et al. (11) found that physically abused delinquents referred to a psychiatric clinic were more likely to commit violent offenses than those who were not abused.

High rates of childhood physical abuse have been documented in the histories of adolescents and adults involved in delinquency, crime, and murder. Alfaro (12) found that 22.8% of adolescents referred to the juvenile courts in New York State in 1971–1972 had had prior contact with child protective agencies. Gutierres and Reich (13) carried out a prospective study of 5392 children referred for child abuse in Arizona. Of this group, 16.2% had subsequently been referred to juvenile court. McCord (14) conducted a follow-up study of 232 males who were divided into groups on the basis of parental treatment in childhood—e.g., abused, neglected, rejected, and loved. Serious crimes were committed during childhood and adolescence by 29% of the rejected children, 10% of the abused children, 15% of the neglected children, and 7% of the loved children. Widom (15) followed a sample of 908 individuals who had been physically abused or neglected and compared them with a group of 667 nonmaltreated controls. She found that abuse or neglect increased the individual's risk for delinquency, adult criminal behavior, and violent criminal behavior. Of the maltreated sample, 26 had been cited for juvenile delinquency, 28% had adult criminal records, and 11.2% had committed a violent crime, as compared with 16.8%, 21.1%, and 7.9% of the controls, respectively, for each of these categories of offenses.

Ressler and Burgess (16) explored the extent of abuse in a sample of 31 sexual murderers. Of these murderers, 13 reported a history of childhood physical abuse, 12 reported childhood sexual abuse, and 23 reported psychological abuse. Lewis et al. (17) found that 7 of 9 young murderers had experienced severe abuse by one or more parents.

Case Illustration: Charles, a 16-year-old adolescent, had been arrested after shooting into a group of teenagers during a rock concert in a park. He told the police that he feared that he and his friend would be attacked by these boys, because they had been taunting and cursing them. Charles had been previously arrested after shooting a teacher in the leg when he was 12. This occurred after the teacher hit Charles as a punishment for his assault of a classmate. Charles had been severely beaten by his mother during the first years of his life, when his mother, herself a victim of physical and sexual abuse, was trying to raise him by herself; she was only 14 years old at the time. Charles exhibited a paranoid, hypervigilant attitude and was constantly preoccupied with being attacked, which was linked to his early and pervasive physical abuse. This prompted his interest in guns and ferocious dogs, which he used as a means of protection from a potential abuser and as a means of retaliation.

IV. PHYSICAL ABUSE LEADING TO SUICIDAL BEHAVIOR

Green (18) documented that 40% of a cohort of physically abused school-age children exhibited self-destructive behavior, including suicidal ideation, suicidal threats, self-mutilation, and suicide attempts. This behavior was often provoked by parental beatings or threatened abandonment by parental figures. Pfeffer (19) reported high rates of physical abuse in children who attempt suicide. Deykin et al. (20) documented a higher incidence of physical abuse in adolescents who attempted suicide than in nonsuicidal adolescents. The adolescent girls and boys were 3.8 and 6.0 times more likely to have been abused than the nonsuicidal girls and boys.

Case Illustration: Cathy, age 8, jumped off a swing with a desire to hurt herself at the command of her mother's "voice." She sustained a broken leg as a result of the fall. Cathy had been scapegoated, physically abused, and chronically rejected by her mother and had clearly internalized and reenacted her mother's hostility towards her with this self-destructive act.

V. PHYSICAL ABUSE LEADING TO ABUSE IN THE NEXT GENERATION

According to Steele (21), "with few exceptions, parents and other caretakers who maltreat babies were themselves neglected and abused in their own childhood." Retrospective studies indicate that physically abusing parents report a high rate of physical and emotional maltreatment during their own childhood (22,23). Egeland et al. (24) followed the child-care practices of women who had been abused in childhood for a period of 3 years. Of these mothers, 70% either maltreated or voided borderline care for their children, whereas all but one of a comparison group of nonabused mothers with a history of good parenting provided adequate care for their children. Herrenkohl et al. (25) determined the incidence rate of child abuse in abusing, neglecting, and nonabusive parents. Fifty-six percent of the abusing parents had one or more abusive caretakers compared with 38% of the parents who denied abusing their children.

Green et al. (26) reported that 51% of 43 mothers of physically abused children referred to an outpatient treatment program for child abuse had also been physically abused during childhood, compared to 8.3% of the mothers of nonabused control children.

This survey of the literature indicates rather unequivocally not only that physically abused and/or neglected children are at risk for engaging in subsequent aggressive and violent behaviors in childhood and adolescence but also that many of them will ultimately become disproportionally involved in delinquent and criminal activities and in crimes of violence. The generational transmission of child battering appears to be another long-term outcome of child abuse. The maltreated children also appear to be at equal risk for self-destructive or suicidal behavior. It is also apparent that the violent outcome for many of these children often represents a direct conscious or unconscious reenactment of their abuse.

Case Illustration: Sally, the young mother who abused Charles, described in the second case illustration, had been physically abused by her own mother until her death, when Sally was 4 years old. Sally was then placed in the home of cousins, where she was physically abused by her female cousin and sexually abused by the cousin's husband. After Sally become pregnant with Charles, at age 13, from a boy in the neighborhood, she was evicted from the cousin's home and lived on her own. She had the fantasy that giving birth to Charles would make her feel worthwhile and make her happy. However, he was an irritable baby and his frequent crying, provoked by hunger and a lack of milk, caused Sally to hit him. According to Sally, "when I hit him he'd start to scream, then I hit him until the screaming stopped, when he feel asleep out of exhaustion." Sally was clearly identifying with her own abusive caretakers as she punished Charles for his inability to "take care" of her.

VI. SEXUAL ABUSE LEADING TO SEXUALLY AGGRESSIVE BEHAVIOR

Just as physically abused children typically manifest dyscontrol of aggression, there has been increasing evidence that many sexually abused children exhibit problems in controlling their sexual impulses. Yates (27) described the eroticization of preschool children by incest that was proportional to the duration and intensity of the sexual contact. These preschoolers were orgastic and maintained a high level of sexual arousal. They were often unable to differentiate affectionate from sexual relationships and were aroused by routine physical or psychological closeness. Friedrich (28) also documented disturbances in sexual behavior in sexually abused children in two controlled studies. One study demonstrated a higher incidence of sexual behavior problems, including hypersexuality, in 20 sexually abused boys between the ages of 4 and 7 than in a comparison group of 23 nonabused boys with a history of conduct disorder. Another study reported frequent sexual behavior problems in sexually abused children of both sexes compared with nonabused children who were psychiatric outpatients and nonabused normal children. These sexual behavior problems also appear in the childhood histories of juvenile sexual offenders.

VII. GENERATIONAL TRANSMISSION OF SEXUAL ABUSE: SEX OFFENDING BY JUVENILES

Studies of juvenile sex offenders often cite prior sexual abuse and other forms of maltreatment. Abel et al. (29) found that 59% of 561 adult male sex offenders reported that their paraphilic behavior commenced during adolescence, but they were rarely apprehended before adulthood. Longo (30) reported that 47% of male adolescent sex offenders in his treatment program had been previously molested. Johnson (31) described the behavior and backgrounds of 13 child molesters, ranging in age from 4 to 13, who were seen in a treatment program. The average age of their victims was 4 years, 4 months. The mean age of their first perpetration was 6 years, 9 months. All of these young perpetrators had been sexually abused. Fehrenbach and Monastersky (32) evaluated a group of 28 female adolescent sexual offenders in an outpatient sexual offender program. The average age of the girls was 13. Half of the girls reported that they had been sexually abused in the past. Hunter et al. (33) described deviant sexual arousal patterns in female adolescent sexual offenders. The majority of these adolescents acknowledged having sexual fantasies about younger children prior to their first sexual offense. These young perpetrators also reported having been sexually aroused during their own previous sexual molestation during childhood. Ray and English (34) evaluated 34 girls and 237 boys who were referred to a treatment program for sexually aggressive youth in the Washington State Department of Social and Health Services. They reported that 93.5% of the girls and 84.9% of the boys had themselves been victims of sexual abuse. Ninety-four percent of the girls and 86.1% of the boys also suffered multiple abuses—e.g. combinations of sexual abuse, physical abuse, emotional abuse, and neglect.

VIII. ADULT SEXUAL OFFENSES AGAINST CHILDREN

A. Male Sex Offenders

Allen (35) reported that 36% of a sample 75 male pedophiles were molested as children. Groth and Burgess (36) found that 32% of a group of 106 child molesters reported sexual trauma during childhood, compared with only 3% of a comparison group of police officers. Langevin et al. (37) documented childhood sexual abuse in 51% of 32 heterosexual pedophiles and in 45% of fathers who committed incest with their daughters, while only 19% of a comparison group of 54 nonoffenders were molested during childhood. Seghorn et al. (38) reported that 57% of 54 incarcerated child molesters and 23% of incarcerated rapists had been victims of child sexual abuse.

Case Illustration: Alan, a 37-year-old man, was accused of molesting Lisa, his 5-year-old daughter. He admitted to fondling Lisa when they showered together at his apartment during weekend visits. He also engaged in mutual masturbation with Lisa and had her perform fellatio. Alan had been a lonely child whose father rarely spent time with him. He often spent weekends going to movies by himself. When he was 8, a man in the next seat fondled his genitals. Alan felt both frightened and sexually aroused but agreed to meet the molester several more times, during which he was fondled and forced to submit to fellatio. Alan recalled that he would have pleasurable fantasies about his own molestation when sexually involved with his daughter, but he was never previously aware of any link between these two events.

B. Female Sex Offenders

Relatively little research has been done with female sexual offenders, most of it taking place during the past decade. However, the few published studies are in complete agreement with the striking prevalence of sexual victimization in their childhood. Mathews et al. (39) reported that 15 of 16 convicted female child molesters had been sexually abused as children, and the remaining offender had been sexually abused in adolescence. McCarty (40) found that 95% of 26 mothers who had maltreated their children had a history of physical or sexual abuse. Knopp and Lackey (41) presented data gathered by 44 providers of treatment to female perpetrators. Among the adult offenders, 93% had been sexually victimized. Green and Kaplan (42) reported that 82% of their sample of female offenders had been sexually abused, and 73% had been physically abused during childhood.

IX. SEXUAL ABUSE LEADING TO DEPRESSION AND SUICIDAL BEHAVIOR

Sgroi (43) described depression, guilt, and low self-esteem, along with a sensation of permanent physical damage or "damaged goods" syndrome" as pivotal issues facing victims of child sexual abuse. Freidrich et al. (44) found that 46% of a sample of 61 sexually abused girls had significantly elevated scores on the internalizing scale of the Child Behavior Checklist, which includes behaviors such as fearful, inhibited, depressed, and overcontrolled. Two studies of sexually abused adolescents admitted to psychiatric inpatient facilities (45,46) reported that the victims of sexual abuse demonstrated a greater severity of depressive symptoms and more suicide attempts than did nonabused inpatients.

Finkelhor (47) maintains that depression is the most commonly reported symptom in adult survivors of child sexual abuse. This has been documented in several studies (48–50). Suicidal behavior has also been frequently documented in adult survivors of child sexual abuse. Briere (51) reported that 51% of adult sexual abuse victims had a history of suicide attempts, compared with 34% of nonabused controls, whereas Sedney and Brooks (50) found that 39% of sexually victimized college students reported suicidal ideation, compared with 16% of a control group.

X. SEXUAL ABUSE LEADING TO REVICTIMIZATION

Females who have been sexually victimized in childhood appear to be vulnerable to revictimization later in life. Russell (1986) reported that between 33 and 68% of sexual abuse victims were subsequently raped, compared with an incidence of rape of 17% for women who had not been sexually abused. Miller et al. (53) compared women who reported a first-time rape with those who had been raped more than once. Of the repeat victims, 18% had incest histories, compared with only 4% of the first-time victims. In addition to rape, victims of child sexual abuse are more likely to be abused by husbands or other adult partners. Russell (52) found that significantly higher numbers of adult female survivors of child sexual abuse had physically violent husbands and were sexually assaulted by them compared with women who had not been victims of child sexual abuse. Briere (51) observed that 49% of his sample of women sexually abused in childhood were battered in adult relationships compared with 18% of a non-victim group.

XI. INDIRECT GENERATIONAL TRANSMISSION OF CHILD SEXUAL ABUSE

A. Mothers of Sexually Abused Children

Although the vast majority of female sexual offenders have been sexually victimized during childhood, most girls who have been molested do not become sexually assaultive. However, there is growing evidence that sexual abuse of a female child might place her at risk for exposing her children to a similar victimization. Faller (54) reported that 49% of mothers in 154 cases of intrafamilial child sexual abuse had experienced sexual abuse as children. Another study of mothers of abused children was carried out by Goodwin et al. (55). They found that 24% of 100 mothers of abused children reported a prior incest experience, compared to 3% of a control group of 500 normal women in the community.

Case Illustration: Cindy had been sexually fondled by her mother's brother-in-law when she was 8 years old. She informed her mother, who replied, "Tell me if he does it again." When Cindy told her mother after a second molestation, her mother ignored her. This man was finally arrested after sexually abusing his own daughter. Cindy's mother trivialized the sexual abuse and maintained that "All Hispanic girls get molested so it's up to them to protect themselves." Cindy's mother had been fondled by her stepfather and vaginally penetrated by three older brothers during her own childhood. She did not disclose these sexual assaults because she feared that her abusive mother would beat her.

Clinical experience with these cases reveals that these mothers appear to be desensitized to the deviancy and negative impact of their own molestation and of the sexual abuse of their children. They denied evidence of their molestation, which was readily visible in the behavior of the perpetrator and the child. These women chose husbands or boyfriends who reminded them of their own abusers. They were often unable to disclose the molestation for fear of an angry, punitive response by their mothers or the perpetrator. If they reported the abuse, their mothers were rejecting or unsupportive. Identification with their own non-protective mothers is a common dynamic in these women.

The violence-related sequelae of sexual abuse in childhood and in adult life described in this section suggests that sexually abused children, like their physically abused counterparts, are highly vulnerable to involvement in subsequent violent behavior during childhood and in adult life. Such behaviors include sexual aggression and sexual offending, suicidality, direct and indirect generational transmission of sexual abuse, and a proneness toward revictimization. However, many or even a majority of abuse victims do not abuse others, nor do they exhibit self-destructive behaviors or contribute to their victimization by others. The remainder of this chapter attempts to seek an explanation for the reenactment of violent behavior by some abuse victims and to explore potential protective factors that neutralize violent behavior in others.

XII. THEORETICAL MODELS

A. Social Learning Model

Social learning theory postulates that behavior can be acquired by observing others (56). Gelles and Straus (57), Hertzberger, (58), and Feshbach (59), using a social learning perspective, hypothesized that abusive parenting behaviors are transmitted by teaching children that aggression is appropriate. Children observe abusive behavior and develop a set of rules that support it. According to Hertzberger, abused children were more likely to form rules supporting abusive behavior if the parent's action is seen as normative, if the abuse is accompanied by rationalizations, and if the abuse is used as a disciplinary measure following an actual wrongdoing. MacEwen (60) maintains that the likelihood of generational transmission of aggression is proportional to the frequency and severity of the family aggression, its negative impact on the family, and the degree to which the observer identifies with the aggressor. The gender of the model and the observer are also important factors—e.g., within-gender modeling is stronger than between-gender modeling, and male models tend to be imitated more than female models.

Becker and Kaplan (61) described an etiological model for the development of deviant sexual behavior in adolescent males in which a series of risk factors operating within the individual, the family, and the social environment act as precursors to the first deviant act. Individual risk factors include an impulse-control or conduct disorder or a history of physical or sexual abuse. Family risk factors include parents who engage in coercive physical or sexual behavior or use poor parenting techniques. Environmental risk factors include social isolation or identification with a peer group engaging in antisocial behavior. According to Becker and Kaplan, the adolescents who reoffend are likely to be those who found the act to be pleasurable, experienced minimal negative consequences in relation to the sexual crime, experienced reinforcement of the deviant sexual behavior through masturbatory activity and fantasy, and were deficient in peer relationships. Adolescents who had supportive parents and received protection and treatment after being molested during childhood were less likely to reenact their victimization with others.

B. Psychoanalytic/Psychodynamic Model

This model emphasizes the importance of psychological trauma inherent in abuse; this initiates pathological defense mechanisms that play a role in perpetuating violent behavior. This model also proposes that internalized mental representations of parental and self objects derived from childhood influence current object relationships.

C. Freud's Concept of Traumatic Neurosis

Freud's concept of traumatic neurosis and the breaching of the stimulus barrier (62) may be useful in understanding the sequelae of abuse. Freud defined the traumatic situation as an experience of helplessness on the part of the ego in the face of cumulative excitation of external or internal origin. Boyer (63) stressed the parent's role as supplementary stimulus barrier; but in case of abuse, the parent not only fails to buttress the stimulus barrier but adds to the trauma. When the barrier is breached, the child's receptive, defensive, and integrative ego functions are overwhelmed, rendering the child helpless. At this point, the repetition compulsion, or the victim's compulsion to repeat the trauma, comes into play. This fixation to the trauma may be regarded as a defensive activity in which passive victimization is replaced by active mastery. According to Green's description of the trauma inherent in child abuse (64), the child uses primitive defenses to deal with the traumatic overstimulation and the emerging core symptoms of anxiety and depression that repression fails to control. Avoidance and distancing behavior—consisting of hypervigilance, gaze aversion, and the raising of sensory thresholds—are initially used to control the traumatic stimulation. These are followed by defenses of denial, projection, splitting, and dissociation, which allow the child to maintain the fantasy of having a "good" parent, whereas the parent's malevolence is displaced onto another person or himself. In cases of severe abuse, these defenses often fail to bind the anxiety generated by the abuse, and the traumatic imagery derived from the physical or sexual assault invades the dreams, fantasies, play, and object relationships of the child victim. Since the internalized object relationships of the abused child are strongly colored by the abuser-victim constellation, prolonged exposure to a harsh and abusive parent promotes a primary identification with the aggressive parent. "Identification with the aggressor" is used as a major defense mechanism in situations of anxiety provoked by fears of attack, helplessness, and humiliation. While this defense is being used, the child's fears of helplessness are replaced by feelings of power, control, and omnipotence. "Identification with the aggressor" appears to be embedded in the child's compulsion to repeat and reenact the trauma. This trauma-induced defense permits the child to displace some of his or her original rage toward the abusive parent onto a substitute and may also serve as a tension-relieving device and as a pathological form of self-esteem regulation. On the other hand, some abused children primarily identify with the role of the victim. They use "identification with the victim" as a primary defense mechanism, which leads to the reenactment of their victim role while they are interacting with others. This may lead to masochistic, provocative behavior designed to provoke maltreatment from others and may be the major determinant of their proneness towards revictimization. The physical and sexual abuse of children is often superimposed upon chronic trauma resulting from ongoing harsh and punitive parenting, rejection and scapegoating, role confusion, maternal deprivation, and threats of abandonment. Prior (65) believes that identification with the aggressor and the reenactment of sadomasochistic relationships are utilized as defenses against isolation and ego disorganization.

D. Attachment Theory

Attachment theory, although derived from psychoanalytic theory, offers a slightly different perspective for explaining the abuse victim's reenactment of his or her victimization. According to Bowlby (66), the transmission of patterns of relating across generations is mediated by an individual's internal working models, which are dynamic representations of self and others that guide the individual's appraisal of and response to others. These models are relatively resistant to change. Maltreated children who become poorly attached to their parents develop internal representations of caretakers as inaccessible, frightening, or unreliable. This results in insecure disorganized/disoriented (type D) attachments to their mothers in the Ainsworth strange situation, as demonstrated by Carlson et al. (67) which differ from Ainsworth's original type A anxious-avoidant, type B, secure, and type C, anxious-ambivalent attachment styles (68). The disorganized/disoriented attachment is characterized by the absence of a coherent coping mechanism to deal with the stress of separation from and reunion with the mother. The maltreated infants displayed contradictory features of strong proximity-seeking followed by strong avoidance, or they appeared dazed and disoriented upon reunion with their caretakers. They also exhibited stilling, slow movements, depressed affect, and apprehension toward the parent. Carlson et al. (67) attribute these behaviors to the simultaneous activation of fear and attachment behavioral systems that produce conflicting motivations—to approach the caregiver for comfort and to retreat from him or her for safety. Chronic abuse by a parent reinforces internal working models of an abusing parent–child victim dyad, which may persist unless it is modified by subsequent contact with benign or supportive parental figures. Maltreated children who become poorly attached to their caregivers later develop insecure attachments to their own children. Fonagy et al. (69), using the Adult Attachment Interview, observed that children whose mothers' internal representation of past relationships were insecure when interviewed in the third trimester of pregnancy tended to develop an insecure relationship with their mothers during the first year of life.

In a previously cited study, Egeland et al. (24) followed mothers who had been abused during childhood for 48 to 54 months postpartum. Of these mothers, 70% were currently maltreating their children. They were compared with a group of mothers who had been victims of physical abuse in childhood but provided adequate care for their children. The following factors appeared to be operating in the mothers who broke the intergenerational continuity of abuse: (a) they had received a less severe form of abuse, (b) they had one parent or caretaker who provided them with love and support, (c) many had been in therapy as adolescents or young adults, (d) they had supportive spouses and adequate living conditions, and (e) they were aware of their own history of having been abused. This suggests that internal working models can be modified by subsequent exposure to positive relationships.

Egeland and Susman-Stillman (70) did a follow-up study with a subsample of the mothers who were abused, comparing those who maltreated their children with those who broke the cycle of abuse. The mothers who were abused and continued to abuse their children were rated higher on idealization, inconsistency, and escapism in their descriptions of their childhood, and they scored higher on Dissociative Experience Scale than mothers who broke the cycle. The authors maintained that the dissociative defenses in mothers who continued to abuse their children interfered with their ability to integrate their traumatic childhood experiences into a coherent view of self. They speculated that dissociation might be related in some way to the internal working models described in attachment theory, in that they both appear to be involved in the transmission of abuse across generations.

Contributions from social learning, psychoanalytic, and attachment theorists have added to our understanding of how many victims of physical and sexual assault utilize their abusers as models for their own violent behavior. Social learning and attachment theories, more easily operationalized than psychoanalytic theory, have informed much of the research on the generational transmission of violence. The concept of internal mental representations underlying psychoanalytic and attachment theories is useful in explaining why some maltreated individuals repeat their traumatic experiences and others can break the cycle of violence. Contact with positive parental role models and the development of supportive peer relationships may alter internal self-object representations in a positive direction and create a receptive climate for the verbal and emotional expression of traumatic experiences.

XIII. PTSD AND THE PSYCHOBIOLOGY OF TRAUMATIC STRESS

Recent research involving traumatized individuals and the impact of trauma on the brain has added another dimension to the understanding of how violent behavior may be repeated. Numerous clinicians have described symptoms of PTSD in physically (71–73) and sexually (43,74) abused children. Kiser et al. (1988) documented PTSD in 9 of 10 children between the ages of 2 and 6 who were molested in a day care setting, while McLeer et al. (1988) diagnosed PTSD in 48% of sexually abused children evaluated at a child psychiatric outpatient clinic. The most frequently observed symptoms associated with PTSD included nightmares and sleep disorders, reexperiencing of phenomena, intrusive memories of the abuse, hypervigilance and autonomic hyperarousal, avoidance of activities reminiscent of the traumatic event, and intensification of symptoms on exposure to events resembling the physical or sexual abuse.

Chronic PTSD has been described in adult female survivors of child sexual abuse. These women displayed sleep disorders, guilt, intrusive imagery of the incest, and feelings of detachment when they were exposed to reminders of their molestation.

Dissociation, or an alteration in consciousness resulting in impairment in identity or memory, has also been observed in child victims of physical and sexual abuse (77,78). Signs of early dissociation in children are forgetfulness with periods of amnesia, excessive fantasizing and daydreaming, trance-like states, sleepwalking, blackouts, and the presence of an imaginary playmate. There appears to be a close relationship between dissociation and PTSD. This was demonstrated by Coons et al., (79), who documented high levels of dissociation in adult survivors of sexual abuse with PTSD, and by Bremner et al. (80), who found a similar correlation between dissociation and PTSD in veterans of combat in Vietnam.

According to van der Kolk et al. (81), the core problem in PTSD consists of a failure to integrate a traumatic event into autobiographical memory. It is likely that memories are registered and consolidated differently under severe stress. van der Kolk et al. (81) suggest that secretion of neurohormones (norepinephrine and oxytocin) promotes a long-term potentiation and overconsolidation of traumatic memories. This is largely mediated by norepinephrine input to the amygdala. Overstimulation of the amygdala will interfere with its function of assigning emotional significance to sensory stimuli arriving from the neocortex and thalamus, which is then passed on to the hippocampus, where the new information is organized and integrated with previously existing sensory information. High levels of stimulation of the amygdala will interfere with the integrative function of the hippocampus, and the memory imprints will be laid down and retrieved as isolated images, bodily sensations, smells, and sounds separate from other life experiences. Brain imaging techniques carried out by Bremner et al. (82) have shown that individuals with chronic PTSD have decreased hippocampal volume and impaired hippocampal functioning. These unintegrated memories appear and cannot be translated into communicable language. A positron emission tomography study by Raush et al. (83) with PTSD patients who were exposed to detailed narratives they had written about their own traumatic experiences demonstrated heightened neuronal activity in the amygdala and in the neighboring limbic system in the right hemisphere, heightened activity in the right visual cortex, and an absence of activity in Broca's area in the left hemisphere. The authors attribute the difficulty that PTSD patients have in putting feelings into words to the suppression of Broca's area.

A. Abnormalities in Catecholamine Activity

The catecholamines—epinephrine, norepinephrine, and dopamine—have been studied in animals and humans exposed to various types of stress. DeBellis et al. (84) found a higher catecholamine functional activity and synthesis in a sample of sexually abused girls who were depressed and suicidal as compared with nonabused controls. Similar high indices of catecholamine activity had been reported in patients with PTSD. Galvin et al. (85) documented significantly lower serum dopamine beta-hydroxylase (DBH) activity in psychiatrically hospitalized boys with a history of childhood maltreatment before the age of 6 than in comparison groups of children maltreated after the age of 6 and hospitalized boys without a history of maltreatment. All of these children had been diagnosed with a form of conduct disorder or disruptive behavior. Low serum DBH was also found in conduct-disordered boys independent of their maltreatment status. Serum DBH, which converts dopamine into norepinephrine, is regarded as an index of sympathetic response to chronic stressors. The authors concluded that maltreatment experienced in early childhood overstimulates the nonadrenergic system, resulting in an initial increase of DBH followed by repression of enzyme activity that is reflected peripherally as low DBH activity. In boys, low serum DBH activity also appears to correlate with conduct disorder, solitary aggressive type.

B. Serotonergic Dysregulation

Decreased serotonin levels were correlated with impulsivity, aggression, and suicidal behavior by Coccaro et al. (86), all of which have been described in maltreated children. Decreased serotonin functioning has been described in male combat veterans with PTSD (87). Studies of serotonergic functioning in maltreated children should be undertaken to assess the contribution of low serotonin to the violent sequelae of physical and sexual abuse.

C. HPA Axis Dysregulation

DeBellis et al. (88) reported attenuated plasma ACTH responses to corticotrophin releasing hormone (CRH) in sexually abused girls. The authors hypothesized that chronic CRH hypersecretion associated with the stress of the traumatic sexual assaults in sexually abused girls lead to an adaptive downregulation of CRH receptors in the anterior pituitary. Kaufman (89) reported abnormalities in cortisol secretion in maltreated children diagnosed with major depression or dysthymia. These children failed to show the expected diurnal drop in cortisol levels.

D. Endogenous Opioids

According to van der Kolk et al. (90), exposure to severe and prolonged stress and reexposure to traumatic situations results in the secretion of endogenous opioids, which produce an anxiolytic and tranquilizing action. When opioid levels drop after the cessation of the stress, an "endogenous" opiate withdrawal ensues. van der Kolk et al. believe that traumatized individuals re-expose themselves to traumatic situations in order to produce an endogenous opioid response and restore higher opioid levels. This might contribute to the tendency of abused children to harm themselves or provoke revictimization from others.

It is likely that the stress-induced maladaptive behaviors and defenses in the abused child and the accompanying psychobiological changes interact synergistically to produce violence-proneness. Alterations in neurotransmitter and hormonal activity, limbic system functioning, and the encoding and retrieval of traumatic memories may all contribute to violent and/or self-destructive behavior and an inability to process the abusive experiences.

XIV. INTERVENTION: BREAKING THE CYCLE OF VIOLENCE

A. Crisis Intervention

The immediate goal of intervention in cases of child maltreatment is to modify the abusive environment so that the child is no longer at risk for physical or sexual abuse—e.g., the abuser should no longer have access to the child. At the same time, one must be certain that the abuse has been reported to child protective services.

Treatment usually begins with crisis intervention to deal with the child's anxiety-related symptoms pertaining to the abuse and the family crisis that often follows the disclosure of maltreatment. The parents, and other relevant caretakers, including the abuser(s), and the siblings of the victim, should all be interviewed in order to assess their caretaking skills and psychological functioning and to determine whether the family will be able to protect their children from further harm. The availability of supportive networks of family and friends and the need for specialized services—e.g., homemaking, financial aid—should be determined during the initial assessment.

B. Intervention with the Children

Individual psychodynamically oriented psychotherapy and play therapy offer the best possibility for effecting changes in the maltreated child's internalized negative self- and object representations that contribute to his or her reenactment of the abuse trauma. The importance of sustained long-term clinical intervention with maltreating families has been cited in the child development literature (91,92). Treatment goals with abused children must initially focus on the child's feelings of betrayal and mistrust of others derived from their abusive experience at the hands of parents and caretakers. This is imperative in the formation of a therapeutic relationship. A crucial component of treatment is to help the child uncover and verbalize painful memories and affects associated with the abuse, which had been denied or dissociated from awareness.

Reintegration of these traumatic experiences into the victim's memory and personal awareness should diminish the need for their repetitive reenactment. Additional treatment issues of importance are the child's sense of stigmatization, shame and guilt, and low self-esteem. These may be alleviated by stressing that the perpetrator and not the child is responsible for the abuse. Impulsivity in physically and sexually aggressive children requires structuring, strict limit setting, and interpretation of their use of "identification with the aggressor" as a primary defense mechanism. Symptoms of depression, suicidal behavior, and PTSD require specialized intervention, including the use of anxiolytic and antidepressant medication. Higher-level defenses, such as repression and sublimation, are strengthened in order to replace primitive defenses of denial, projection, splitting, and dissociation. Ultimately, the therapist must convey to the child that pathological defenses designed to master abusive experiences and protect against further assault are maladaptive in nonabusive environments.

Short-term treatment models have also been reported to be useful in treating abused children, such as cognitive behavioral therapy, (93) group psychotherapy, (94), and family therapy (95). Abused infants and preschool children may be treated in a therapeutic nursery designed to assess and improve the pathological parent-child interaction (96).

Establishing a positive, supportive relationship with a therapist perceived as being dependable, understanding, and trustworthy should gradually lead to a positive change in the child's internalized self- and object representations. This is likely to be more important in reversing the child's tendency to reenact violent experiences than the therapeutic modality itself.

C. Intervention with the Parents

The major goal of intervention is to improve the quality of parenting so that further maltreatment is less likely to occur. This requires a blend of psychotherapy and parenting education, the former dealing with current psychopathology and unresolved issues from the parent's own childhood traumas and the latter focused on improving the current parent-child interaction.

Psychotherapy is designed to interpret the link between current abusive practices and the parent's childhood experiences of maltreatment, and to reverse the parent's misperception of the child that leads to scapegoating and role reversal. The therapist also provides the parent with a positive child-rearing model for identification.

Therapeutic groups for mothers may be used as an adjunct to individual psychotherapy. Parenting education focuses on the implementation of nonabusive disciplinary and child-rearing techniques and dispenses information about parenting and child development. The parent is also taught to be more sensitive to the child's cues. In cases of maltreatment associated with family disorganization and poverty, the families will require special advocacy and outreach, consisting of the provision of social services, home visits, assistance with housing and finances, and the monitoring of medical care. This multifaceted intervention with the parents should effect positive changes in the parent's internalized mental representations of negative childhood experiences that formed the model for the reenactment of their own victimization.

XV. SUMMARY

This chapter describes how many child abuse victims are driven to repeat and reenact their violent experiences during childhood and as adults. Their identification with abusive models, their use of pathological defense mechanisms that interfere with the processing of traumatic events, and their re-involvement with negative object relationships derived from the past contribute to their violence-proneness. A coexisting psychobiological substrate for perpetuating violence was discussed, consisting of pathological alterations in catecholamine and serotin release, abnormalities in the functioning of the HPA axis and limbic system, and fluctuating levels of endogenous opioids. These biological changes are generated by the traumatic stress accompanying child maltreatment.

While childhood physical and sexual abuse are definite risk factors for subsequent violent behavior, the progression from abuse victim to an abuser of self or others is not inevitable. The availability of supportive and nonviolent relationships that can neutralize pathological internal mental representations acts as a protective factor against the transmission of violence. Interventions designed to protect the child from further maltreatment, provide a positive role model, enhance the reintegration of split-off traumatic memories and affects into personal awareness, and strengthen parental functioning have been successful in breaking the cycle of violence.

REFERENCES

1. *Current Trends in Child Abuse Reporting and Fatalities: The Results of the 1995 Annual Fifty State Survey*, National Committee to Prevent Child Abuse, Chicago, 1996.
2. C. George and M. Main, Social interactions and young abused children, *Child Dev. 50*:306 (1979).
3. D.M. Bousha and C.T. Twentyman, Mother-child interactional style in abuse, neglect, and control groups: Naturalistic observations in the home, *J. Abnorm. Psychol. 93*:106 (1984).

4. A.H. Green, Psychopathology of abused children, *J. Am. Acad. Child Psychiatry 17*:579 (1978).
5. R. Livingston, Sexually and physically abused children, *J. Amer. Acad. Child Psychiatr. 26*:413 (1987).
6. R. Famularo, R. Kinscherr, and T. Fenton, *J. Am. Acad. Child Adolesc. Psychiatry 31*:863 (1992).
7. A.S. Scerbo and D.J. Kolko, Child physical abuse and aggression: Preliminary findings on the role of internalizing problems. *J. Am. Acad. Child Psychiatry 34*:1060 (1995).
8. D. Truscott, Intergenerational transmission of violent behavior in adolescent males. *Aggress. Behav. 18*:327 (1992).
9. D. Lewis, S. Shanok, J. Pincus, and F. Glaser, Violent juvenile delinquents: Psychiatric, neurological, and abuse factors. *J. Am. Acad. Child Psychiatry 18*:307 (1979).
10. M. Geller and L. Ford-Somma, Violent homes, violent children: *A Study of Violence in the Families of Juvenile Offenders* (New Jersey State Department of Corrections, Trenton), Report prepared by the National Center on Child Abuse and Neglect, Department of Health and Human Services, Washington, DC, 1984.
11. R.E. Tarter, A.M. Hegedus, N.E. Winsten, and A.I. Alterman, Neuropsychological, personality, and familial characteristics of physically abused delinquents, *J. Am. Acad. Child Psychiatry 23*:688 (1984).
12. J.D. Alfaro, *Report on the Relationship Between Child Abuse and Neglect and Later Socially Deviant Behavior*, New York State Assembly Select Committee on Child Abuse, New York, NY, 1977.
13. S. Gutierres and J.A. Reich, A developmental perspective on runaway behavior: Its relationship to child abuse. *Child Welfare 60*:89 (1981).
14. J. McCord, A forty year perspective on effects of child abuse nd neglect. *Child Abuse Neglect 7*:265 (1983).
15. C.S. Widom, Does violence beget violence? A critical examination of the literature. *Psychol. Bull. 106*:3 (1989).
16. R.K. Ressler and A.W. Burges, The men who murdered, *FBI Law Enforce. Bull. 54*:2 (1985).
17. D.O. Lewis, E. Moy, L.D. Jackson, et al., Biopsychological characteristics of children who later murder: A prospective study, *Am. J. Psychiatry 142*:1161 (1985).
18. A.H. Green, Self-destructive behavior in battered children, *Am. J. Psychiatry 135*:579 (1978).
19. C. Pfeffer, *The Suicidal Child*, Guilford Press, New York, 1985.
20. E. Deykin, J. Alger, and J. McNamara, A pilot study of the effect of exposure to child abuse or neglect on suicidal behavior. *Am. J. Psychiatry 112*:299 (1985).
21. B.H. Steele, The effect of abuse and neglect on child development, *Frontiers of Infant Psychiatry* (J.D. Call, E. Galenson, and R.L. Tyson, eds.), Basic Books, New York, 1983.
22. B.J. Steele and C.B. Pollock, A psychiatric study of parents who abuse infants and small children, *The Battered Child* (R.E. Helfer and C.H. Kempe, eds.), University of Chicago Press, Chicago, 1968, p. 103.

23. A.H. Green, R.W. Gaines, and A. Sandgrund, Child abuse: Pathological syndrome of family interaction, *Am. J. Psychiatry 133*:882 (1974).
24. B. Egeland, D. Jacobvitz, and K. Papatola. Intergenerational continuity of parental abuse, *Biosocial Aspects of Child Abuse* (J. Lancaster and R. Gelles, eds.), Jossey-Bass, San Francisco, 1987, p. 255.
25. E.C. Herrenkohl, R.C. Herrenkohl, and L.J. Toedter, Perspectives on the intergenerational transmission of abuse, *The Dark Side of Families* (D. Finkelhor, R.J. Gelles, G.T. Hotaling, and M.A. Straus, eds.), Sage Publications, Beverly Hills, CA, 1983, p. 305.
26. A.H. Green, E. Toledo, and H. Eckholdt, Generational transmission of maltreatment in mother-child dyads attending a child abuse clinic, unpublished manuscript, 1996.
27. A. Yates, Children eroticized by incest, *Am. J. Psychiatry 139*:482 (1982).
28. W.N. Friedrich, Behavior problems in sexually abused children: An adaptational perspective, *Lasting Effects of Child Sexual Abuse*, (G.E. Wyatt and G.J. Powell, eds.), Beverly Hills, CA, 1988.
29. G.G. Abel, M. Mittelman, and J.V. Becker, Sex offenders: Results of assessment and recommendations for treatment, *Clinical Criminology: Current Concepts* (H. Ben-Aron, S. Hucker, and C. Webster, eds.) M&M Graphics, Toronto, 1985.
30. R.E. Longo, Sexual learning and experience among adolescent offenders, *Int. J. Offend. Ther. Comp. Criminol. 26*:235 (1982).
31. T.C. Johnson, Female child perpetrators: Children who molest other children, *Child Abuse Neglect 13*:571 (1989).
32. P.A. Fehrenbach and C. Monastersky, Characteristics of female adolescent sexual offenders, *Am. J. Orthopsychiatry 58*:148 (1988).
33. J.A. Hunter, L.J. Lexier, B.A. Goodwin, et al. Psychosexual, attitudinal, and developmental characteristics of juvenile female sexual perpetrators in a residential treatment setting, *J. Child Fam. Stud. 2*:317 (1993).
34. J. Ray, *Comparison of Female and Male Children with Sexual Behavior Problems,* Dept. of Social and Health Services, Office of Children's Administration Research, Olympia, WA, 1992.
35. C.M. Allen, *Women and Men Who Sexually Abuse Children: A Comparative Analysis,* The Safer Society Press, Orwell, VT, 1991.
36. A.N. Groth and A. Burgess, Sexual trauma in the lives of rapists an child molesters, *Victimol. Int. J. 4*:10 (1979).
37. R. Langevin, L.Handy, H. Hook, et al. Are incestuous fathers pedophilic and aggressive? *Erotic Preference, Gender Identity, and Aggression* (R. Langevin, ed.), Erlbaum, Hillsdale, NJ, 1985.
38. T.K. Seghorn, R.A. Prentky, and R.J. Boucher, Childhood sexual abuse in the lives of sexually aggressive offenders, *J. Am. Acad. Child Adolesc. Psychiatry 26*:262 (1987).
39. R. Mathews, J. Matthews, and K. Speltz, *Female Sexual Offenders: An Exploratory Study*, The Safer Society Press, Orwell, VT, 1989.
40. L. McCarty, Mother-child incest: Characteristics of the offender, *Child Welfare 65*:457 (1986).
41. F.H. Knopp and L.B. Lackey, Female sexual abusers: A summary of data from 44

treatment providers, *The Safer Society Program of the New York Council of Churches*, Orwell, VT, 1987.
42. A.H. Green and M.S. Kaplan, Psychiatric impairment and childhood victimization experiences in female child molesters, *J. Am. Acad. Child Adolesc. Psychiatry 33*: 954 (1994).
43. S. Sgroi, *Handbook of Clinical Intervention in Child Sexual Abuse*, Lexington Books, Lexington, MA, 1982.
44. W.N. Friedrich, A.J. Urquiza, and R.J. Beilke, Behavior problems in sexually abused young children, *J. Pediatr. Psychol. 11*:47 (1986).
45. A. Cavaiola and M. Schiff, Behavioral sequelae of physical and/or sexual abuse in adolescents, *Child Abuse Neglect 12*:181 (1988).
46. H. Sansonnet-Hayden, G. Haley, K. Marriage, and S. Fine, Sexual abuse and psychopathology in hospitalized adolescents, *J. Am. Acad. Child Adolesc. Psychiatry 26*:753 (1987).
47. D. Finkelhor, *A Sourcebook on Child Sexual Abuse,* Sage, Beverly Hills, CA, 1986.
48. C. Bagley and R. Ramsay, Sexual abuse in childhood: Psychosocial outcomes and implications for social work practice, *J. Soc. Work Hum. Sexual. 4*:33 (1986).
49. S.D. Peters, Child sexual abuse and later psychological problems, paper presented at the meeting of the American Psychological Association, Los Angeles, August 1985.
50. M.A. Sedney, and B. Brooks, Factors associated with a history of childhood sexual experiences in a nonclinical female population, *J. Am. Acad. Child Psychiatry 23*:215 (1984).
51. J. Briere, The long-term effects of childhood sexual abuse: Defining a post-sexual abuse syndrome, Paper presented at the Third National Conference on Sexual Victimization of Children, Washington, DC, 1984.
52. D. Russell, *The Secret Trauma: Incest in the Lives of Girls and Women*, Basic Books, New York, 1986.
53. J. Miller, D. Moeller, A. Kaufman, et al. Recidivism among sexual assault victims, *Am. J. Psychiatry 135*:1103 (1978).
54. K.C. Faller, Why sexual abuse? An exploration of the intergenerational hypothesis, *Child Abuse Neglect 8*:543 (1989).
55. J. Goodwin, K. Cheevers, and V. Connell, Defining a syndrome of severe symptoms in survivors of extreme incestuous abuse, *Sexual Abuse: Incest Victims and their Families* (J. Goodwin, ed.), Year Book, Chicago, 1989.
56. A. Bandura, *Aggression: A Social Learning Analysis*, Prentice-Hall, Englewood Cliffs, NJ, 1973.
57. R. Gelles and M. Straus, Determinants of violence in the family: Towards a theoretical integration, *Contemporary Theories About the Family* (W. Burr, R. Hill, F. Nye, and I. Reiss, eds.), Free Press, New York, 1972.
58. S.D. Hertzberger, Social cognition and the transmission of abuse, *The Dark Side of Families* (D. Finkelhor, R.J. Gelles, G.T. Hotaling, and M.A. Straus, eds.), Sage, Beverly Hills, CA, 1983, p. 317.
59. S. Feshbach, Child abuse and the dynamic of human aggression and violence, *Child*

Abuse: An Agenda for Action (J. Gerbner, C.J. Ross, and E. Zigler, eds.), Oxford University Press, New York, 1980.
60. K.E. MacEwen, Refining the intergenerational hypothesis, *J. Interpers. Violence 9*:350 (1994).
61. J.V. Becker and M.S. Kaplan, Assessment and treatment of the male sex offender, *Child Sexual Abuse: A Handbook for Health Care and Legal Professionals* (D.H. Schetky and A.H. Green, eds.), Brunner/Mazel, New York, 1988, p. 136.
62. Freud, S. Beyond the pleasure principle, *The Standard Edition of the Complete Psychological Works of Sigmund Freud*, Vol. 18, Hogarth Press, London, 1968, p. 7.
63. L.B. Boyer, On maternal overstimulation and ego defects, *Psychoanal. Study Child 11*:236 (1956).
64. A.H. Green, Child abuse: Dimensions of psychological trauma in abused children, *J. Am. Acad. Child Psychiatry 22*:231 (1983).
65. S. Prior, *Object Relations in Severe Trauma*, Jason Aronson, Northvale, NJ, 1996.
66. J. Bowlby, *Attachment and Loss:* Vol. 3. *Loss*, Basic Books, New York, 1980.
67. V. Carlson, D. Cicchetti, D. Barnett, and K. Braunwald, Disorganized/disoriented attachment relationships in maltreated infants. *Dev. Psychol. 25*:525 (1989).
68. M.D.S. Ainsworth, M.C. Blehar, E. Waters, and S. Wall, *Patterns of Attachment: A Psychological Study of the Strange Situation*, Erlbaum, Hillsdale, NJ, 1978.
69. P. Fonagy, M. Steele, G. Moran, et al. Measuring the ghost in the nursery: An empirical study of the relation between parents' mental representations of childhood experiences and their infants' security of attachment, *J. Am. Psychoanal. Assoc. 41*:957 (1993).
70. B. Egeland and A. Susman-Stillman, Dissociation as a mediator of child abuse across generations, *Child Abuse Neglect 16*:1123 (1996).
71. A.H. Green, Children traumatized by physical abuse, *Posttraumatic Stress Disorder in Children* (S. Eth and R.S. Pynoos, eds.), American Psychiatric Press, Washington, DC, 1985, p. 135.
72. R. Kempe and C.H. Kempe, *Child Abuse*, Harvard University Press, Cambridge, MA, 1978.
73. C. Ounstead, R. Oppenheimer, and J. Lindsay, Aspects of bonding failure: The psychotherapeutic treatment of families of battered children, *Dev. Med. Child Neurol. 16*:446 (1974).
74. J. Goodwin, Post-traumatic symptoms in incest victims, *Post-traumatic Stress Disorder in Children* (S. Eth and R.S. Pynoos, eds.), American Psychiatric Press, Washington, DC, 1985, p. 157.
75. L.J. Kiser, B.J. Ackerman, E. Brown, et al., Post-traumatic stress disorder in young children: A reaction to purported sexual abuse, *J. Am. Acad. Child Adolesc. Psychiatry 27*:645 (1988).
76. S.V. McLear, E. Deblinger, M.S. Atkins, et al., Post-traumatic stress disorder in sexually abused children, *J. Am. Acad. Child Adolesc. Psychiatry 27*:650 (1988).
77. R. Kluft, *Childhood Antecedents of Multiple Personality*, American Psychiatric Press, Washington, DC, 1985.
78. F.W. Putnam, J.J. Guroff, E.K. Silberman, et al., The clinical phenomenology of

multiple personality disorder: Review of 100 recent cases, *J. Clin. Psychiatry 47*:285 (1996).
79. P.M. Coons, E.S. Bowman, T.A. Pellow, and P. Schneider, Post-traumatic aspects of the treatment of victims of sexual abuse and incest, *Psychiatr. Clin. North Am. 12*:325 (1989).
80. J.D. Bremner, S.M. Southwick, E. Brett, et al., Dissociation and posttraumatic stress disorder in Vietnam combat veterans, *Am. J. Psych. 149*:328 (1992).
81. B.H. van der Kolk, Trauma and memory, *Traumatic Stress* (B.H. van der Kolk, A. C. McFarlane, and L. Weisaeth, eds.) Guilford Press, New York, 1996, p. 279.
82. J.D. Bremner, P. Randall, T. Scott, et al., MRI-based measures of hippocampal volume in patients with PTSD, *Amer. J. Psychiat. 152*:973 (1995).
83. J.L. Raush et al., *Am. J. Psych. 147(10)*:1308 (1990).
84. M.D. DeBellis, L. Lefter, P.K. Trickett, et al., Urinary catecholamine excretion in sexually abused girls, *J. Amer. Acad. Child Adolesc. Psychiatr. 33*:320 (1994).
85. J.E. Galvin et al., *Ann Neurol. 42*:595 (1997).
86. E.F. Coccaro et al., Serotonergic studies in patients with affective and personality disorders, *Arch. Gen. Psych. 46*:587 (1989).
87. R.C. Arora, C.G. Fichtner, F. O'Connor, and J.W. Crayton, Paroxetine binding in the blood platelets of post-traumatic stress disorder patients, *Life Sci 53*:929 (1993).
88. M.D. DeBellis, G.P. Chrousos, L.D. Dorn, et al., Hypothalamic-pituitary-adrenal axis dysregulation in sexually abused girls, *J. Clin. Endocrinol. Metab. 78*:249 (1994).
89. J. Kaufman, Depressive disorders in maltreated children, *J. Am. Acad. Child. Adolesc. Psychiatry 30*:257 (1991).
90. B.H. van der Kolk, M.S. Greenberg, S.P. Orr, and R.K. Pitman, Endogenous opioids and stress induced analgesia in post traumatic stress disorder, *Psychopharmacol. Bull. 25*: 108 (1989).
91. D. Cicchetti and F.A. Rogosch, The toll of child maltreatment on the developing child: Insights from developmental psychopathology, *Child Adolesc. Psychiatr. Clin. North Am. 3*:759 (1994).
92. P.M. Crittenden, Treatment of anxious attachment in infancy and early childhood, *Dev. Psychopathol. 4*:575 (1992).
93. J.A. Cohen and A.P. Mannarino, A treatment model for sexually abused preschoolers, *J. Interpers. Violence 8*:115 (1993).
94. K. Sturkie, Group treatment for sexually abused children, *Child Adolesc. Psychiatr. Clin. North Am. 3*:813 (1994).
95. J.T. Pardeck, Family therapy as a treatment approach to child abuse. *Fam. Ther. 16*:113 (1989).
96. A.H. Green and P.F. Meersand, Therapeutic nursery interventions for abused preschoolers, *Child Adolesc. Psychiatr. Clin. North Am. 3*:831 (1994).

18

The Clinician's Legal Duties When the Patient May Be Violent

James C. Beck
Harvard Medical School and Cambridge Hospital, Cambridge, Massachusetts

Pat Cerundolo
Foley, Hoag & Eliot, L.L.P., Boston, Massachusetts

I. INTRODUCTION

A. General Issues

Violent patients raise unique clinical and legal issues for physicians. *Clinical issues are fundamental* and legal issues are secondary, but the physician must understand the legal issues if these are to be kept in perspective. The purpose of this chapter is to provide sufficient information about legal issues relating to violence so that the physician will put them in perspective and focus primarily on the clinical issues in dealing with the patient. Readers impatient with the discussion of legal duties may want to read only the last section (Sec. III) of this chapter, on practical implications.

1. Violence

Violence refers to acts that physically injure or pose the threat of serious injury to another person. Our discussion excludes violence to self and destruction of property. The person who throws dishes or hits walls is not our concern unless he or she is throwing the dishes *at* someone. Our concern is with people who physically attack others—e.g., stalkers or firesetters. At the margin the definition blurs. People who put others at risk of serious harm, such as HIV-positive persons who have unprotected sex, pose a risk of physical harm. Men who expose themselves to strangers and psychotherapists who have sex with their patients create a foreseeable risk of psychological harm to others.

2. Whose Duty

This chapter applies to all health care professionals, but not all legal duties apply equally to all health care professionals. Clinicians in all 50 states have a duty to report violence toward children. Physicians may have legal duties that other clinicians do not—for example, the duty to report gunshot wounds. Psychotherapists may have a duty under certain circumstances to prevent their patients' violent behavior. In this chapter, we refer generically to clinicians when duties apply across professional lines. When duties apply primarily or only to physicians, we limit the discussion accordingly.

3. The Duty to Protect

In 1974, a California Court held that the existence of a psychotherapist-patient or doctor-patient relationship creates a duty for the clinician (1). This duty may require the clinician to warn persons foreseeably endangered by a patient. Mental health professionals immediately saw a conflict between the duty to warn and the duty to maintain the patient's confidentiality. Since 1974 this conflict has been a subject of many court cases and of legal and psychiatric commentary.

4. Statutory Law, Case Law, and Regulations

Statutory law is enacted by the legislature. The judiciary creates case law. The executive branch promulgates regulations that have the force of law. There are federal and state statutes as well as federal and state case law. Most of the laws and regulations governing clinical practice are state laws and regulations. The clinician should be familiar with or at least know of the statutes, case law, and regulations governing practice in his or her state. The practical way to obtain this knowledge is through consultation with the attorney retained by one's professional association.

B. Confidentiality and Privilege

1. Confidentiality

Patients' have a right to confidentiality unless one of the specific exceptions to that right is present.

The following exceptions *require* the clinician to disclose information about the patient:

When the patient consents to release information to someone who requests it—for example, an insurer

When gunshot or knife wounds are involved (may apply only to medical personnel)
When certain contagious diseases are involved (may apply only to medical personnel)
When the patient is abusing identifiable children or elderly persons
When a hospital emergency service that treats a rape victim is required to report the rape to the police department

In Massachusetts, such reports must be made to the police in the city where the rape occurred. If the victim agrees, all relevant information is reported. If the victim does not agree, the emergency room notifies the police only that a rape occurred in their city on a particular day.

A statutory exception permits but does not require the physician (or psychologist in some states) to disclose information. This exception applies when failure to hospitalize the patient would create a likelihood of serious harm to the patient or to another person by reason of mental illness. The law in most states is written to give the physician discretion; that is, the physician may (not shall) commit under these circumstances. As a practical matter, it is difficult to decide not to commit a patient who meets the standard. If the physician does not commit a patient who meets the standard, it is especially important to document the basis for the decision.

The following laws permit or provide that a judge may require the clinician to disclose information:

In a divorce proceeding, when the judge determines that disclosure is in the child's best interest
In a contested will, when the patient is deceased
In any legal proceeding in which the patient introduces his or her mental condition as an element of the case and the judge orders the health care professional to disclose
When the patient sues the physician for malpractice

2. Privilege

Many physicians are confused about the distinction between confidentiality and privilege. *Confidentiality* refers to the patient's right and the physician's duty to keep private what the patient has communicated, including the bare fact that that the person is a patient. *Privilege* is a legal term, referring specifically to the right to release information in a legal proceeding. Privilege lies with the patient. That is, the patient has the right to say in a legal proceeding what information shall be disclosed and to whom, absent one of the above exceptions.

Many physicians believe that authorship and physical custody of a record confer privilege. Because physicians have written most or all of a patient's record and have physical custody of it, they think it is their record, but it is not. The patient has the privilege of disclosing, and the physician almost always has the legal duty to obey the patient's directives in this matter.

The physician has an independent legal right to refuse to disclose privileged material in the limited case in which the physicians claims that it would be seriously damaging to the patient's health to disclose what is asked for. In that situation, a judge will hear the physician's argument in a closed hearing and rule on what is to be disclosed. As a practical matter, this is an exception that the physician should invoke rarely, and only for very clear and compelling reasons.

C. Past and Future Violence, Confidentiality, and the Duty to Protect

Suppose that a patient reveals to his clinician that he has raped or killed someone in the past. What is the doctor's legal duty? If the clinician has no reason to be concerned about potential future violence, the clinician's duty is to maintain the patient's confidentiality. If a clinician is concerned that a patient may be violent in the future, there may exist a duty to protect third parties. This duty may override the duty to maintain confidentiality.

The relationship between the duty to protect and the duty to maintain confidentiality has vexed clinicians for a generation. Currently, the law on this subject is changing rapidly, as we discuss below. Note that this simple example highlights the importance of good clinical assessment. The question of the likelihood of future violence can be answered only by careful clinical assessment, a topic discussed at length elsewhere in this book.

D. Social Role

The clinician's legal duty to third parties follows from the relationship of the clinician to the patient. If there is no clinician-patient relationship, there is no duty to protect. However, there are differences in how courts have interpreted the duty, depending on certain parameters of the relationship. Is the clinician a physician? And if a physician, a psychiatrist or not? Is there a treatment relationship, or has only an evaluation been made? Is the patient ambulatory or hospitalized? If hospitalized, voluntarily or involuntarily?

E. Diagnosis

Diagnosis is a critical parameter. Physicians have unique responsibilities regarding violence related to mental illness. In all 50 states, physicians have the statutory authority to hospitalize patients involuntarily who meet the commitment standard. These statutes always include the provision that the patient is mentally ill and almost always require some estimate of future dangerousness.

For purposes of applying a commitment standard, psychiatrists disagree as to whether a personality disorder is a mental illness. Our strongly held opinion is that personality disorders are not mental illnesses within the meaning of commitment statutes. For commitment to meet legal standards, there must be an Axis I mental disorder according to DSM-IV—that is, a symptomatic mental disorder such as depression or schizophrenia (2).

If the patient is dangerous but not mentally ill, our legal duties do not permit us to hospitalize involuntarily. Patients who are not mentally ill but who have histories of antisocial and violent behavior raise special problems for physicians.

F. Legal Duty and Moral Duty

Legal duty and moral or ethical duty overlap to a great extent but are not always congruent. Violent patients raise both legal and moral dilemmas, and the clinician should not confuse one with the other. For example, if I see a blind person about to walk in front of a car, I have a moral obligation to warn that person. I have no legal obligation to that person, because I have no *special relationship* to that person. In law, one person has a duty to another only if a special relationship exists. Landlord-tenant, parent-child, train-passenger, doctor-patient are examples of a special relationship. The special relationship may include the duty to control the behavior of the other person so as to prevent injuries to third parties. A parent has a duty to control a child so as to prevent the child from injuring others, at least in certain circumstances. The question of whether doctors have a special relationship to patients that requires them to act to prevent the patient from injuring third parties has been the subject of case law at least since 1955.

II. TORT LAW

A. Introduction

Tort law refers to civil wrongs, not criminal wrongs. Civil wrongs cannot be punished by imprisonment. The legal penalty for committing a civil wrong—that is, a tort—is limited to monetary damages. When a defendant in a tort suit is found to be negligent, he or she or his or her insurer may have to pay money to the plaintiff. Torts are either negligent or intentional—i.e., the wrong was committed either inadvertently or on purpose. A negligent act is one in which the actor fails to use the care that a reasonably prudent person would use under the same circumstance.

Malpractice is medical negligence—that is, the failure of the physician or clinician to provide the care that a reasonably prudent practitioner would provide in the same circumstances. Most malpractice cases involve negligent rather than intentional torts. An example of an intentional tort that can lead to a suit occurs when a clinician engages in sexual behavior with a patient.

Fear of a malpractice suit can cloud clinical judgment. Malpractice suits are common, and violent patients pose special risks of potential suit. The clinician who understands what is involved in such a suit is better able to act to prevent one. Here we discuss the legal standards and the practical issues that determine whether a suit is likely to be filed, and if filed, whether it is likely to be successful.

Tort law includes the doctrine of unfortunate medical outcome. That is, the mere fact that a case turned out badly is not sufficient basis to find that the clinician was negligent. A certain degree of risk is assumed to exist in the clinician-patient relationship. The risk is reasonable if the clinician meets the standard of care—that is, if he or she exercises the usual degree of skill and knowledge of someone practicing in that profession at that place and time. If the clinician practices within the standard of care, there is no negligence. If the clinician does not meet the standard of care, the clinician is derelict in his or her duty.

To find negligence, a plaintiff must prove more than dereliction. The plaintiff must prove that the defendant owed a duty to the plaintiff, that the defendant was derelict in that duty, and that the plaintiff was damaged as a direct result of the defendant's dereliction. This is sometimes referred to as "the four D's" of negligence: *duty*, *dereliction*, and *direct damage* must all be proved in a negligence action.

B. Case Example

A 36-year-old single woman with a diagnosis of paranoid schizophrenia is seen for medication and support by a psychiatrist. She lives with her parents and is compliant with antipsychotic medication.

The psychiatrist refers the patient to a gynecologist. Over the course of several years, the gynecologist becomes the patient's primary care physician. The psychiatrist retires and the patient asks the gynecologist to continue prescribing her antipsychotic medication. The gynecologist agrees.

Time passes and the patient develops sufficient trust in her doctor to reveal her belief that strangers had removed her uterus and were trying to implant an electronic monitor into her brain. She revealed that, several years earlier, she had pushed a man in front of an oncoming subway train when she became afraid that he was part of the plot against her. She has told no one else about this, and she denies other episodes of violence. Several months later she commits an unprovoked assault on her father and seriously injures him.

1. First Scenario

The notes reveals that the patient stopped taking her medication but continued to see her doctor. The doctor urged the patient to take medication, but she refused. The doctor's notes contain no evidence that he ever asked her about alcohol or drug use. When he tried to discuss her past violence, she became angry and threatened to leave the office.

2. Second Scenario

The patient continued to take her medication. The notes document that the patient denies alcohol or drug use and that the doctor obtained a consultation from a psychiatric colleague. He then records a description of her delusional beliefs. He learns that she no longer believes that strangers are actively trying to harm her. She believes there was a plot in the past, but this no longer is a source of concern to her. She denies any current anger at anyone and denies intent to harm anyone.

C. The Plaintiff's Attorney's Perspective

The victim decides to sue the doctor, and he goes to a plaintiff's attorney. What happens next? The plaintiff s attorney listens to the story and explains that he needs more information. He also explains that if he takes the case it will be on a contingency basis—the attorney will charge no fee to prepare the case but will take as his fee 33% or more of any settlement or jury award.

Preparing a case like this for trial will cost between $50,000 and $75,000. Trying the case will cost approximately that much again. The attorney's decision to take a malpractice case represents, at a minimum, a $50,000 gamble. The successful plaintiff s attorney must be very conservative in accepting new cases. His first step is to subpoena's the patient's records documenting a doctor-patient relationship. However, the plaintiff's attorney is not an expert on medical dereliction. His or her next step is to hire a physician who will review the record and give an opinion as to whether the doctor's care and treatment fell below the standard of care. One of the present authors (J.C.B.) does these evaluations. On the facts of scenario one, the gynecologist did not do an adequate job of assessing this woman's potential for violence and did not consider appropriate courses of action. In the second scenario, the gynecologist met the standard of care and there was no basis for suit.

In the first scenario, the plaintiff's attorney files suit. In the second scenario, no suit is ever filed and the plaintiff's attorney meets with the client and tells him that this is an example of an unfortunate medical outcome—sad but not the doctor's fault.

The point is that the plaintiff's attorney has made a decision almost entirely on the basis of the adequacy of the doctor's notes. Assuming that a physician is reasonably well trained and practices reasonably competently, *the question of whether he or she will be sued after a bad outcome depends almost entirely on the adequacy of the notes.*

Note that the usual advice on how to avoid suit—do not make patients angry, be sure to spend enough time with them—is irrelevant in cases of violence. The doctor had no relationship with the victim. Uniquely in these cases, notes are all.

Suppose now that scenario 2 is correct. The plaintiff's attorney sues. On the facts, it could be argued the doctor fell below the standard of care for a psychiatrist treating such a patient. But is a primary care gynecologist held to the same standard of care as a psychiatrist? Did the doctor owe a duty to the plaintiff? Was the father a foreseeable victim? The answers may vary from state to state, and we turn now to a discussion of relevant case law.

D. The Duty to Protect

The dilemma the physician faces when dealing with potential violence is often formulated as a conflict between the duty to maintain the patient's confidentiality and the duty to protect third parties. The physician worries that if he or she maintains confidentiality and the patient is violent, the victim may sue. Conversely, breaching confidentiality in order to prevent foreseeable harm may lead the patient to sue for breach of confidentiality. In practice, as we hope to show by the end of this chapter, good clinical work can usually resolve this potential conflict.

In deciding whether a clinician owes a duty to a victim, courts rely on the case law that already exists, and they apply the law to the facts of the case. The relevant case law begins with *Tarasoff v. Regents of the University of California* (1).

Tatiana Tarasoff was a student at the University of California at Berkeley in the late 1960s when she met Prosanjit Poddar, an engineering student. He was a native of India and a member of the untouchable caste. They kissed on New Year's Eve. When she told him later that she had no romantic interest in him he became depressed, retreated to his room, and stopped going to classes. Later he began psychotherapy.

The following summer, Ms. Tarasoff left the country and Mr. Poddar talked to his therapist about hurting or even killing Ms. Tarasoff. His therapist became convinced that he was a danger to her and attempted to have him involuntarily hospitalized. This attempt failed because Mr. Poddar convinced the police that he was not a danger, so they left him in his apartment. The therapist had not discussed his concerns with his patient, nor had he mentioned that he was planning to commit him. Not surprisingly, Mr. Poddar quit treatment.

Later, Mr. Poddar moved in with Tarasoff's brother. When Ms. Tarasoff returned in the fall, Mr. Poddar went to her home and threatened her. She fled and he pursued. He shot her in the back with a pellet gun and then stabbed her to death with a butcher knife. He was convicted of second-degree murder and was imprisoned. After his release he returned to India. Several years later, he reported to an inquiring psychiatrist that he was married and feeling well.

Ms. Tarasoff's parents sued, claiming that the therapist knew or should have known that Poddar was dangerous to Tatiana and that the therapist had a duty to warn Ms. Tarasoff of her peril. The California Supreme Court, divided 4 to 3, found that a duty existed. The court said that there is a special relationship between a doctor or a psychotherapist and a patient which imposes a duty to warn endangered third parties. The dissent argued that there were sound social policy reasons for preserving patient confidentiality, that there were no standards for predicting dangerousness, and that the majority opinion was vague on why the duty existed or what obligations it imposed and to whom.

The case aroused a firestorm of protest. Earlier courts had found a duty to third parties only when a psychiatrist had released a patient from the hospital. In two such cases, psychiatrists were sued for failing to use due care in releasing a patient who went on to kill or injure a third party (3,4). *Tarasoff* was so troubling because it potentially expanded the class of potential plaintiffs to include anyone whom any patient seriously injured.

Uniquely, the professional organizations of psychiatrists, psychologists, social workers, and private psychiatric hospitals agreed to collaborate. They filed briefs with the court arguing that this case imposed an unreasonable duty on psychotherapists and physicians.

The court agreed to hear the case again. In the second *Tarasoff* decision, the court essentially agreed with itself (5). It said, "When a therapist determines or pursuant to the standard of his profession should determine, that his patient presents a serious danger of violence to another, he incurs an obligation to use reasonable care to protect the intended victim against such danger. The discharge of this duty may require the therapist to take one or more of various steps depending upon the nature of the case. Thus it may call for him to warn the intended victim or others likely to apprise the intended victim of danger, to notify the police, or to take whatever steps are reasonably necessary under the circumstances" (5, p. 346).

Creating a duty is one thing; proving malpractice, as we have seen, is quite another. In fact, there have been relatively few suits against physicians based on the duty to protect. There have been fewer than ten published cases in which physicians have been found liable for breach of the duty to protect. The physicians in these cases have almost all been psychiatrists who worked in state or Veterans Administration hospitals.

Since *Tarasoff*, there have been approximately 70 published cases involving allegations that a health care professional breached the duty to protect. Until recently, no court has rejected the duty to protect on social policy grounds; that is, no court has disagreed with the *Tarasoff* court when it put the duty to protect above the duty to maintain confidentiality.

Holding that there is a legal duty does not imply that a court finds that the duty applies to the facts of the case before it. Courts find that a duty exists when the violence was foreseeable and when the clinician had a duty to control the patient. Courts are likely to find that violence is foreseeable when two or three of three facts are present: there is a clearly identifiable victim, the patient has a plausible motive for violence, and there is a past history of violence. Courts have found that there is a duty to control in cases involving discharge of a hospital patient, although some recent courts have found that doctors and hospitals have no duty to control voluntary patients. Doctors do have the capability and therefore the legal duty to control involuntary patients.

Some courts find that a clinician has a duty to control ambulatory patients; others do not. There is no discernible basis on which to distinguish the ambulatory patient cases in which courts said control was present from those in which they did not (6).

Mental health professionals acting through their local professional societies have proposed legislation to limit the duty to protect. Laws have been enacted in one form or another in some states. These laws state that a mental health professional has a duty to protect in the limited situation in which the patient has made a credible threat to a named or otherwise clearly identifiable person or the patient has a history of violence and the professional has reason to believe the patient may be violent. The duty is discharged by warning the victim or the appropriate law enforcement agency or taking steps to hospitalize the patient. These laws provide that no liability shall attach to the professional under these conditions.

In 1991, for the first time, a court rejected the *Tarasoff* duty (7). The court said flat out, "Although other jurisdictions have followed the lead of the California Supreme Court in the landmark decision of *Tarasoff*, we reject that 'enlightened approach'" (7, p. 448). The facts involved an outpatient who shot and killed someone. The victim's family sued the psychiatrist, claiming that the doctor failed to hospitalize the patient and failed to warn the victim. The Florida Court affirmed a lower court's dismissal of the suit, saying it would not impose liability based on defendant's failure to control the patient. Further, the court questioned the wisdom of applying a duty that seemed to require clairvoyance on the part of the psychiatrist, acknowledging that psychiatry is an inexact science and that psychiatric predictions of violence are often inaccurate.

Recently, other courts have also begun to limit the duty to protect. A Michigan court found that a general hospital emergency room physician had no duty to protect (8). After a fight with her boyfriend, a young woman overdosed. She was treated at a general hospital emergency room and admitted. The admitting doctor cared for her in the hospital. She refused to see a psychiatrist. After she was discharged, she shot and killed her boyfriend and herself. His survivors sued. The court said that without a psychiatric consultation, the doctor had no way to assess her dangerousness; it found that the doctor was not negligent. Further, the court noted that the boyfriend knew she was dangerous, so there was no duty to warn.

Another Michigan Court found no duty to protect because the patient had been hospitalized for only a few days (9). A paranoid man was hospitalized for a few days on a psychiatric ward in a general hospital. The hospital personnel saw the patient choke his girlfriend. Later, he signed out AMA. Nine days later he raped his former girlfriend. He was arrested and released on bail. Two weeks later, he kidnapped her and shot and killed three people: his girlfriend, a security guard, and himself. Although there was a motive, an identified victim, and a recent history of serious violence, the court declined to find this psychiatrist and this hospital liable after a brief, voluntary hospitalization.

A Virginia court held that the *Tarasoff* duty did not apply in Virginia when a doctor and/or a hospital had a voluntary treatment relationship with the patient (10). The court declined to find a duty to warn in spite of the fact that the patient held a gun to his girlfriend's head, then admitted himself voluntarily to the hospital. There, he was under the care of his long-time psychiatrist who knew of his violent history. He signed out after a few days and no one told the girlfriend that he was out. He went to her house and shot and killed her and himself. The court held that the doctor-patient relationship did not involve any degree of control sufficient to create a special relationship. Therefore, there was no duty to protect in Virginia based on this fact alone.

A man with a history of psychiatric hospitalization shot and killed a stranger who was making too much noise. The survivors sued, and South Carolina courts dismissed the case, finding for the defendant. The court said that South Carolina did not recognize a *Tarasoff* duty to warn, and the court declined to do so on these facts (11). The court distinguished these facts from those of *Tarasoff* because the victim was not clearly identifiable.

Several other courts have held that clinicians have no duty to protect in cases involving an injury caused by a patient who was hospitalized voluntarily (12–14). These courts hold that voluntary hospitalization does not imply any duty to control the patient so as to prevent harm to third parties. These same courts and others have held that there is no duty to warn when the victim has prior knowledge of the patient's violent propensities.

A Kansas court found no negligence in a case in which a man discharged from a voluntary hospitalization returned home and seriously assaulted his uncle (15). The court rejected the plaintiff's claim on two grounds: there was not sufficient basis to control a voluntary patient, and the uncle knew his nephew was violent, so a warning would have been superfluous.

A federal court made a similar holding in a case involving a V.A. hospital patient. After the patient seriously injured his father, the father sued (12). The court found no negligence, holding first that there was no duty to control a voluntary patient and second that because the father had ample prior knowledge of his son's dangerousness, there was no duty to warn.

A Georgia court similarly held that when victims had prior knowledge of a patient's dangerousness, there was no duty to warn. (13).

An Ohio court found that, because the mother knew her assailant-son was dangerous, she assumed some risk in taking care of him (16). While he was home on a pass from the hospital, he threatened to kill her. Although a police officer visited her at home to warn her about potential violence, she took no action. Five days later her son killed her. Surviving family members sued, but the court said she had contributed to the bad outcome by refusing to call for help.

After a paranoid schizophrenic man shot and killed his mother and brother, a Michigan court found that the treating psychiatrist had a duty to protect the brother but not the mother (12). There was no history of violence and no threats were made against the mother, so the court said her death was not foreseeable. An old record from another facility documented that the patient had threatened to kill his brother, apparently because he believed his brother had given him a hernia. The court said this violence was foreseeable based on the existence of this record. This is the fourth published case in which courts have held psychiatrists responsible for reviewing old records. *These four cases speak to the critical importance of obtaining old records.*

A recent Supreme Court case is not directly on point, but the decision is one that should have considerable influence on future *Tarasoff* cases (17). The court considered whether a therapist could be required to testify in a civil suit against the wishes of the patient. The patient was a police officer who had shot and killed someone in the line of duty and who subsequently entered psychotherapy. The victim's family sued and attempted to compel the officer's therapist to testify. The therapist refused.

The Supreme Court stated for the first time a psychotherapy patient's right to privilege under federal law. Although all states have such laws, there was not, until this decision, federal law on psychotherapist-patient privilege. The decision was noteworthy because it specifically stated that privilege belongs to patients of social workers as well as to patients of physician or psychologist psychotherapists. Further, the court wrote at length about the importance of confidentiality in the psychotherapeutic relationship. Because Supreme Court decisions carry great weight with state courts, the effect of this case is likely to be that other courts will limit the duty to breach confidentiality in future cases. This should limit clinicians' potential future liability in *Tarasoff* suits.

III. PRACTICAL IMPLICATIONS

A. General Remarks

This section represents the authors' perspective on how to manage potentially violent patients successfully. *Success* is defined clinically and legally. Successful clinical management minimizes the likelihood of violence and maximizes the probability of maintaining a therapeutic alliance with the patient. If violence occurs, a successful strategy minimizes the likelihood of being sued. If a suit occurs, a sound strategy maximizes the likelihood of a successful defense. We do not discuss the specifics of assessment and management. Those are discussed elsewhere. Here we note only that a thorough evaluation should include both psychiatric and general medical evaluations of the patient. Our discussion assumes that a medical evaluation has ruled out organic causes of violence. Absent organic causes, management of the patient becomes primarily an interpersonal task.

B. Patients with Mental Disorders

Patients are rarely unconflicted about their violent impulses. The callous psychopath or career criminal is far less common in clinical practice than the person with a mental or personality disorder. It is an oversimplification, but one that serves here, to say that the final common psychological pathway for violence is frustration and anger. Someone important in the patient's life has refused to gratify a patient's wish or has done something the patient did not want him or her to do, and the patient is angry. When the patient's efforts fail to get what he or she wants, violence may occur.

The basic clinical imperative is to discuss the potential violence with the patient. It is not in the patient's interest to be violent. A responsible clinician should try equally hard to prevent a patient's violence toward others as toward self. The clinician's discussion of potential violence should convey concern for the patient as well as for the potential victim. When the clinician does so, the patient understands that the clinician has the patient's interests at heart, and this strengthens the therapeutic alliance. With this approach, the clinician can almost always reach an agreement with the patient on a nonviolent solution to the current problem. Often patients will agree that the clinician should speak with the victim or invite the victim in to meet with the clinician and the patient. When the patient agrees, involvement of third parties does not breach confidentiality. In the rare case where the clinician cannot reach agreement with the patient and must breach confidentiality or initiate commitment, the patient at least will appreciate that the clinician is acting in the patient's interest.

C. Patients with No Mental Disorder

These patients create unique problems for clinicians. The duty to protect is triggered by the clinician-patient relationship, regardless of whether the patient has a mental disorder. If the patient has a mental disorder and the potential for violence warrants it, the physician can always commit. Clinicians without the statutory authority to commit can seek help to initiate commitment proceedings.

When the patient has no mental disorder, this ultimate sanction does not exist. Here it is important to remember that clinical practice provides a highly biased sample of violent behavior. In clinical practice, most violence is associated with mental disorder, but in the population as a whole, most violence is not associated with mental disorder. Best estimates are that approximately 3% of violence in this country is associated with mental disorder (18) exclusive of alcohol and drug abuse. The clinician's capacity for preventing this latter violence is limited. Fortunately, most of our patients do have mental disorders, so we can commit when we think it is indicated.

In managing potential violence in these patients, as with all patients, the clinical imperative applies. Talk with the patient. Do what you can to prevent violence. But if all fails and the patient leaves with the potential for imminent violence unchanged, it is essential to notify appropriate parties and to write careful notes.

D. Survival Strategies in a Litigious World

1. What You Should Know

You should know the statute law in your jurisdiction on duty to report certain violent acts (see Section I.B). Your professional society should be able to give you this information.

2. Make Careful Notes

For the reasons discussed earlier in this chapter, good notes prevent suits. Good notes on a potentially violent patient document a psychiatric and general medical evaluation: history, mental status, physical examination, impression, and plan.

If the patient refuses any of these or they are not possible for any reason, document that as well as what information is obtained.

In recording a mental status exam, it is good practice to include direct quotes from the patient. To do this, the clinician must take notes while talking with the patient. A quote such as "The neighbors are trying to electrocute me," gives the reader useful information. Conclusory statements like, "Patient appears paranoid and delusional" convey almost nothing useful.

In writing up a diagnostic impression and treatment plan, it is worthwhile to record what is ruled out as well as what is ruled in. That is, explain why the patient is given one diagnosis rather than another, especially if one diagnosis would permit commitment and another would not. Discuss the alternative treatment plans considered; why one was selected, and, equally important, what other plans were considered and ruled out and why they were not chosen. Notes like these convey that the clinician made thoughtful decisions.

3. Get a Consultation

If the clinician is seriously concerned about potential violence and is unsure of the best course to follow, it is often good policy to obtain a consultation. This can be informal—a quick telephone consult is better than a more formal one scheduled days later. Document that the consultation has occurred and the consultant's opinion.

4. Protect Yourself

The point of all this—careful notes and consultation—is to demonstrate that the clinician was thoughtful in evaluating and treating the patient. In the worst, rare case that violence does occur, the question may reasonably be asked whether the violence occurred in spite of the clinician's good practice or because the clinician failed to do a careful job. When violence has occurred, any evidence that the clinician was careful and thoughtful will lead observers to conclude that this was an unfortunate medical outcome, not a case of malpractice.

Malpractice attorneys say, "If it wasn't written down, it didn't happen." This is pretty close to the truth. It is a tragic error to spend 2 hours evaluating a patient, then 5 minutes writing a sketchy note before rushing on to the next patient. If violence occurs, no one will be interested in after-the-fact statements of how carefully an evaluation was done. Notes are all that will matter. Self-protection requires the clinician to take the time to write careful notes when potential violence is an issue.

Note that this section contains no suggestion that the clinician should alter his or her ideas of good practice in order to prevent suits. If one practices well and records carefully, one has done what one can.

Some clinicians believe that they can protect themselves by writing minimal notes so that they will not be identified or held accountable for a bad outcome. This is a dangerous strategy and one that rarely works. Plaintiffs' attorneys are smart and resourceful. They know well how to find out who has done what, and when violence has occurred, they will.

E. The Worst-Case Scenario

If violence occurs and suit follows, first and foremost, never lie. Do not attempt to alter any record. Never postdate a record—that is, write it on one date and date it earlier. It is good practice after a violent episode to write as detailed a note as possible about the events and the evaluation that occurred before the violence. This is not because it will aid your defense in court; it will not. The purpose is to provide useful background for the defense attorney and to aid your memory if you are deposed. Always date such a note accurately.

If you are deposed, tell the truth. Lying witnesses are almost always caught. Anyone can make a clinical mistake that may be deemed negligent. That does not imply moral turpitude. Lying under oath or falsifying a record is evidence of moral turpitude, and this carries potentially far more serious penalties than malpractice. Lying under oath is perjury, which is a felony. Moral turpitude is grounds for loss of a professional license in most if not all jurisdictions.

In the usual malpractice case, the insurance company's interest and the defendant's interest are close to identical. The defendant can count on the insurance company's lawyer to defend his or her interests. Occasionally this is not the case—for example, if one company defends several doctors in a single suit. It is beyond the scope of this chapter to discuss specifics, but if a defendant in a malpractice suit is concerned that the insurance company lawyer is not representing his or her interests adequately, that is a reason to get legal consultation. Usually, the issues can be worked out, but occasionally a defendant should retain independent counsel.

REFERENCES

1. *Tarasoff v. Regents of the University of California*, 529 P.2d 553, 118 Cal Rptr 129 (Cal Sup Ct 1974).
2. *Diagnostic and Statistical Manual of Mental Disorders*, 4th ed., American Psychiatric Association, Washington, DC, 1994.
3. *Fair v. United States*, 234 F. 2d 288 (5th Cir. 1956).
4. *Underwood v. United States*, 356 F. 2d (5th Cir. 1966).
5. *Tarasoff v. Regents of the University of California*, 551 P.2d 334, 17 Cal 3d 425 (Cal Sup CT 1976).

6. J C Beck, The Psychotherapist's duty to protect third parties from harm, *Men. Phys. Disabil. Law Rep. 11*:141 (1987).
7. *Boynton v. Burglass*, 490 So2d 446 (Fla. App. 1991).
8. *Paul v. Plymouth General Hospital*, 408 NW 2d 492 (Mich Ct App 1987).
9. *Hinkelman v. Borgess Medical Center*, 403 NW 2d 547 (Mich App 1987).
10. *Nasser v. Parker et al.*, 249 Va 172, 455 SE 2d 502, 1995.
11. *Sharpe v. So Carolina Dept. of Mental Health*, 354 SE 2d 778 (S.C.App. 1987).
12. *Bardoni v. Kim*, 390 NW2d 3128 (Mich App 1986).
13. *Moye v. Milton Ray Moye, Adm.*, 735 F.Supp. 179 (D.N.C. 1990).
14. *Jacobs v. Taylor*, 379 SE 2d 563 (Ga.App. 1989).
15. *Boulanger v. Pol*, 900 P.2d 823 (Kan. 1995).
16. *McDonald v. Toledo Mental Health Center*, 587 NE 2d 350 (Ohio App. 1990).
17. *Jaffee v. Redmond*, 116 S.Ct. 1923 (U.S. 1996).
18. J.W. Swanson, C.E. Holzer, V.K. Ganju, and R.T. Jono, Violence and psychiatric disorder in the community: evidence from the epidemiologic catchment area surveys, *Hosp. Commun. Psychiatry 41*:761 (1990).

19
Violence Prevention at Work

Carol W. Wilkinson
IBM Corporation, Armonk, New York

I. INTRODUCTION

Violence at work is an area of increasing concern and interest. This awareness has been fueled, at least in part, by high profile incidents when disgruntled employees come back with a gun "to get even" (1). Though these incidents are rare, they heighten awareness for both employees and employers of the potential for violence at the workplace. Actually, most cases of homicides at work are related to robbery, and the injury or killing involved was incidental to the primary act of robbery (2).

Violence at work has different meaning for different people. At the very least it includes nonfatal assaults as well as homicide. For most people, it also includes the potential for violence as expressed in both direct and indirect threats. Some would consider that verbal abuse is another form of violence. This chapter focuses on violence at work as defined by homicide, assaults, and threats. It discusses the magnitude of the problem, the development of a workplace violence prevention program, the role of security, and legal issues. In addition, it touches upon special concerns of high-risk occupations, how to handle separations and layoffs, and what to do if one has a serious incident of violence at work.

II. MAGNITUDE OF THE PROBLEM

First, how significant is the problem? NIOSH (National Institute of Occupational Safety and Health), using Bureau of Labor statistics data, has found that homicide at work is among the leading causes of occupational death, second only to motor vehicle accidents. In 1994, a total of 1071 people were killed at work and almost 1 million are estimated to have been assaulted (3). The types of violence at work range from terrorism to robbery, disgruntled employees attacking managers and coworkers, and domestic spillover. In this country, terrorism is a rare occurrence. At work, a little over 80% of homicides are related to robbery. In addition to robbery, business disputes account for 9 to 10% of workplace homicides, police and security in line of duty account for 6%, and personal disputes for about 4% (4). Though over 80% of workplace homicides involve men rather than women, homicide is the leading cause of death at work for women (5,6). In addition, more workplace homicides for women may involve personal disputes such as domestic spillover (3). The pattern of workplace homicide differs from that in the community. Most community homicides are personal disputes, while robbery accounts for less than 10% of homicides in the community.

Violence at work includes assaults as well as homicides. Overall, the data on nonfatal assaults are less reliable than those for homicides. Not only is there underreporting, but there is a lack of agreement as to what constitutes a nonfatal assault. The National Crime Victimization Survey, an annual household-based survey of over 100,000 individuals, estimates that nearly 1 million persons were assaulted at work on duty, with 16% of these assaults resulting in injury (7). This would mean there were 1000 assaults for each death and about 170,000 people injured in workplace assaults.

Other estimates have been lower or higher. The Bureau of Labor Statistics' Annual Survey of Occupational Injuries and Illnesses reported 18,500 assaults in 1996 where employees lost 1 or more days at work. This survey is restricted to 165,000 private establishments but excludes self-employed and government workers (8). Northwestern National Life Insurance Company (9) surveyed 600 employees and estimated, based on a 3% positive response, that there were 2.2 million workplace assaults. This study was questioned as not having been based on a representative sample of the workplace population (9). Violence at work is estimated to account for 15% of violence experienced by Americans (7).

The characteristics of those assaulted at work differ significantly from those of victims of workplace homicide. Though there are four times as many men than women murdered at work, the ratio of men to women for nonfatal assaults is more equal. Also, though over 80% of workplace homicides are associated with robbery, only about 8% of nonfatal assaults are so associated. In addition, the assailant had a weapon in only one-third of workplace assaults. It is of note that about half of assaults at work were not reported to the police, highlighting the problem of underreporting (7).

Finally, threats are the most common occurrences of violence at work. At the same time, it is difficult to get agreement on a definition for threats, and there are no good statistics. Their import is twofold. First, threats are indicators of possible violence; second, threats make employees feel unsafe at work. Threats vary as to their seriousness and are usually not tracked. Despite the prevalence of threats as the most common expression of violence at work, they have been the least studied and most poorly characterized. Not only do we lack a typology of threats, but we know little about their motivation, history, and outcome (10). What little work has been done suggests that threats usually precede more overt acts of violence. Threats are seen as the early warning sign of violence. The assessment and management of threats is the basis of most violence prevention programs.

III. INDUSTRIES AND OCCUPATIONS AT GREATEST RISK OF HOMICIDE AND ASSAULT

Analysis of Bureau of Labor Statistics (BLS) data identifies the service and retail industries as having the highest risk of workplace homicide, accounting for over 50% of homicides at the workplace. These occupations include taxicab drivers and employees of liquor stores, gas service stations, grocery stores, jewelry stores, hotels and motels as well as employees of eating and drinking establishments (3,11). In all of these industries there is extensive contact with the public and the provision of service for money. Therefore, employees are at risk when robbers are looking for an accessible source of money or other valuables. An ongoing challenge of these industries is to balance service to the public with protection of their employees. Some businesses have successfully reduced robberies and thereby reduced the risk for violence. This is an area of continued interventions and research (12).

Similarly, law enforcement occupations, both public and private, are at increased risk of homicide and assault by virtue of the kind of work they do. Over the past 10 to 15 years, there has been a decrease in the rate of workplace homicide for public law enforcement officers. There are a number of reasons for this, including the increased use of bulletproof vests, changes in firearms training exercises, and greater emphasis on violence avoidance, combined with better verbal techniques to diffuse potentially violent situations. Unfortunately, this trend has been offset by an increase in the homicide rate for private law enforcement officers. They are often less experienced than public law enforcement officers and do not have access to the same level of training (3).

Though health care workers are not at risk of fatal attacks, they are at increased risk of nonfatal assaults in emergency rooms, nursing homes, and mental hospitals. This occupational risk is only recently getting the attention of regulatory organizations. In the past, such hazards were often seen as "part of the job" and blame was attributed to the employee who "brought it on by his or her behavior." Also, restraining, disciplining, and otherwise limiting aggressive and assaultive patients was seen at odds with a commitment to "patient's rights." This interpretation made intervention more difficult and at times disregarded the right of health care workers to be safe at work (13).

IV. WHY HAVE A PROGRAM?

Increasingly, businesses are coming to recognize the value of having a violence prevention policy and program. Often, management's objections to having such a policy and program are based on denial, superstitious fear, or economics. Management believe that "We don't have this kind of problem with our employees or our workplace" and "It could never happen here." Or they fear that even discussing the potential for violence increases the risk of something happening. Finally, there is concern that proposed changes will not be cost-effective.

Realistically, based on statistics, the probability of a workplace fatality is remote. Therefore, with the exception of certain high-risk occupations and industries, management's view that the likelihood of a workplace homicide is very low is correct. Nevertheless, it is often prudent to have a plan in place for handling such uncommon incidents, since the potential cost, if and when something happens, is high. Additionally, though the risk of homicides is low, assaults, threats, and other inappropriate behavior and language do occur and can negatively impact employee morale and productivity. Threats can be found with any group of people, in any workplace, particularly if there are no sanctions against that kind of behavior.

When management is silent on the issue of violence and threats at work there is the possibility of creating confusion and uncertainty among employees as to exactly what the company's position is. It is important to give careful thought to the wording of a workplace violence prevention policy and to integrating this into the company's culture. It is naive to believe that not talking about violence somehow will ensure that violence will not occur. Such evasive behavior does not reduce the risk; it only means that the organization is less prepared to respond when incidents occur.

All businesses should carefully review their experience and their potential for risk so that they can determine the type of policy and program that will be helpful in ensuring employee safety. Though there are costs associated with ensuring a safe workplace, employers often find out, belatedly, that those costs are generally much less than the costs of restoring and maintaining security after an incident occurs. Regulations and legal ruling are increasingly making the employer responsible for maintaining a workplace that is safe with respect to personal safety as well as the traditional occupational safety and health hazards. This is reflected in increased support for proposed regulation at both the state and federal levels (14,15).

Discussions with corporations that have had to deal with a workplace fatality uniformly concur on the value and importance of having a plan in place before an incident happens. It is difficult if not impossible to manage workplace violence without a well-thought-out and coordinated plan. There is not time, in the heat of the moment, to do many of the things that can minimize the impact of such events on the workplace, employees, and customers. In addition, there is the very real concern that deaths might have been prevented or injuries lessened had there been a program in place. The planning and development of a program provides both good insurance and a positive impact on employee morale through the emphasis on a safe workplace (16–18).

V. VIOLENCE PREVENTION PROGRAM

Components of a workplace-based violence prevention program include a policy of zero tolerance, executive support, establishment of cross-functional teams, development of an early notification system, identification of appropriate support resources, training for managers and employees, and coordination with other policies and practices.

A policy of zero tolerance for violence is an important cornerstone of any workplace violence program. This means that the business will not tolerate any violence in words or action. Ambiguity as to acceptable workplace behavior and language makes it more difficult to both identify and address inappropriate situations in a timely fashion. Many episodes of workplace violence have been preceded by warning signs, where a person is angry and threatening (19). At times the organization's response to the threatening behavior at work is either nonexistent or ineffectual. People often find it easier to deny or justify problematic behavior than to address it directly. Coworkers and management may excuse threatening behavior and language by saying "Joe really didn't mean it" or "That's the way Joe is." Unfortunately, with this nonresponse, the employee comes to believe, at least implicitly, that he or she can continue to make threats. Some people use threatening words or behavior to express their feelings and to get attention or gain control of situations. They may find that threatening words and behavior are an effective means to get desired changes made at work. Therefore, without sanctions, they may, when stressed, escalate their behavior and language such that coworkers are even more afraid but unsure of what to do. At that point management and employees are faced with the problem of having to address threatening behavior in the context of what may have been long-standing tacit acceptance of similar words and behavior. Therefore, a policy of zero tolerance that does not allow for threatening words is a valuable means to set limits early and clearly.

However, if there is not clear executive support, coworkers may choose not to report threats and assaults because of a belief that "management won't do anything." Employees need to know that threatening language and behavior is unacceptable and will not be tolerated. Communication and implementation of this policy requires both executive and management support. Management needs to know that decisions to address threats and discipline employees are both expected and supported. Employees need to know that management is committed to enforcing this policy both fairly and consistently. When incidents occur and are identified, employees are checking to see how they are handled. Is it consistent with policy? Is it fair? Without employee trust and confidence, management may not even be aware of problematic situations.

Companies with well-established violence prevention programs ensure that employees have a means to report incidents and concerns immediately, 24 hours a day, 7 days a week. Early identification allows for early intervention. In many companies these calls go to security; in other companies human resources is the first contact. Regardless of where the call is received, there needs to be a process to evaluate the incident, involve appropriate resources, and respond in a timely fashion. Cross-functional teams are an important component of the process, since they ensure representation from all areas that have concern and need to be involved. These teams need to include security, human resources, medical (when available), legal, line management, and, when necessary, communication. This team will have been involved in the development and implementation of the company's violence prevention program. They will be prepared to meet and respond to threats and incidents as needed. They will be able to provide the expertise and support that is critical to management of these incidents.

Management needs to carefully investigate incidents to understand as well as possible what happened and then base their response on the facts. Just as there are problems with underresponding, there are likewise problems with overreacting. Management may find that threats are part of that employee's cultural or personal background and may not be intended as they are heard by others. The employee needs to be told and to understand what is unacceptable in the workplace. The employee can reasonably be expected to change his or her threatening language and behavior so that others feel safe. The degree of detail and involvement in threat assessment will vary. At times, the threat investigation may consist of a conversation between the supervisor and the employee, where the supervisor confirms that the employee said or did what was alleged, hears the employee's explanation, and reinforces that "threats, no matter how inconsequential, are not acceptable at work." At other times, the investigation may need the experience and resources of others, such as human resources, security, legal, and medical (20). The assessment of risk needs to be done quickly. Members of the cross-functional team will have information about the employee as well as access to resources that can contribute to the assessment. The process of risk assessment is covered in more detail elsewhere in this book. It includes a careful history of the incident (what happened, who said what, in what context) as well as any history of prior episodes at work. It will take into consideration other information, such as any nonwork episodes of violence, military service, access to and fascination with weapons, etc. (21). At times, it may be necessary to go to the local law enforcement organization to determine if the employee has any prior convictions that may be related to violence. At other times, it is necessary to get an assessment of the imminent potential for violence from a psychiatrist or psychologist who is experienced in the assessment and management of potentially violent people. In this process, the value of planning and the development of resources and contacts is most evident. The company with a workplace violence prevention program will already have identified professionals who can provide a violence assessment when needed. The company will have had the opportunity to evaluate their qualifications and determine whether they are comfortable with the person's approach to violence assessment. Similarly, they will have established relationships with local law enforcement that can facilitate management of the case and awareness of episodes outside of work.

Once the company has put together their cross-functional team and developed their violence prevention program and policy, this needs to be communicated to managers and employees. The training needs to clearly state the policy and possible consequences of failure to adhere to the policy, which may include disciplinary action such as suspension, termination, or even legal action. Managers and employees need to know how to report incidents. They need to know that incidents will be investigated and addressed. The policy and program needs to be integrated in the overall culture and policies of the company. During training, management needs to learn about the warning signs for violence and where to go for help. Managers need to know that there are resources both within and outside of the company to help them assess the potential for violence. Unlike much of management, in these situations managers are expected to ask for help and should not be acting independently. Employees in positions of increased risk—such as receptionists, sales personnel or security—need to receive more training tailored to the particular exposures of their jobs. For example, receptionists need to know how to control access to the workplace, how to get help if a person is threatening, and how to handle difficult telephone callers, who can range from angry customers to mad bombers. Similarly, people who deal with money need to learn procedures to minimize the availability of money and to protect themselves and others if they are faced with demands for their cash. This training needs to be done both upon starting the job and at regular intervals. Since threatening incidents occur infrequently, employees will need periodic reminders of how to avoid risk. It is easy to become complacent and comfortable with behavior that can make one more vulnerable.

No violence prevention program can function independently of company policies and practices if it is to be successful. Effective programs are most successful in a climate where there are good employee relations—where employees feel supported and fairly treated by management in all aspects of their work. There needs to be an environment of trust and respect. The violence prevention program is just one aspect of good human resource management within a company.

VI. ROLE OF SECURITY

Security personnel are among the key resources in violence prevention. Their responsibilities include assessment and maintenance of a safe workplace through staffing and assurance of physical security (22). All companies need to review the layout of the worksite to ensure that they are providing physical safety for their employees. This includes having adequate lighting and protection in parking lots and public places. Landscaping needs to be designed so that it does not provide a place for perpetrators to hide. Entrances to buildings need to be well lit and with clear sight lines. The company needs to decide how to handle access to the workplace. An unmonitored, unrestricted workplace can be a problem. Limiting the ability to enter the building and having employees and visitors wear identification is a way to manage site security. Employers who deal with the public—such as retail, food and health care—have additional challenges on how to ensure the safety of their employees. Similarly, employees who travel to provide services need assistance and advice on how to ensure their safety. This review of site security can be done internally or can use external consultants, depending on the nature of resources available within the company.

The security staff needs to be trained in handling a range of situations as well as in early recognition of situations that are beyond their ability to handle and how to get help. One of the problems is having unrealistic expectations of security support. At times, these employees may have limited training and experience. The organization needs to consider how to provide the additional resources when warranted. This can include calling for local law enforcement assistance or other security professionals. This will depend on the nature of the relationship with community enforcement and the level of community expertise available. Experts agree that at times a show of force can be helpful in managing difficult situations. Hospital emergency rooms long ago learned the value of having security guards present as a violence deterrent. On the other hand, it is important not to aggravate and escalate a situation that is only potentially threatening to one which is directly threatening. This can happen with inexperienced security people who misread the cues and may react inappropriately.

The development of good relations with local law enforcement starts long before any incident and is part of any good violence prevention program. A good understanding of each other's organization and good relations are a valuable foundation when problems arise. With good working relations, there is better communication and cooperation. Finally, in some situations there may appear to be a need for surveillance. The decision to initiate surveillance needs to be carefully thought out, since there are both legal and practical ramifications to this.

VII. LEGAL CONSIDERATIONS

In the development and implementation of a violence prevention program, there are a number of legal considerations, including compliance with the Americans With Disabilities Act (ADA) and balancing the need for a safe workplace with individual rights (23). This section cannot be a substitute for legal advice, it is meant only to increase the reader's awareness of legal issues. ADA legislation states that one cannot remove an employee from the workplace unless there is an imminent threat of danger. That is, an employer cannot decide to terminate anyone or keep people from work because there is a "vague possibility" of violence. The employer needs to have evidence that a threat to employee safety is both highly likely and expected to occur in the near future. This is a situation when a professional assessment can be helpful. Even though its long-term predictive value may be limited, a good evaluation can help an employer decide if the employee poses an imminent threat. Similarly, a professional evaluation will support management's decision to restrict access to work. ADA also has guidelines that pertain to the hiring process and that limit what the employer can ask and how much can be investigated. Employers would like to avoid hiring employees who are known to have a potential for violence. They would like to have a screening questionnaire that can identify those people who are at risk of violence, so they do not have to be hired. Unfortunately, these questionnaires are very imprecise tools at best. The best predictor of violence is past behavior, and even that is of limited value. Personality profiles that purport to screen out violence-prone employees are even more problematic. Usually, the profile of an offender is too general and too inclusive to be useful (24). It is impossible to successfully predict which individual will be violent given the constellation of associated risk factors. Even in a population of psychiatric patients, where detailed clinical histories were available, it was difficult to predict the likelihood of violence (25). Elsewhere in this book are more detailed discussions of the limitations in predicting violence. Finally, one of the most severe limitations of using any hiring profile is that it will not address the possibility of risk associated with current employees. As one looks at the experience of workplace violence, perpetrators are often current employees. Therefore, one is better served by having an integrated approach to violence that is alert to the potential for violence—that identifies incidents early and intervenes effectively.

VIII. OCCUPATIONS WITH INCREASED RISK OF VIOLENCE

There are some occupations with increased risk of violence, such as retail and food service, security, and health care. Below, we briefly discuss some of their concerns and challenges and the solutions that have been developed to address and reduce the risk of violence in the workplace.

Since most workplace violence is associated with money, service establishments that are open late and are in high-crime areas are at greater risk of violence. Food establishments, convenience stores, liquor stores, and gasoline stations are all subject to robbery and thereby the possibility of violence. Workplace modifications that have helped reduce this risk include drop safes, which reduce the amount of money available; increased lighting around buildings; and landscaping so that there is more visibility around both front and back entrances.

Employees who travel to provide service are also at risk of robbery and violence. Employee awareness and training are important components of violence prevention. Taxi drivers continue to be targets of robbery and thereby violence, since they carry cash, work at all hours, and travel to all areas of a city. Safety features for taxicabs have had some success; however, these are costly, are only partially effective and are not in most cars.

Law enforcement officers are at risk by virtue of their work. The use of personal protective wear—i.e., bulletproof vests—has helped to save officers' lives. Equally important has been the combination of improved firearms training and emphasis on conflict-resolution skills. At this point the greatest problem lies with private security staff. Their training and experience is more limited than that of public security officers. As a result, they are not always adequately prepared to handle threatening or potentially violent situations without putting themselves at risk. Hopefully, over the next few years, experience from the private sector can be applied to the area of private security and can thus reduce the risk (26).

There is increased recognition of the risk of assault to health care workers, particularly in emergency rooms, nursing homes, and psychiatric institutions. Again, a preventive approach is best. This combines understanding of the nature of the risk and identifying and instituting appropriate protective measures.

Components of a program includes the use of employee identification and maintenance of access control to buildings. In some inner-city emergency rooms, metal detectors have been installed to enforce the policy of no weapons. Where patients can be assaultive and violent, health care workers need to be trained in violence identification, avoidance, and assault management techniques. Some hospitals have systems to identify violence-prone patients on the medical record. Most have established ways to summon help quickly when needed, whether it be a panic alarm or an emergency code word. Certainly there needs to be an incident review process both to incorporate any changes as well as to provide support to involved employees. Guidelines for preventing violence to health care workers are being developed by a number of organizations, including the government (15,27) and professional medical associations (28).

IX. SEPARATIONS AND LAYOFFS

Violence at work can be associated with involuntary separations, whether it be individual termination or layoffs involving a number of employees. For any termination, the management team needs to be sensitive to maintaining the individual's dignity. Loss of job can also mean loss of self-esteem, since for many people their work is one of the most important part of their identity (29). If the termination is seen as demeaning or insulting, the person may feel more anger and there may be more risk of violence. In the termination process, the emphasis needs to be on the behavior and performance that are unacceptable and not on the person. The goal is to help the person maintain his or her dignity and to facilitate moving on to constructive solutions of the current problems—looking for a job, etc. There are particular concerns if an employee has already had a history of violent and threatening behavior. In those situations there needs to be increased sensitivity to nuances of threats and at times additional precautions, such as limiting access to the workplace and perhaps an effort to provide additional support measures.

Layoffs differ from individual separations. As a group process, there is the benefit of group support. A number of people are affected and the reason for the layoff is economic rather than an individual's performance. It can be easier for an employee not to see the job loss as a personal rejection. Of course, the concern is that this may not always be the case, and there is the risk that someone will decide to react violently. With preparation and coordination, employers can reduce this risk. It is important to have organizational planning and cooperation throughout the process. Human resources, line management, legal, security, medical (if available), and communications units need to work together both in development and implementation. It helps to have psychological assistance and job transition resources available to the employees being terminated. Similarly, when management identifies fragile or at-risk employees, it helps them be better prepared for the reactions and questions of the employee. If management can understand the emotional states of the employee (denial, anger, bargaining, sadness, and acceptance), it will help them with employees as well as to better understand their own reactions and feelings. If management can acknowledge the employee's feelings without taking them personally, it will help the employee come to accept the termination and move on toward whatever is the next step. This will involve considering options and taking action to pursue possible job opportunities.

X. CRITICAL INCIDENT DEBRIEFING

Despite all efforts, one may have to deal with a death or traumatic event at work. Again, both preparation and identification of qualified resources are invaluable. The two important components of postincident management are psychological support for the victims and coworkers as well as an effective communication plan (1).

Early on in an incident, the confusion, emotional turmoil, and uncertainty all contribute to making it difficult for anyone to find out what the present situation is and what is being done. Rumors and misinformation are common. Management needs to identify a spokesperson and establish a regular communication schedule with update bulletins (30). This is important for the employees, their families, and the public as well as the media. During communication, management should take care not to make unsubstantiated, conjectural statements. It is better to acknowledge that answers are not known and that the situation is being investigated. Follow-up reports at regular intervals are important, even if there is no new information available. These reports are a means of providing information access and reassurance and to counter rumors. It is important to address rumors quickly and directly.

At the same time that management is communicating with the general public and employee population, those people who were involved in the incident need special attention and support. Early intervention has been shown to reduce long-term emotional distress and to facilitate earlier return to work (31). The experience of violence at work attacks the very foundation of people's trust and their belief in the safety of the work environment. After episodes of violence, employees experience emotions ranging from fear, anger, and guilt to depression. They may also experience physical reactions, flashbacks, panic attacks, and problems sleeping and eating. There is a need to relive the experience, but with it can come self-blame: "I should have . . ." or anger at the company, "They should have. . . ."

There is conflict between relief at being alive and a sense that perhaps the incident could have been prevented. People need to know that these feelings and thoughts are normal reactions to a traumatic event. Without that awareness, employees can begin to question their own sanity and even become more disturbed and impaired. Another benefit of early intervention is that employees can share the experience with each other. It is common for people to have only a limited awareness of what happened. In discussion, they get both a fuller picture of what happened and a realization that despite their feelings, they were not alone. With retelling, the events become more familiar and less distressing. Coworkers can also be an important source of support and healing to one another. The objective of critical incident management is to assist employees in dealing with the experience and associated feelings so that they can return more quickly to normalcy (32). Finally, with early intervention, it becomes easier to identify those employees who are having more problems and need referral for additional professional help.

XI. SUMMARY

Violence at work has different meanings depending on the nature of the workplace and the kind of work done. Though most fatal and nonfatal assaults at work are associated with robbery, a significant percentage of nonfatal assaults arise from coworker–manager relations. Overall, threats are the most common expression of workplace violence. These reflect the personalities, culture, and emotions of the employees. The development of a violence prevention policy and program will provide a structure to deal with both threats as well as the less common though more serious expressions of violence, such as assault and homicide. Any violence prevention program needs to start with a review of a business's past experience as well as its potential for violence. This will determine the appropriate extent and nature of a program. Components of a violence prevention program include a policy of zero tolerance, executive support, and management and employee education. There needs to be a means to identify and assess the potential for violence when an incident occurs, as well as a plan to respond. Physical security measures such as lighting and access control are important features in increasing safety at work. When dealing with potentially violent situations at work, one needs to be aware of legal implications of one's actions so that one is not inadvertently making a situation worse. Similarly, as management takes job actions such as terminations and layoffs, they need to strive to maintain the individual's dignity and self-respect so as to avoid having employee anger turn into violence against the company. Finally, when faced with serious violence at work, the company can manage the trauma through support of involved employees as well as ensuring coordinated and effective communication. Though most companies will never have to deal with homicide or assault, they can ensure a safer workplace by having a violence prevention program in place. Their commitment to employee safety will increase employees comfort and be invaluable in the more effective management of a fatal or nonfatal assault at work, should it occur.

REFERENCES

1. E. Johnson, When disaster strikes, *Safety Health*, Feb. 1992, pp. 28–32.
2. E. Larsen, Trigger Happy: How workplace violence became a hot issue, *Wall Street Journal*, Oct. 12, 1994, p. A1–10.
3. NIOSH, *Violence in the Workplace, Risk Factors and Prevention Strategies, Current Intelligence Bulletin #57*, DHHS (NIOSH) Publication 96–100, Washington, DC, 1996.
4. J. Windaw and G. Toscano, *Workplace Homicides in 1992. Compensation and Working Conditions*. U.S. Department of Labor, Bureau of Labor Statistics, Washington, D.C., 1994.
5. E.L. Jenkins and L.A. Layne, Homicide in the workplace: The U.S. experience, 1980–88, *Am. Assc. Occup. Health Nurses J.* 40:215 (1992).
6. C.A. Bell, Female homicide in United States workplaces, 1980–85, *Am J Public Health*, 81:729 (1991).
7. R. Bachman, Violence and theft in the workplace, *U.S. Department of Justice Crime Data Brief*, U.S. Government Printing Office, Washington, D.C., NCJ-148199, 1994.
8. U.S. Bureau of Labor Statistics, *Lost-Worktime Injuries and Illnesses: Characteristics and Resulting Time Away from Work, 1996*. U.S. Department of Labor, 98-157, April 23, 1998.
9. Northwestern National Life Insurance Co., *Fear and Violence in the Workplace*, Northwestern National Life Insurance Co., Minneapolis, MN, 1993.
10. H.G. Macioszek, The Use and Misuse of Threats in Business, speech delivered before Executives in the Food Industry, Barcelona, Spain, Oct. 6, 1992. *Vital Speeches*, 81 (1992).
11. D.N. Castillo and E.L. Jenkins, Industries and Occupations at High Risk for Work-Related Homicides, *J. Occup. Med. 36*:125 (1994).
12. L.J. Warshaw and J. Messite, Workplace Violence: Preventive and Intervention Strategies, *J. Occup. Med. 38*:993 (1996).
13. J.A. Lipscomb and C.C. Love, Violence toward health care workers. *Am. Assc. Occup. Health Nurses J. 40*:219 (1992).
14. CAL/OSHA Consultative Services. (California Division of Occupational Safety and Health), *Model Injury and Illness Preventive for Workplace Security*. Department of Industrial Relations, Los Angeles, 1995.
15. Occupational Safety and Health Administration, *Guidelines for Preventing Workplace Violence for Health Care and Social Service Workers*, Washington, D.C., DOL, OSHA.

16. M. Braverman and S.R. Braverman, Seeking Solutions to Violence on the Job. *USA Today*, May 1994, pp. 29–31.
17. C. Grainger, Occupational "Violence": managing the risk of assault in the workplace. *J. Occup. Health Safety Aust N.Z. 9*:43 (1993)
18. D.C. Johnson, J.B. Kiehlbauch, and J.A. Kinney, Breaking the cycle of violence, *Security Management*, Feb. 1994, pp. 24–28.
19. D.C. Johnson and J.A. Kinney, *Breaking Point*, National Safe Workplace Institute, Chicago, 1993.
20. J.A. Kinney, When domestic violence strikes the workplace, *HR Magazine*, Aug. 1995, pp. 74–78.
21. K. Tardiff, *Assessment and Management of Violent Patients*, 2d ed., American Psychiatric Press, Washington, D.C., 1996.
22. International Association of Chiefs of Police, *Combating Workplace Violence; Guidelines for Employees and Law Enforcement*, International Association of Chiefs of Police, Alexandria, VA, 1996.
23. Littler, Mendelson, Fastiff, Tichy, and Mathiason, Terror and violence in the workplace, *Lawyer's Brief*, Business Laws, Chesterland, OH, 1993, pp. 2–32.
24. L.P. DiLorenzo and D.J. Carroll, The Growing menace: Violence in the workplace, *N.Y. State Bar J.* Jan. 1995, pp. 24–30.
25. C.W. Lidz, E.P. Mulvey, and W. Gardner, The accuracy of predictions of violence to others. *J.A.M.A. 269*:1007 (1993).
26. E. Brondolo, *Leader Guide: Agent Conflict Resolution Training*, St. Johns University, Dept. of Transportation, New York City, 1995.
27. State of California, *Guidelines for Security and Safety of Healthcare and Community Service Workers*. Division of Occupational Safety and Health. Department of Industrial Relations, Sacramento, CA, 1993.
28. AMA, Young Physicians Section, *Violence in the Medical Workplace Prevention* Strategies, A.M.A., Chicago, IL, 1995.
29. C.R. Leana and D.C. Feldman, Individual responses to job loss: Perceptions, reactions and coping behaviors, *J. Mgmt. 14*:375 (1988).
30. G.W. Lewis, Managing crises and trauma in the workplace. *Am. Assc. Occup. Health Nurses J. 41*:124 (1992).
31. R.J. Friedman, M.B. Framer, and D.R. Shearer, Early response to posttraumatic stress, *EAP Digest*, Sept./Oct. 1988, pp. 45–49.
32. G.W. Lewis, *Critical Incident Stress and Trauma in the Workplace*, Accelerated Development Bristol, PA, 1994.

20
Violence and Suicidal Behavior: What is the Link?

Peter M. Marzuk
Cornell University Medical College, New York, New York

I. INTRODUCTION

The link between violent and suicidal behavior has only begun to be fully appreciated. For thousands of years, the public has observed that many violent individuals ultimately kill themselves, all the while deriving a sense of justice from this fact. In contrast, the notion that many individuals who are suicidal have histories of violence has been realized only in the last several decades. While suicide is seen as aggression turned inward, it has been difficult to conceive that suicidal people could be capable of directing aggression outward. At the most basic level, our lack of understanding of the link between violent and suicidal behavior arises from our failure to see self-destructive behavior for what it really is—aggression. It is certainly hard to see aggression in the face of the hopeless depressed person who hangs himself or the political martyr who immolates herself. Even the peaceful sleep of the terminally ill patient who dies of barbiturate poisoning does not seem aggressive. Yet we humans are very adept at disguising aggression. Thus, I submit that the two behaviors are linked because they arise from aggressive impulses. Understanding the link between violence and suicide is important not only in the clinical management of these individuals but also because it may lead to new clues as to the sources of our aggressiveness.

In this chapter, we examine the evidence that suggests an association between violent and suicidal behavior. The data come largely from surveys of psychiatric patients and criminal populations. Second, we examine possible etiologies behind the link, focusing on developmental precursors and social risk factors of both behaviors, shared underlying neurobiological substrates, and psychiatric disorders common to both. Finally, we conclude with a brief discussion of the clinical implications of assessing both these behaviors in patients. At the outset, it should be mentioned that violent behavior in this chapter is defined as interpersonal assault, not merely destruction of property or the threat of violence. Likewise, suicidal behavior is considered to comprise self-destructive acts with intent to die, not merely self-mutilation.

II. EVIDENCE OF THE LINK

It should be recognized that many suicidal people have never been and never will be violent. Likewise, there are many violent individuals who have not been self-destructive. The two groups constitute separate but overlapping populations. It has been estimated, for example, that at least 30% of violent persons have a history of self-destructive behavior and 10 to 20% of suicidal person have a history of violence (1). Moreover, the previous notion that suicide and homicide are inversely correlated is false. There are some countries, for instance, where both suicide and homicide rates are relatively high, e.g., the United States, and others where both are low, e.g., Ireland (1).

Most of the evidence linking these two rare behaviors is longitudinal, but it must, of necessity, be retrospective. In one type of design, researchers assess patients who are admitted to psychiatric hospitals for suicidal behavior and then determine whether the fraction of these patients with a history of violence exceeds the fraction of those with violence who had been admitted for reasons other than suicide. In a variant of this design, the researchers assess the past history of suicidal behaviors of patients admitted for violent behaviors in comparison with patients who were admitted for reasons other than violence. These strategies focus exclusively on those individuals whom society has, in effect, labeled as having "psychiatric problems."

An alternative strategy involves the comparison of the prevalence of suicidal behavior among individuals arrested, jailed, or incarcerated for the commission of violent offenses with that of individuals detained for nonviolent crimes. In this design the focus is on individuals whom society has labeled as "criminal." Both strategies have their pitfalls because they rely on a retrospective assessment of a socially undesirable behavior in a group that has already been labeled as "deviant." It must be remembered that many violent and self-destructive acts occur in the community but never come to the attention of either mental health or criminal justice authorities. However, a longitudinal, prospective, naturalistic study of the relationship of these two rare events would require the assessment of so many thousands of individuals for so many years as to be unfeasible. Nevertheless, much has been learned from surveys of psychiatric patients and forensic populations.

A. Psychiatric Patients

Surveys of psychiatric populations have shown an association between violence and suicidal behavior. In a comprehensive survey of 9365 patients admitted to public hospitals on Long Island, New York, Tardiff and Sweillam (2) found that among 597 male patients with assaultive behavior, 15.1% had a history of suicidal behavior, compared with only 8.7% of 4635 male patients without assaultive behavior. Men who were assaultive were twice as likely to have had suicidal problems as men who were not. Among females, 18.4% of the 326 assaultive patients had suicidal behavior, compared with 15.2% of 3806 without assaultive behavior—a nonsignificant difference.

In another study, Tardiff and Sweillam (3) examined the factors related to the risk of assaultive behavior in suicidal patients. Among the 667 suicidal male patients admitted to Long Island hospitals, 14% were assaultive to persons just prior to admission; of the 893 suicidal female patients, 7% were assaultive. For both sexes compared with nonassaultive suicidal patients, those who were assaultive and suicidal were more likely to have delusions, hallucinations, belligerence, and antisocial behavior. Interestingly, there was no significant difference in regard to the frequency of depressive symptoms between assaultive and nonassaultive patients. Female assaultive suicidal patients were more likely to be younger than 34 years and to have a diagnosis of paranoid schizophrenia, alcohol or drug abuse, or organic brain syndrome. In contrast, for men, there were no differences in primary diagnoses relating to assaultive behavior.

In a study of 94 inpatients who had been hospitalized for a longer term, many for years, all of whom had attempted suicide while hospitalized, Tardiff (4) found that 45% had also been assaultive to other persons in the hospital at least once. Only young age was associated with the risk of being assaultive. There were no differences in regard to gender, race, length of stay, primary psychiatric diagnoses, or legal status. Neither the presence of psychotic nor depressive symptoms differentiated the assaultive from the nonassaultive patients. In a study of patients presenting to an emergency room, Skodal et al. (5) found that 30% of violent patients were also judged to be suicidal.

Studies of adolescents have yielded similar findings. Inamdar et al. (6) found that among 51 adolescent inpatients, 66% had been violent, almost half had been suicidal, and 28% had been both—a finding that was more marked in boys than in girls. In another study, Grosz et al. (7) compared 40 adolescent inpatients with histories of frequent interpersonal violent behavior with 36 hospitalized adolescents without histories of overt violence. Violent adolescents had made more suicide attempts and had significantly higher family histories of attempted and completed suicide. There was also a high intercorrelation among risk of violence, suicide, and impulsivity. A 30-year follow-up of former child psychiatric patients showed that aggressiveness was most often observed among those who committed suicide (8).

In a study comparing a forensic population of violent individuals and a municipal hospital population that was nonviolent, Apter et al. (9) found different correlates with suicide risk. In the forensic group, there was a highly significant correlation between suicide risk and anger, whereas in the municipal hospital population, suicide risk was strongly correlated with sadness. The study suggests that suicide risk should be managed differently in violent patients than in those who do not have a history of violence.

B. Forensic Populations

Both jails and prisons have been found to have high rates of suicide that are several-fold higher than that of the general population (10–13). Among such suicides, individuals changed with violent or sexual offenses are overrepresented (14). In a study of the Maryland prison system, the suicide rate of prisoners was almost twice that expected in a demographically adjusted community population (15). Moreover, the suicide rate of men who had committed violent crimes against persons (e.g., murder, manslaughter, rape, assault, kidnapping) was more than three times that of men who committed crimes against property. Another study found that inmates in an urban jail who had been charged with murder or manslaughter were 19 times more likely to commit suicide than were inmates with other charges (16). Likewise, a Dutch study found that the rate of suicide in jails was higher for men charged with murder or manslaughter than for those charged with other crimes, but it also revealed that the lengths of sentences, which are longer for violent crimes, could be a confounding variable (17).

C. Murder-Suicide

In contrast to the longitudinal assessment of violent behavior in suicidal people or suicidal behavior in violent people, the study of murder-suicide offers a unique perspective because both violent and self-destructive behaviors occur virtually simultaneously. Murder-suicide is a violent event in which an individual commits homicide and shortly thereafter commits suicide. It occurs with an annual incident of 0.2 to 0.3 per 100,000 persons in the United States (18–21) and worldwide (22). In the United States alone, these events account for an annual loss of 1000 to 1500 lives to homicide and suicide (23).

Marzuk et al. proposed that murder-suicide occupies a distinct epidemiological domain that overlaps with simple suicide, domestic homicide, and mass murder. Most of these events in the United States involve amorous jealousy (23). Typically, a man between the age of 18 and 60 years develops suspicions, either real or perceived, of his girlfriend's or wife's infidelity, becomes enraged, murders her, and then commits suicide shortly thereafter. Usually the relationship had been chronically chaotic and characterized by jealousy, verbal abuse, and previous violence or threats. Often, the triggering event is the woman's rejection of her lover and her threat of withdrawal, estrangement, or divorce. In a much rarer variant, the depressed senior male of a household commits familicide and then suicide. In this scenario, the senior male—who is depressed, paranoid, or intoxicated—kills every member of his family including spouse and children and sometimes pets. Precipitants often include marital, financial, or other social stresses on the family. In some cases, suicide notes have suggested that the perpetrator is delivering the family from continued hardships in a "spirit of altruism" (24). In other cases, marital infidelity is suspected (25).

The second most common type of murder-suicide, after amorous jealousy, involves filicide (23). In these cases, a parent, often a mother, murders her children and then commits suicide. The children are typically infants or preadolescents. The parents are typically depressed and despondent. Sometimes the mother is psychotic, sacrificing her children in a deluded altruism to save herself and them from a ruinous existence (26–30).

Murder-suicides usually involve family members. A rarer type, which often receives extensive news coverage, involves a disgruntled individual who has narcissistic and paranoid traits. Dismissed from a job, passed over for promotion, denied insurance money, loans, or disability, such individuals see themselves as humiliated by others and deprived of recognition. In a vengeful act, they often murder employers, bankers, teachers, physicians, or others with firearms prior to turning the gun on themselves. Bystanders are often killed. Individuals who murder police officers are also at high risk of committing suicide (31).

The intent of perpetrators of murder-suicide ranges from predominantly homicidal to predominantly suicidal. In the spousal and extrafamilial types, homicidal motives arising from jealousy and revenge are strong. The murder of blood relatives and children often represents an "extended" suicide in which the family is seen as an extension of the perpetrator (32,33).

There are no studies that have been able to assess the diagnosis of the perpetrators systematically. Nonetheless, depression appears to be common among perpetrators of spousal murder-suicide, filicide-suicide, and familicide-suicide (25,26,34–37).

Other studies have stressed the role of psychosis, particularly delusions of jealousy (38,39), paranoia (40), or rescue (24,27,32). Murder-suicide is also reported in the culture-bound syndrome of amok (41).

III. ETIOLOGY

The reasons for a link between violent and suicidal behavior are unknown. Several possible etiologies warrant consideration. In one scenario, these two behaviors can be seen as arising from developmental precursors or socioeconomic environments that are independently associated with each. For example, numerous studies have linked early family disorganization with later violence; other studies have shown a link between family chaos and suicidal behavior. Another possibility is that both behaviors arise from a common underlying genetic, neuroanatomic, or neurochemical substrate. Serotonin, for example, is widely considered the neurotransmitter involved in both behaviors.

Third, as most suicides are among persons with serious mental illnesses and violence has also been linked with mental illnesses, it is possible that the link between these behaviors occurs because such individuals have a mental disorder that has symptomatological features of both.

A. Early Developmental and Socioenvironmental Risk Factors

One reason suicidal and violent behaviors may be found in the same person is that some developmental and socioenvironmental risk factors for suicide are similar to those for violence. Thus an individual who experienced bad child-rearing practices or certain misfortunes in adulthood might be expected to behave violently or self-destructively later in life, depending on circumstances. Risk factors for antisocial behavior have included poor parenting, antisocial and alcoholic parents, and early separation (42). Among adolescent suicides, loss of a parent, parental psychopathology and substance abuse, parental suicidal behavior, and family violence have been found to be common (43). Early parental loss through death and early exposure to violence in the family are related to both the risk of violence and the risk of suicide (44).

In adulthood, certain socioenvironmental risk factors are common to both behaviors. For example, poverty and crowding are more closely linked to violence than to self-destructive behavior. However, unemployment has been correlated with both homicide and suicide rates in men (45). Others have postulated that as the population grows within a given stratum, more individuals need to compete for limited resources (46). This competition results in aggression, which may be expressed as outward violence or self-destruction.

While violence is likely to be strongly influenced by social factors, the likelihood that suicide is principally explained by social forces, a view first proposed by Durkheim, is somewhat questionable. Although suicide occurs in a "social group" and has communicative value for the surviving group left behind, it remains a highly individual matter. Social and environmental circumstances may increase the likelihood of suicide in someone who is suicidal, but they are unlikely to be causative themselves. Suicide is more likely to result from an individual's decision rather than to represent a behavior induced by group dynamics.

B. Neurobiological Substrates

One promising explanation for the link between violent and suicidal behavior is the notion that these behaviors share a common genetic, neurobiochemical, or neuroanatomic substrate. The neurological underpinnings of violence have been extensively studied, owing to the vast possibilities of experimental control offered by animal models. In contrast, the neurobiology of suicide is much less understood.

The most extensive literature posits serotonin as the key neurotransmitter in both aggression and suicide. Asberg (47), for example, found that unipolar, depressed patients with the lowest levels of cerebrospinal fluid (CSF)-5-hydroxyindoleacetic acid (5HIAA), the principal metabolite of serotonin, were more likely to attempt or commit suicide, particularly by using violent means, compared with patients who had higher levels. This finding was subsequently confirmed in other patient groups, including those with schizophrenia and personality disorders (48,49). A number of other studies using platelet models, fenfluramine challenge, or postmortem brain receptor–binding assays have found low serotonergic functioning in suicidal persons (50). Brown (51), and then subsequent studies, have found a strong negative correlation between CSF 5-HIAA and lifetime aggression score.

The low levels of serotonin found in violent and suicidal groups seem to be associated more with impulsivity than violence per se. For example, in a comparison of impulsive fire setters, age, sex-matched violent offenders, and healthy volunteers, the CSF 5-HIAA concentrations were lowest among the arsonists and intermediate among the violent offenders (52). Likewise, in a study of persons incarcerated for murder or attempted murder, impulsive offenders had lower CSF 5-HIAA concentrations than nonimpulsive offenders. Those impulsive offenders with a history of attempted suicide had even lower 5-HIAA concentrations than those who had not made such an attempt (53). Whether low serotonin is a persistent enduring characteristic of some violent and suicidal individuals (i.e., a trait), a more transient state, or perhaps a little of both is not certain. Likewise, many individuals who are violent or suicidal do not have low serotonin. Thus, it is still not clear whether the relationship is causative or merely epiphenomenal. Nonetheless, the low-serotonergic system continues to be studied extensively in these populations in the quest for causes, biological markers, and pharmacological "cures" for such behaviors.

Suicidal and violent behavior may be linked because they share common genetic underpinnings. Recently, a tryptophan hydroxylase polymorphism was found to be associated with suicidal behavior in alcoholic violent offenders (54). However, another study found no link between the tryptophan hydroxylase gene and suicidal behavior (55). Another study found that impulsive aggression, arson, attempted rape, and exhibition were associated with a point mutation in the structural gene for monoamine oxidase A, which resulted in a complete deficiency in this enzyme's activity (56).

Other psychobiological variables that may link suicidal and violent behavior have not been studied as extensively. For example, low blood glucose concentrations during an oral glucose tolerance test have been found in recurrently violent individuals (57). Insulin resistance has also been found in severely depressed and suicidal patients (58).

There is also a controversy about whether drugs that lower cholesterol also increase the risk of suicide, homicide, and accidents (59). It should be pointed out, however, that in these studies, the term *homicide* refers to being a victim rather than a perpetrator of violence.

The neuroanatomic pathways for aggression have been extensively studied. There is strong evidence to implicate the orbitofrontal cortex, amygdala, septum, hippocampus, thalamus, hypothalamus, and brainstem in mediating aggression (60). Because of the evolutionary and survival value of well-directed, "appropriate" aggression, it would not be surprising if most regions of the brain played some role in modulating goal-directed aggression. Likewise, the devastation of species that would result from unchecked aggression makes it likely that multiple brain centers are responsible for inhibiting intra-species violence. Unfortunately, the neuroanatomic pathways of suicide are not understood. However, a number of postmortem studies have suggested that the brains of people who committed suicide had alterations in the serotonergic and beta-adrenergic function of the prefrontal cortex (50). These data, together with evidence that patients with frontal lobe dysfunction display heightened impulsivity and aggressiveness (61), suggest that the frontal lobe may prove to be a common substrate for both behaviors. It is possible that suicidal acts result from a strong counterbalance of cognitive facilitators and inhibitors that arises from the prefrontal cortex and emotional input that arises from the limbic system. It is thus conceivable that there are similar neuroanatomic pathways for aggression, be it outwardly or inwardly directed.

C. Diagnostic Commonalities

Studies estimate that almost 95% of all suicides have a mental illness (62). Because violence is a feature of a number of psychiatric disorders, it is possible that suicidal and violent behaviors are correlated merely because they are features of certain mental disorders.

The most common disorders that are likely to involve both behaviors are alcoholism and substance abuse. The literature on the association of interpersonal violence with alcohol use is extensive (63). At least 25% of all suicides are among alcoholics and at least 15% of alcoholics will die by suicide (64). In a study of male alcoholics, Bergman et al. (65) found that those who had violent behaviors were twice as likely to have attempted suicide as those who were nonviolent. Other studies have also shown a strong correlation of violence and suicide risk with alcoholism (66). Some have also argued that alcoholism results in a low serotonergic state, which is associated with both violence and self-destructive acts (67). Other sedative hypnotics, and stimulants such as cocaine and amphetamines, have been associated with both types of behaviors (68). Phencyclidine, an arylhexamine with both stimulant and hallucinogenic properties, has also been associated with violence and suicide (69).

The cluster B personality disorders, particularly borderline and antisocial personality disorders, have also been linked with both behaviors (70). Some schizophrenic patients, particularly those who have the paranoid or disorganized subtypes, may be at risk for both violence and suicidality (71).

Although depression per se has generally not been linked with violence for the most part with the exception of murder-suicide and mania is typically not linked with suicide, bipolar patients are likely to have a history of *both* violence and suicidal behavior. Moreover, the mixed state characterized by depressive mood and hopeless cognition combined with motor restlessness and agitation may predispose to both violence and suicidality simultaneously.

Among adolescents, suicide and violence share diagnostic commonalities. Alessi et al. (72) used a structured interview to assess 71 juvenile delinquents who had been arrested for violent behaviors or assaults. Some 60% had made suicide attempts, including individuals with major affective and psychotic disorders. Psychological autopsy studies of children who committed suicide (73–75) have also found a high percentage of cases of antisocial personality disorder. In a study of 43 adolescent suicide victims and 43 community controls, the cluster B and C disorders were more common among suicide victims than among controls (76). Suicides also had higher scores on lifetime aggression even after controlling for differences in psychopathology between suicides and controls. In addition, homicidal ideation was noted to be prominent in the week before completed suicide in adolescents (77).

Diagnoses are, of course, construed in categorical terms—i.e., present or absent. The diagnostic commonality between suicide and violence may be better conceived in the dimensional terms of the symptomatic states they produce. Seen this way, all of these disorders may lead to increased impulsivity, poorly modulated affect, or disturbed reasoning—i.e., hallucinations and delusions, each of which contributes to the joint risk of suicide and violence. The underlying symptoms conducive to aggression may be more important than a diagnostic label per se.

IV. CLINICAL ASSESSMENT OF THE RISK OF VIOLENCE AND SUICIDE

The clinical assessment of violence is described in another chapter. However, the association of violence and suicide behooves the clinician to consider the risk of both behaviors in psychiatric, emergency, and forensic settings. All patients who present with recent violence or violent ideation should have careful clinical histories taken for past suicidal behavior or ideation, current suicidal ideation, intent, or plan, and family history of suicide. Likewise, individuals who present with suicidal plans or who have recently made a suicide attempt should be carefully questioned about recent and past violence, circumstances, targets, and degree of injury.

The careful, regular assessment of suicide risk in individuals who are jailed or incarcerated cannot be stressed enough, given the high rate of suicide among prison populations. Within jails, the maximum risk for suicide appears to be in the first few days, especially the first 24 hours of incarceration (78). Felthous (79) outlined six principles for preventing jailhouse suicides; these include immediate screening of new inmates, psychological support, surveillance and "disarming" of suicidal inmates, establishment of clear and consistent precautionary measures, and the possible transfer of inmates to psychiatric hospitals for more intensive evaluation and treatment.

Within psychiatric hospitals, patients who are violent should be carefully questioned about suicidal behavior and vice versa, as either behavior may be a prelude to the other in the hospital. Individuals with substance abuse or alcoholism, personality disorders, bipolar disorder—mixed, or schizophrenia are particularly likely to display both types of behaviors.

Suicide should be carefully assessed among persons who present as either the victims or perpetrators of domestic violence. In couples who present with chronic marital discord, the clinician should seek to determine whether amorous jealousy is a significant contributor. The presence of obsessional or delusional jealousy in a young or middle-aged man should raise concerns about the possibility of murder-suicide. The presence of depression and despondency in a young mother should raise the concern about a filicide-suicide. Likewise, individuals who are paranoid or vengeful and feel slighted should be carefully questioned about both violent motives and suicidal intent.

As Tardiff (80) has pointed out, assessments of violence and suicide are very similar. Both involve appreciation of the epidemiological risk factors, past personal and family history of the behavior, and evaluation of current ideation and plans. Likewise, both involve clinician and patient safety as well as increased patient surveillance, and both may involve seclusion or restraint when indicated.

V. SUMMARY

There is not as yet a unifying model that would explain the underlying causal links between outward-directed aggression and suicidal behavior. Plutchik et al. (81) have postulated a common aggressive drive that results in manifest behavior when a threshold is surpassed. Aggressive impulses may arise from threat, challenge, insult, or loss of control. At the first stage, variables act to amplify or attenuate the aggressive drive.

In the second stage, variables correlated selectively and positively with risk of violence or suicide direct the "vector" of aggression outward or inward, respectively. Variables correlated with suicide, for instance, might include depression, life stressors, or hopelessness. Variables correlated with violence might include impulsivity, recent stresses, and so on. Negatively correlated variables act to reduce the risk of violence; thus the final action, in effect, represents the product of competing vectorial forces. While this mode is useful descriptively and for heuristic purposes, the field awaits a more detailed model that will relate behaviors more closely to neuroanatomic and neurochemical pathways.

In conclusion, violence and suicidal behaviors appear to be closely related. Additional studies are needed to sort out the sociological, neurobiological, and diagnostic factors that underlie the links between aggressive behavior. Studies are also needed to provide better management and treatment guidelines for individuals who manifest both behaviors.

REFERENCES

1. H.M. Van Praag, R. Plutchik, and A. Apter, (eds.), *Violence and Suicidality: Perspective in Clinical and Psychological Research*, Brunner/Mazel, New York, 1990.
2. K. Tardiff and A. Sweillam, Factors related to increased risk of assaultive behavior in suicidal patients, *Acta Psychiatr. Scand. 62*:63 (1980).
3. K. Tardiff and A. Sweillam, Assault, suicide, and mental illness, *Arch. Gen. Psychiatry 37*:614 (1980).
4. K. Tardiff, The risk of assaultive behavior in suicidal patients. II. An inpatient survey, *Acta Psychiatr. Scand. 64*:295 (1981).
5. A.G. Skodal and T.B. Karasu, Emergency psychiatry and the assaultive patient, *Am. J. Psychiatry 135*:202 (1978).
6. S.C. Inamdar, D.D. Lewis, G. Siomopoulous, S.S. Shanack, and M. Lamela, Vio-

lent and suicidal behavior in psychotic adolescents, *Am. J. Psychiatry 139*:932 (1982).
7. D.E. Grosz, D.S. Lipschitz, S. Eldar, G. Finkelstein, N. Blackwood, G. Gerbino-Rosen, G.L. Fuedda, and R. Plutchik, Correlates of violence risk in hospitalized adolescents, *Comp. Psychiatry 35*:296 (1994).
8. P. Dechatcau, Mortality and aggressiveness in a 30-year follow-up study in child guidance clinics in Stockholm, *Acta Psychiatr. Scand. 81*:472 (1990).
9. A. Apter, M. Kotler, S. Sevy, et al., Correlates of risk of suicide in violent and nonviolent psychiatric patients, *Am. J. Psychiatry 148*:883 (1991).
10. L.M. Hayes, And darkness closes in . . . a national study of jail suicides, *Crim. Justice Behav. 10*:461 (1983).
11. W.E. Stone, Jail suicide, *Corrections Today 46*:84 (1984).
12. J.E. Smialek and W.V. Spitz, Death behind bars, *J.A.M.A. 240*:2563 (1978).
13. L.F. Novick and E. Remmlinger, A study of 128 deaths in New York City correctional facilities (1971–76): Implications for prisoner healthcare, *Med. Care* 16:749 (1978).
14. E. Dooley, Prison suicide in England and Wales, 1972–87, *Br. J. Psychiatry 156*:40 (1990).
15. M.E. Salive, G.S. Smith, and T.F. Brewer, Suicide mortality in the Maryland state prison system, 1979 through 1987, *J.A.M.A. 262*:365 (1989).
16. C.J. Durand, G.J. Burtka, E.J. Federman, J.A. Haycox, and J.W. Smith, A quarter century of suicide in a major urban county jail: implications for community psychiatry, *Am. J. Psychiatry 152*:1077 (1995).
17. A.J.F.M. Kerkhof and W. Bernasso, Suicidal behavior in jails and prisons in the Netherlands: incidence, characteristics, and prevention, *Suicide Life Threat. Behav. 20*:123 (1990).
18. S. Currens, T. Fritsch, D. Jones, et al., Homicide followed by suicide—Kentucy, 1985–1990, *M.M.W.R. 40*:652 (1991).
19. S. Palmer and J.A. Humphrey, Offender-victim relationships in criminal homicide followed by offender's suicide, North Carolina, 1972–1977, *Suicide Life Threat. Behav. 10*:106 (1980).
20. N.H. Allen, Homicide followed by suicide: Los Angeles, 1970–1979, *Suicide Life Threat. Behav. 13*:155 (1983).
21. M.E. Wolfgang, An analysis of homicide-suicide, *J. Clin. Exp. Psychopathol. 19*:208 (1958).
22. J. Coid, The epidemiology of abnormal homicide and murder followed by suicide, *Psychol. Med. 13*:855 (1983).
23. P.M. Marzuk, K. Tardiff, and C.S. Hirsch, The epidemiology of murder-suicde, *J.A.M.A. 267*:3179 (1992).
24. J. Selkin, Rescue fantasies in homicide-suicide, *Suicide Life Threat. Behav.* 6:79–85.
25. R.D. Goldney, Family murder followed by suicide, *Forens. Sci. 9*:219 (1977).
26. D.J. West, *Murder Followed by Suicide*, Harvard University Press, Cambridge, MA, 1967.
27. S.A. Myers, Maternal filicide, *Am. J. Dis. Child, 120*:534 (1970).

28. M. Rodenburg, Child murder by depressed parents, *Can. Psychiatr. Assoc. J. 16*:41 (1971).
29. P.J. Resnick, Child murder by parents: a psychiatric review of filicide, *Am. J. Psychiatry 126*:73 (1969).
30. L.K. Somander and L.M. Rammer, Intra- and extra-familial child homicide in Sweden, 1971–1980, *Child Abuse Negl. 15*:45 (1991).
31. D. Lester, Murder followed by suicide in those who murder police officers, *Psychol. Rep. 60*:1130 (1987).
32. W.J. Browne and A.J. Palmer, A preliminary study of schizophrenic women who murdered their chidren, *Hosp. Commun. Psychiatry 26*:71 (1975).
33. P.T. D'Orban, Women who kill their children, *Br. J. Psychiatry 134*:560 (1979).
34. S. Hirose, Depression and homicide, *Acta Psychiatr. Scand. 59*: 211 (1979).
35. M. Rosenbaum, The role of depression in couples involved in murder-suicide and homicide, *Am. J. Psychiatry 147*:1036 (1990).
36. D. Lester, W. Perdue, and D. Brookhart, Murderers who have attempted suicide, *Psychol. Rep. 35*:238 (1974).
37. D.A. Fishbain, V.J. Rao, and T.E. Aldrich, Female homicide-suicide perpetrators: A controlled study, *J. Forens. Sci. 30*:1148 (1985).
38. T.L. Dorpat, Suicide in murderers, *Psychiatr. Dig. 27:*51 (1966).
39. M. Shepherd, Morbid jealousy: Some clinical and social aspects of a psychiatric symptom, *J. Ment. Sci. 107*:687 (1961).
40. P.A. Lesco, Murder-suicide in Alzheimer's disease, *J. Am. Geriatr. Soc. 37*:167 (1989).
41. J.I. Teoh, The changing psychopathology of amok, *Psychiatry 35*:345 (1972).
42. I. Kolvin, F.J.M. Miller, M. Fleeting, and P.A. Kolvin, Risk/protective factors for offending with particular reference to deprivation, *Studies of Psychosocial Risk: The Power of Longitudinal Data* (M. Rutter, ed.), Cambridge University Press, Cambridge, UK, 1988, pp. 77–95.
43. C.R. Pfeffer, Life stress and family risk factors for youth fatal and nonfatal suicidal behavior, *Suicide Among Youth: Perspectives on Risk and Prevention* (C.R. Pfeffer, ed.), American Psychiatric Press, 1991, Washington, DC, pp. 143–164.
44. A.J. Botsis, R. Plutchik, M. Kotter, and H.M. Van Praag, Parental loss and family violence as correlates of suicide and violence risk, *Suicide Life Threat. Behav. 25*:253 (1995).
45. S. Platt, Unemployment and suicidal behavior: A review of the literature, *Soc. Sci. Med. 19*:93 (1984).
46. P. Holinger, *Violent Deaths in the United States*, Guilford Press, New York, 1987.
47. M. Asberg, L. Traskmen and P. Thoren, 5-HIAA in the cerebrospinal fluid: A suicide predictor, *Arch. Gen. Psychiatry 33*:1193 (1976).
48. H.M. Van Praag, CSF 5-HIAA and suicide in nondepressed schizophrenics, *Lancet 2*:977 (1983).
49. P.T. Ninan, D.P. van Kammen, M. Scheinin, et al., CSF 5-hydroxyindoleacetic acid levels in suicidal schizophrenic patients, *Am. J. Psychiatry 141*:566 (1984).
50. J.J. Mann, P.M. Marzuk, V. Arango, P.A. McBride, A.C. Leon, and H. Tierney, Neu-

rochemical studies of violent and nonviolent suicide, *Psychopharmacol. Bull. 25*:407 (1989).
51. G.L. Brown, M.H. Ebert, P.F. Goyer, et al., Aggression, suicide and serotonin: Relationships to CSF amine metabolites, *Am. J. Psychiatry 139*:741 (1982).
52. M. Virkkunnen, A. Nuutila, F.K. Goodwin, et al. Cerebrospinal fluid monoamine metabolite levels in male arsonists, *Arch. Gen. Psychiatry 44*:241 (1987).
53. M. Linnoila, M. Virkkunnen M. Scheinin M, et al., Low cerebrospinal fluid 5-hydroxyindoleacetic acid concentration differentiates impulsive from non-impulsive violent behavior, *Life Sci. 33*:2609 (1983).
54. D.A. Neilsen, D. Goldman, M. Virkkunen, R. Tohola, R. Rawlings, and M. Linnoila, Suicidality and 5-hydroxy indoleacetic acid concentrations associated with a tryptophan hydroxylase polymorphism, *Arch. Gen. Psychiatry 51*:34 (1994).
55. M. Abbar, P. Courtet, S. Amadeo, Y. Caer, J. Mallet, M. Baldy-Moulinier, D. Castelnau, and A. Malfosse, Suicidal behaviors and the tryptophan hydroxylase gene, *Arch. Gen. Psychiatry 52*:846 (1995).
56. H.G. Brunner, N. Nelen, X.O. Breakefield, H.H. Ropers, and B.A. van Oost, Abnormal behavior associated with a point mutation in the structural gene for monoamine oxidase A, *Science 262*:578 (1993).
57. M. Virkkunen and M.D. Huttunen, Evidence for abnormal glucose tolerance test among violent offenders, *Neuropsychobiology*, *8*:30 (1982).
58. G. Heninger, P. Mueller, and L. Davis, Progressive symptoms and the glucose tolerance test and insulin tolerance test, *J. Nerv. Ment. Dis. 161*:421 (1975).
59. M.F. Muldoon, S.B. Manuck, and K.A. Matthews, Lowering cholesterol concentrations and mortality: A quantitative review of primary prevention trials, *Br. Med. J. 301*: 309 (1990).
60. F.A. Elliot, Violence, the neurologic contribution: An overview, *Arch. Neurol. 49*:595 (1992).
61. J.M. Fuster, *The prefrontal Cortex*, Raven Press, New York, 1989.
62. D.W. Black and G. Winokin, Suicide and psychiatric diagnoses, *Suicide Over the Life Cycle: Risk Factors, Assessment and Treatment of Suicidal Patients* (S.J. Blumenthal and D.J. Kupfer, eds.), American Psychiatric Press, Washington, DC, 1990, pp. 135–153.
63. R.N. Norton and M.Y. Morgan, The role of alchol in mortality and morbidity from interpersonal violence, *Alcohol Alcoholism 24*:565 (1989).
64. G.E. Murphy, Suicide in alcoholism, *Suicide* (A. Roy, ed.), Williams & Wilkins, Baltimore, 1986, pp. 89–96.
65. B. Bergman and B. Brismar, Characteristics of violent alcoholics, *Alcohol Alcoholism 29*:451 (1994).
66. D.J. Greenwald, M. Reznikoff, and R. Plutchik, Suicide and violence risk in alcoholics: Predictors of aggressive risk, *J. Nerv. Ment. Dis. 182*:31 (1994).
67. M. Linnoila and M. Virkkunen, Aggression, suicidality, and serotonin, *J. Clin. Psychiatry 53(suppl 1)*:46 (1992).
68. P.M. Marzuk and J.J. Mann, Suicide and substance abuse, *Psychiatr. Ann. 18*:639 (1988).
69. A. Poklis, M. Graham, D. Maginn, C.A. Branch, and G.E. Gantnev, Phencyclidine

and violent deaths in St. Louis, Missouri: A survey of medical examiners' cases from 1977 through 1986, *Am. J. Drug. Alcohol Abuse 16*:265 (1990).

70. A. Frances, M.R. Fyer, and J. Clarkin, Personality and suicide, *Ann. N.Y. Acad. Sci. 487*:281 (1986).
71. M. Krakowski, J. Volavka, and D. Brizer, Psychopathology and violence: A review of the literature, *Compr. Psychiatry 27*:131 (1986).
72. N.E. Alessi, M. McManus, A. Brickman, and L. Grapentine, Suicide behavior among serious juvenile offenders, *Am. J. Psychiatry 141*:286 (1984).
73. M. Shafii, S. Carrigan, L. Whillinghil, and A. Derrick, Psychological autopsy of completed suicide in children and adolescents, *Am. J. Psychiatry 142*:1061 (1985).
74. M.J. Marttunen, H.M. Aro, M.M. Henrikssen, and J.K. Lonnqvist, Antisocial behavior in adolescent suicide, *Acta Psychiatr. Scand. 89*:167 (1994).
75. D. Shaffer, Suicide in childhood and adolescence, *J. Child Psychol. Psychiatry 15*:275 (1974).
76. D.A. Brent, B.A. Johnson, J. Perper, J. Connoly, J. Bridge, S. Bartle, and C. Rather, Personality disorder, personality traits, impulsive violence, and completed suicide in adolescents, *J. Am. Acad. Child Adolesc. Psychiatry 33*:1080 (1994).
77. D.A. Brent, J.A. Perper, G. Mortiz, et al., Psychiatric risk factors for adolescent suicide: A case-control study, *J. Am. Acad. Child Adolesc. Psychiatry 32*:521 (1993).
78. L.M. Hayes, National study of jail suicides: seven years later, *Psychiatr. Q. 60*:7 (1989).
79. A.R. Felthous, Preventing jailhouse suicides, *Bull Am Acad Psychiatry Law 22*:477 (1994).
80. K. Tardiff, *Assessment and Management of Violent Patients*, American Psychiatric Press, Washington, DC, 1996.
81. R. Plutchik, H.M. Van Praag, and H.R. Conte, Correlates of suicide and violence risk: III. A two-stage model of countervailing forces, *Psychiatry Res. 28*:215 (1989).

Index

About the Editor

KENNETH TARDIFF is a Professor of Psychiatry and Public Health at Cornell Medical College, and Attending Psychiatrist at New York Presbyterian Hospital, New York, New York. The author, coauthor, editor, or coeditor of over 150 journal papers, books, and book chapters on violence and suicide, he is a member of the American Psychiatric Association and the American Academy of Psychiatry and the Law. Dr. Tardiff received the M.D. degree (1969) from the Tulane University School of Medicine, New Orleans, Louisiana, and the M.P.H. degree (1973) from the Harvard University School of Public Health, Boston, Massachusetts.